# CRASH COURSE
# Internal Medicine

# Internal Medicine

# Ragavendra Baliga, MD

Clinical Professor of Internal Medicine
Ohio State University
Director of Cardiology
Ohio State University Hospitals East
Columbus, OH

Student authors
**Daniel Becker, David Corteville, and Michael D. Nauss**

UK edition authors
**Rachel Hough and Iftikhar Haq**

UK series editor
**Wilf Yeo**

**ELSEVIER**
**MOSBY**

**ELSEVIER**
**MOSBY**

1600 John F. Kennedy Blvd.
Ste 1800
Philadelphia, PA 19103-2899

CRASH COURSE: INTERNAL MEDICINE
**Copyright 2006, Elsevier, Inc. All right reserved.**

ISBN-13: 978-0-323-03565-1
ISBN-10: 0-323-03565-5

---

### Notice

Knowledge and best practice in this field are constantly changing. As new research and experience broaden our knowledge, changes in practice, treatment and drug therapy may become necessary or appropriate. Readers are advised to check the most current information provided (i) on procedures featured or (ii) by the manufacturer of each product to be administered, to verify the recommended dose or formula, the method and duration of administration, and contraindications. It is the responsibility of the practitioner, relying on their own experience and knowledge of the patient, to make diagnoses, to determine dosages and the best treatment for each individual patient, and to take all appropriate safety precautions. To the fullest extent of the law, neither the Publisher nor the Author assumes any liability for any injury and/or damage to persons or property arising out or related to any use of the material contained in this book.

The Publisher

---

Adapted from Crash Course Internal Medicine by Rachel Hough and Iftikhar Haq, ISBN 0-7234-3114-0.
© Mosby International Limited 1999.

The rights of Rachel Hough and Iftikhar Haq to be identified as the authors of this work have been asserted by them in accordance with the Copyright, Designs and Patents Act, 1988

**Library of Congress Cataloging-in-Publication Data**
Baliga, R. R.
   Internal medicine / Ragavendra Baliga—1st ed.
      p. ; cm.—(Crash course)
   ISBN 0-323-03565-5
   1. Internal medicine.   I. Title.   II. Series.
   [DNLM: 1.  Internal Medicine. WB 115 B186i 2006]
RC48.B35 2006
616–dc22

2005053002

Commissioning Editor: *Alex Stibbe*
Project Development Manager: *Stan Ward*
Project Manager: *David Saltzberg*
Design: *Andy Chapman*
Cover Design: *Antbits Illustration*
Illustration Manager: *Mick Ruddy*

Printed in the United States of America

Last digit is the print number:
9  8  7  6  5  4  3  2  1

# Preface

*Crash Course Internal Medicine* is designed to help medical students in their internal medicine and clinical clerkship. In addition it will help students preparing for the USMLE Steps 2 and 3.

Part I of this book is focused on approach to a patient depending on their symptoms. Part II includes history, clinical examination, and common investigations in patients seen by internists, and Part III discusses specific diseases including diagnosis and treatment. The strengths of this text include the liberal use of diagrams and "hints" to highlight essential information that is expected from every medical student.

The book is best used soon after examining a patient. This approach allows students to go back to the patient to compare their clinical findings with this text. In my experience clinical medicine is best learnt using the 4-step Baliga **ERRD** technique (**e**licit, **r**ead, **r**eview, and **d**iscuss):

- **E**licit the history, clinical features, and relevant investigations.
- **R**ead relevant medical literature immediately.
- **R**eview history, clinical features and diagnostic tests.
- **D**iscuss with peers, seniors or the attending physician.

Therefore, I encourage all students to take this book to the hospital with them during their internal medicine clinical clerkship, so that it is readily available for use soon after they have examined a cardiovascular patient. Finally, this book is a primer. Follow-up texts for further reading are the third edition of *250 Cases in Clinical Medicine*, 3rd ed., by R. R. Baliga (W.B Saunders) and *Cecil's Textbook of Medicine*, 22nd ed. (W.B. Saunders).

**Ragavendra R. Baliga, MD, MBA, FRCP (Edin), FACC**

# Acknowledgments

I thank Rachael Hough and Iftikhar Haq for allowing me to adapt their British book for U.S. medical students.

I thank Daniel Becker, David Corteville, and Michael Nauss for critically reviewing this book and giving me three separate perspectives from the view of a medical student. They were third- and fourth-year medical students at University of Michigan Medical School when they worked on this project. Dan is now a resident at Brigham & Women's Hospital & Harvard Medical School, Dave is a resident at University of California, San Francisco (UCSF) and Mike is a resident at University of Cincinnati. I have no doubt that they all will continue to excel in their field of endeavor. It was a pleasure to work with them.

Finally, I thank my wife Jay for doing my share of the domestic chores and to my children Anoop and Neena for their patience when I worked on this book.

# Dedication

This book is dedicated to the memory of my father, R. K. Baliga (who founded the Electronic City in Bangalore, India). It is also dedicated to my mother, Shanthi Baliga (whom I applaud for work on social causes, including women's emancipation in India); my wife, Jayashree; my children, Anoop and Neena; and my siblings, Narendra and Lathika.

# Contents

**34. Central Nervous System** . . . . . . . . . . . . . **309**
Cerebrovascular disease . . . . . . . . . . . . . . 309
Management of conditions causing
headache . . . . . . . . . . . . . . . . . . . . . . . 314
Parkinsonism . . . . . . . . . . . . . . . . . . . . . 317
Multiple sclerosis . . . . . . . . . . . . . . . . . 320
Meningitis . . . . . . . . . . . . . . . . . . . . . . . 322
Epilepsy . . . . . . . . . . . . . . . . . . . . . . . . 325
Intracranial tumors . . . . . . . . . . . . . . . . 328
Miscellaneous neurologic disorders . . . . . . 329

**35. Metabolic and Endocrine Disorders** . . . . . . **333**
Diabetes . . . . . . . . . . . . . . . . . . . . . . . 333
Lipid disorders . . . . . . . . . . . . . . . . . . . . 339
Metabolic bone disease . . . . . . . . . . . . . . 341
Hyperparathyroidism . . . . . . . . . . . . . . . . 345
Hypoparathyroidism . . . . . . . . . . . . . . . . 346
Crystal arthropathy . . . . . . . . . . . . . . . . . 346
Hypercalcemia . . . . . . . . . . . . . . . . . . . . 347
Pituitary disorders . . . . . . . . . . . . . . . . . 348
Thyroid disorders . . . . . . . . . . . . . . . . . . 352
Disorders of the adrenal glands . . . . . . . . . 357
Miscellaneous endocrine conditions . . . . . . 360

**36. Musculoskeletal and Skin Disorders** . . . . . . **361**
Arthritis . . . . . . . . . . . . . . . . . . . . . . . . 361
Systemic lupus erythematosus . . . . . . . . . . 367

Polymyalgia rheumatica . . . . . . . . . . . . . . 369
Other connective tissue disorders . . . . . . . . 370
Primary skin diseases . . . . . . . . . . . . . . . . 373
Skin manifestations of systemic disease . . . . 376
Malignant skin tumors . . . . . . . . . . . . . . . 377

**37. Hematologic Disorders** . . . . . . . . . . . . . . **379**
Anemia . . . . . . . . . . . . . . . . . . . . . . . . . 379
Leukemias . . . . . . . . . . . . . . . . . . . . . . . 387
Multiple myeloma . . . . . . . . . . . . . . . . . . 391
Malignant lymphomas . . . . . . . . . . . . . . . 393
Bleeding disorders . . . . . . . . . . . . . . . . . . 395
Disseminated intravascular coagulation . . . . 397
Thrombotic disorders . . . . . . . . . . . . . . . . 398

**38. Infectious Diseases** . . . . . . . . . . . . . . . . **401**
HIV and AIDS . . . . . . . . . . . . . . . . . . . . . 401
Malaria . . . . . . . . . . . . . . . . . . . . . . . . . 406

**39. Drug Overdose** . . . . . . . . . . . . . . . . . . . **409**
Epidemiology . . . . . . . . . . . . . . . . . . . . . 409
Etiology . . . . . . . . . . . . . . . . . . . . . . . . . 409
Presentation . . . . . . . . . . . . . . . . . . . . . 409
Investigations . . . . . . . . . . . . . . . . . . . . . 410
Management . . . . . . . . . . . . . . . . . . . . . . 410

Index . . . . . . . . . . . . . . . . . . . . . . . . . . . . . 413

# PART I: THE PATIENT PRESENTS WITH

# 1. Chest Pain

Chest pain is a common cause for admission to hospital. Taking a clear history is essential in making the correct diagnosis. Different diseases present with different types of chest pain.

## Differential diagnosis of chest pain

### Pleuritic chest pain
This is a sharp pain that is worse on deep inspiration, coughing, or movement. The differential diagnosis includes the following:
- Pneumothorax.
- Pneumonia.
- Pulmonary embolus (PE).
- Pericarditis: retrosternal.
- Bornholm disease (Coxsackie B unilateral infection of respiratory muscles).

### Dull central chest pain
The differential diagnosis of dull central pain includes the following:
- Angina: crushing.
- Myocardial infarction (MI): crushing.
- Dissecting aortic aneurysm: tearing interscapular pain.
- Esophagitis: burning.
- Esophageal spasm.
- Esophageal tear (Boerrhave's syndrome).

### Chest wall tenderness
The differential diagnosis of chest wall tenderness includes the following:
- Rib fracture.
- Shingles (herpes zoster): pain precedes rash.
- Costochondritis (Tietze's syndrome).
- Nerve root compression.

### Atypical presentations (or any of the above)
The differential diagnosis in atypical presentations (or in any of the above) includes anxiety and referred pain from vertebral collapse, causing nerve root irritation or intra-abdominal pathology (e.g., pancreatitis, peptic ulcer, or the biliary tree). In addition, any of the above diagnoses can present in an atypical manner. For instance, MI can present as epigastric or jaw pain. For this reason, the most serious causes of chest pain should always be added to the differential diagnosis and considered to avoid missing a potentially life-threatening problem.

## History in the patient with chest pain

A careful history of the chest pain will generally be suggestive of the likely underlying problem. It is important during the history to take note of any procedures that have been done and what doctors the patient has seen over the past few years. In addition, social history (drug use and occupation) and psychiatric history can provide insight into the nature of chest pain (e.g., anxiety disorder, cocaine-induced MI). The focus should then turn to any associated symptoms and risk factors.

### What type of chest pain does the patient have?
#### Onset and progression of pain
Cardiac ischemic pain typically builds up over a few minutes and may be brought on by exercise, emotion, or cold weather. In angina the pain resolves on resting or with sublingual nitroglycerin (NTG). In unstable angina the pain may come on at rest and commonly waxes and wanes, becoming severe at times. In MI the pain is severe, often associated with systemic symptoms such as nausea, vomiting, and sweating, and lasts for at least 30 minutes. Spontaneous pneumothorax and pulmonary embolism usually causes sudden onset of pleuritic pain (patients often remember exactly what they were doing at the time). Pain that follows an episode of vomiting, especially if hematemesis is present, suggests esophageal disease.

Always ask the patient what he or she was doing when the pain came on. This generally gives valuable information!

## Site and radiation of pain

Cardiac ischemia and pericarditis cause retrosternal pain. In ischemia, the pain often radiates to the jaw, neck, or arms, while dissecting aortic aneurysm causes a tearing interscapular pain, and pulmonary disease causes unilateral pain which the patient can often localize specifically. Esophageal disease can also cause retrosternal pain and may mimic cardiac pain. Referred pain from vertebral collapse or shingles will follow a dermatome pattern.

A note about shingles: Lesions never cross the midline except in patients with immunocompromise, which may be iatrogenic (e.g., steroid use) or due to another cause. In addition, the pain of shingles can begin before the rash appears. Patients complain of "electrical" type pain. Treatment with acyclovir is effective only if given within 24 hours of the initial rash.

## Nature of pain

The precise nature of the pain gives important clues as to the underlying diagnosis—for instance, crushing, sharp, pleuritic, burning, or stabbing (see above).

## Are there any associated symptoms?

Important associated symptoms include:
- Dyspnea: pulmonary embolism, pneumonia, pneumothorax, pulmonary edema in cardiac ischemia, hyperventilation in anxiety.
- Cough: purulent sputum in pneumonia, hemoptysis in pulmonary embolism, frothy pink sputum in pulmonary edema.
- Rigors: pneumonia (particularly lobar pneumonia).
- Calf swelling: has PE arisen from deep vein thrombosis? Bilateral swelling suggests heart failure.
- Palpitations: arrhythmia can cause angina or result from cardiac ischemia, PE, or pneumonia.
- Clamminess, nausea, vomiting, and sweating are features of myocardial infarction or massive pulmonary embolism.

Do not forget about anginal equivalents, such as those listed above, or jaw pain/tightness or indigestion. Anginal equivalents may be the only presenting symptoms of an MI, especially in elderly and diabetic patients. When in doubt, get an ECG and cardiac enzymes.

## Are risk factors present?

Important risk factors include:
- Ischemic heart disease: smoking, family history, cholesterol, hypertension, diabetes, male sex, age over 50 years.
- PE: recent travel, immobility, or surgery, family history, pregnancy, malignancy.
- Pneumothorax: spontaneous (young, thin men), trauma, emphysema, asthma, malignancy, staphylococcal pneumonia, cystic fibrosis.

## Examining the patient with chest pain

Vital signs are *vital* and therefore should be checked first. Get in the habit of checking the vital signs yourself to avoid error. The examination should focus on determining the cause of the pain and then looking for risk factors and consequences of the underlying problem. A schematic guide to examining the patient with chest pain is given in Fig. 1.1.

## What is the cause of the pain?

Pay particular attention to:
- Pulse: tachycardia or arrhythmia.
- Blood pressure: discrepancy between left and right arms in aortic dissection.
- Chest wall tenderness: rib fracture, costochondritis, anxiety, shingles.
- Chest examination: pneumothorax, consolidation, pleural rub.
- Cardiac examination: fourth heart sound (PE or MI), rub (pericarditis).

## Are there risk factors?

The following risk factors may be present:
- Abnormal lipids: xanthelasma, tendon xanthoma.
- Nicotine-stained fingers: predisposition to ischemic heart disease.
- Hot, edematous, tender calf, suggesting deep vein thrombosis.
- Hypertension: ischemic heart disease.

**Fig. 1.1** Examining the patient with chest pain.

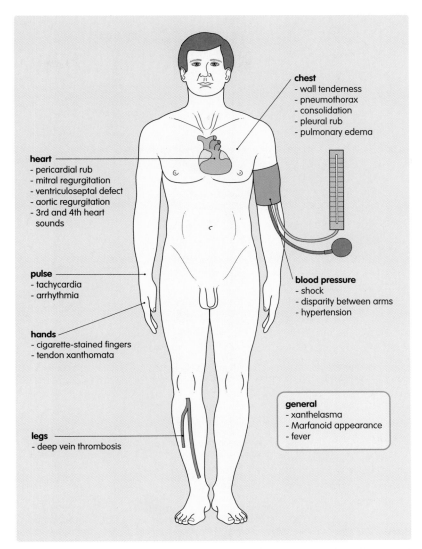

**chest**
- wall tenderness
- pneumothorax
- consolidation
- pleural rub
- pulmonary edema

**heart**
- pericardial rub
- mitral regurgitation
- ventriculoseptal defect
- aortic regurgitation
- 3rd and 4th heart sounds

**pulse**
- tachycardia
- arrhythmia

**hands**
- cigarette-stained fingers
- tendon xanthomata

**legs**
- deep vein thrombosis

**blood pressure**
- shock
- disparity between arms
- hypertension

**general**
- xanthelasma
- Marfanoid appearance
- fever

Also look for signs of venous stasis and arterial insufficiency in the lower extremities. Is there a brown discoloration (hemosiderin staining due to blood pooling) of the ankles? Does the patient have palpable lower extremity pulses.

## What are the complications?

Complications may include:

- Pulse: arrhythmia, tachycardia.
- Blood pressure: shock in tension pneumothorax, massive pulmonary embolism, MI.
- Heart failure: pulmonary edema and 3rd heart sound.
- Murmurs: acute mitral regurgitation and ventricular septal defect after MI; aortic regurgitation in dissecting aortic aneurysm.

## Investigating the patient with chest pain

All patients with chest pain should have an electrocardiogram (ECG), chest x-ray (CXR), and cardiac enzymes (see Fig. 1.5). Further investigation will be directed by findings in these tests in conjunction with the history and clinical examination. An algorithm for the investigation of the patient with chest pain is given in Fig. 1.2.

## Electrocardiogram

ST depression and elevation (Fig. 1.3) on ECG are suggestive of myocardial ischemia and acute MI,

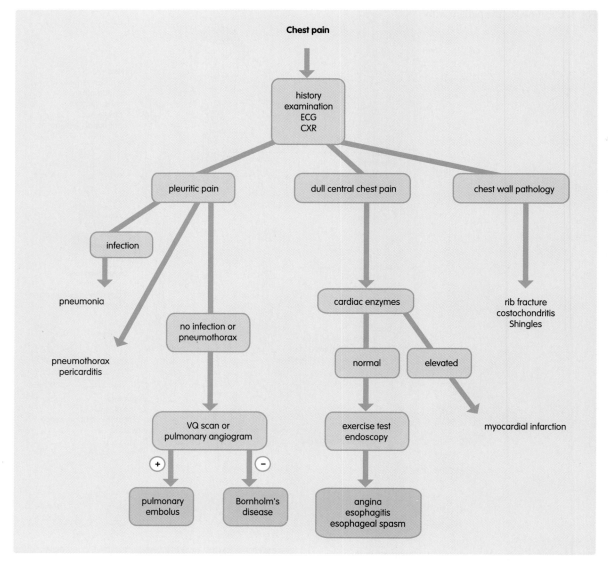

**Fig. 1.2** Algorithm for the investigation of the patient with chest pain. (CXR, chest x-ray; ECG, electrocardiogram; V/Q, ventilation–perfusion.)

respectively. Changes suggestive of PE are shown in Fig. 1.4. Arrhythmia may also be detected on ECG.

## Chest x-ray

Pneumothorax, consolidation (pneumonia, PE), widened mediastinum (aortic dissection), pulmonary edema (myocardial ischemia/infarction) and fractured ribs may be detected on CXR.

## Cardiac enzymes

Serial cardiac enzymes should be assessed every 8 hours for 24 hours if MI is considered (see Fig. 1.5).

## Stress test

An exercise test may be diagnostic when angina is suspected. Patients walk, ride a bike, or receive medication to increase the heart rate. These tests are done in conjunction with ECG monitoring, and a rest and stressed echocardiogram may also be used during this exam. Any sign of ischemia, such as ST elevation/depression, a drop in blood pressure, chest pain, or arrhythmia, is grounds for stopping the exam. Of note, exercise stress tests with ECG monitoring have a high false-negative rate in women. Therefore, it is often advantageous for a female

| Causes of ST elevation | |
|---|---|
| **Cause** | **Distribution of ST elevation** |
| myocardial infarction | right coronary artery (inferior): $aV_f$, II, III left anterior descending artery (anterior): I, $aV_l$, $V_{4-6}$ circumflex artery (anteroseptal): $V_{1-4}$ (overlap between territories may be seen) |
| pericarditis | across all leads (saddle-shaped ST change) |
| Prinzmetal's angina | leads of affected coronary artery (spasm) |
| aortic dissection | only if coronary artery involved |
| left ventricular aneurysm | persistent changes following infarct, persistently elevated ST segment |

**Fig. 1.3** Causes of ST elevation.

**ECG changes associated with pulmonary embolus**

- sinus tachycardia
- atrial arrhythmia, e.g. atrial fibrillation
- right heart strain
- right axis deviation
- right bundle branch block
- $S_1 Q_3 T_3$, i.e. deep S wave in I, Q wave in III, T wave inversion in III

**Fig. 1.4** Electrocardiogram (ECG) changes associated with pulmonary embolus. Note that sinus tachycardia may be the only abnormality present.

**Fig. 1.5** Cardiac enzyme elevation following myocardial infarction. (CK, creatine kinase; Myo, myoglobin; Tn, troponin.)

| Cardiac enzyme elevation after myocardial infarction | | | |
|---|---|---|---|
| **Enzyme** | **Begins to rise (hours after infarct)** | **Peak (hours after infarct)** | **Returns to normal (days after infarct)** |
| CK | 6 | 24 | 2–3 |
| $M_{yo}$ | 1–4 | 6–7 | 1 |
| $T_n$ | 3–12 | 24–48 | 6 |

patient either to undergo a nuclear medicine test, such as an adenosine/thallium stress test, or to go directly to catheterization. In the adenosine/thallium stress test, the heart is medically stressed and a radiolabeled tracer (thallium or sestimibi) is introduced to detect areas of low flow during stressed conditions.

## Coronary angiography

Coronary angiography allows direct visualization of the coronary arterial tree. It should be used in severe angina to determine whether angioplasty or coronary artery bypass grafting might be beneficial. Angiography is becoming more and more common as the number of centers with interventional cardiologists increases. Patients with equivocal or positive findings on exercise stress tests, along with those who have "good stories" (i.e., risk factors for coronary artery disease) are taken to catheterization

regularly. Patients should undergo catheterization if they have two of the following three characteristics:
- Good clinical picture of angina/MI.
- Positive cardiac markers (troponin, CK-MB).
- ST segment changes on ECG or new left bundle-branch block (LBBB).

## Arterial blood gases

The assessment of arterial blood gases is useful in determining the severity of PE, pneumonia, or pulmonary edema, showing hypoxia and occasionally hypocapnia. In hyperventilation related to anxiety, the $pO_2$ will be elevated while there will be hypocapnia and a respiratory alkalosis.

## Ventilation-perfusion scan

Ventilation-perfusion scan is used to diagnose PE. In some circumstances (e.g., when there is pre-existing obstructive airways disease) interpretation of this test can be difficult, so pulmonary angiography should then be performed. PE protocol CT can be used in addition to angiography in evaluating the patient with pre-existing pulmonary disease.

## Echocardiogram

The presence of a dissecting aortic aneurysm should be confirmed by urgent echocardiography (particularly transesophageal echocardiography) or by computed tomography scan. Urgent echocardiography is now used to help detect cardiac effusions and tamponade. Echocardiography also can be used to assess for possible sequelae of MI, such as myocardial dyskinesia, papillary rupture, or ventricular thrombus.

## Upper gastrointestinal endoscopy

Upper gastrointestinal endoscopy will confirm esophagitis and should be considered when the cause of chest pain is unclear.

# 2. Shortness of Breath

Shortness of breath (dyspnea) is the subjective sensation of breathlessness which is excessive for any given level of activity.

It is important to remember that any component of the respiratory system can cause dyspnea. Therefore, in making a differential diagnosis for dyspnea, think from the respiratory drive of the brain all the way to the individual alveoli. For example, remember that the peripheral nerves, respiratory muscles, lung parenchyma, airways, heart, and red blood cell (RBC) count are separate entities, each of which can cause shortness of breath.

Dyspnea may be due to any of the following:
- Pulmonary disease: disorders of the airways, lung parenchyma, pleura, respiratory muscles, or chest wall (pulmonary embolus, COPD, pneumonia, pneumothorax, pleural effusion, neoplasm, aspiration, ARDS, asthma, interstitial lung disease, any chest wall disease or neurologic disorder that affects respiratory drive).
- Cardiac disease: when it is the result of left ventricular failure (LVF) from any cause, such as coronary artery disease, valvular heart disease (aortic stenosis/regurgitation, mitral stenosis/regurgitation, pulmonary stenosis), or arrhythmia (ventricular tachycardia, supraventricular tachycardia).
- Metabolic disease (e.g., thyrotoxicosis, ketoacidosis, sepsis, drug overdose).
- Anemia.
- Psychogenic causes (e.g., anxiety or hyperventilation [psychogenic dyspnea]).

## History in the patient with shortness of breath

How breathless is the patient (severity)? Try to quantify exercise tolerance (e.g., distance walked on the flat or on hills, while dressing, climbing stairs).

Orthopnea is breathlessness on lying down. It is characteristic of heart failure but can occur with airways obstruction or, more rarely, with bilateral diaphragmatic paralysis. Paroxysmal nocturnal dyspnea is breathlessness that wakes the patient from sleep and is generally a symptom of cardiac disease. Ask patients where they slept last night; if the answer is in a chair, the patient has severe orthopnea. Also ask about how many pillows the patient uses at night.

The onset of breathlessness will often give a clue to its etiology:
- Acute onset may be due to a foreign body, pneumothorax, pulmonary embolism, asthma, or acute pulmonary edema.
- Subacute onset is more suggestive of parenchymal disease (e.g., alveolitis; pleural effusion; pneumonia; carcinoma of the bronchus or trachea).
- Chronic onset is associated with chronic obstructive pulmonary disease (COPD), cryptogenic fibrosing alveolitis, occupational fibrotic lung disease, nonrespiratory causes (e.g., LVF, anemia, or hyperthyroidism).

 Determining the patient's exercise tolerance gives a useful marker of the progression of symptoms.

In addition to the above, the following factors should be assessed when taking a history from a patient with breathlessness:
- Is the breathlessness associated with a cough? A chronic persistent cough may be due to smoking, asthma, COPD, drugs (especially angiotensin-converting enzyme [ACE] inhibitors), occupational agents, cardiac failure, or psychogenic factors.
- How long has the cough been present?
- Is the cough worse at any particular time of day?

- Are there any precipitating factors?
- If there is sputum, ask what it looks like.
- Does the patient have hemoptysis? This is coughing up blood—either frank blood or blood-tinged sputum. It needs to be distinguished from hematemesis and nasopharyngeal bleeding (see Chapter 5 for the causes of hematemesis).
- Ask about stridor (a harsh sound caused by turbulent airflow through a narrowed airway). Inspiratory stridor suggests extrathoracic obstruction, expiratory stridor suggests intrathoracic obstruction, and inspiratory and expiratory stridor suggests a fixed obstruction.
- Does the patient wheeze? These are whistling noises caused by turbulent airflow through narrowed intrathoracic airways. The most common cause is asthma.
- Does the breathlessness affect the activities of daily living and quality of life?
- Occupational history, including exposure to dusts or allergies. Dyspnea only during the working week may be suggestive of occupational lung disease.

## Examining the patient with shortness of breath

The findings on examination of common respiratory conditions are listed in Fig. 2.1, and the examination approach in the patient with breathlessness is summarized in Fig. 2.2. A more detailed description showing examination findings in respiratory disease can be found in Chapter 26.

## Inspection

Note the respiratory rate from the end of the bed or while feeling the pulse.

Look for cyanosis; a blue color in the mouth and tongue due to inadequate oxygenation (i.e., 5g reduced hemoglobin (Hb) per 100ml of blood). It is commonly associated with lung disease and cardiac disease and hypoventilation from other causes (note that severely anemic patients are not cyanotic—they don't have enough Hb to break the 5g/100ml barrier).

Cyanosis is an unreliable guide to the degree of hypoxemia. Peripheral cyanosis is due to poor peripheral circulation (e.g., in cardiac failure, peripheral vascular disease, or arterial obstruction) and physiologic when due to cold. Cyanosis is rarely seen in anemic patients.

The following factors should also be looked for when assessing the patient with shortness of breath:
- Anemia.
- Clubbing: respiratory causes include carcinoma of the bronchus; pus in any part of the respiratory tract (e.g., empyema, lung abscess, bronchiectasis, cystic fibrosis; fibrosing alveolitis; chronic suppurative pulmonary tuberculosis; pleural mesothelioma).
- Chest movements on inspiration and expiration: an abnormality is normally found on the side of diminished movements.

| Findings on examination of common respiratory conditions | | | | | |
|---|---|---|---|---|---|
| Condition | Movement on side of lesion | Position of trachea | Percussion | Tactile fremitus | Breath sounds vocal |
| pleural effusion | ↓ | central or deviated away from effusion if massive | ↓ ["stony dull"] | ↓ | ↓ with bronchial breathing at top of effusion |
| pneumothorax | ↓ | central or deviated away | ↑ | ↓ | ↓ |
| pneumonia | ↓ | central or deviated towards if associated with collapse | ↓ | ↑ | bronchial breathing (absent if obstruction of bronchus) |
| pulmonary fibrosis | ↓ | central or deviated towards if upper lobe involvement | ↓ | ↑ | bronchial breathing |

**Fig. 2.1** Findings on examination of common respiratory conditions.

**Fig. 2.2** Examining the patient with breathlessness.

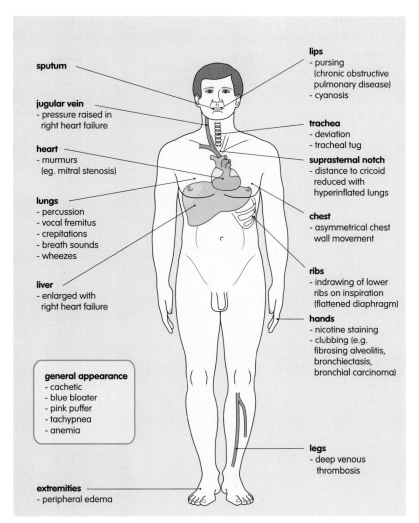

**sputum**

**jugular vein**
- pressure raised in right heart failure

**heart**
- murmurs (eg. mitral stenosis)

**lungs**
- percussion
- vocal fremitus
- crepitations
- breath sounds
- wheezes

**liver**
- enlarged with right heart failure

**general appearance**
- cachetic
- blue bloater
- pink puffer
- tachypnea
- anemia

**extremities**
- peripheral edema

**lips**
- pursing (chronic obstructive pulmonary disease)
- cyanosis

**trachea**
- deviation
- tracheal tug

**suprasternal notch**
- distance to cricoid reduced with hyperinflated lungs

**chest**
- asymmetrical chest wall movement

**ribs**
- indrawing of lower ribs on inspiration (flattened diaphragm)

**hands**
- nicotine staining
- clubbing (e.g. fibrosing alveolitis, bronchiectasis, bronchial carcinoma)

**legs**
- deep venous thrombosis

- Accessory muscles: patients with COPD typically have overexpansion of the lungs. Because the diaphragm provides less lung expansion, they often rely on chest and neck muscles to respire.
- Barrel-shaped chest: emphysema.
- Kyphoscoliosis: can decrease chest size and expansion.
- Ankylosing spondylitis: can "fix" the chest.
- Rhythm of respiration: Cheyne–Stokes respiration describes periods of fast and deep inspiration followed by periods of apnea due to depression of the central respiratory center in the medulla. This may occur with severe chest infections, metabolic acidosis, opiate overdose, and raised intracranial pressure.

Don't forget to look at the sputum:
- Purulent, moderate quantity—bronchitis or pneumonia.
- Purulent, copious quantity—bronchiectasis or pneumonia.
- Pink and frothy—pulmonary edema.
- Blood-stained—causes of hemoptysis.
- Rust-colored—pneumococcal lobar pneumonia.

## Palpation

- Feel for lymphadenopathy secondary to malignant disease or infections.
- Palpate the trachea: displacement may indicate underlying chest disease or cardiac disease.
- Check the movement of the rib cage.
- Feel for tactile vocal fremitus.

- Compare both sides anteriorly and posteriorly.
- Percuss for signs of consolidation.

## Auscultation

- Expiration: may be prolonged in COPD.
- Bronchial breathing: consolidation, cavitation, or at the top of an effusion.

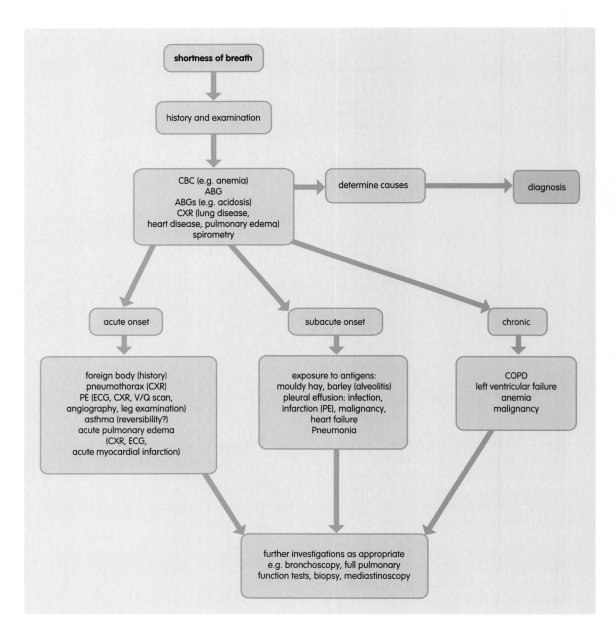

**Fig. 2.3** Algorithm for the investigation of the breathless patient. Note that more than one cause of shortness of breath may be apparent. (COPD, chronic obstructive pulmonary disease; CXR, chest x-ray; ECG, electrocardiogram; CBC, complete blood count; PE, pulmonary embolus; V/Q, ventilation-perfusion ratio; ABG, arterial blood gases.)

- Breath sounds: diminished over an effusion, pneumothorax, and in the obese.
- Rhonchi or wheezes: partially obstructed bronchi; found in asthma, bronchitis, and occasionally LVF.
- Crackles (sudden opening of small closed airways): pulmonary congestion (fine crackles in early inspiration); fibrosing alveolitis (fine crackles in late inspiration); bronchial secretions (coarse crackles).
- Friction rub: pleural disease.

To simulate the sound of bronchial breathing, place the stethoscope over your own trachea and listen.

## Investigating the patient with shortness of breath

An algorithm for the investigation of the patient with breathlessness is given in Fig. 2.3. The following investigations should be performed:

- Complete blood count: anemia leading to breathlessness, leukocytosis in pneumonia.
- Basic metabolic panel: renal failure secondary to dehydration, sepsis, or acidosis, producing breathlessness; hyponatremia of fluid overload.
- D-dimer: if negative in a patient with low probability for having PE, PE is ruled out.
- BNP: can help distinguish between heart failure and pulmonary causes.
- Chest x-ray: examine methodically (see p. 194).
- CT scan: the gold standard for parenchymal disease. CT has been used increasingly to evaluate for PE in patients with structural lung disease. In addition, high-resolution CT scans can be used to evaluate interstitial lung disease.

- Electrocardiogram (ECG): $S_1 Q_3 T_3$ pattern in PE (see Fig. 1.4), p pulmonale (tall p waves >2.5mm in lead II) in COPD with cor pulmonale; cardiac conditions leading to breathlessness (e.g., myocardial infarction with consequent pulmonary edema).
- Arterial blood gases: pH, partial pressures of oxygen and carbon dioxide, and hydrogen ion concentration (see respiratory failure, Chapter 29).
- Spirometry: to distinguish between obstructive and restrictive lung pathology, to test reversibility to treatments, and to gauge decline/improvement in patients with pre-existing results.
- Transfer factor ($D_2 CO$) and lung volume.
- Ventilation–perfusion scan: suspected pulmonary emboli.
- Bronchoscopy with or without transbronchial biopsy.

Metabolic acidosis leads to "deep sighing" breathlessness (Kussmaul respiration). Causes include uremia, diabetic ketoacidosis, salicylate ingestion, methanol ingestion, and lactic acidosis

The classic $S_1 Q_3 T_3$ pattern on the ECG with pulmonary emboli is rare. The ECG commonly shows sinus tachycardia, but other changes include right bundle-branch block, right ventricular strain, and atrial fibrillation.

# 3. Palpitations

Always check what the patient means by "palpitations" or clarify what you mean, as the word means different things to different people. It is usually understood as an awareness of the heartbeat. The most common cause is an arrhythmia, although other causes include conditions causing an increase in stroke volume (e.g., regurgitant valvular disease) or conditions causing an increase in cardiac output, often noncardiac causes (e.g., exercise, thyrotoxicosis, anemia, or anxiety). If an arrhythmia is suspected, try to determine whether there is an underlying cause.

## Differential diagnosis by description of the rhythm

### Regular rhythm
The differential diagnosis of regular palpitations includes the following:
- Heavy heart beats with normal rate: most often cardiac consciousness with sinus rhythm. It tends to be worse at rest, especially when lying in bed at night and during periods of stress.
- Fast heart rate: sinus tachycardia, atrial flutter with block, or ventricular tachycardia.
- Bursts of fast beats: paroxysmal atrial tachycardia. There is often a very long history dating back years, with a single attack followed by a long interval before the next attack. Other causes include atrial flutter, junctional rhythm, or ventricular tachycardia.
- Slow heart rate: sinus bradycardia (look for signs of hypothyroidism), atrioventricular block.

### Irregular rhythm
The differential diagnosis of irregular palpitations includes the following:
- Missed beats, "thumps": multiple ectopics from the atrium or ventricle. The symptoms are more troublesome at rest and may disappear during exercise.

- Fast (or normal if treated): atrial flutter with variable block, atrial fibrillation (may be worse with exercise), multiple premature beats with sinus tachycardia.

## History

Obtain a full description of the palpitations. Are they continuous or intermittent? Are they fast, normal rate, or slow? Are they regular or irregular? When did the palpitations start?—this can vary from a few minutes to decades. Generally, if the onset dates back years and there have been no serious complications (e.g., syncope), the palpitations are usually benign. Often it can be helpful if the patient can tap the heart rate with a finger to represent what the patient feels.

How often do the palpitations occur and how long do they last for? They may last for days or seconds, with intervals between episodes of a few hours to years. The patient may fear serious underlying cardiac disease, although there is usually a benign cause.

 Ask the patient to tap out the heart rhythm on the desk top. This will often give a good guide to rate and rhythm.

Are there any associated features? These may be related to the underlying cause (e.g., angina, features of hyperthyroidism) or a consequence of the palpitations (e.g., faintness or dizziness). Always obtain a full drug history as medication is often the culprit. Ask the patient to include over-the-counter drugs and herbal supplements. This is important given the number of over-the-counter weight loss pills and other medications that contain stimulants such as caffeine or ephedra (recently banned in the U.S.).

## Causal and contributory factors

Ask about smoking, alcohol, and caffeine (tea, coffee, cola) intake. These may contribute to extrasystoles. Myocardial ischemia may lead to any supraventricular or ventricular arrhythmia. Digoxin, which is commonly used to control atrial fibrillation, may also cause any arrhythmia, especially in the presence of hypokalemia. Note that most antiarrhythmic agents also have a proarrhythmic effect. Ask about rheumatic heart disease as atrial fibrillation often accompanies mitral stenosis.

Noncardiac causes of sinus tachycardia and causes of sinus bradycardia are outlined in Figs. 3.1 and 3.2, respectively.

Noncardiac causes of palpitations include the following:

- Thyrotoxicosis: may cause sinus tachycardia, paroxysmal atrial tachycardia, atrial flutter/

| Non-cardiac causes of sinus tachycardia |
| --- |
| • exercise<br>• fever<br>• anemia<br>• thyrotoxicosis<br>• pregnancy<br>• arteriovenous fistulae<br>• anxiety<br>• cigarettes, alcohol, caffeine<br>• sympathomimetic drugs<br>• heavy metals<br>• gastroesophageal reflux disease |

**Fig. 3.1** Noncardiac causes of sinus tachycardia.

| Causes of sinus bradycardia |
| --- |
| • athletes<br>• hypothyroidism<br>• obstructive jaundice<br>• raised intracranial pressure<br>• hypopitutarism<br>• hypothermia<br>• cardiac causes include ischemia, drugs (e.g. digoxin and β-blockers), inflammation, degeneration/fibrosis |

**Fig. 3.2** Causes of sinus bradycardia.

fibrillation. Ask about hyperthyroid symptoms such as sweating, tachycardia, weight loss, and tremor.
- Anemia: ask about anticoagulant usage, recent history of hematemesis, melena, heavy menorrhea.
- Myxedema: may be responsible for sinus bradycardia.
- Anxiety: a very common cause of palpitations.

## Consequences of palpitations

Palpitations may not affect the patient or may just be a minor nuisance. If a benign arrhythmia is present, reassurance that the condition is not serious is often all that is required. Changes in rate may be more serious, compromising coronary blood supply and leading to symptoms of myocardial ischemia or cardiac failure.

Tachycardia or bradycardia may lead to a reduction in cardiac output and cause dizziness or collapse (e.g., Stokes-Adams attacks in complete heart block).

## Examining the patient with palpitations

Always start with the vital signs:

### Inspection

A guide to examining the patient with palpitations is given in Fig. 3.3. Look for signs of anemia and hypo/hyperthyroidism (tremor, nervousness). Examine the limbs for signs of DVT, since PE can cause arrhythmias.

### Cardiovascular system

Next feel the pulse. Note the following:
- Rate: beats per minute.
- Rhythm: regular, regularly irregular (e.g., Wenckebach second-degree heart block), irregularly irregular (e.g. multiple ectopic beats or atrial fibrillation).
- Volume (e.g., a collapsing pulse of hyperdynamic circulation or a slow volume pulse of shock or aortic stenosis).

If the patient is symptom free at the time of examination, the pulse may be normal.

**Fig. 3.3** Examining the patient with palpitations. (CHB, complete heart block.)

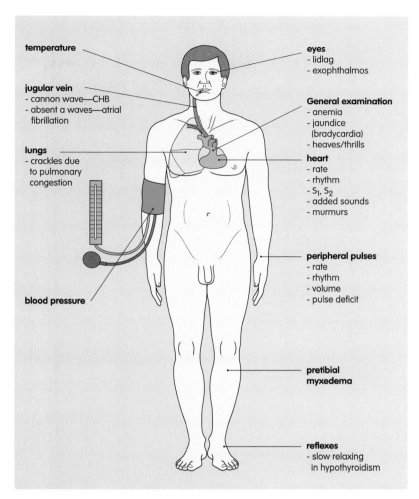

temperature

jugular vein
- cannon wave—CHB
- absent a waves—atrial fibrillation

lungs
- crackles due to pulmonary congestion

blood pressure

eyes
- lidlag
- exophthalmos

General examination
- anemia
- jaundice (bradycardia)
- heaves/thrills

heart
- rate
- rhythm
- $S_1$, $S_2$
- added sounds
- murmurs

peripheral pulses
- rate
- rhythm
- volume
- pulse deficit

pretibial myxedema

reflexes
- slow relaxing in hypothyroidism

The blood pressure will be low if the arrhythmia leads to a reduction in cardiac output. Hypertension may predispose to atrial fibrillation.

The jugulovenous pressure may be elevated if cardiac failure is present. Cannon a waves are visible with complete heart block, and a waves are absent in atrial fibrillation.

An irregularly irregular pulse (e.g., in atrial fibrillation) is irregular in rhythm *and* volume.

Feel for heaves and thrills with associated right ventricular enlargement and valvular heart disease. Assess the rate and rhythm by auscultation. The peripheral pulse rate may be slower than the apical rate in atrial fibrillation (pulse deficit). The first heart sound is of variable intensity in heart block and atrial fibrillation. Listen for cardiac murmurs, e.g., evidence of mitral valve disease predisposing to atrial fibrillation. Focus on any abnormal findings (see Chapter 4).

## Investigating the patient with palpitations

An algorithm for the investigation of the patient with palpitations is given in Fig. 3.4. The following tests should be performed:

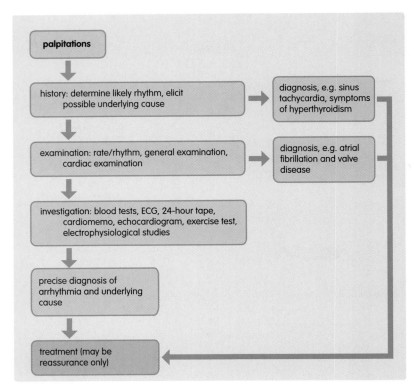

**Fig. 3.4** Algorithm for the investigation of the patient with palpitations. (ECG, electrocardiogram.)

## Blood tests

- Complete blood count: anemia.
- Metabolic panel: especially disturbances of potassium; less commonly, magnesium deficiency may contribute to refractory arrhythmias.
- D-dimer: to rule out PE.
- Thyroid function tests: hypo/hyperthyroidism.
- Drug concentration if appropriate (e.g., digoxin levels).

## Other tests

- Electrocardiogram (ECG): mandatory for anyone with palpitations and can often reveal the precise nature of the palpitations if present.
- 24-hour ECG: for intermittent symptoms. It should be carried out with a diary of symptoms to see if they correlate with any rhythm disturbances found.
- Palpitations memo: if symptoms do not occur every day, a palpitations memo can record the heart rhythm by phone at the press of a button.
- Echocardiogram: to exclude any underlying valvular disease.
- Holter monitor: if symptoms do not occur every day, a Holter monitor or event monitor can record the heart rhythm by phone at the press of a button or for a set duration of time.
- Chest x-ray: can show cardiomegaly, suggesting heart failure; also shows pulmonary causes.
- Stress test: the induction of symptoms, under controlled conditions with ECG monitoring, may be appropriate.
- Electrophysiologic studies: more rarely, patients may be referred for specialized studies. These can be used to induce arrhythmias, locate the origin of the arrhythmic focus, and to assess the response to drug treatment.

# 4. Heart Murmurs

Heart murmurs are due to vibrations caused by turbulent flow within the heart. The most common causes are due to left-sided valvular heart disease and tricuspid regurgitation. Nonvalvular causes include:

- Innocent "flow" murmurs, especially in children.
- High-output states (e.g., pregnancy, thyrotoxicosis, and fever).
- Congenital heart disease, such as atrial septal defects (ASD), ventricular septal defects (VSD), patent ductus arteriosus (PDA), and coarctation of the aorta.

## Differential diagnosis of heart murmurs

The differential diagnosis of heart murmurs includes ejection systolic murmurs, holosystolic murmurs, diastolic murmurs, and continuous murmurs.

## Ejection systolic murmurs
These usually originate in the right or left ventricular outflow tracts. They reach a crescendo in mid-systole and die down before the second heart sound.

Causes of ejection systolic murmurs in the aortic area (second right intercostal space) include the following:

- Supravalvular (e.g., supra-aortic stenosis or coarctation of the aorta).
- Valvular (e.g., aortic stenosis or aortic sclerosis).
- Subvalvular (e.g., hypertrophic obstructive cardiomyopathy).
- Hyperkinetic states due to increased flow across the valves.

Causes of ejection systolic murmurs in the pulmonary area (second left intercostal space) include the following:

- Supravalvular (e.g., pulmonary arterial stenosis).
- Valvular (e.g., pulmonary valve stenosis).
- Subvalvular (e.g., infundibular stenosis).

- Flow murmurs, hyperkinetic states, and left-to-right shunts (e.g., ASD).

Causes of ejection systolic murmurs at the apex include flow murmurs and aortic stenosis (radiation from the aortic area).

## Holosystolic murmurs
These murmurs are of uniform intensity and are heard throughout systole, merging with the second heart sound.

Causes of holoystolic murmurs at the lower left sternal edge include tricuspid regurgitation and VSD, and causes of those at the apex include mitral regurgitation.

## Diastolic murmurs
These are never normal or physiologic. Causes of early diastolic murmurs at the left sternal edge include aortic regurgitation and pulmonary regurgitation, and causes of mid-diastolic murmurs include tricuspid stenosis and increased flow across a nonstenotic tricuspid valve (e.g., ASD and tricuspid regurgitation).

Causes of diastolic murmurs at the apex include the following:

- Mitral stenosis.
- Carey Coombs murmur (due to thickening of mitral valve leaflets in acute rheumatic fever).
- Austin Flint murmur (due to fluttering of the anterior mitral valve cusp in aortic regurgitation by the regurgitant stream).
- Increased flow across a nonstenotic mitral valve (e.g., VSD and mitral regurgitation).
- Graham Steell murmur: pulmonary regurgitation secondary to pulmonary hypertension (also heard at left sternal edge).

## Continuous murmurs
Continuous murmurs are heard during systole and diastole, such as in PDA, coronary arteriovenous

19

fistula, ruptured aneurysm of the sinus of Valsalva, cervical venous hum, or ASD with mitral stenosis.

Pure diastolic murmurs are ALWAYS pathologic.

## History in the patient with heart murmurs

There are no symptoms of cardiac murmurs *per se*. Therefore, the history should focus on possible causes of the murmur or consequences of the responsible lesion. Ask about the following:

- Rheumatic fever: particularly affecting the mitral valve.
- Ischemic heart disease (e.g., mitral regurgitation). Due to papillary muscle damage or heart dilation.
- Congenital heart disease.
- Hypertension: flow murmurs.
- Family history: hypertrophic cardiomyopathy is inherited as an autosomal dominant condition.
- Aortic regurgitation (AR) may be associated with rheumatoid arthritis or seronegative arthropathies (e.g., ankylosing spondylitis, Reiter's syndrome, colitic and psoriatic arthropathy, Marfan's syndrome, syphilitic aortitis, or coarctation of the aorta). If you suspect any of these, question further about joint symptoms, gastrointestinal symptoms, neurologic symptoms, etc. In addition, AR is much more common in patients with a known bicuspid valve.
- Mitral regurgitation may be caused by connective tissue disorders (e.g., systemic lupus erythematosus, rheumatoid arthritis), ankylosing spondylitis, or congenital conditions (e.g., Marfan's syndrome, Ehlers-Danlos syndrome, pseudoxanthoma elasticum, or osteogenesis imperfecta).
- Social history: drug and alcohol use may predispose to dilated cardiomyopathy. IV drug abuse suggests infective endocarditis, and smoking is a risk factor for CAD.
- Risk factors for endocarditis, especially a history of rheumatic fever (particularly affecting the mitral valve) or prior infective endocarditis; prosthetic heart valves; recent dental, GI, or respiratory invasive procedures; or known valvular damage.

## Consequences

The following consequences of a heart murmur may be noted:

- None: aortic valve disease and mitral regurgitation may remain asymptomatic for years.
- Fatigue and weakness: low cardiac output.
- Palpitations: especially atrial fibrillation.
- Angina: especially in coronary heart disease or aortic stenosis.
- Symptoms of right ventricular failure (secondary to pulmonary hypertension): congestion may result in anorexia, ankle and leg swelling, and hepatic pain.
- Symptoms of left ventricular failure: shortness of breath on exertion, cough and hemoptysis (especially mitral stenosis), orthopnea, and paroxysmal nocturnal dyspnea (PND).
- Syncope due to poor cardiac output in conditions obstructing the outflow tract (e.g., severe aortic stenosis).
- Symptoms of systemic emboli (e.g., transient ischemic attacks or stroke); often a complication in mitral stenosis.
- Symptoms of enlarged left atrium pressing on other structures (especially in mitral stenosis), such as recurrent laryngeal nerve leading to hoarseness (Ortner's syndrome), esophagus leading to dysphagia, left main bronchus leading to left lung collapse.
- Symptoms of infective endocarditis: fever, malaise, weight loss.

In patients with pulmonary hypertension, pulmonary edema may be precipitated by the following:

- Onset of uncontrolled atrial fibrillation.
- Chest infection.
- Anesthesia.
- Exercise.
- Pregnancy.

## Examining the patient with heart murmurs

Always follow the examination routine—inspection, palpation, then auscultation. Many clues can be gained about the nature of the murmur before the stethoscope is placed on the chest.

## Mitral stenosis

Mitral stenosis usually occurs in women with a history of rheumatic fever. The incidence has declined with the decline in rheumatic fever.

### Clinical symptoms

Resistance in blood flow from the left atrium to the ventricle causes symptoms of left heart failure and eventual dilatation of the left atrium. Dyspnea on exertion is an early symptom, and may progress to orthopnoea and PND. Breathlessness often worsens considerably with the onset of atrial fibrillation, and is often accompanied by palpitations. Cough and hemoptysis may occur because of bronchitis, pulmonary infarction, pulmonary congestion, and bronchial vein rupture. Systemic emboli may occur in patients, particularly in atrial fibrillation. Fatigue and cold extremities are late symptoms, probably secondary to a low cardiac output. Chest pain occurs in a few people and may be due to coronary artery embolism or severe pulmonary hypertension. The patient may have coexistent coronary artery disease.

### Clinical signs

The clinical signs of mitral stenosis are given in Fig. 4.1.

### Differential diagnosis

The differential diagnosis of mitral stenosis includes the following:

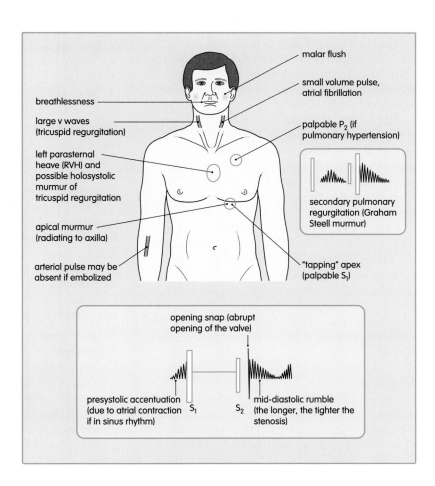

**Fig. 4.1** Mitral stenosis. (RVH, right ventricular hypertrophy.)

- Inflow obstruction (e.g., hypertrophic cardiomyopathy or left atrial myxoma).
- Aortic regurgitation.
- Tricuspid stenosis.

## Investigations

The electrocardiogram (ECG) may show atrial fibrillation or "p" mitrale in sinus rhythm. There may be signs of right ventricular hypertrophy (RVH)—e.g., a dominant R wave in $V_1$—and right axis deviation.

The murmur of mitral stenosis is louder after exercise. Ask the patient to jog on the spot or do sit-ups on the examination couch if the murmur is soft.

The chest x-ray (CXR) shows left atrial enlargement visible as a double shadow behind the heart. Valve calcification may be seen in lateral projections. There may also be signs of pulmonary edema and a splayed carina.

Echocardiography can be used to assess the area of the mitral valve orifice, and the gradient across the mitral valve. It can also be used to assess left ventricular function and measure the size of the left atrium, and the right-sided heart chambers. This is important in deciding who is eligible for mitral ballon valvotomy.

Cardiac catheterization is usually reserved for patients with suspected coronary artery disease but can be used to measure the pulmonary capillary wedge pressure as an indirect gauge of left atrial pressure, and the left ventricular end diastolic pressure (LVEDP), and hence the gradient across the mitral valve. The measurements should be repeated after exercise if the right-sided heart pressures are normal.

## Treatment

For patients without symptoms, it is important to provide prophylaxis against endocarditis. For patients with any symptoms or signs of right ventricular hypertension, it is essential that the stenosis be relieved with balloon mitral valvotomy or surgery.

# Mitral regurgitation

In a group of patients referred for surgery, mitral regurgitation (MR) was thought to be secondary to mitral valve prolapse (20–70%), ischemia (13–30%), rheumatic fever (3–40%), and endocarditis (10–12%).

## Clinical symptoms

Most patients with MR are without symptoms. Symptomatic patients may have progressive exertional dyspnea; palpitations, and fatigue are common, with symptoms of pulmonary edema if severe. Atrial fibrillation, systemic emboli, and chest pain are less common than in mitral stenosis.

## Clinical signs

The clinical signs of mitral regurgitation are given in Fig. 4.2.

## Differential diagnosis

The differential diagnosis of mitral regurgitation includes the following:
- Aortic stenosis.
- Hypertrophic cardiomyopathy.
- VSD.
- Tricuspid regurgitation.

## Investigations

The CXR shows cardiomegaly with enlargement of the left ventricle and left atrium. In acute mitral regurgitation the heart size is normal with signs of pulmonary edema.

The ECG may show signs of left ventricular hypertrophy (LVH), "p" mitrale associated with left atrial hypertrophy, and occasionally atrial fibrillation.

Echocardiography may reveal a cause for the regurgitation and can be used to assess the degree of left ventricular dilatation, which is useful for following the progress of the regurgitation.

## Treatment

Usually patients remain asymptomatic and do not require any intervention. Medical therapies have proved of little benefit for patients with MR. Patients with severe MR or with an acute presentation secondary to infectious endocarditis or ischemia often need mitral valve repair or replacement.

**Fig. 4.2** Mitral regurgitation.

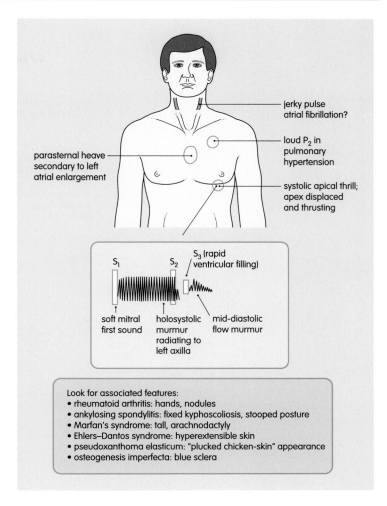

jerky pulse
atrial fibrillation?

loud $P_2$ in
pulmonary
hypertension

systolic apical thrill;
apex displaced
and thrusting

parasternal heave
secondary to left
atrial enlargement

$S_1$ $S_2$ $S_3$ (rapid
ventricular filling)

soft mitral
first sound

holosystolic
murmur
radiating to
left axilla

mid-diastolic
flow murmur

Look for associated features:
• rheumatoid arthritis: hands, nodules
• ankylosing spondylitis: fixed kyphoscoliosis, stooped posture
• Marfan's syndrome: tall, arachnodactyly
• Ehlers–Dantos syndrome: hyperextensible skin
• pseudoxanthoma elasticum: "plucked chicken-skin" appearance
• osteogenesis imperfecta: blue sclera

## Aortic stenosis
### Clinical symptoms
Initially the patient may be asymptomatic. Classically late symptoms are angina pectoris, syncope, and signs of heart failure (dyspnea). With these symptoms, the mean survival time is 5, 3, and 2 years, respectively, Sudden death may occur, probably secondary to ventricular dysrhythmias.

### Clinical signs
Clinical signs in aortic stenosis are given in Fig. 4.3.

### Investigations
The ECG shows signs of LVH with increased QRS voltages and ST/T segment changes.

The CXR usually shows a normal heart size. The ascending aorta may be prominent due to poststenotic dilatation, and the valve may be calcified.

Echocardiography may show a calcified valve and can be used to estimate the valve area. Cardiac chamber dimensions can be assessed, and doppler studies can be used to assess the gradient across the valve.

Cardiac catheterization is usually only necessary to exclude coexisting coronary disease but can determine the systolic gradient across the valve.

## Aortic regurgitation
### Clinical symptoms
The patient is usually asymptomatic until the ventricle fails, giving rise to symptoms of heart failure. Angina rarely occurs.

23

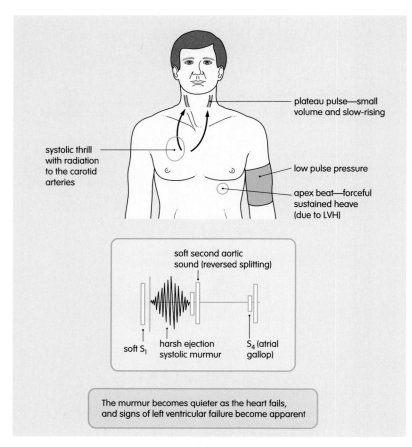

**Fig. 4.3** Aortic stenosis. (LVH, left ventricular hypertrophy.)

plateau pulse—small volume and slow-rising

systolic thrill with radiation to the carotid arteries

low pulse pressure

apex beat—forceful sustained heave (due to LVH)

soft second aortic sound (reversed splitting)

soft S$_1$

harsh ejection systolic murmur

S$_4$ (atrial gallop)

The murmur becomes quieter as the heart fails, and signs of left ventricular failure become apparent

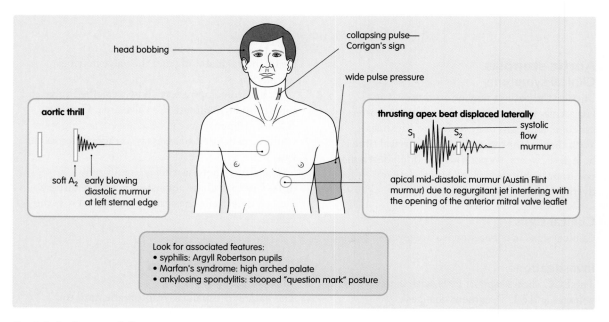

head bobbing

collapsing pulse— Corrigan's sign

wide pulse pressure

**aortic thrill**

soft A$_2$

early blowing diastolic murmur at left sternal edge

**thrusting apex beat displaced laterally**

S$_1$      S$_2$

systolic flow murmur

apical mid-diastolic murmur (Austin Flint murmur) due to regurgitant jet interfering with the opening of the anterior mitral valve leaflet

Look for associated features:
• syphilis: Argyll Robertson pupils
• Marfan's syndrome: high arched palate
• ankylosing spondylitis: stooped "question mark" posture

**Fig. 4.4** Aortic regurgitation.

When listening for aortic regurgitation, ask the patient to sit up and hold his or her breath in expiration.

## Clinical signs

Clinical signs in aortic regurgitation are given in Fig. 4.4. The pulse has a sharp rise and fall ("collapsing" or "water hammer") with a wide pulse pressure. Other manifestations of this are visible pulsation in the nail bed (Quincke's sign), visible arterial pulsation in the neck (Corrigan's sign), head bobbing (de Musset's sign), "pistol shot" femoral artery sound (Traube's sign), and a diastolic murmur following distal compression of the artery (Duroziez's sign).

## Differential diagnosis

The differential diagnosis of aortic regurgitation includes the following:

- Pulmonary regurgitation.
- PDA.
- VSD and aortic regurgitation.
- Ruptured aneurysm of the sinus of Valsalva.

## Investigations

The ECG shows signs of LVH and the CXR reveals cardiomegaly. Echocardiography can assess chamber size and may give a clue to the etiology. Cardiac catheterization can be used to assess the severity of the regurgitation, assess ventricular function, and for coronary arteriography.

# 5. Cough and Hemoptysis

Coughing is a nonspecific reaction to irritation anywhere in the respiratory tract from the pharynx to the lungs, and it is the most common manifestation of lower respiratory tract disease. Any cough that persists for over 3 weeks merits further investigation in the absence of an obvious cause.

## Differential diagnosis of cough and hemoptysis

### Cough
The differential diagnosis of cough includes:
- Postnasal drip: sinusitis.
- Upper respiratory tract infections (e.g., pharyngitis, laryngitis, tracheobronchitis).
- Pressure on the trachea (e.g., from a goiter): this may be associated with stridor.
- Croup and laryngitis.
- Lower respiratory tract causes: almost any lung pathology may be associated with cough, in particular asthma (suspect if there is a nocturnal cough), chronic obstructive pulmonary disease (COPD), bronchiectasis, and left ventricular failure.
- Drugs (e.g., angiotensin-converting enzyme [ACE] inhibitors) and irritants, especially occupational agents.
- Psychogenic cough.
- Nonrespiratory causes (e.g., pericardial irritation, gastroesophageal reflux).
- Causes of hemoptysis.

### Hemoptysis
Common causes of hemoptysis include the following:
- Acute infections (e.g., exacerbations of COPD).
- Bronchiectasis: can be responsible for massive hemoptysis.
- Bronchial carcinoma: secondary deposits and benign tumors can also lead to hemoptysis but are less common.
- Pulmonary tuberculosis: a common cause worldwide.
- Pulmonary embolus with infarction.
- Left ventricular failure can lead to the production of pink, frothy sputum.
- Mitral stenosis.
- Other infections, such as lobar pneumonia ("rusty" sputum) or, less commonly, lung abscess.
- Trauma (e.g., contusions to the chest, inhalation of foreign bodies, or after intubation).

Rare causes of hemoptysis include the following:
- Bleeding diatheses.
- Vasculitis (e.g., Goodpasture's syndrome and Wegener's granulomatosis).
- Diffuse interstitial fibrosis.
- Idiopathic pulmonary hemosiderosis.
- Arteriovenous malformations (Osler-Weber-Rendu disease [hereditary hemorrhagic telangiectasia], a favorite in exams but rare in practice).
- Eisenmenger's syndrome.
- Sarcoidosis and amyloidosis.
- Primary pulmonary hypertension.
- Cystic fibrosis.
- Invasive aspergillosis.

Note that in up to 15% of cases no cause for hemoptysis is found.

Be aware that Osler-Weber-Rendu disease occurs more often on exams than in clinical practice.

## History in the patient with cough and hemoptysis

The nature of the cough may help in the diagnosis (Fig. 5.1). The following factors should be assessed in the patient with cough or hemoptysis:

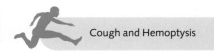

| Details of coughs that may be important for diagnosis |
| --- |
| • If the cough is productive, look at the sputum (see Chapter 2)<br>• A "brassy" cough, described as hard and metallic, may be associated with pressure on the trachea<br>• A cough associated with retrosternal pain, "like a hot poker" occurs in tracheitis<br>• A bovine cough results from laryngeal paralysis, usually from bronchial carcinoma infiltrating the left recurrent laryngeal nerve<br>• Croup is a hard and hoarse cough of laryngitis<br>• Associations with stridor may occur with whooping cough and in the presence of laryngeal or tracheal obstruction<br>• Ask about other associated symptoms, e.g. a wheeze may occur with asthma or left ventricular function; there may be orthopnea or paroxsymal nocturnal dyspnea (see Chapter 2)<br>• If associated with pleuritic pain, suspect pulmonary embolus<br>• A hacking, irritating frequent cough occurs in pharyngitis<br>• Associations with hemoptysis should trigger the differential diagnosis of hemoptysis |

**Fig. 5.1** Details regarding the nature of the cough that may be important for diagnosis.

- How long has the cough been present? A chronic cough is more commonly associated with tuberculosis, foreign bodies, and asthma.
- Has the patient been in contact with any person with infection or traveled anywhere that has endemic tuberculosis?
- How severe is the cough? Complications include worsening of bronchospasm, vomiting, rib fractures, urinary incontinence, and syncope.
- Does the patient smoke? This can often cause a cough in its own right by acting as an irritant but may also be associated with malignancy.
- Ask about drug history, in particular treatment with ACE inhibitors. Of people on ACE inhibitors, 10–20% will have a dry, tickly cough. It is more common in women than men. The patient may find the cough tolerable once reassured that there is no serious underlying condition, and the ACE inhibitor may be continued if needed. (Note: Angiotensin receptor blockers [ARBs] do not have this side effect.]
- Are there any occupational agents or exposure to dust which might account for the cough?
- Has there been any weight loss? Think of carcinoma or lung abscess. Ask about other features of malignancy if suspected, such as change in bowel habit.
- Has there been a history of trauma to the chest?
- Is there a family history of bleeding disorders?
- Ask about a past history of rheumatic fever— hemoptysis in mitral stenosis.
- If a diagnosis is suspected, ask more leading questions.

- If the patient is a lung transplant recipient or has cystic fibrosis, additional causes need to be considered (acute vs. chronic rejection, cytomegalovirus [CMV] pneumonitis).
- Don't forget nonrespiratory causes. For example, are there any symptoms suggestive of gastroesophageal reflux disease?

## Examining the patient with cough and hemoptysis

A full general and respiratory examination should be carried out (Fig. 5.2, and see Chapters 2 and 27). Assess the following:

### Inspection
- If the patient appears breathless, assess the severity and count the respiratory rate.
- Check for anemia: if present think of malignancy, connective tissue diseases, or chronic infection.
- If clubbing is present, suspect bronchial carcinoma, lung abscess, mesothelioma, bronchiectasis, cystic fibrosis, or fibrosing alveolitis.
- If the patient is cyanosed, suspect COPD or Eisenmenger's syndrome.
- Examine for lymphadenopathy, caused by infections or malignancy.
- Look at the sputum cup if the cough is productive.
- Examine for a goiter. Is there retrosternal extension?

**Fig. 5.2** Examining the patient with cough and hemoptysis.

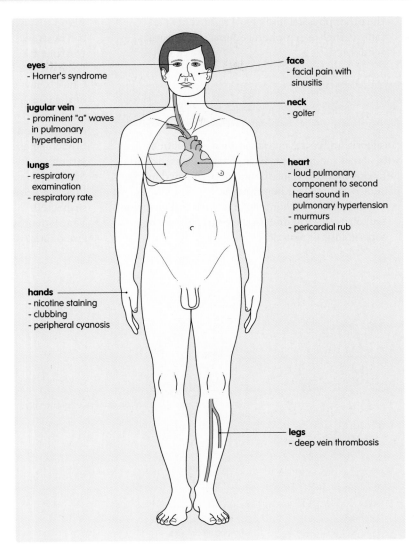

eyes
- Horner's syndrome

face
- facial pain with sinusitis

jugular vein
- prominent "a" waves in pulmonary hypertension

neck
- goiter

lungs
- respiratory examination
- respiratory rate

heart
- loud pulmonary component to second heart sound in pulmonary hypertension
- murmurs
- pericardial rub

hands
- nicotine staining
- clubbing
- peripheral cyanosis

legs
- deep vein thrombosis

- Examine specifically for signs of bronchial carcinoma (e.g., Horner's syndrome, paraneoplastic syndromes).
- Examine the legs for DVT, with pulmonary embolus as a cause for hemoptysis.
- Look at the skin. Punctate lesions on mucus membranes are present with Osler-Weber-Rendu disease.
- Check for facial pain in sinusitis.

## Auscultation
- Proceed to a full respiratory examination, including auscultation for murmurs over the lung fields with arteriovenous malformations, bronchial breathing in lobar consolidation, fine crackles with left ventricular failure and fibrosing alveolitis, and the coarser crackles in bronchiectasis.
- A localized wheeze, not disappearing on coughing, suggests a blocked major airway from a carcinoma or a foreign body.

## Other systems
- Auscultate the heart for the murmur of mitral stenosis or a pericardial rub.
- Listen for the pleural rub of pulmonary infarction.
- In pulmonary hypertension, there will be a loud pulmonary component of the second heart sound, a right ventricular heave, a pulmonary systolic murmur, and prominent a-waves in the jugulovenous pressure. This also may lead to

29

the other physical findings of right ventricle failure, such as peripheral edema and hepatic tenderness.

## Investigating the patient with cough and hemoptysis

An algorithm for the investigation of the patient with cough and hemoptysis is given in Fig. 5.3. The following investigations should be performed in the patient with cough or hemoptysis:

- Complete blood count: anemia with malignancies, leukocytosis with infection, eosinophils with aspergillosis or allergies.

- Blood cultures: help define infection. Viral titers can be drawn but probably will not influence treatment.
- Basic metabolic panel.
- Chest x-ray: this may reveal the pulmonary cause of the cough (e.g., pneumonia, a straight left heart border with mitral stenosis, infiltrative lung diseases, honeycombing or cyst formation with bronchiectasis, bilateral hilar lymphadenopathy in sarcoidosis).
- Sputum: microscopy, culture, and cytology.
- Pharyngoscopy: if an upper respiratory cause is suspected.
- Ventilation/perfusion scan: if a pulmonary embolus is suspected.

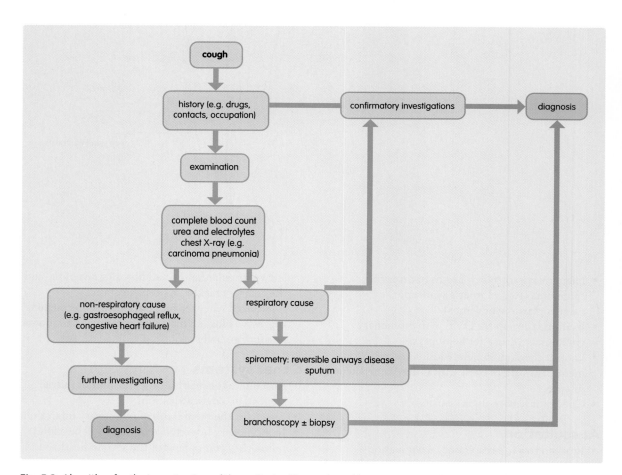

**Fig. 5.3** Algorithm for the investigation of the patient with cough and hemoptysis. Confirmatory investigations include sputum and blood cultures for pneumonia, and a ventilation-perfusion scan for pulmonary emboli.

- Bronchoscopy with or without biopsy—if infection is still unknown or if neoplasm/interstitial lung disease is suspected.
- Specific lung function tests: if the cause has not been found after the above tests have been carried out (see Chapter 29).

- High-resolution computed tomography: to confirm the presence of interstitial disease; it is useful in confirming bronchiectasis.
- Gastroscopy or barium meal: to investigate possible gastroesophageal reflux disease.

# 6. Fever of Unknown Origin

Most fevers are due to viral illnesses and are self-limiting. Fever of unknown origin (FUO) is a persistent and unexplained fever that lasts more than 3 weeks.

## Causes

The causes of FUO depend largely on the patient population and previous medical history. For instance, an HIV-positive patient has a much larger differential diagnosis that starts with infections and lymphomas as a possible cause for fever.

In general, FUO may be caused by the following:
- Infections: 20–40%.
- Connective tissue disorders: 20%.
- Malignancy: 10–20%.
- Undiagnosed: 20%.
- Drugs (e.g., phenytoin): rare.

## History in the patient with FUO

This should be thorough. Note especially:
- Foreign travel: the incubation period of many tropical diseases may mean that the fever starts some time after arrival back home.
- Contact with animals (zoonoses), such as leptospirosis, Q fever, salmonellosis, cat-scratch fever, psittacoses and ornathoses, toxoplasmosis, hydatid disease, toxocariasis, meningitis, anthrax.
- Contact with infected people (e.g., tuberculosis).
- Sexual history.
- Alcohol intake.
- Previous illnesses.
- Previous surgery or accidents.
- Recent hospitalization or recent dental, GI, GU, or respiratory work.
- Previous known valvular disease or prosthetic material.
- Rashes.
- Diarrhea.

- Ask about illicit drug use, especially any IV use, because this greatly increases the risk for bacterial endocarditis.
- A full history of medication, including over-the-counter drugs.
- Immunization history.
- Symptoms such as sweats, weight loss, and itching (these suggest a hematologic malignancy).
- Immunosuppression (transplant patient, previous autoimmune disease, HIV).
- Lumps.
- Familial disorders (e.g., familial Mediterranean fever).

Every symptom should be explored in detail. The diagnosis should be made by going over the history repeatedly to look for additional or missed clues.

 The temperature and pulse should be recorded at least 4-hourly when a patient is admitted with FUO.

## Examining the patient with FUO

The examination of a patient with FUO is shown in Fig. 6.1. It should be especially thorough and may need to be repeated several times. Particular attention should be given to:
- Teeth and throat.
- Temporal artery tenderness (if this is suspected, ask about jaw claudication or any visual changes that the patient has experienced).
- Eye signs (e.g., conjunctival petechiae).
- Skin lesions (e.g., rashes, petechiae, and infarctions). Look for Janeway lesions and Osler's nodes (which are painful).
- Lymphadenopathy and organomegaly.

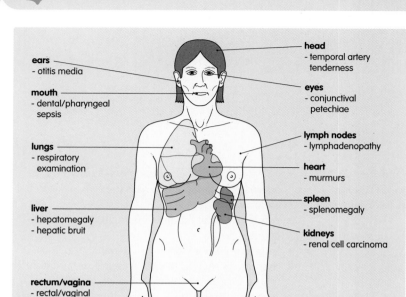

**Fig. 6.1** Examining the patient with fever of unknown origin (FUO).

ears
- otitis media

mouth
- dental/pharyngeal sepsis

lungs
- respiratory examination

liver
- hepatomegaly
- hepatic bruit

rectum/vagina
- rectal/vaginal masses and infections

legs
- deep venous thrombosis

head
- temporal artery tenderness

eyes
- conjunctival petechiae

lymph nodes
- lymphadenopathy

heart
- murmurs

spleen
- splenomegaly

kidneys
- renal cell carcinoma

hands
- nail-fold infarcts

skin
- rashes

- Cardiac murmurs.
- Rectal and vaginal examinations.

## Investigating the patient with FUO

An algorithm for the investigation of the patient with FUO is given in Fig. 6.2. Investigations are best directed from the history and examination. For example, if the patient has just returned from a part of the world where malaria is endemic, thick and thin blood films should be requested. Often there will be no clue, and the best way to proceed is to ask for general nonspecific screening tests, which may then suggest an area to focus on.

## Complete blood count and differential white cell count

Complete blood count and differential white cell count may yield information on the following:

- Neutrophil leukocytosis: bacterial infections, myeloproliferative disease, malignancy (e.g., hepatic metastases), collagen vascular diseases.
- Leukopenia: viral infections, lymphoma, systemic lupus erythematosus, brucellosis, disseminated tuberculosis, drugs.
- Monocytosis: subacute bacterial endocarditis, inflammatory bowel disease, Hodgkin's disease, brucellosis, tuberculosis.

**Fig. 6.2** Investigation of the patient with fever of unknown origin (FUO).

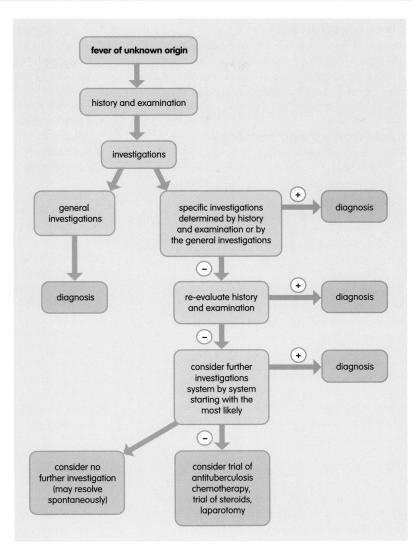

- Abnormal mononuclear cells: glandular fever, cytomegalovirus infection, toxoplasmosis.
- Eosinophilia: parasitic infections such as trichiasis, hydatid disease (infection with the echinococcus tapeworm), malignancy (especially Hodgkin's disease), pulmonary eosinophilia.

Always go over the history and examination repeatedly, even when investigations are in progress.

## Erythrocyte sedimentation rate

A very high erythrocyte sedimentation rate suggests the following:
- Multiple myeloma.
- Rheumatic fever.
- Lymphoma.
- Subacute bacterial endocarditis.
- Autoimmune diseases, most of which have an elevated ESR (e.g., SLE, temporal arteritis, polymyalgia rheumatica, Juvenile rheumatoid arthritis (Still's disease)).

## Basic metabolic panel

Assessment of urea and electrolytes may reveal renal impairment or hyponatremia due to pneumonia.

35

## Liver function tests

Abnormal results may lead to more detailed investigations of the liver. Note, however, that alkaline phosphatase may also be raised in metabolic bone disease, Hodgkin's disease, Still's disease, and in patients with bony metastases.

## Bacteriology and serology

Microscopy and culture from every site possible:

- Urine: bacteria (infections), hematuria (may suggest subacute bacterial endocarditis or hypernephroma).
- Blood cultures: several samples are needed from different veins at different times of the day.
- Feces microscopy for ova, cysts, and parasites.
- Vaginal and cervical swabs.
- Urethral swabs in men.
- Sputum microscopy and culture.
- Throat swab cultures.
- Amylase/lipase: will show pancreatitis.
- Liver function tests: will show hepatitis.
- Throat swab cultures.

With regard to serology, many specific tests are available (e.g., glandular fever, psittacosis, brucellosis). A second sample must be taken 2–3 weeks later to show a rising antibody titer or IgM titers may signal acute infection.

## Chest x-ray

Chest x-ray should be performed to show, for example, tuberculosis, subphrenic abscess, and bilateral hilar lymphadenopathy (sarcoidosis).

## Further investigations

Further investigations should be directed by the results of previous investigations. For example, if a renal problem is suspected, further tests might include an intravenous pyelogram and renal ultrasound. If a pulmonary problem is suspected, a ventilation/perfusion scan or pulmonary angiography may be useful to exclude multiple pulmonary emboli as the cause of FUO.

If there are no clues from previous investigations, the following further investigations should be considered:

- Echocardiography: to rule out endocarditis (needs to be transesophageal echocardiography).
- Immunoglobulins: raised immunoglobulin (IgG) suggests SLE or chronic hepatitis; raised IgM suggests viral hepatitis; raised IgA suggests Crohn's disease.
- Rheumatoid factor.
- Intradermal PPD test for tuberculosis.
- Bone marrow aspiration.
- Lumbar puncture.

All nonessential drugs should be stopped on admission. It may be necessary to withhold other drugs at this stage, one at a time for 48 hours each.

If there is still no clue as to the cause of the fever, the system most likely to be responsible should be investigated. Thus, to investigate the abdominal system, the following investigations should be considered:

- Abdominal ultrasound (e.g., subphrenic or pelvic abscess).
- Abdominal computed tomography scan (e.g., retroperitoneal lymphadenopathy, lymphoma).
- Barium studies (e.g., malignancy or abscess).
- Liver biopsy (e.g., granulomatous diseases or brucellosis).

Very rare causes should be considered if not already investigated. These include hyperthyroidism, pheochromocytoma, and familial Mediterranean fever.

Factitious fever is caused by the deliberate manipulation of the thermometer. This is classically said to occur in young women. The diagnosis should be suspected if other causes have been excluded; if there is no evidence of a chronic illness and no increase in pulse rate during fever; or if the patient looks inappropriately well despite fever.

If all else fails, it may be necessary to carry out an exploratory laporotomy, although the postoperative complication rate is 15–20%. Consideration should also be given to treating tuberculosis with antituberculosis chemotherapy, endocarditis with antibiotics, and vasculitides with steroids.

# 7. Hematemesis, Hematochezia, and Melena

Hematemesis is the vomiting of fresh (bright red) or altered ("coffee ground") blood. Melena is the production of black, tarry stools and is due to bleeding from the upper gastrointestinal (GI) tract of more than 100mL of blood. GI bleeding is an emergency, and treatment may need to be initiated before a diagnosis has been made (Chapter 32). Always remember that since blood is a cathartic, hematochezia may be caused by an upper GI bleed. When in doubt place a nasogastric tube and aspirate the contents of the stomach. This will help differentiate between lower and upper GI bleeding in the acute setting.

## Differential diagnosis of hematemesis, hematochezia, and melena

### Upper GI bleed (hematemesis/melena)

- Peptic ulcer disease: the most common cause, accounting for about half of major upper GI bleeds. The acute mortality rate is about 10%.
- Erosive gastritis: implicated in about 20% of upper GI bleeds, although they are an unusual cause of severe GI bleeding unless associated with other pathology.
- Mallory-Weiss tears: lacerations of the gastroesophageal junction accounting for about 10% of upper GI bleeds. Often due to retching after an alcohol binge.
- Esophagitis/hiatus hernia: secondary to chronic gastroesophageal reflux.
- Ruptured esophageal varices: secondary to portal hypertension, accounting for 10–20% of upper GI bleeds. The acute mortality rate is up to 40%.
- Vascular abnormalities: may cause upper or lower GI bleeding. The most common abnormalities are vascular ectasias or angiodysplasias.
- Dieulafoy's ulcer: an eroded gastric artery, often with pulsatile bleeding on EGD.
- Boerhave's syndrome: similar to a Mallory-Weiss tear except that it is a full-thickness esophageal tear. Often the result of persistent vomiting.
- Gastric neoplasms: about 5% of upper GI bleeds.
- Rarer causes include esophageal or stomal ulcers, esophageal tumors, blood dyscrasias, aortoenteric fistula complicating an abdominal aortic graft, pancreatic tumor, pseudoaneurysm.

### Lower GI bleed (hematochezia/melena)

- Diverticulosis: diverticuli are small outpouchings, usually of the sigmoid colon, that are prone to bleeding. They are thought to be related to the Western low fiber diet.
- Hemorrhoids: the most common cause of frank drops of blood with defecation. Associated with straining on defecation and a low fiber diet.
- Mesenteric ischemia: emboli or atherosclerosis causes necrosis of a portion of bowel that can then bleed. Usually this is associated with significant pain as well.
- Arteriovenous malformations (AVMs): common causes of acute massive bleeding. AVMs are more common in elderly patients.
- Inflammatory bowel disease: bleeding is more likely with ulcerative colitis, in which bloody diarrhea is common.
- Radiation colitis: the GI epithelium is highly sensitive to radiation, given its frequent regeneration, and can slough and bleed.
- Colonic neoplasm/polyp: often a common cause of occult bleeding, although it can present with frank blood as well. More common in older patients or patients with a family history of polyps and cancer.

## History in the patient with hematemesis, hematochezia, and melena

The history may have to be taken after initial resuscitation procedures (i.e., placement of two large-bore IV lines, NG tube, Foley catheter, and blood typing and screen). It is important to determine whether the blood has been vomited or coughed. In cases of difficulty, the presence of food mixed with the blood or an acid pH is suggestive of hematemesis, although the vomitus may not be acidic in patients with carcinoma of the stomach.

Hematemesis may be due to blood swallowed from the nasopharynx or mouth.

You must ask about the following:

- Nonspecific symptoms of GI blood loss: faintness, weakness, dizziness, sweating, palpitations, dyspnea, pallor, collapse. These symptoms may precede the actual hematemesis/melena. Also ask about the time frame of these symptoms. If the patient has fatigue and pallor, are they acute or chronic?
- Weight loss and anorexia: carcinoma.
- Current drugs: aspirin, nonsteroidal anti-inflammatory drugs, and excessive alcohol are suggestive of gastric erosions; iron therapy causes black stools, but this is not melena. Clopidogrel and warfarin are also associated with GI bleeds.
- Symptoms of chronic blood loss: suggests gastric carcinoma if associated with anorexia and weight loss.
- Heartburn: esophagitis.
- Intermittent epigastric pain relieved with antacids: peptic ulceration.
- Sudden severe abdominal pain: perforation.
- Dysphagia or odynophagia (pain on swallowing): esophageal carcinoma.
- Chronic excessive alcohol intake: esophageal varices.
- Inquiry into the causes of liver failure (Chapter 10): esophageal varices.
- Retching, especially after an alcohol binge: Mallory-Weiss tear.
- Family history: inherited bleeding disorders.
- A past history of GI bleeds and their cause.

## Examining the patient with hematemesis, hematochezia, and melena

The approach to examining the patient with hematemesis and melena is given in Fig. 7.1. Step back from the patient for a few seconds. Does the patient look well or pale and clammy? An initial common-sense impression affects the immediacy of subsequent management.

**Remember:** Vital signs are vital, and the ABCs (airway, breathing, circulation) should be attended to first. Tachycardia, low blood pressure, or orthostastic blood pressure often indicates a patient who needs immediate attention. In any patient with a suspected GI bleed, two large-bore IV lines should be placed and input/output should be monitored.

If hemoptysis is suspected, a full respiratory examination should be carried out.

### General examination

The general examination should assess the following:

- Anemia: mucous membranes. If clinically anemic, this may indicate chronic blood loss.
- Jaundice: may indicate portal hypertension.
- Clubbing of fingers: inflammatory bowel disease, cirrhosis.
- Lymphadenopathy: especially Virchow's node (left supraclavicular lymph node), which is associated with gastric carcinoma (Troisier's sign).
- Pulse: tachycardia can be the first warning of a large GI bleed and may precede a blood pressure fall. A young and healthy patient may lose more than 500mL of blood before a rise in heart rate or fall in blood pressure occurs.
- Blood pressure: if hypotensive, intravenous fluids should be given. The pulse and blood pressure measurements should be repeated frequently to monitor hemodynaimc trends.
- Skin: bruises, purpura (bleeding disorders); telangiectasia (Osler-Weber-Rendu disease [hereditary haemorrhagic telangiectasia—autosomal dominant]); neurofibromata.
- Mouth: pharyngeal lesions; pigmented macules (Peutz-Jeghers syndrome).
- Cachexia.

### Specific examination

This includes a search for signs related to the differential diagnosis:

**Fig. 7.1** Examining the patient with hematemesis and melena.

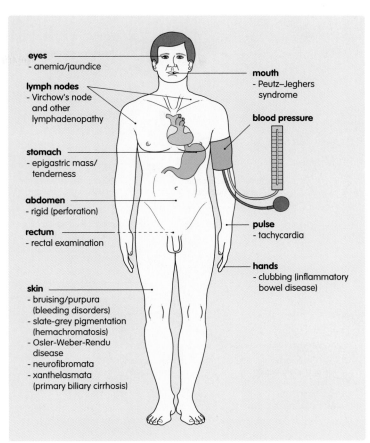

eyes
- anemia/jaundice

lymph nodes
- Virchow's node
  and other
  lymphadenopathy

stomach
- epigastric mass/
  tenderness

abdomen
- rigid (perforation)

rectum
- rectal examination

skin
- bruising/purpura
  (bleeding disorders)
- slate-grey pigmentation
  (hemachromatosis)
- Osler-Weber-Rendu
  disease
- neurofibromata
- xanthelasmata
  (primary biliary cirrhosis)

mouth
- Peutz–Jeghers
  syndrome

blood pressure

pulse
- tachycardia

hands
- clubbing (inflammatory
  bowel disease)

- A rigid abdomen suggests perforation.
- Epigastric tenderness suggests peptic ulcer disease, esophagitis, hiatus hernia, or gastric carcinoma.
- Epigastric mass: gastric carcinoma.
- If malignancy is suspected, examine for metastases.
- Signs of chronic liver failure (Chapter 10), including those suggesting specific diagnoses: xanthelasmata in primary biliary cirrhosis; slate-gray pigmentation in hemochromatosis; Kayser-Fleischer rings in Wilson's disease, elevated prothrombin time and Dupuytren's contracture in chronic alcohol abuse.
- A rectal examination is essential. This will confirm the presence of melena, which may be present despite hemodynamic stability.

## Investigating the patient with hematemesis, hematochezia, and melena

An algorithm for the investigation of the patient with hematemesis and melena is given in Fig. 7.2. The following investigations should be carried out:
- A complete blood count should be performed as part of the investigation. The hemoglobin may be normal in the acute phase, despite a large GI bleed, as it takes some hours for hemodilution to occur. A low hemoglobin on initial presentation suggests chronic blood loss, and the white cell count may be raised after a GI bleed. Platelet count may be reduced after an acute bleed, or increased after chronic blood loss. A very low

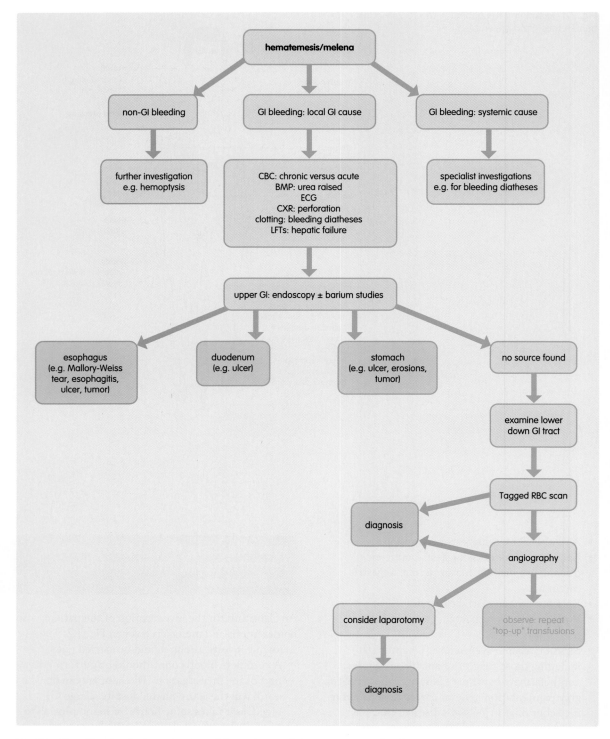

**Fig. 7.2** Algorithm for the investigation of the patient with hematemesis and melena. (ECG, electrocardiogram; CXR, chest x-ray; CBC, complete blood count; GI, gastrointestinal; RBC, red blood cell; LFTs, liver function tests; BMP, basic metabolic panel.)

platelet count should raise suspicion of a bleeding diathesis.

- Type and cross even if there is only a small GI bleed and the patient is hemodynamically stable. Blood should be cross-matched for more significant bleeding.
- Coagulation studies should also be performed since the prothrombin time is raised in liver disease. More specific investigations may be indicated (e.g., in patients with hemophilia or von Willebrand's disease).
- Urea is raised due to the absorption of protein when blood reaches the small bowel. Chronic renal failure can be associated with GI bleeding.
- On erect chest x-ray, the presence of gas under the right hemidiaphragm indicates perforation.

Further investigations are done to confirm the site of the bleeding and to make a definitive diagnosis:

- Endoscopy allows direct visualization of the pathology and can identify the source of the bleeding. It will determine the most appropriate form of medical therapy. The risk of rebleeding may be estimated; for example, Mallory-Weiss tears or erosive gastritis have a low risk of rebleeding with appropriate management, whereas esophageal varices have a much higher risk of rebleeding. Treatment may be given endoscopically (e.g., banding of the varices, injection of a sclerosant into a bleeding varix, or cautery of a bleeding vessel). New treatments for variceal bleeding include octreotide and vasopressin. Remember, however, that octreotide must be given with nitroglycerin because its

vasoconstricting effects occur in the coronary arteries as well as in the portal and splenic beds.

- Barium examinations are becoming rarer as endoscopy is becoming more widely available, although they may be useful when endoscopy is contraindicated (e.g., in patients with an unstable cervical spine).
- Abdominal ultrasound should be performed to determine whether liver cirrhosis is present or to look for metastases if carcinoma is suspected. Abdominal computed tomography scanning may be helpful if a mass is present.
- Tagged red blood cell scans require active bleeding to be present. They may be useful for continued bleeding despite a thorough search of the GI tract and help the surgeon if resection of the bleeding segment is considered.
- Mesenteric angiography again requires active bleeding to localize the source. It can also be used to visualize the portal venous system.

Despite extensive investigation, a small minority of patients will remain undiagnosed. If bleeding is severe laparotomy may be required, but if it is not severe the patient may attend for repeat "top-up" transfusions as required.

Elevated blood urea with normal serum creatinine suggests gastrointestinal bleeding.

Always ask about the patient's normal bowel habit as there are considerable differences between people, usually varying from three times a day to once every 3 days. It is important to note a change in bowel habit as this is more commonly associated with pathology.

## Differential diagnosis of a change in bowel habit

### Diarrhea

Infective causes of changes in bowel habit include the following:

- Bacterial: *Staphylococcus aureus* (from dairy products and meat), *Bacillus cereus* (fried rice), *Clostridium perfringens* (meat), *Escherichia coli* (meat), *Vibrio parahemolyticus* (seafood), *Campylobacter* (poultry), *Salmonella* (meat, poultry, and dairy), and *Shigella* (fecal–oral transmission). Less common bacteria include *Yersinia enterocolitica*, *Chlamydia*, and *Neisseria gonorrhoeae*. Note that the first two causes of diarrhea result in symptom within hours (4–8) while the remainder take much longer.
- Viral: rotavirus, Norwalk virus, cytomegalovirus (Norwalk and rotavirus are famous for their cruise ship outbreaks).
- Protozoa: *Giardia lamblia*, *Cryptosporidium*, *Entamoeba histolytica*.

Osmotic causes of diarrhea include:

- Medications (e.g., antacids and lactulose).
- Lactose intolerance.
- Factitious diarrhea (e.g., laxative abuse).

Secretory causes of diarrhea include:

- Infections.
- Endocrine causes: VIPoma, carcinoid syndrome, Zollinger-Ellison syndrome.
- Factitious diarrhea.
- Villous adenoma.
- Bile salt malabsorption.

Inflammatory causes of diarrhea include:

- Ulcerative colitis.
- Crohn's disease.
- Malignancy (e.g., lymphoma).
- Radiation enteritis (e.g., following radiotherapy).

Causes of malabsorption include:

- Celiac sprue
- Tropical sprue and Whipple's disease.
- Lymphatic obstruction (e.g., lymphoma, carcinoid syndrome, Kaposi's sarcoma, sarcoidosis).
- Pancreatic disease (e.g., cystic fibrosis and chronic pancreatitis).
- Bacterial overgrowth (e.g., blind loop syndrome).

Many medications other than laxatives can also cause diarrhea (e.g., antibiotics, motility drugs), as can heavy metals, herbs, and plant toxins.

Increased motility may be caused by irritable bowel syndrome and systemic disorders such as hyperthyroidism, scleroderma, and diabetes mellitus.

Chronic infections should also be considered in a patient with a change of bowel habit (e.g., giardiasis or amebiasis).

### Constipation

Ask what is meant by constipation. It usually means that the bowels are only opened infrequently and that the feces are hard, with pain on defecation.

Make sure that by "constipation" and "diarrhea" you and the patient mean the same thing.

Medical causes of constipation include the following:

- Low-fiber diet.
- Poor bowel habit.

- Endocrine causes: hypothyroidism and hyperparathyroidism.
- Metabolic causes: hypokalemia, hypercalcemia, and uremia.
- Neurologic causes: paraplegia and multiple sclerosis.
- Irritable bowel syndrome (often a mixed picture with diarrhea and constipation).
- Medications: anticholinergic agents, opiates, diuretics, verapamil, psychotropics, and disopyramide.
- Prolonged bed rest or immobility.
- Dehydration.
- Psychogenic causes (e.g., depression, agitation).
- Others: amyloidosis and scleroderma.

Surgical causes of constipation include:
- Perianal disease (e.g., fissure, thrombosed hemorrhoids).
- Intestinal obstruction due to a mass (e.g., carcinoma of the rectum/sigmoid colon).
- Pelvic mass, including pregnancy.
- Outlet delay: rectocele, rectal intussusception, rectal prolapse.
- Colonic stricture (e.g., diverticulitis and Crohn's disease).
- Hirschsprung's disease (aganglionic segment of the rectum, usually presenting in the first years of life).
- Postgastrectomy (although this usually causes diarrhea).
- Postoperative pain.

Note the features of acute gastrointestinal (GI) obstruction: absolute constipation, vomiting, pain, and abdominal distention.

## History in the patient with a change in bowel habit

Ask about the following:
- Normal bowel habit (note interindividual variation).
- Onset: sudden or chronic. Infectious diarrhea is usually of acute onset.
- Frequency of defecation.

- Stool appearance: formed, loose or watery; color—normal, red (blood from low in the GI tract), black (melena), yellow (mucus and slime), "redcurrant jelly" (intussusception), putty-colored (obstructive jaundice); volume. Do the stools float? If so, they have high fat content—think of malabsorption.
- Drugs: antacids, laxatives, cimetidine, digoxin, antibiotics, alcohol.
- Tenesmus (a sense of incomplete voiding).
- Smell: offensively malodorous in malabsorption; characteristic smell of melena.
- Foreign travel.
- Contact with diarrhea sufferers.
- Relationship to food.
- Stress.
- Associated features (e.g., pain, fever, vomiting, weight loss).
- Symptoms of thyrotoxicosis.
- Nocturnal diarrhea: autonomic neuropathies from diabetes mellitus.
- Sexual history: gay bowel syndrome—suspect this if multiple or unusual organisms are cultured.

## Examining the patient with a change in bowel habit

It is always important to estimate volume status first. Changes in vital signs will not occur until 5–10% of intravascular volume has been lost. The examination approach in the patient with a change in bowel habit is given in Fig. 8.1.

## Investigating the patient with a change in bowel habit

An algorithm for the investigation of the patient with change in bowel habit is given in Fig. 8.2. The following investigations should be performed in this type of patient:
- Complete blood count.
- Basic metabolic panel, including calcium.
- Thyroid function tests.
- Blood glucose: diabetes.
- Liver function tests.
- Albumin: decreased in malabsorption, protein-losing enteropathies, inflammatory diseases.

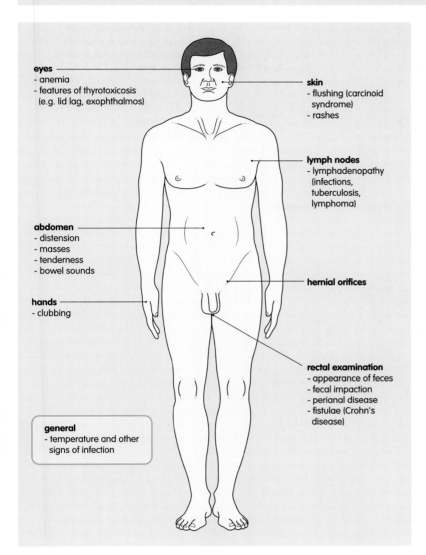

**Fig. 8.1** Examining the patient with a change in bowel habit.

**eyes**
- anemia
- features of thyrotoxicosis (e.g. lid lag, exophthalmos)

**skin**
- flushing (carcinoid syndrome)
- rashes

**lymph nodes**
- lymphadenopathy (infections, tuberculosis, lymphoma)

**abdomen**
- distension
- masses
- tenderness
- bowel sounds

**hernial orifices**

**hands**
- clubbing

**rectal examination**
- appearance of feces
- fecal impaction
- perianal disease
- fistulae (Crohn's disease)

**general**
- temperature and other signs of infection

- In malabsorption: anemia—vitamin $B_{12}$, folate, iron; hyponatremia in profound secretory diarrhea; increased prothrombin time due to malabsorption of fat-soluble vitamins; hypocalcemia.
- Specialized tests: serum vasoactive intestinal polypeptide; serum gastrin (Zollinger-Ellison syndrome); calcitonin (medullary thyroid carcinoma); cortisol (Addison's disease); urinary 5-hydroxyindoleacetic acid (carcinoid syndrome); culture and microscopy for ova, cysts, and parasites.
- Stool: if weight > 300g per 24 hours, consider a secretory process; if fat content > 10g per 24 hours, consider malabsorption; laxative screen; leucocytes in inflammatory processes.
- Abdominal x-ray: pancreatic calcification suggests chronic pancreatitis, distended intestinal loops and fluid levels suggest obstruction, and gross dilatation of the colon suggests Hirschsprung's disease.
- Fiberoptic sigmoidoscopy with or without biopsy: inflammatory bowel disease.
- Barium enema.
- Colonoscopy: carcinoma, melanosis coli, or inflammation.
- Colonic transit study: to confirm constipation and measure the transit time.

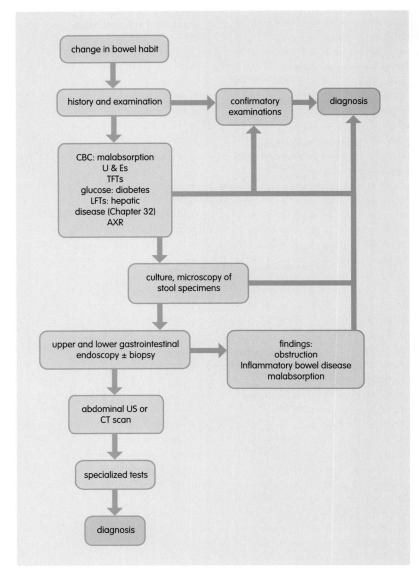

**Fig. 8.2** Algorithm for the investigation of the patient with a change of bowel habit. (AXR, abdominal x-ray; CT, computed tomography; CBC, complete blood count; LFT, liver function test; U&Es, urea and electrolytes; US, ultrasound; TFTs, thyroid function test.)

- Studies of pelvic floor function: defecography and anal manometry.
- Upper GI series: Crohn's disease, lymphoma, carcinoid syndrome.
- Upper GI endoscopy with or without duodenal biopsy (malabsorption).
- Abdominal ultrasound: suspected mass.
- Abdominal CT scan: pancreatitis, tumors.

# 9. Weight Loss

Weight loss is due to decreased energy intake, increased energy output, loss of energy in stool or urine, or a combination of these factors. Involuntary weight loss is a common manifestation of physical or psychological illness and always warrants further investigation. It should be confirmed objectively with records of previous weights. If this is not possible, a change in clothes size gives a useful clue. Family members may be able to give a more objective history.

## Differential diagnosis of weight loss

Weight loss has been defined as an involuntary loss of 5lb or more of body weight, or ten pounds within 6 months. Always distinguish deliberate from involuntary weight loss from the outset. The differential diagnosis of weight loss includes the following causes.

## Psychiatric/psychological causes
- Anorexia nervosa: typically young Caucasian females, with disturbance of body image and fear of weight gain, weight loss of > 15% body mass, and amenorrhea. (Note that bulimic patients will often be of normal weight. They engage in bouts of binging and purging which keep their weight near normal).
- Depression or agitation.
- Catatonia.
- Schizophrenia.
- Laxative or diuretic abuse.
- Anxiety disorders: agoraphobia, panic disorder, social phobias.
- Neglect (e.g., "tea and toast" diet in widowhood); also predisposes to folate and other vitamin deficiencies.

## Physiologic factors
- Dieting or food fads.
- Smoking.
- Increase in exercise.

## Endocrine causes
- Uncontrolled diabetes mellitus: often with increased appetite.
- Hyperthyroidism: weight loss despite an increased appetite.
- Adrenal insufficiency.
- Hypothyroidism: due to diminished appetite; although this more commonly presents with weight gain.
- Pheochromocytoma.
- Hypopituitarism.
- Severe diabetes insipidus.

## Drugs
- Anorectics.
- Theophylline.
- Amphetamines.
- Metformin.
- Digoxin.
- Opiates.
- Laxative or diuretics.
- Tobacco smoking.
- Herbal stimulants (e.g., ephedra).
- Psychiatric medications, selective serotonin reuptake inhibitors, atypical antipsychotics.
- Alcohol.

## Infections
- Tuberculosis.
- Human immunodeficiency virus.
- Other chronic infections and infestations.

## Chronic illnesses
- Cardiac cachexia (seen in advanced heart failure).
- Chronic obstructive pulmonary disease.
- Metastatic carcinoma.
- Connective tissue diseases.

## Gastrointestinal causes
- Peptic ulcer disease or mesenteric ischemia: pain on eating leading to decreased appetite.
- Dysphagia.
- Malabsorption: decreased absorption of nutrients and diarrhea (e.g., inflammatory bowel disease).

- Celiac disease.
- Liver disease.

## Neurologic causes
- Motor neuron disease.
- Myopathies.
- Poliomyelitis.

## Renal causes
Renal pathologies leading to chronic renal failure and uremia.

Malignancies anywhere that produce a high metabolic rate ("hungry tumors") or that lead to anorexia or dysphagia (e.g., esophageal carcinoma) will result in weight loss.

## History in the patient with weight loss

Weight loss can be a complication of disease in any physiologic system.

Try to confirm weight loss objectively with records of previous weights. Ask if the weight loss was voluntary or involuntary. Ask members of the family or friends if they have noticed weight loss. Ask about the amount of weight loss, its duration, and any accompanying symptoms such as anorexia or increased appetite.

In assessing the past medical history, it is important to evaluate any previous malignancy, GI disorder, or autoimmune disease. Remember to include sexual and psychiatric history within the past medical history. Past surgeries can also cause obstructions, dysmotility, and fistulas that can lead to weight loss. Also ask questions about family history of weight loss, malignancy, autoimmune disease, and endocrine disorders.

Further factors to assess, if the cause is not apparent, include the following:
- Diet: detailed intake and any recent changes in diet history.
- Physical activity: any changes in level.
- Full drug history: including over-the-counter and illegal medicines.
- GI symptoms: diarrhea, constipation, hematemesis, hematochezia, melena, nausea,

vomiting, dysphagia. Abdominal pain also may prevent food intake, as in mesenteric ischemia. The appearance of stools can be helpful; for example, floating stools suggest steatorrhea (malabsorption). Is hepatosplenomegaly present?
- Alcohol intake: with and without associated liver disease.
- Smoking: if recent onset, this may lead to eating less; if chronic, assess its association with malignancies.
- Symptoms of chronic infection or malignancy: fever and sweats, rashes, general malaise, anorexia, change in bowel habit, floating stools (malabsorption), hemoptysis, hematemesis, hematuria, melena (or bleeding from any other site), "lumps and bumps," joint or muscle tenderness, contacts with infected people, dysphagia.
- Symptoms of renal insufficiency: anorexia, general malaise and lethargy, bruising, urinary symptoms (e.g., polyuria and nocturia), vomiting, hiccoughs.
- Cardiorespiratory symptoms: cardiac cachexia.
- Neurologic symptoms.

Finally, the symptoms of endocrinopathies include the following:
- Diabetes: polyuria and polydipsia, weakness and fatigue, blurred vision, pruritus or thrush, nocturnal enuresis.
- Adrenal insufficiency: dizziness and collapses, weakness, nausea and diarrhea, pigmentation.
- Thyrotoxicosis: tremor, diarrhea, irritability, heat intolerance, palpitations.
- Pheochromocytoma: paroxysmal (or sustained) hypertension, panic, pain (abdominal or headache), palpitations, perspiration, pallor, paroxysmal thyroid swelling (remember the "Ps"), nausea, tremor.
- Panhypopituitarism: pallor, dizziness, loss of body hair, loss of libido, amenorrhea, visual field defects, symptoms of hypothyroidism.

## Examining the patient with weight loss

### Vital signs
Look for signs of hypovolemia (low blood pressure), which suggests water loss; tachycardia, which may suggest hyoperthyroidism, infection, etc.; tachypnea,

which suggests respiratory infections such as tuberculosis; fever, which suggests infections; autoimmune disorders, and endocrinopathies. Determine the patient's body mass index (BMI).

## General observation

The examination approach in the patient with weight loss is given in Fig. 9.1. Does the patient look like they have lost weight (loose skin, loose clothes)? Check the temperature. Does the patient look well or ill?

## Hands

The hands should be examined in the patient with weight loss, and the following should be noted:
- Clubbing: malignancy, cirrhosis, inflammatory bowel disease, and infections (pus in the lungs).

- Leukonychia: liver disease.
- Koilonychia: iron-deficiency anemia (dietary, malabsorption).
- Pigmentation: increased in Addison's disease but decreased in anemia.

## Other signs

Other signs include the following:
- Joint swelling and decreased range of movement: connective tissue diseases.
- Tremor: hyperthyroidism.
- Uremia: yellow discoloration of the skin.
- Jaundice and other signs of liver failure (e.g., spider nevi).
- Muscle wasting.
- Goiter.

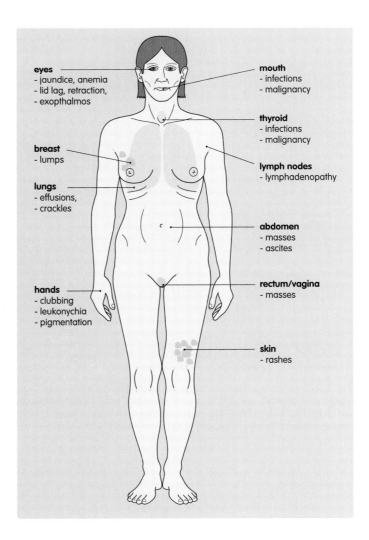

**Fig. 9.1** Examining the patient with weight loss.

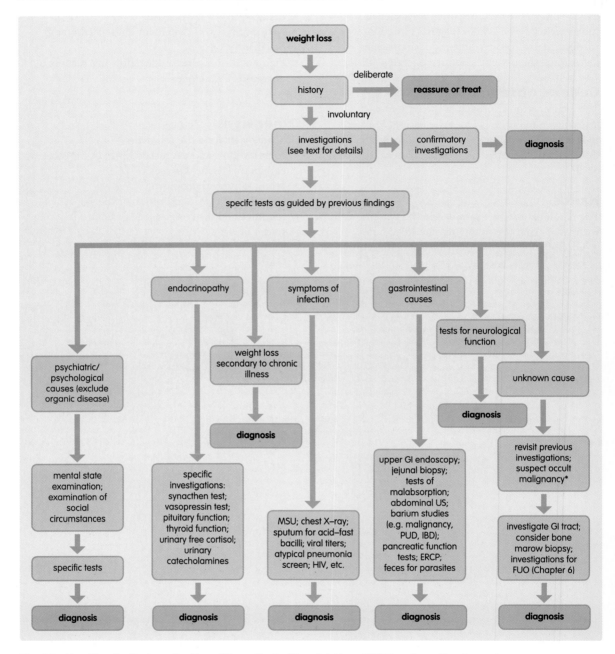

**Fig. 9.2** Algorithm for the investigation of the patient with weight loss. (ECRP, endoscopic retrograde cholangiopancreatography; GI, gastrointestinal; HIV, human immunodeficiency virus; IBD, inflammatory bowel disease; MSU, mid-stream urine; PUD, peptic ulcer disease; FUO, fever of unknown origin; US, ultrasound.) * Investigate site under suspicion (e.g., endoscopy for GI tract); look for metastases.

- Skin rashes: different rashes can represent vitamin deficiencies.
- Subacute bacterial endocarditis: splinter hemorrhages, Osler's nodes, and Janeway's lesions.
- Blood pressure: pheochromocytoma.
- Fundi: diabetic retinopathy.
- Mouth: infections and malignancies.
- Dental exam: very important in the elderly. Poorly fitting dentures or lack of teeth may inhibit feeding.
- Lymphadenopathy.

## Examination of individual systems

The following individual systems should be examined:
- Head, eyes, ears, nose, throat (HEENT): lymphadenopathy. Look for Roth spots due to infective endocarditis.
- Respiratory system: infection or malignancy. Don't forget to look for Horner's syndrome.
- Cardiac system.
- Gastrointestinal system: including careful palpation for abdominal masses, rectal examination, and organomegaly (e.g., liver metastases).
- Breast lumps.
- Vaginal examination: pelvic malignancy.

## Investigating the patient with weight loss

An algorithm for the investigation of the patient with weight loss is given in Fig. 9.2. The following investigations should be carried out:
- Complete blood count: anemia with malignancy, iron deficiency, vitamin $B_{12}$ deficiency, or folate deficiency, with inadequate dietary intake.
- Urea and electrolytes for uremia.
- Liver function tests (LFTs): liver failure or metastases, although LFTs may be normal with metastases.
- Blood glucose: diabetes, low glucose in liver failure, Addison's disease.
- Thyroid function tests.
- Chest x-ray: infection or tuberculosis, and malignancy.
- Blood cultures: infection. Remember to send viral, fungal cultures if necessary.
- ESR: to look for signs of inflammation.
- ANA, RF, and other serologic studies if looking for autoimmune disease.
- PPD placement, AFB of sputum, and sputum if tuberculosis is suspected.
- Chest x-ray: infection or tuberculosis and malignancy.
- Other investigations depend on the history and examination.

# 10. Jaundice

Jaundice (icterus) is the yellow discoloration of the skin, sclera, and mucosae, which is detectable when serum bilirubin concentrations exceed approximately 2.5mg/dL. Normal bilirubin metabolism is summarized in Fig. 10.1. Jaundice can arise as a result of increased red blood cell (RBC) breakdown, disordered bilirubin metabolism, or reduced bilirubin excretion. It is important to remember the two types of bilirubin: direct and indirect. The indirect (or unconjugated) bilirubin has yet to be transformed by the liver. The direct (or conjugated) bilirubin has already undergone post-production modification in the liver. This post-production processing in the liver provides a way to differentiate between pre- and intra-/post-hepatic causes of hyperbilirubinemia.

## Differential diagnosis of jaundice

### Prehepatic
Prehepatic jaundice results from increased bilirubin production, caused by abnormal RBC breakdown (hemolysis). Chronic TPN can also cause hyperbilirubinemia. For more on this, see Chapter 25.

### Intrahepatic
Disordered bilirubin metabolism resulting from hepatocyte dysfunction may also cause jaundice. Hepatocellular damage can arise as a consequence of the following acute insults or chronic pathologies.

#### Acute hepatocellular damage
- Viral infection (e.g., hepatitis A, B, C and E; Epstein–Barr virus [EBV]; cytomegalovirus [CMV]).
- Nonviral infection (e.g., *Leptospira icterohaemorrhagiae*).
- Drugs (e.g., acetaminophen poisoning, halothane).
- Alcohol.
- Pregnancy.
- Autoimmune liver disease.
- Shock.

#### Chronic hepatocellular damage
- Chronic active hepatitis (e.g., autoimmune disease, hepatitis B, hepatitis C).
- Cirrhosis (e.g., alcohol, chronic active hepatitis, primary biliary cirrhosis, Wilson's disease, hemochromatosis, $\alpha_1$-antitrypsin deficiency).
- Metastatic carcinoma.

### Posthepatic
Posthepatic jaundice is caused by reduced bilirubin excretion. This may be due to intrahepatic or extrahepatic biliary obstruction.

#### Extrahepatic obstruction
- Gallstones.
- Carcinoma of the head of the pancreas, ampulla of Vater or bile duct.
- Sclerosing cholangitis.
- Stricture (e.g., postendoscopic retrograde cholangiopancreatography [post-ERCP]).
- Pancreatitis.
- Parasitic infections (*Stronglyoides* sp.).
- Biliary atresia.

#### Intrahepatic obstruction
- Primary biliary cirrhosis.
- Alcohol.
- Viral hepatitis.
- Drugs (e.g., oral contraceptive pill).
- Pregnancy.
- Sepsis causing intrahepatic cholestasis.
- Postsurgical cholestasis.

## History in the patient with jaundice

The following factors should be assessed when obtaining a history in a patient with jaundice:
- Pruritus, dark urine, and pale stools: underlying cholestasis.
- Duration of illness: a short history of malaise, anorexia and myalgia are suggestive of viral

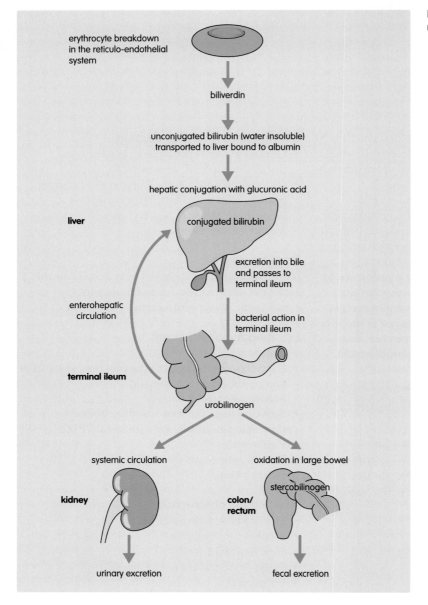

**Fig. 10.1** Normal bilirubin metabolism.

hepatitis. If there is a prolonged history of weight loss and anorexia in an elderly patient, carcinoma is more likely.

- Abdominal pain: the episodic, colicky, right upper quadrant pain of biliary colic will commonly be due to gallstones. A dull, persistent epigastric or central pain radiating to the back may suggest a pancreatic carcinoma.
- Fevers or rigors: cholangitis.
- Full recent drug history: particularly acetaminophen, oral contraceptive pill.

- Alcohol consumption: acute alcoholic hepatitis, cirrhosis.
- Infectious contacts: hepatitis A.
- Recent foreign travel to areas of high hepatitis risk. Malaria can also cause a hemolytic anemia. Parasitic infection can cause liver abscesses and obstruction of the biliary system.
- Recent surgery: halothane exposure, surgery for known malignancy, biliary stricture due to previous ERCP.

- Intravenous drug abuse, tattoos, homosexuality: increased risk of hepatitis B and C.
- Occupation: sewage workers are at an increased risk of leptospirosis.
- Family history of recurrent jaundice: inherited hemolytic anemias, Crigler-Najjar syndrome, and Gilbert's syndrome, which can cause an increase in indirect bilirubin, and Rotor syndrome and Dubin-Johnson syndrome, which lead to direct hyperbilirubinemia.

## Examining the patient with jaundice

There are three important groups of abnormalities that should be looked for in the jaundiced patient:
- How severe is the jaundice? Is there any evidence of encephalopathy?
- Is this an acute or chronic problem? (Are there any signs of chronic liver disease?)
- Are there any signs of specific disorders?

This approach is summarized in Fig. 10.2.

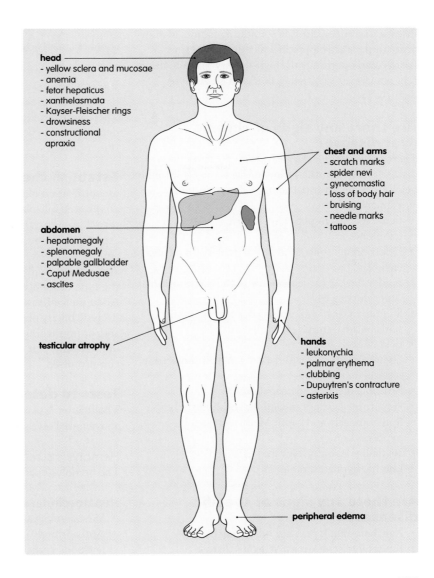

**head**
- yellow sclera and mucosae
- anemia
- fetor hepaticus
- xanthelasmata
- Kayser-Fleischer rings
- drowsiness
- constructional apraxia

**chest and arms**
- scratch marks
- spider nevi
- gynecomastia
- loss of body hair
- bruising
- needle marks
- tattoos

**abdomen**
- hepatomegaly
- splenomegaly
- palpable gallbladder
- Caput Medusae
- ascites

**testicular atrophy**

**hands**
- leukonychia
- palmar erythema
- clubbing
- Dupuytren's contracture
- asterixis

**peripheral edema**

**Fig. 10.2** Examining the patient with jaundice.

## Is there evidence of encephalopathy?

The following factors suggest the presence of encephalopathy:

- Drowsiness: this will eventually progress through stupor to coma.
- Slurred speech.
- Asterixis: flapping tremor of outstretched hands.
- Seizures.
- Constructional apraxia (inability to perform purposeful movements): test by asking the patient to copy a five-pointed star.
- Hepatic fetor (patient smells like a freshly opened corpse—a smell that all medical students surely know).

Hepatic encephalopathy can arise as a result of fulminating acute liver failure or when chronic disease decompensates. Precipitating factors include acute upper gastrointestinal bleeding, infection (particularly peritoneal), high-dietary protein, drugs (e.g., diuretics, sedatives), fluid and electrolyte disturbance.

## Are there any signs of chronic liver disease?

There are few clinical signs specific to acute liver disease. However, the following signs may commonly be found when liver pathology is longstanding:

- Palmar erythema.
- Leukonychia: hypoalbuminemia.
- Clubbing.
- Dupuytren's contractures: particularly in alcoholic cirrhosis.
- Spider nevi: greater than five in the distribution of superior vena cava.
- Scratch marks: cholestasis (deposition of bile acids in the dermis leads to pruritus).
- Loss of body hair.
- Gynecomastia: elevated estrogen, spironolactone, testicular atrophy.
- Bruising: disordered coagulation.
- Hepatomegaly: not in well-established cirrhosis.
- Splenomegaly and caput Medusae: portal hypertension.
- Testicular atrophy: elevated estrogen.
- Edema: hypoalbuminemia.

## Are there any signs of specific diseases?

- Xanthelasmata: primary biliary cirrhosis.
- Kayser-Fleischer rings: Wilson's disease.
- Slate-gray pigmentation: hemochromatosis.
- Hard, irregular hepatomegaly: malignant metastases.
- Palpable gallbladder: carcinoma of head of pancreas (Courvoisier's law).
- Splenomegaly: portal hypertension, viral infection.
- Needle marks or tattoos: hepatitis B, C.

Test for constructional apraxia by asking the patient to copy a five-pointed star without lifting the pen off the paper.

## Investigating the patient with jaundice

The investigation of jaundiced patients falls into two stages. Firstly, the type of jaundice must be determined (prehepatic, intrahepatic, posthepatic). Then more detailed tests should be performed to determine the specific etiology. Fig. 10.3 summarizes this approach.

### Establish the type of jaundice

Quantification of urinary urobilinogen and conjugated bilirubin, along with measurement of serum liver enzymes—alanine aminotransferase, aspartate aminotransferase, alkaline phosphatase, and $\gamma$-glutamyltransferase and bilirubin (both direct and indirect) will give a reasonable indication as to the type of abnormality present (Fig. 10.4). Abdominal ultrasound scan is then essential to exclude biliary obstruction. Albumin measurement and/or prothrombin time will show how dramatically, if at all, the liver's synthetic function is compromised.

### Tests to determine specific etiology

The following tests should be used as guided by the above initial investigations.

#### Hemolysis screen

The hemolysis screen is detailed in Chapter 25.

#### Hepatocellular screen

- Viral serology: hepatitis A, B, and C; EBV, CMV.
- Autoantibody screen: antimitochondrial antibodies, antinuclear antibodies, ESR.

**Fig. 10.3** Investigation of the patient with jaundice. (CT, computed tomography; ERCP, endoscopic retrograde cholangiopancreatography; PTC, percutaneous transhepatic cholangiography.)

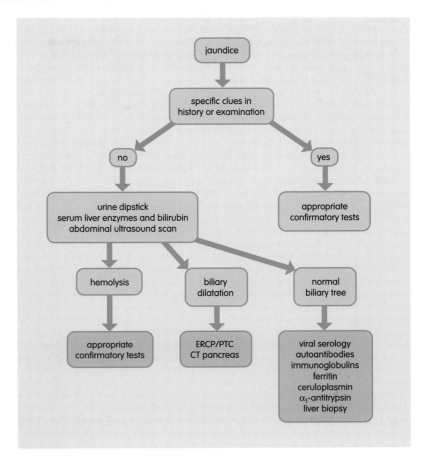

| Biochemical abnormalities in different types of jaundice | | | | |
|---|---|---|---|---|
| Specimen | Test | Hemolysis | Hepatocellular | Cholestasis |
| urine | urobilinogen<br>conjugated bilirubin | raised<br>absent | normal or raised<br>present | decreased or absent<br>raised |
| feces | stercobilinogen | raised | normal | decreased or absent |
| serum | bilirubin<br>liver enzymes raised | unconjugated<br>normal | unconjugated and conjugated<br>AST, ALT | conjugated<br>alkaline phosphatase, GGT |

**Fig. 10.4** Biochemical abnormalities in different types of jaundice (ALT, alanine aminotransferase; AST, aspartate aminotransferase; GGT, γ-glutamyltransferase.)

- Ferritin: hemochromatosis.
- Serum ceruloplasmin and urinary copper excretion: Wilson's disease.
- $\alpha_1$-antitrypsin.
- Liver biopsy: definitive diagnostic test for intrinsic liver disease.

## Cholestasis screen

- ERCP and percutaneous transhepatic cholangiography: detailed information regarding the biliary tree; also used to perform therapeutic maneuvers such as stent insertion.

- RUQ ultrasound/Doppler should always be performed to look for signs of portal vein thrombosis, gallstones, liver parenchyma, and signs of ascites.

- Computed tomography scan: good images of the pancreas, which is often poorly visualized on an ultrasound scan.

# 11. Abdominal Pain

Abdominal pain is a common cause for consultation (and therefore is often found in examinations). The underlying problem can often be identified by considering which structures normally lie at the site of the pain.

It is important to remember that the visceral organs are innervated imprecisely and can initially present with diffuse or midline pain. Pain can be localized only when an area of inflammation, such as a ruptured appendix in one quadrant, interacts with the pain receptors in the bowel wall.

 Be aware that there is a long list of possible differential diagnoses for abdominal pain.

## Differential diagnosis of abdominal pain

Depending on the specific area affected, abdominal pain may result from the following causes:

### Epigastric pain
- Lower esophagus: esophagitis, malignancy.
- Stomach: peptic ulcer, gastritis.
- Pancreas: pancreatitis, malignancy.

### Right upper quadrant pain
- Biliary tree: biliary colic, cholecystitis, cholangitis.
- Liver: hepatitis, malignancy, abscess, right ventricular failure.
- Subphrenic space: abscess.

### Left upper quadrant pain
- Spleen: traumatic rupture, infarction (sickle cell disease), splenic vein thrombosis.
- Pancreas: pancreatitis, malignancy.
- Subphrenic space: abscess.

### Central abdominal pain
- Pancreas: pancreatitis, malignancy.
- Small/large bowel: obstruction, perforation, intussusception, ischemia, Crohn's disease, lymphoma, irritable bowel syndrome, adhesions.
- Lymph nodes: mesenteric adenitis, lymphoma.
- Abdominal aorta: ruptured aortic aneurysm.

### Right lower quadrant pain
- Terminal ileum: Crohn's disease, infection (tuberculosis), Meckel's diverticulum.
- Appendix: appendicitis, carcinoid syndrome, tumor.
- Cecum/ascending colon: diverticulitis, paracolic abscess, ulcerative colitis, malignancy.
- Ovary/fallopian tubes: malignancy, ectopic pregnancy, pelvic inflammatory disease.

### Left lower quadrant pain
- Sigmoid/descending colon: diverticulitis, paracolic abscess, ulcerative colitis, malignancy, sigmoid volvulus
- Ovary/fallopian tubes: malignancy, ectopic pregnancy, cyst (bleeding or torsion), pelvic inflammatory disease.

### Groin pain
- Kidneys: malignancy, pyelonephritis, polycystic disease.
- Ureters: colic due to stone or clot.

### Suprapubic pain
- Bladder: urinary tract infection, acute urinary retention.
- Uterus/adnexae: pelvic inflammatory disease, endometriosis.

### Other causes of abdominal pain
Occasionally, other medical problems can present with abdominal pain. These should be considered when some of the more common diagnoses listed above have been ruled out:

- Constipation.
- Anxiety.
- Myocardial infarction: usually inferior myocardial infarction causing epigastric pain.
- Lower lobe pneumonia: ipsilateral upper quadrant or sometimes groin discomfort.
- Porphyria.
- Diabetic ketoacidosis.
- Addison's disease.
- Sickle cell crisis.
- Lead poisoning.
- Henoch–Schönlein purpura.
- Hypercalcemia.

## History in the patient with abdominal pain

When a patient presents with abdominal pain, the first priority is to determine whether he or she has an acute abdomen requiring urgent admission to hospital. The history should focus on the pain itself and then associated symptoms. It is also very important to ask about previous surgeries. Small bowel obstructions secondary to abdominal adhesions are quite common, especially in patients who have undergone multiple intra-abdominal surgeries.

### The pain itself

The onset, course, nature, and site of the pain must be accurately assessed.

Sudden onset of sustained severe pain is often due to perforation or rupture of a viscus, such as the bowel, spleen, or abdominal aorta.

Colicky pain is a griping pain that comes and goes. It is due to muscular spasm in a viscus wall, such as the bowel, ureters, and gallbladder. The muscles contract in an attempt to overcome obstruction caused by a stone, tumor, foreign body, strictures, strangulated hernias, or intussusception.

Gradual onset with sustained pain can be seen in inflammatory conditions, such as ulcerative colitis or Crohn's disease, infection including abscess formation, or gastroenteritis and malignancy.

The site and radiation of pain may help to determine the organ involved (as above)—pancreatic and aortic pain may radiate to the back, ureteric pain often radiates from "loin to groin," and diaphragmatic irritation caused by subphrenic

pathology such as an abscess causes referred shoulder tip pain.

## Associated symptoms

The history should now assess other symptoms that may suggest the cause of pain or the consequence of the disease.

Vomiting is common. Hematemesis is seen in upper gastrointestinal bleeding from ulcers or varices, projectile vomiting is seen in pyloric stenosis, and feculent vomiting results from severe large bowel obstruction.

Rigors suggest sepsis (e.g., abscess, cholangitis, or urinary tract infection). Rigors are particularly common with Gram-negative septicemia.

Change in bowel habit may be an important symptom. Absolute constipation (no feces or wind passed rectally) indicates complete bowel obstruction, whereas gastroenteritis or diverticulitis often cause diarrhea. Constipation alternating with diarrhea is a feature of colonic malignancy but is also seen in irritable bowel syndrome.

Rectal bleeding may indicate malignancy, inflammatory bowel disease, diverticulitis, dysentery, and angiodysplasia. Dark-red bleeding is a feature of bowel infarction.

Dysuria, hematuria, and urinary frequency indicate urinary infection. Renal stones are occasionally passed per urethra.

Vaginal discharge will often be present in pelvic inflammatory disease.

Do not forget constipation as a cause of abdominal pain in the elderly.

## Examining the patient with abdominal pain

The first question that must be asked is, "Is the patient acutely ill?" Signs of shock and peritonitis should be looked for. The examination should then focus on specific signs. Fig. 11.1 summarizes the examination approach.

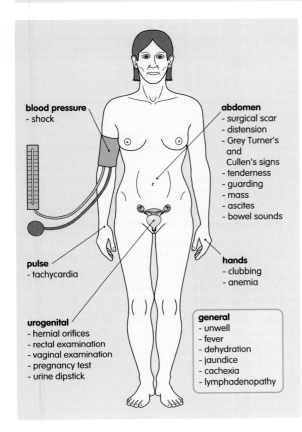

**blood pressure**
- shock

**abdomen**
- surgical scar
- distension
- Grey Turner's and Cullen's signs
- tenderness
- guarding
- mass
- ascites
- bowel sounds

**pulse**
- tachycardia

**hands**
- clubbing
- anemia

**urogenital**
- hernial orifices
- rectal examination
- vaginal examination
- pregnancy test
- urine dipstick

**general**
- unwell
- fever
- dehydration
- jaundice
- cachexia
- lymphadenopathy

**Fig. 11.1** Examining the patient with abdominal pain.

| Causes of peritonitis | |
|---|---|
| **Cause** | **Examples** |
| infection | spread from paracolic/ subphrenic abscess following surgery or paracentesis bowel perforation |
| chemical irritation | bile feces gastric acid pancreatic enzymes |
| transmural inflammation | Crohn's disease salpingitis |

**Fig. 11.2** Causes of peritonitis.

rebound tenderness, guarding) are often referred to as peritoneal signs suggestive of an acute abdomen. In this situation the patient will need acute surgical consultation and, most likely, operative intervention.

A quick way of differentiating whether a patient has signs of peritonitis vs. colic abdominal pain is to observe the patient in bed. Patients with peritonitis lie still because any movement causes pain, while those with colic will constantly be adjusting their position to find a comfortable way to lie.

## What is the underlying cause?
- Fever: high temperatures indicates infection; low-grade fever can be found in malignancy, bowel infarction, inflammatory bowel disease, and pancreatitis.
- Jaundice: hepatitis or pancreatitis (causing periampullary edema).
- Dehydration: rapid fluid loss.
- Cachexia: suggests a chronic pathology, particularly malignancy.
- Clubbing: inflammatory bowel disease or small bowel lymphoma.
- Lymphadenopathy: lymphoma; or may be due to metastases.
- Cullen's sign (periumbilical or central bruising) and Grey Turner's sign (bruising in the flanks): severe hemorrhagic pancreatitis; rarely, a leaking abdominal aortic aneurysm.
- Recent surgical scar: may indicate a source of peritoneal sepsis, such as an anastomotic leak.
- Abdominal distention: if marked, indicates bowel obstruction and is accompanied by a resonant

## Is the patient acutely ill?
### Pulse and blood pressure
Tachycardia and hypotension indicate shock. Consider septicemia (particularly gram-negative), severe bleeding (ruptured abdominal aortic aneurysm, spleen), fluid loss (vomiting, diarrhea, pancreatitis) and, rarely, acute addisonian crisis. Signs of hypovolemia may be common since a large amount of third spacing can occur with abdominal obstruction and volume loss secondary to GI bleeds.

### Peritonitis
The patient often lies still as movement exacerbates the pain. Look for rebound tenderness and guarding (involuntary spasm of the abdominal wall on palpation). When the peritonism becomes generalized the abdomen will be rigid and bowel signs will be absent due to paralysis of peristalsis. Causes of peritonism are summarized in Fig. 11.2. The physical exam findings listed above (e.g.,

percussion note. Occasionally, visible peristalsis may be present.

- Tenderness: it is important to consider what structures lie at the site of tenderness. As discussed, rebound tenderness indicates peritonitis.
- Mass: this can be malignant or inflammatory as in Crohn's disease.
- Ascites: malignancy, peritoneal sepsis, pancreatitis.
- Bowel sounds: high-pitched (tinkling) suggests obstruction; absence indicates an ileus (paralysis of bowel) from whatever cause.
- Hernial orifices (inguinal and femoral): these must be examined, particularly if obstruction is suspected.
- Pelvic and rectal examination: pelvic inflammation, cervical excitation, ectopic pregnancy, rectal mass or bleeding, stool consistency.
- Urine dipstick: should be used to determine the presence of white blood cells (infection), RBCs (stone, tumor or infection), glucose, and ketones.

## Investigating the patient with abdominal pain

All patients admitted to hospital with abdominal pain should have a complete blood count (CBC) and serum biochemistry performed. The use of radiology and other tests will depend on a focused differential diagnosis. The diagnostic pathway is outlined in Fig. 11.3:

- Complete blood count: leukocytosis is seen in infection and occasionally inflammation and malignancy. Anemia may be due to acute blood loss or chronic pathology such as malignancy.
- Serum amylase: very high in acute pancreatitis, but may also be raised in perforated peptic ulcer, diabetic ketoacidosis, cholecystitis, abdominal trauma, and myocardial infarction.
- Metabolic panel: dehydration, renal failure as a consequence of obstructive uropathy or shock.
- Serum calcium: hypercalcemia may cause renal stones and pancreatitis; hypocalcemia may be a consequence of pancreatitis.

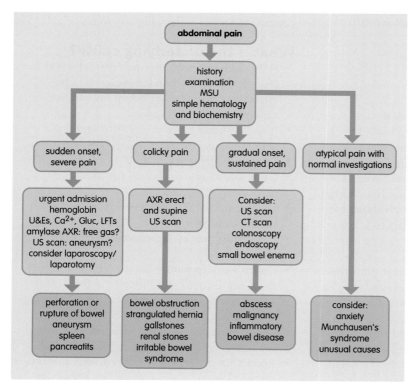

Fig. 11.3 Diagnosis in the patient with abdominal pain. (AXR, abdominal x-ray; CT, computed tomography; Gluc, glucose; LFTs, liver function tests; MSU, midstream urine; U&Es, urea and electrolytes; US, ultrasound.)

- Blood glucose: hypoglycemia will result from liver failure or Addison's disease; hyperglycemia will be present in ketoacidosis and may complicate acute pancreatitis.
- Liver function tests: abnormal in acute hepatitis, biliary disease, and shock.
- Microscopy, culture, and sensitivity of mid-stream urine: to exclude infection.
- Abdominal x-ray: erect and supine films should be performed if the following are suspected: perforation—air beneath the diaphragm representing free gas; obstruction—dilated loops of bowel with fluid level; pancreatitis—sentinel loop due to ileus in overlying loop of small bowel; infarction—"thumb printing" representing mucosal oedema; renal stone—90% of such stones are radiopaque.
- Abdominal ultrasound scan: dilatation of biliary tree and ureters; intra-abdominal mass; ascites; abscess.
- Diagnostic pericentesis: if ascites, fluid can be sent for CBC, amylase, culture, Gram stain, and glucose measurement.

When there is difficulty in making the diagnosis, a computed tomography scan, laparoscopy/laparotomy, or diagnostic tests for the unusual causes of abdominal pain should be considered.

# 12. Polyuria and Polydipsia

Polyuria is the passing of excessive volumes of urine. Urine output depends on fluid intake and body losses, and typically ranges from 1–3.5 L/day. Polydipsia, the ingestion of excessive volumes of fluid, is usually a consequence of polyuria.

Water is normally reabsorbed from the loop of Henle as it passes through the hyperosmolar renal medulla. Fluid in the collecting ducts enters the hyperosmolar renal medulla, with water reabsorption being controlled by antidiuretic hormone (ADH) (Fig. 12.1). The secretion of this is controlled by the hypothalamus in response to osmolality changes in the blood. A rise in osmolality leads to an increase in ADH secretion, and a fall results in a decrease in ADH secretion.

The renin-aldosterone feedback cycle is also responsible for water retention. Cells in the juxtaglomerular complex are responsive to changes in the blood pressure coming into the afferent arteriole. When blood pressure is low, the cells secrete renin, which is cleaved to form angiotensin I, which in turn is cleaved in the lungs by angiotensin-converting enzyme (ACE) to form angiotensin II. Angiotensin II is a powerful vasoconstrictor and promotes the absorption of Na and water by acting on the tubules themselves and also through the stimulation of aldosterone secretion.

## Differential diagnosis of polyuria

The differential diagnosis of polyuria includes the following.

### Insufficient secretion of ADH
Central diabetes insipidus (DI) may be secondary to lesions of the hypothalamic/pituitary axis and includes the following:
- Idiopathic: often familial and the most common form.
- Surgery or irradiation to the pituitary gland.
- Trauma: especially head injury.
- Malignancy (e.g., craniopharyngioma, pinealoma, glioma, and secondary deposits).
- Anorexia nervosa.
- Ischemia.
- Infections (e.g., meningitis and pneumonia).
- Infiltrations (e.g., sarcoid and histiocytosis X).

### Inhibition of ADH release
This leads to increased thirst and thus polydipsia. Examples include psychogenic DI and lesions affecting the thirst center.

### Inability of the kidney to respond to ADH
This is nephrogenic DI and may be congenital or acquired. The familial form is due to a primary renal tubular defect. The secondary defect may be due to an inability to maintain renal medullary hyperosmolality and includes electrolyte imbalances such as hypercalcemia and hypokalemia, lithium toxicity, and secondary to longstanding pyelonephritis or hypdronephrosis, and renal papillary necrosis (analgesic nephropathy).

### Chronic renal failure
Chronic renal failure may occur as a result of the depressed ability of the kidneys to concentrate urine. The volume of urine may therefore increase to excrete the same osmotic load.

### Acute renal failure
Polyuria occurs in the diuretic phase of acute renal failure and in postobstructive uropathy.

### Osmotic diuresis
Incomplete reabsorption in the tubules of substances in the glomerular filtrate leads to osmotic diuresis, i.e., increased solute per nephron. This occurs with glucose in diabetes mellitus (DM), hypercalcemia in chronic renal failure, and in intravenous infusion with hypertonic solutions (mannitol).

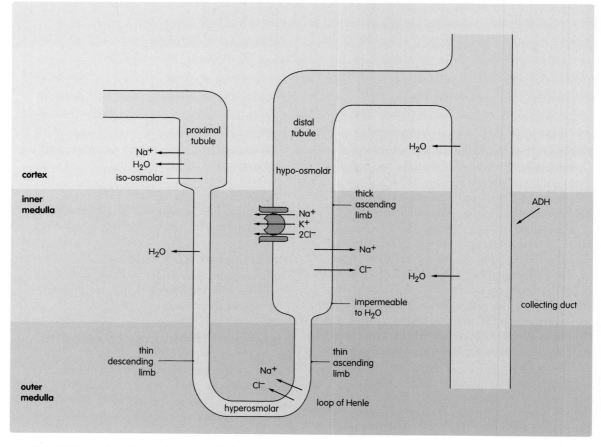

**Fig. 12.1** Water and electrolyte balance in the loop of Henle. (ADH, antidiuretic hormone.)

## Other causes

- Drugs (e.g., lithium carbonate, diuretics, amphoterecin B).
- Psychogenic polydipsia (e.g., schizophrenia).
- Excessive hypertonic fluid intake.

## History in the patient with polyuria or polydipsia

After asking general questions, focus on suspected causes. The following should be ascertained:

- Differentiate between polyuria (an increase in urine production) and frequency (the frequent passage of small amounts of urine).
- Weight loss: think of diabetes; malignancies (especially of the brain—does the patient have headaches?); myeloma leading to renal failure; ectopic production of adrenocorticotrophic hormone (ACTH); and bony metastases. Look for signs of anorexia nervosa (<15% of ideal body weight).
- General features of infection: a history of recurrent infection should suggest diabetes.
- Psychiatric symptoms: especially if thirst appears to dominate the picture, patients may resent investigations, especially a water deprivation test, and may drink surreptitiously. There may be an inconsistency or variation in the severity of the symptoms, and an absence of nocturnal symptoms. There may also be other neurotic symptoms.
- Symptoms of renal failure: such as hematuria, nausea and vomiting; likely precipitating factors.
- If renal failure is suspected, consider associated systemic conditions, such as collagenoses (e.g., systemic lupus erythematosus and polyarteritis nodosa), gout, subacute bacterial endocarditis, amyloid, Wegener's granulomatosis, and Goodpasture's syndrome.

- Hypercalcemia: produces symptoms of nausea, vomiting, constipation, abdominal pain, and, if severe, confusion and coma (Chapter 35).
- Hypokalemia: leads to muscle weakness and paralysis (Chapter 33).
- Drug history: analgesic abuse may cause renal papillary necrosis; lithium may cause nephrogenic DI; vitamin D or milk-alkali syndrome may lead to hypercalcemia; steroids and nephrotoxic drugs.
- History of head injury or childhood meningitis?
- History of hypertension? If so, suspect hypertensive renal disease.
- Family history (e.g., in DI, DM, and nephrogenic DI).

## Examining the patient with polyuria or polydipsia

The examination approach in the patient with polyuria or polydipsia is summarized in Fig. 12.2. The general appearance of the patient should be noted:

- Yellow-brown skin: renal failure, liver failure.
- Skin manifestations: DM (e.g., necrobiosis lipidica diabeticorum, granuloma annulare, infections).
- Wasting: malignancy or diabetes.
- Anemia: malignancy or chronic renal failure.
- Clubbing: bronchogenic carcinoma leading to excess ACTH or parathyroid hormone (PTH) production.

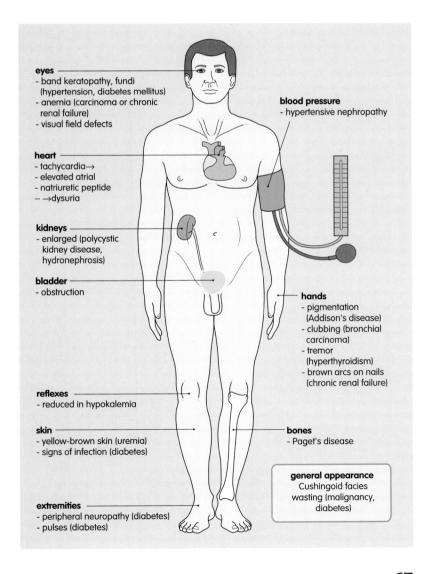

**eyes**
- band keratopathy, fundi (hypertension, diabetes mellitus)
- anemia (carcinoma or chronic renal failure)
- visual field defects

**blood pressure**
- hypertensive nephropathy

**heart**
- tachycardia→
- elevated atrial
- natriuretic peptide
- →dysuria

**kidneys**
- enlarged (polycystic kidney disease, hydronephrosis)

**bladder**
- obstruction

**hands**
- pigmentation (Addison's disease)
- clubbing (bronchial carcinoma)
- tremor (hyperthyroidism)
- brown arcs on nails (chronic renal failure)

**reflexes**
- reduced in hypokalemia

**skin**
- yellow-brown skin (uremia)
- signs of infection (diabetes)

**bones**
- Paget's disease

**general appearance**
Cushingoid facies
wasting (malignancy, diabetes)

**extremities**
- peripheral neuropathy (diabetes)
- pulses (diabetes)

**Fig. 12.2** Examining the patient with polyuria or polydipsia.

- Brown arcs on nails: chronic renal failure.
- Optic signs: band keratopathy or subconjunctival calcification in hypercalcemia; visual defects in tumors of the hypothalamus or pituitary; fundal changes of hypertension or diabetes.

## Cardiovascular system

Check for tachycardias (producing atrial natriuretic peptide) and peripheral vascular disease in DM. Also, check the blood pressure for hypertensive nephropathy.

## Abdominal examination

Palpate the kidneys as they may be palpable in polycystic kidney disease or hydronephrosis. A large bladder may indicate urinary tract obstruction.

## Neurologic examination

The neurologic examination should assess the following:

- Other signs of drug toxicity (e.g., diplopia, dizziness, nausea)
- Diabetic peripheral neuropathy.
- Hypotonia and areflexia with hypokalemia.
- Wasting in malignancy.
- Paraneoplastic syndromes.

## Investigating the patient with polyuria and polydipsia

An algorithm for the investigation of the patient with polyuria and polydipsia is given in Fig. 12.3. The following investigations should be carried out:

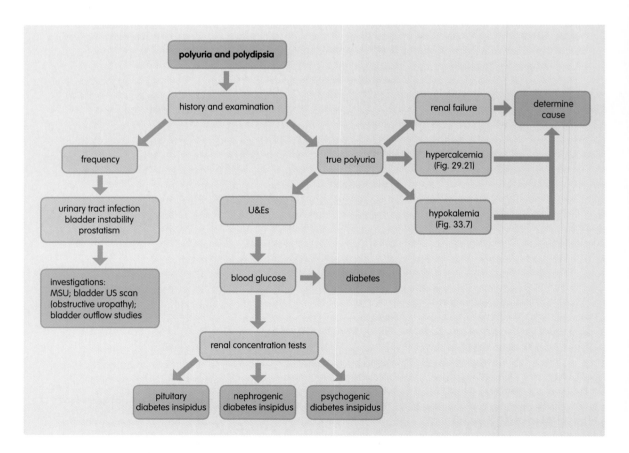

**Fig. 12.3** Algorithm for the investigation of the patient with polyuria and polydipsia. (MSU, mid-stream urine; U&Es, urea and electrolytes; US, ultrasound.)

- Collect 24-hour urine and confirm polyuria if any doubt exists.
- Urinalysis: specific gravity with or without osmolality.
- Urea and electrolytes: renal failure and hypokalemia. If renal impairment is found, further investigations may include creatinine clearance, tests for systemic diseases associated with renal failure, and an ultrasound scan of the kidneys. (If hypokalemia is found, go through the differential diagnosis—see Fig. 33.7—to look for causes. Remember simple things like drugs—is the patient on diuretics?).
- Dehydration test—does the patient appropriately concentrate urine?
- Blood glucose: DM.
- Administer vasopressin. If the patient responds to exogenous ADH, central diabetes insipidus is confirmed. If the patient is still unable to respond, nephrogenic diabetes insipidus is confirmed.
- Complete blood count: anemia with chronic renal failure, or malignancy (e.g., leukemia), and reticuloses.
- Serum calcium corrected for plasma proteins: if raised, further tests to elucidate the cause will be required, such as PTH assay, tests of pituitary function, bone scan, myeloma screen, alkaline phosphatase, and bone x-rays for Paget's disease, thyroid function tests, and serum angiotensin-converting enzyme for sarcoidosis, and synacthen test to exclude adrenal insufficiency.
- Chest x-ray (CXR): bilateral hilar lymphadenopathy with sarcoidosis, and bronchial neoplasm with ectopic PTH secretion. If there are any abnormalities on the CXR it may be necessary to proceed to bronchoscopy with or without biopsy.
- Skull x-ray: brain tumor (e.g., craniopharyngioma or secondary deposits).

If either a hypothalamic or pituitary cause or renal tubular dysfunction is suspected, it may be appropriate to proceed with renal concentration tests. It is mandatory to exclude other potential causes for polyuria, as renal concentration tests may be dangerous.

The patient is told to drink nothing from 4 PM the day before attending the outpatient department. If the urine osmolality the next morning is not above 800mmol/kg, inpatient tests are required (Figs. 12.4 and 12.5).

---

**Procedure for testing outpatients with polyuria and polydipsia**

- weigh the patient
- deprive of all fluids the night before the tests
- the next morning, weigh the patient every 2 hours (a decrease in weight by >3% indicates dehydration, so stop the test)
- collect urine and blood for osmolality
- if the urine osmolality fails to reach 800mmol/kg give intramuscular DDAVP (DDAVP is synthetic vasopressin which acts in the same way as ADH)
- collect blood and urine for osmolality

**Fig. 12.4** Procedure for testing outpatients with polyuria and polydipsia. (ADH, antidiuretic hormone; DDAVP, desmopressin.)

---

**Fig. 12.5** Interpretation of outpatient test results. (DI, diabetes insipidus; *may be some acquired resistance to ADH; ↑ increase in osmolality; → no significant change in osmolality.)

| Interpretation of outpatient test results | | | | |
|---|---|---|---|---|
| | **Fluid deprivation** | | **i.m. DDAVP** | |
| | plasma osmolality | urine osmolality | plasma osmolality | urine osmolality |
| pituitary DI | ↑ | → | ↑ | ↑ |
| psychogenic DI* | ↑ | ↑ | ↑ | ↑ |
| nephrogenic DI | → | → | → | → |

# 13. Hematuria and Proteinuria

Hematuria and proteinuria are common presentations of renal disease, although both may also be due to systemic conditions. Hematuria is abnormal if there are more than 2 red blood cells per high-power field; proteinuria is defined as more than 150mg of protein per 24-hour collection of urine. Red-colored urine may also be due to hemoglobinuria (hemolysis), porphyria, drugs (e.g., rifampicin), or even the ingestion of beets.

Patients need to be stratified by the quantity of hematuria, age, symptoms, past medical history, and family history in addition to whether proteinuria is also present. It is important to rule out life-threatening causes since urologic cancers are the cause of 5% of cases of microscopic hematuria.

## Differential diagnosis of hematuria and proteinuria

### Hematuria

This is best classfied by the site of pathology. Causes of isolated hematuria are summarized in Fig. 13.1.

### Systemic conditions
- Clotting disorders and anticoagulants.
- Thrombocytopenia.
- Sickle cell disease.
- Endocarditis.
- Exercise-related.
- Vasculitides.

### Kidneys/ureters
- Glomerulonephritis and its associated conditions (e.g., Hodgkin's disease, subacute bacterial endocarditis, systematic lupus erythematosus, polyarteritis nodosa, Wegener's granulomatosis, Goodpasture's syndrome).
- Infections (e.g., pyelonephritis, tuberculosis).
- IgA nephropathy.
- Alport's syndrome.
- Benign familial hematuria.

- Tumors: carcinoma, nephroblastoma, angioma, adenoma, papilloma.
- Cystic disease: polycystic kidney disease, medullary sponge kidney.
- Sudden release of retained urine (e.g., after catheterization for urinary retention).
- Drugs (e.g., sulfonamides, warfarin).
- Hydronephrosis.
- Papillary necrosis.
- Hydatid disease.

When thinking of causes of hematuria, think of the site of pathology along the renal tract. At each site, tumors, calculi, and infection are possible.

### Bladder/urethra
- Cystitis: infection, chemical-induced cystitis, postradiation cystitis.
- Tumors: carcinoma, papilloma, hemangioma, sarcoma.
- Trauma.
- Calculi.
- Infections: tuberculosis.
- Foreign bodies (e.g., urinary catheters)
- Schistosomiasis.

### Prostate
- Prostatic carcinoma.
- Tuberculosis.

### Other sites
Hematuria may result from lesions in adjacent organs (by fistula formation or inflammation) such as:
- Colonic diverticulitis.
- Inflammatory bowel disease.
- Acute appendicitis in a pelvic appendix.
- Acute salpingitis.

**Fig. 13.1** Causes of isolated microscopic hematuria by site of origin. Disorders are listed roughly in order of decreasing frequency. (Adapted from Cohen RA, Brown RS: Microscopic hematuria. N Engl J Med 348:2230–2338, 2003.)

## Causes of isolated microscopic hematuria by site of origin

### A. In patients <50 years old
**Glomerular**
- IgA nephropathy (increased incidence in Asians)
- Thin basement membrane disease (benign familial hematuria)
- Hereditary nephritis (Alport's syndrome)
- Mild focal glomerulonephritis due to other causes

**Upper urinary tract**
- Nephrolithiasis
- Pyelonephritis
- Polycystic kidney disease
- Medullary sponge disease
- Hypercalciuria, hyperuricosuria, or both without stones
- Renal trauma
- Papillary necrosis
- Ureteral strictures and hydronephrosis
- Sickle cell trait or disease (Afro-Americans)
- Renal infarction or arteriovenous malformation
- Renal tuberculosis (associated with endemic areas and HIV infection)

**Lower urinary tract**
- Cystitis, prostatitis, urethritis
- Benign bladder and ureteral polyps, tumors
- Bladder cancer
- Prostate cancer
- Urethral and meatal strictures
- Schistosomiasis (North Africans)

**Of uncertain origin**
- Exercise hematuria
- Benign hematuria
- Excessive anticoagulation (e.g., warfarin)
- Factitious hematuria (usually gross rather than microscopic)

### B. In patients >50 years old
**Glomerular**
- IgA nephropathy
- Hereditary nephritis (Alport's syndrome)
- Mild focal glomerulonephritis due to other causes

**Upper urinary tract**
- Nephrolithiasis
- Renal cell cancer
- Polycystic kidney disease
- Pyelonephritis
- Transitional cell cancer of the kidney-pelvis or ureter
- Papillary necrosis
- Renal infarction
- Ureteral stricture and hydronephrosis
- Renal tuberculosis

**Lower urinary tract**
- Cystitis, prostatitis, urethritis
- Bladder cancer
- Prostate cancer
- Benign bladder and ureteral polyps/tumors
- Of uncertain origin
- Exercise hematuria
- Excessive anticoagulation (e.g., warfarin)

- Pelvic inflammatory disease.
- Carcinoma of the colon or genital tract.

## Proteinuria

Benign proteinuria may result from the following:
- Functional proteinuria: fever, strenuous exercise, congestive heart failure, acute medical illnesses, pregnancy.
- Idiopathic transient proteinuria: intermittent.
- Orthostatic proteinuria: common in patients under 30 years of age; significant proteinuria when upright but normal when supine.

Other differential diagnoses include:
- Urinary tract infections.
- Vaginal mucus.
- Diabetes mellitus.
- Glomerulonephritis.
- Causes of nephrotic syndrome (Fig. 13.2).
- Myeloma: Bence Jones protein in urine (light chain dimers).
- Obstructive nephropathy.
- Analgesic abuse.

| Causes of nephrotic syndrome | |
|---|---|
| **Cause** | **Examples** |
| renal disease | glomerulonephritis, renal artery stenosis, renal vein thrombosis, transplant rejection |
| systemic disease | amyloidosis, SLE, polyarteritis nodosa, Henoch-Schönlein purpura |
| metabolic disease | diabetes mellitus, hypothyroidism |
| neoplastic disease | lymphoma, plasma cell myeloma, carcinoma, e.g. lung, GI tract |
| infections | malaria, schistosomiasis, hepatitis B, infective endocarditis, cytomegalovirus, infectious mononucleosis |
| drugs | heavy metals, gold and mercury compounds, captopril, peniciliamine, probenecid |
| familial disorders | congenital nephrotic syndrome, Alport's syndrome, sickle cell anemia |
| allergy | bee stings, poison oak, pollen, vaccines |

**Fig. 13.2** Causes of nephrotic syndrome. (GI, gastrointestinal; SLE, systemic lupus erythematosus.)

In addition to the above, tubular proteinuria, due to tubular or interstitial damage, may occur. Proteinuria results from failure of the tubules to reabsorb some of the plasma proteins that have been filtered by the normal glomerulus. The loss of protein is usually mild and may result from the following:
- Congenital disorders: Fanconi's syndrome (a proximal tubular defect), cystinosis, renal tubular acidosis.
- Heavy metal poisoning: lead, cadmium, Wilson's disease.
- Recovery phase of acute tubular necrosis.
- Chronic nephritis and pyelonephritis.
- Renal transplantation.

Finally, overflow proteinuria may occur. This is when abnormal amounts of low molecular mass proteins (filtered at the glomerulus) are neither reabsorbed nor catabolized completely by the renal tubular cells (e.g., as in acute pancreatitis [amylase]). The following may be responsible:
- Multiple myeloma: Bence Jones protein.
- Hemolytic anemia and march hemoglobinuria: hemoglobin. March hemoglobinuria is due to repeated trauma and was first reported in soldiers after a long march.
- Myelomonocytic leukemia: lysozyme.
- Myoglobinuria and crush injuries: myoglobin.

## History in the patient with hematuria and proteinuria

Bear the differential diagnosis in mind.

If hematuria is present in a woman, ensure that she is not menstruating.

The following factors should be determined when obtaining a history in the patient with hematuria or proteinuria:
- Ask about associated urinary symptoms, such as frequency (urinary tract infection, bladder calculus, prostatism), hesitancy, strangury (the desire to pass something that will not pass, e.g., a calculus), and dysuria (painful micturition reflecting urethral or bladder inflammation).

- Has the patient recently had an upper respiratory infection? A positive answer may suggest IgA nephropathy or post-streptococcal GN.
- Does the patient have a history of hypercalcemia, taking calcium, or parathyroid disorders?
- Is the hematuria worse with exercise? This suggests tumor or calculus.
- Ask about groin pain. This suggests pyelonephritis or renal calculi.
- Ask about colicky pain (especially flank pain). This suggests a ureteric calculus.
- Has there been a history of fever (e.g., with pyelonephritis)?
- Are there generalized features of carcinoma (e.g., anorexia and weight loss)?
- Ask about drugs, such as analgesics (nephropathy) or sulphonamides.
- Is there a history of trauma?
- Is there a past history of radiotherapy?
- Does the urine contain crystals or stones?
- Are there any signs of systemic or chronic illness, such as recurrent infections and polyuria with diabetes mellitus?
- Has there been recent foreign travel (e.g., schistosomiasis or tuberculosis)?
- Is there a positive family history? African Americans should be asked about a family history of sickle cell trait or disease.
- Are there clotting disorders—does the patient bruise easily? Is there a history of renal problems (e.g., polycystic kidney disease)?

The following factors should be assessed, particularly if proteinuria is suspected:
- Ask about the appearance of the urine. Heavy proteinuria turns the urine dark and frothy. However, the urine may appear normal, and proteinuria may only be picked up on formal testing.
- Are there symptoms of urinary tract infection (e.g., frequency, dysuria, urgency, or incontinence)?
- Does the patient have a vaginal or penile discharge?
- Are there signs of systemic disease (e.g., diabetes mellitus)?
- Does the patient have a temperature or other signs of acute illness?
- Are there symptoms of congestive heart failure (e.g., shortness of breath, orthopnea, ankle swelling)?

- Ask about heavy metal exposure and other drugs (e.g., analgesic abuse).
- Is the proteinuria only present after vigorous exercise?
- Is the proteinuria absent in early morning specimens (orthostatic proteinuria)?
- Ensure that the patient is not pregnant.
- Do not forget to keep the causes of nephrotic syndrome in mind (Fig. 13.2).

Ask about the appearance of the urine:
- If the urine is blood stained at the start of micturition and clear later on, the site of pathology is likely to be the urethra or prostate.
- If the urine is more blood stained toward the end of micturition, the site of pathology is likely to be the bladder.
- If the urine is evenly blood stained throughout micturition, the site of pathology is likely to be the kidney or ureter.

## Examining the patient with hematuria and proteinuria

The examination approach is summarized in Fig. 13.3.

## Investigating the patient with hematuria and proteinuria

An algorithm for the investigation of the patient with hematuria and proteinuria is given in Fig. 13.4. Ultimately, it may be necessary to proceed to a renal biopsy, but, initially, urine, blood, and radiologic tests should be performed.

### Urine
It is important to note that the urine dipstick detects predominantly albumin, *not* light chains and other smaller proteins. In addition, it takes >300–500mg/day before the test becomes

**Fig. 13.3** Examining the patient with hematuria and proteinuria. (SBE, subacute bacterial endocarditis.)

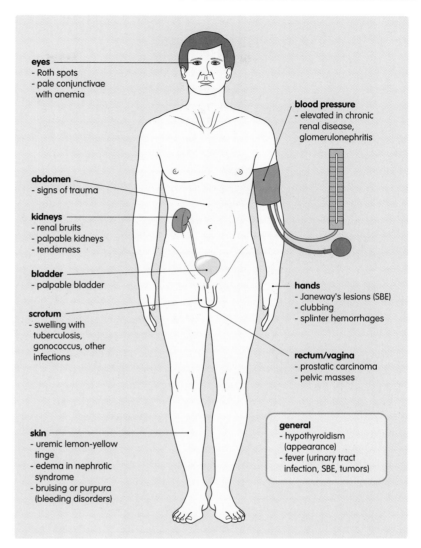

**eyes**
- Roth spots
- pale conjunctivae with anemia

**blood pressure**
- elevated in chronic renal disease, glomerulonephritis

**abdomen**
- signs of trauma

**kidneys**
- renal bruits
- palpable kidneys
- tenderness

**bladder**
- palpable bladder

**scrotum**
- swelling with tuberculosis, gonococcus, other infections

**hands**
- Janeway's lesions (SBE)
- clubbing
- splinter hemorrhages

**rectum/vagina**
- prostatic carcinoma
- pelvic masses

**skin**
- uremic lemon-yellow tinge
- edema in nephrotic syndrome
- bruising or purpura (bleeding disorders)

**general**
- hypothyroidism (appearance)
- fever (urinary tract infection, SBE, tumors)

---

positive. The following urinary tests should be performed:

- Albumin.
- Glucose.
- Urobilinogen: jaundice.
- Porphyrins: porphyria.
- Microscopy: red blood cells, white blood cells, casts, crystals, protein.
- Culture: infection.
- Early morning urine: acid-fast bacilli, if tuberculosis is suspected.
- Cytology: malignancy.

Urine may be tested for protein at different times in the day. Protein is normally absent in orthostatic proteinuria first thing in the morning before getting up. (The patient is asked to void the bladder before sleep). It may also be tested after exercise.

## 24-hour collection of urine for protein
24-hour collection of urine for protein is useful for distinguishing mild to moderate proteinuria, in which the loss is not sufficient to cause protein depletion, from severe proteinuria, in which the loss is usually 5–10g. More benign causes of proteinuria usually result in excretion of less than 1–2g/day. In patients under the age of 30 years, the urine should be split into "upright" and "supine" specimens to aid in the diagnosis of orthostatic proteinuria.

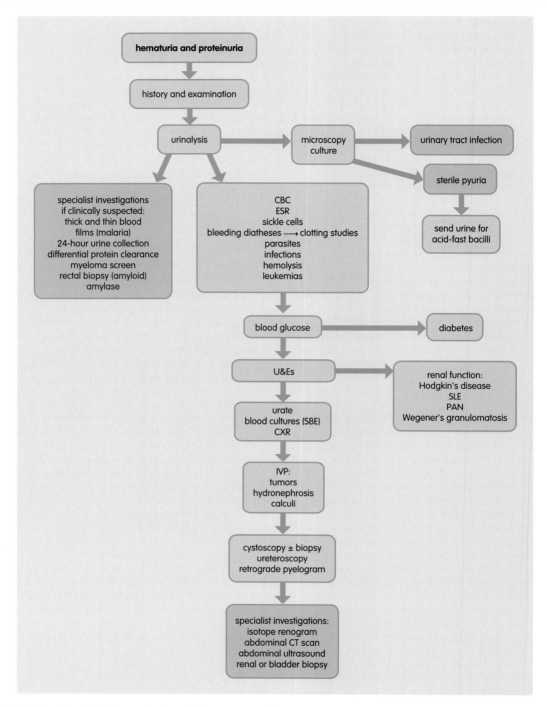

**Fig. 13.4** Algorithm for the investigation of the patient with hematuria and proteinuria. (CT, computed tomography; CXR, chest x-ray; CBC, complete blood count; ESR, erythrocyte sedimentation rate; IVP, intravenous pyelogram; PAN, polyarteritis nodosa; SBE, subacute bacterial endocarditis; SLE, systemic lupus erythematosus.)

## Differential protein clearance

Differential protein clearance (selectivity) is occasionally performed in patients with nephrotic syndrome. Patients with selective proteinuria (small molecular mass proteins are cleared more rapidly than large proteins) are more likely to respond to steroid therapy.

## Kidney biopsy

This is performed for patients who have 2–3g/day of urine protein on a 24-hour collection. The renal biopsy can be helpful in nephritic syndrome to differentiate among causes and to direct treatment.

Causes of a sterile pyuria:
- Tuberculosis.
- Tumors.
- Analgesic nephropathy.

## Blood

The following blood tests should be performed:
- Complete blood count: platelet deficiency in bleeding disorders, sickle cells, parasites, leukocytosis with infections.
- Erythrocyte sedimentation rate.
- Clotting studies: bleeding diathesis.
- Blood glucose: diabetes mellitus.
- Urea and electrolytes: renal function.
- Urate: gout.
- Blood cultures: infective endocarditis.
- Specialized investigations according to clinical suspicion: thick and thin films for malaria; serum complement and autoantibodies for glomerulonephritis.

- Myeloma screen: immunoelectrophoresis; urine for Bence Jones protein.
- Hepatitis B, cytomegalovirus, and Epstein-Barr virus serology: potential causes of nephrotic syndrome.

## Kidney biopsy

For isolated cases of red cell casts with preserved renal function, biopsy is usually not required. The patient should be referred for close follow-up. Most cases of glomerulonephritis can be ascertained by history and systemic symptoms. Kidney biopsy is definitely indicated for patients who have an undetermined diagnosis.

Remember: urea and electrolytes may be normal despite significant renal disease.

## Radiology

The following radiologic tests should be performed:
- Chest x-ray: primary and secondary tumors, tuberculosis, polyarteritis.
- Abdominal x-ray: renal outline and stones. Ninety per cent of renal calculi are opaque; urate, cysteine, and xanthine stones may be radiolucent.
- Intravenous pyelogram: excretory function, stones, shape of the calyces, ureters and bladder.
- Cystoscopy: bladder lesions.
- Ureteroscopy: ureter lesions.
- Retrograde pyelogram: stones or obstructive lesions in the ureters are suspected.
- Abdominal CT scan: to visualize the kidneys, adjacent organs, and other abdominal masses.

# 14. Hypertension

The level of blood pressure above which someone is "hypertensive" is controversial and varies among different countries. However, most clinicians would consider treatment when blood pressure is persistently elevated above 160/90mmHg. This is an arbitrary cut-off point and is influenced by age, end-organ damage, and other risk factors.

The most recent Joint National Committee (JNC-7) guidelines for definition and treatment of hypertension have redefined blood pressure goals and treatment algorithms. Normal blood pressure is still defined as below 120/80mmHg, but a new category prehypertension, has been introduced. This group of people, with blood pressure between 120–139/80–89mmHg, should be given strong encouragement for lifestyle modification (e.g., weight loss, cessation of smoking) so that they do not progress into the newly defined stage 1 or stage 2 groups of hypertension.

Stage 1 hypertension includes blood pressures of 140–159/90–99mmHg; the initial treatment recommendation is monodrug therapy.

Stage 2 hypertension is defined as blood pressure >160/>100mmHg; the new treatment guidelines recommend initial therapy with a two-drug combination consisting of a thiazide diuretic with an ACE inhibitor, angiotensin receptor blocker (ARB), calcium channel blocker (CCB), or beta blocker.

Approximately 95% of all hypertensive patients have "essential" or "primary" hypertension and have no underlying disease. Secondary hypertension can be the result of a range of different pathologic processes.

Hypertension is present in 20–30% of the population, depending on ethnic background. African-Americans have higher blood pressures than Hispanic and Caucasian populations. The incidence increases with age; hypertension is present in 55–80% of the population over the age of 60 years.

## Differential diagnosis of hypertension

### Essential hypertension
Essential hypertension accounts for 95% of cases. There is no underlying cause.

### Secondary hypertension
Secondary hypertension accounts for 5% of cases. Factors leading to secondary hypertension are:

### Lifestyle
- Obesity.
- High alcohol intake.
- Lack of exercise.
- High salt intake.

### Renal
- Renal parenchynmal disease (e.g., chronic pyelonephritis, glomerulonephritis, polycystic disease, tumor, tuberclosis).
- Renal artery disease (e.g., atherosclerosis, fibromuscular dysplasia, vasculitis).
- Obstructive uropathy (e.g., hydronephrosis due to a stone or tumor).

### Cardiovascular
- Congenital (e.g., coarctation of the aorta).

### Drugs
Examples include:
- Combined oral contraceptive pill.
- Nonsteroidal anti-inflamatory drugs [NSAIDs]).

### Endocrine
- Pheochromocytoma.
- Conn's syndrome.
- Secondary hyperaldosteronism.
- Cushing's syndrome.
- Hyperthyroidism.

- Hypercalcemia.
- Obesity.

**Other**
- Raised intracranial pressure.
- Obstructive sleep apnea.

95% of patients with hypertension have no underlying disease.

## History in the patient with hypertension

Hypertension is usually asymptomatic and is often found incidentally. The history should be approached in three parts:
- Firstly, how long has the patient had hypertension and what treatments have been given so far?
- Secondly, how severe is the hypertension and has it resulted in complications?
- Finally, are there any risk factors suggesting that an underlying pathology may be present?

### Presentation and history of hypertension

Important questions to address are as follows:
- How was the hypertension discovered? For example, at a routine preoperative assessment or with malignant (accelerated) hypertension. When was the last time that the patient had a normal blood pressure reading?
- For how long has the blood pressure been monitored? Unless severe (>160/100mmHg), the diagnosis should not be made until blood pressure is persistently elevated for at least 6 months.
- What treatments, if any, has the patient been given so far? If blood pressure control is poor, despite taking correct doses of three antihypertensive agents, the patient is said to have "resistant hypertension."

### How severe is the hypertension? Are there complications?

Mild hypertension is asymptomatic. However, when hypertension is severe or chronic and associated with complications, the following symptoms may occur:
- Headaches (mostly frontal).
- Dyspnea.
- Symptoms of frank heart failure.
- Angina pectoris or myocardial infarction.
- Transient ischemic attacks or stroke.
- Visual disturbance.

### Is the history suggestive of an underlying cause?

Ask about the following:
- Lifestyle history, paying particular attention to alcohol and smoking (atherosclerosis). Stimulants such as cocaine and amphetamines can also cause hypertension.
- Precise drug history.
- Previous medical history (e.g., recurrent pyelonephritis, nephrectomy).
- Family history may suggest underlying polycystic disease.
- Symptoms of pheochromocytoma are rare but include episodic pallor, headache, tremor, palpitations, and nausea.

## Examining the patient with hypertension

Patients with uncomplicated mild essential hypertension will have no associated clinical signs. However, when a patient is found to be hypertensive, one should search for evidence of complications or an underlying cause (Fig. 14.1).

### Evidence of an underlying cause
- Palpable kidneys: polycystic disease, renal tumor.
- Peripheral vascular disease and xanthelasmata: renal artery stenosis.
- Renal bruit (throughout both systole and diastole): renovascular disease.
- Radiofemoral delay: coarctation of the aorta.
- Neurofibromatosis: renal artery stenosis.
- Cushing's disease.

### Evidence of complications
- Atrial fibrillation.
- Displaced, thrusting PMI, indicating left ventricular hypertrophy.
- Frank heart failure.

**Fig. 14.1** Examining the patient with hypertension.

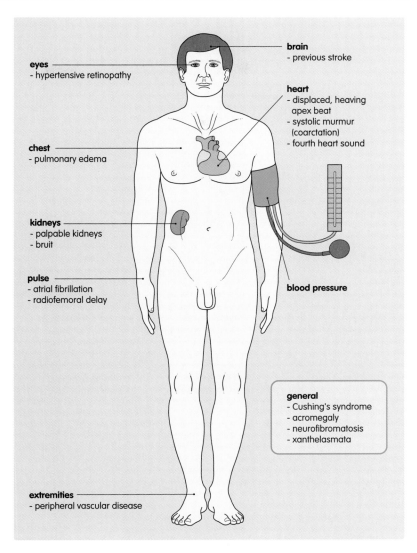

**eyes**
- hypertensive retinopathy

**brain**
- previous stroke

**heart**
- displaced, heaving apex beat
- systolic murmur (coarctation)
- fourth heart sound

**chest**
- pulmonary edema

**kidneys**
- palpable kidneys
- bruit

**pulse**
- atrial fibrillation
- radiofemoral delay

**blood pressure**

**general**
- Cushing's syndrome
- acromegaly
- neurofibromatosis
- xanthelasmata

**extremities**
- peripheral vascular disease

- Retinopathy.
- Previous stroke.

## Investigating the patient with hypertension

An algorithm for the investigation of the patient with hypertension is given in Fig. 14.2. At presentation all hypertensive patients should have the following tests:

- Urine dipstick: parenchymal disease, urinary tract infection, stone, associated diabetes.
- Metabolic panel: renal impairment suggests underlying disease.

- Lipid profile: to rule out metabolic syndrome.
- Electrocardiogram: significant hypertension may result in left ventricular hypertrophy (LVH).
- Echocardiogram. Most patients have an echocardiogram to look for LVH. While the ECG is helpful, an echocardiogram can give information not only about LVH but also about any wall motion abnormalities.

Fig. 14.3 shows patients who should then be investigated further. This group includes patients diagnosed with hypertension at an early age and patient initially resistant to multiple antihypertension medication. The following tests may be used:

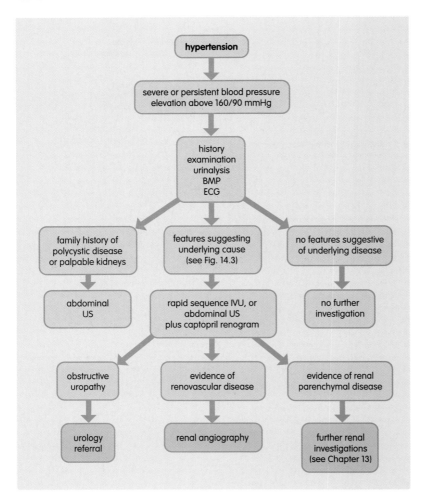

**Fig. 14.2** Algorithm for the investigation of the patient with hypertension. (ECG, electrocardiogram; IVU, intravenous urogram; BMP, basic metabolic panel.)

| Indications for detailed investigation of hypertension |
| --- |

- recent onset or worsening of hypertension
- malignant (accelerated) hypertension
- uncontrolled hypertension despite three antihypertensive drugs
- abdominal bruit
- proteinuria, hematuria, or abnormal renal function
- hypokalemia not otherwise explained, e.g. by diuretic therapy
- renal failure caused by angiotensin-converting enzyme (ACE) inhibitors
- young age (<30 years)
- severe generalized atherosclerosis
- unexplained pulmonary oedema

**Fig. 14.3** Indications for detailed investigation of hypertension.

- 24-hour urinary vanilly mandelic acid (VMA) and catecholamine excretion: pheochromocytoma.
- Radiologic investigations: renovascular disease, renoparenchymal disease, obstructive uropathy. This should be either rapid sequence intravenous urogram, or abdominal ultrasound scan plus captopril renogram.
- Renal angiography: renal artery disease; this is a definitive test and should be performed if indicated by the radiologic tests or clinical circumstances.

All hypertensive patients should have urine dipstick, urea and electrolytes, and an electrocardiogram. Only a few need any further tests.

# 15. Headache and Facial Pain

Headache is one of the most common presenting symptoms. There are often few clinical signs, and the history is the main diagnostic tool. Many different pathologic processes can result in headache or facial pain.

## Differential diagnosis of headache and facial pain

### Headache

The differential diagnosis of headache includes the following:

- Tension headache.
- Migraine.
- Tumor: primary, secondary.
- Infection: abscess, meningitis, encephalitis, sinusitis, herpes zoster.
- Bleeding: subdural, extradural, intracerebral hematoma, subarachnoid hemorrhage.
- Vasculitic: temporal arteritis.
- Thrombosis: dural sinus thrombosis.
- Skull: fracture, tumor, Paget's disease.
- Drugs: nitrates.
- Others: benign intracranial hypertension, hydrocephalus, post-traumatic, coital cephalgia, withdrawal from coffee.

### Facial pain

Diseases affecting the teeth, temporomandibular joint, cervical spine, sinuses, eye, ear, nose, and even heart (myocardial ischemia) can cause pain which radiates to the face. Other causes are disease of the trigeminal nerve such as trigeminal neuralgia and postherpetic neuralgia.

## History in the patient with headache or facial pain

The onset, nature, and subsequent pattern of pain will usually provide a good short list of likely causes.

The presence of additional symptoms and risk factors may add further weight to this list.

It is important to rule out the most dangerous causes of headache below. Danger signs include acute onset with extreme pain, headache after strenuous exercise, the "first" or "worst" headache of the patient's life, any signs of increased intracranial pressure, any associated neurologic deficits (including vision), concurrent infection at another site, and association with trauma.

### Solitary acute episode

This pattern is seen in infection, hemorrhage, or thrombosis. (Note that it may also be the first presentation of the other causes of headache).

*Subarachnoid hemorrhage* presents with a sudden onset of severe pain. It may be described as "the worst headache of my life" or "as if someone had hit me on the back of the head." Nausea, vomiting, neck stiffness, and photophobia result from meningeal irritation. Altered consciousness level and focal neurologic deficits may also occur depending on the site and size of the bleed. Fig. 15.1 lists the causes of subarachnoid hemorrhage.

Patients with *infective meningitis* present with a short history of headache, symptoms of infection (malaise, fever, and rigors) and symptoms of meningeal irritation (vomiting, photophobia, and neck pain and stiffness). However, tuberculous and malignant meningitis have a more subacute presentation which can be easily missed.

*Cerebral abscess* causes headaches, seizures, symptoms of infection, and symptoms of raised intracranial pressure as the lesion expands (see below). The infection may have spread from a primary focus, such as the lung in bronchiectasis, middle ear, or paranasal sinuses.

Seizures, focal neurologic symptoms, and symptoms of raised intracranial pressure can also result from *dural venous sinus thrombosis*. This is a rare complication of pregnancy, oral contraceptive

| Causes of subarachnoid hemorrhage |
| --- |
| • berry aneurysm (70%)<br>• arteriovenous malformation (10%)<br>• no underlying lesion (15–20%)<br>• bleeding disorders<br>• mycotic aneurysm (endocarditis)<br>• tumor<br>• arteritis<br>• trauma |

**Fig. 15.1** Causes of subarachnoid hemorrhage. Note that berry aneurysms may be associated with coarctation of the aorta and polycystic kidney disease.

| Symptoms of raised intracranial pressure |
| --- |
| • headache worse on coughing, sneezing, stooping down<br>• headache worse in the morning<br>• visual disturbance due to papilledema<br>• nausea and vomiting<br>• diplopia (false localizing 6th cranial nerve palsy) |

**Fig. 15.2** Symptoms of raised intracranial pressure.

pill use, dehydration, paranasal sinus infection, and severe intercurrent illness.

## Progressive headache

A headache that comes on gradually over days or weeks and increases in severity is often a feature of a tumor, benign intracranial hypertension, or hydrocephalus. In all three the headache results from raised intracranial pressure and has the characteristic features shown in Fig. 15.2. Temporal arteritis also presents gradually, but the nature of the headache is very different.

*Cerebral tumors* can be primary or secondary. The patient may have a history of malignancy elsewhere. The most common tumors to metastasize to the brain are those of the thyroid, bronchus, and breast, as well as gastric, renal and prostate tumors. In addition to headache, the patient may also develop seizures and focal neurologic deficits related to the site of the lesion.

*Benign intracranial hypertension (pseudotumor cerebri)* is most common in young women. Headache, nausea, and visual disturbance are the presenting symptoms. There is an association with obesity, empty sella turcica, and certain drugs. If left untreated, the patient may become blind due to infarction of the optic nerve.

*Temporal arteritis* (TA) affects predominantly the elderly. It is extremely rare before the age of 50 years. The patient presents with a superficial headache overlying the temporal arteries. The pain may be exacerbated by brushing or combing the hair. Jaw claudication may arise as a consequence of inflammation of the branches of the external carotid artery. Visual loss may be temporary (amaurosis fugax) or permanent if the ciliary or central retinal

artery is affected. Weight loss, anorexia, fever, and proximal muscle pain may also occur. Treatment with high-dose IV steroids should begin as soon as TA becomes number one on the differential diagnosis. If you plan to get a TA biopsy, the steroids should be started before the procedure because they can be vision-sparing.

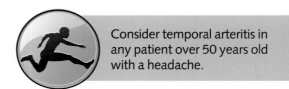

Consider temporal arteritis in any patient over 50 years old with a headache.

## Episodic headache or facial pain

Migraine and cluster headaches present with episodes of pain (often severe) interspersed with long symptom-free periods. Paroxysms of pain are also a feature of trigeminal neuralgia.

*Classic migraine* usually starts with a prodrome lasting 5–60 minutes, characterized by a sense of ill health and visual abnormalities (fortification spectra, scotomata, or teichopsia). A throbbing headache then develops, which tends to be unilateral but can become generalized. This is associated with nausea, vomiting, photophobia, and phonophobia. The attack resolves spontaneously after several hours and is often followed by sleep. In uncommon variants of migraine, headache may be accompanied by hemiplegia, ophthalmoplegia, ataxia, vertigo, or unilateral facial palsy.

Migraine is more common in women. Provoking factors include menstruation, fatigue, cheese, and red wine.

*Cluster headache* (migrainous neuralgia) is a severe unilateral pain centered around one eye. The pain lasts for around an hour and occurs daily for several weeks, often waking the patient from sleep. There is ipsilateral nasal congestion, and the eye becomes watery. Horner's syndrome can develop and is occasionally permanent. Symptom-free periods of many months occur between attacks. Cluster headaches are more common in men and may be precipitated by alcohol.

*Trigeminal neuralgia* (tic douloureux) is characterized by paroxysms of lancinating pain in the distribution of the 5th cranial nerve. It is stimulated by touching "trigger zones" on the face such as the lips, or by eating or drinking. The pain lasts for up to 1 minute and does not occur during sleep. Spontaneous remissions can last several months. While there is usually no underlying cause, trigeminal neuralgia may occasionally be secondary to multiple sclerosis (MS) in the young patient or to tumors affecting the cerebellopontine angle or 5th cranial nerve.

## Chronic headache or facial pain

Persistent pain is a feature of postherpetic neuralgia, post-traumatic headache, or tension headache.

Following *zoster* of the trigeminal nerve (usually the ophthalmic division), a persistent burning pain, known as postherpetic neuralgia, may develop. Facial scarring is usually apparent, and the pain may disturb sleep. It is uncommon in the young.

*Tension headaches* are the most common cause of headaches presenting to doctors. The feeling is often described as a "tight band around the head," being most common in the frontal and occipital regions, or as a "pressure" behind the eyes. It is a constant pain, which tends to be worse toward the end of the day or at times of particular stress. There may be coexistent depression.

Following *head injury*, which may not necessarily be severe, a few patients develop persistent headache, similar to a tension headache. It is associated with poor memory and concentration, dizziness, irritability, and symptoms of depression. The patient may be involved in litigation related to the accident responsible.

## Examining the patient with headache or facial pain

The diagnosis is often clear from the history. On examination look for evidence of the pathologic processes, such as raised intracranial pressure and meningism. Focal neurologic deficits, if present, help to determine the site of the lesion. Fig. 15.3 summarizes the examination approach. Measure blood pressure to rule out hypertensive encephalopathy.

## Signs of raised intracranial pressure
- Papilledema: commonly, the only sign.
- False localizing sign (ipsilateral, then bilateral 6th cranial nerve palsy).
- Altered level of consciousness, bradycardia, hypertension if acute or severe, which can progress to decerebrate posturing and death.

## Signs of meningism
- Irritability: with a preference for a quiet, darkened room.
- Neck stiffness.
- Positive Kernig's sign: spasm and pain in hamstrings on knee extension.
- Positive Brudzinski's sign: neck flexion causes leg flexion.
- Delirium, fever, and petechial rash: may also be present in infectious meningitis.

If subarachnoid hemorrhage is suspected, look for subhyaloid (retinal) hemorrhage, bruit of an arteriovenous malformation, and a 3rd cranial nerve palsy caused by direct pressure from a posterior communicating artery aneurysm.

When meningitis is suspected clinically, treat with antibiotics first and then complete investigations. Patients can die awaiting confirmation of the diagnosis.

## Signs of temporal arteritis
- Temporal artery tenderness.
- Loss of temporal artery pulsation—there may be overlying erythema.
- Optic atrophy.
- Low-grade fever.

## Focal neurologic deficit
Focal neurologic signs will help to determine the site of the lesion (see Chapter 20) and may be found in

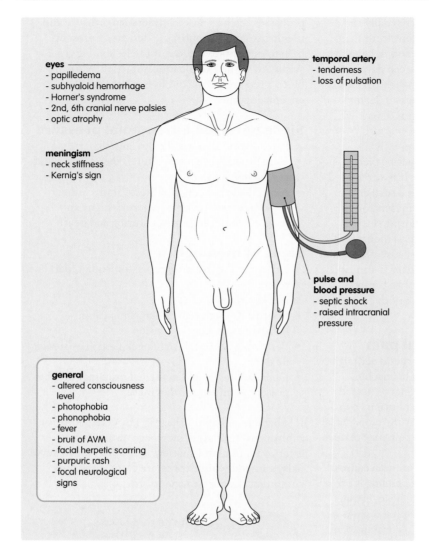

**Fig. 15.3** Examining the patient with headache and facial pain. (AVM, arteriovenous malformation.)

**eyes**
- papilledema
- subhyaloid hemorrhage
- Horner's syndrome
- 2nd, 6th cranial nerve palsies
- optic atrophy

**meningism**
- neck stiffness
- Kernig's sign

**temporal artery**
- tenderness
- loss of pulsation

**pulse and blood pressure**
- septic shock
- raised intracranial pressure

**general**
- altered consciousness level
- photophobia
- phonophobia
- fever
- bruit of AVM
- facial herpetic scarring
- purpuric rash
- focal neurological signs

addition to other signs, such as meningism or raised intracranial pressure.

## Investigating the patient with headache or facial pain

An algorithm for the investigation of the patient with headache or facial pain is given in Fig. 15.4. Investigations used in this type of patient include:
- Complete blood count: normochromic normocytic anemia suggests chronic pathology (e.g., temporal arteritis, tuberculous meningitis); leukocytosis will be seen in infection.
- Erythrocyte sedimentation rate: high in temporal arteritis but may also be raised in infection and malignancy.
- Temporal artery biopsy: temporal arteritis. This is a definitive test, but as there is often patchy vascular involvement, a negative result does not exclude the diagnosis.
- Computed tomography scan or magnetic resonance imaging of the head: presence of blood, space-occupying lesion (tumor, abscess), or hydrocephalus. Contrast enhancement should be used if tumor is suspected.
- Lumbar puncture: this should never be performed when raised intracranial pressure is a possibility, as

**Fig. 15.4** Algorithm for the investigation of the patient with headache or facial pain. (CSF, cerebrospinal fluid; CT, computed tomography; ESR, erythrocyte sedimentation rate.)

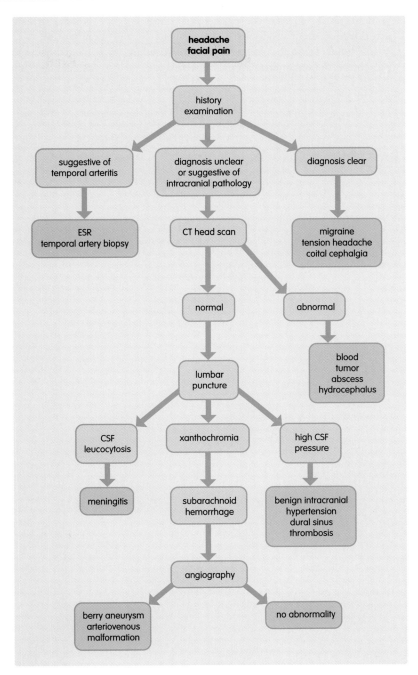

it causes cerebral herniation. Cerebrospinal fluid (CSF) examination is invaluable in the diagnosis of meningitis. CSF should be sent to the laboratory for assessment of glucose and protein, microscopy, culture, and cytology.

- Head CT scan should be done for all cases of trauma, especially in the elderly, patients taking anticoagulants, and patients with mental status changes.
- MRI should be done to look for signs of ischemia. MRA can be done to look for signs of vasculitis.
- Cerebral angiography: should be performed if surgery is considered in subarachnoid hemorrhage.

It identifies and localizes berry aneurysms and arteriovenous malformations.

- Visual fields: these should be serially measured in patients with benign intracranial hypertension, which carries a serious risk of optic nerve infarction.
- Electroencephalography: herpes simplex encephalitis shows characteristic features.

# 16. Joint Disease

## Differential diagnosis of joint disease

It is important to distinguish accurately cases that need emergent care. These include hot/swollen joints, associated systemic symptoms (e.g., weight loss, malaise), neurologic symptoms, and weakness.

### Common causes
- Rheumatoid arthritis (RA).
- Osteoarthritis (OA).
- Gout.
- Seronegative arthritides: ankylosing spondylitis, Reiter's syndrome, and psoriatic arthritis.
- Septic arthritis.

The causes of a single, hot, red joint are as follows:
- Septic arthritis, possibly secondary to rheumatoid arthritis, osteoarthritis, osteomyelitis, or injury.
- Trauma.
- Gout.
- Pseudogout.
- Hemarthrosis.
- Gonococcal arthritis.
- Rheumatoid arthritis.

Arthritis may also be a feature of connective tissue diseases, especially systemic lupus erythematosus (SLE) and polyarteritis nodosa (PAN).

### Less common causes
- Enteropathic arthropathies (e.g., inflammatory bowel disease, Whipple's disease).
- Behçet's syndrome.
- Leukemia and lymphoma.
- Metastases: bronchial, breast, thyroid, kidney, and prostate carcinomas.
- Hypertrophic pulmonary osteoarthropathy: bronchial carcinoma.
- Viral, bacterial, and fungal infections.
- Endocrine causes: acromegaly, myxedema, hyperparathyroidism, idiopathic hyperparathyroidism.
- Metabolic diseases: Wilson's disease, hemochromatosis, chondrocalcinosis, ochronosis, pyrophosphate arthropathy.
- Psychiatric causes: fibromyalgia, depression.
- Others: familial Mediterranean fever, sarcoidosis, amyloidosis, sickle cell disease, Wegener's granulomatosis.

## History in the patient with joint disease

The different types of joint disease have many features in common, and examination will provide further additional important clues to the etiology. Ask about the following:
- Onset: rapid or slowly progressive.
- Persistent or relapsing. Gout has a classic history of recurrent attacks or inflammation.
- Association with movement. OA improves with movement and worsens with rest.
- Early morning stiffness: classically RA is worse first thing in the morning and OA is worse at the end of the day, although there is considerable overlap.
- Weakness: with or without wasting of muscles.
- Distribution of the affected joints, monoarticular vs. polyarticular (see below).
- Patient's age: RA classically affects women aged 25–55 years, and OA usually occurs in patients over 40.

- Any history of trauma.
- Drug history: procainamide, hydralazine, isoniazid, and methydopa can cause a lupus-like syndrome; thiazide diuretics cause a predisposition for gout.
- Recent infection (e.g., viral illness and reactive arthritis, septic arthritis, or neutropenia).
- Features associated with different arthropathies: inflammation of the eye (RA and seronegative arthropathies), shortness of breath (fibrosis or aortic regurgitation in RA, and ankylosing spondylitis), paresthesias (entrapment neuropathies), gastrointestinal symptoms (enteropathic arthropathies), and rarer causes of arthropathies (e.g., endocrine causes).
- In patients with chronic arthritis it is important to explore the extent of loss of function. How limited are the activities of daily living?
- Chronic arthritis can lead to feelings of helplessness and depression. Assessment of these features is also an important part of the history.

## Examining the patient with joint disease

Remember: "Look, feel, move, and measure":
- **Look:** inspect for joint swelling, redness, muscular atrophy.
- **Feel:** palpate for warmth, joint effusion, and tenderness.
- **Move:** move the joint passively and ask the patient to move the joint actively. Look for limitation in the range of motion, tenderness, and joint subluxation.
- **Measure:** use a tape measure to determine muscular atrophy of large joints or decrease in size of limbs, etc.

### Rheumatoid arthritis

RA is a systemic connective tissue disorder, the joints being one of many body parts affected. Look for the following (see Fig. 36.1):
- Symmetrical deforming arthropathy.
- Swelling of the proximal interphalangeal (PIP) and metacarpophalangeal (MCP) joints. For diagnosis, swelling must be present in 3 or more joints for 6 weeks.
- Wasting of the small muscles of the hand.
- Nodules on the elbows and extensor tendons. They are nonfixed and several millimeters in diameter.

- Ulnar deviation of the fingers: subluxation and dislocation at the MCP joints.
- Swan neck deformity: hyperextension of the PIP joints and flexion of the MCP and distal interphalangeal (DIP) joints.
- Boutonnière deformity: flexion of the PIP joints and extension of the DIP and MCP joints.
- Swollen or deformed knees.
- Cervical spine disease.
- Anemia.
- Systemic symptoms: weight loss, malaise, low-grade fever, depression. Usually on acute presentation.
- Arteritic lesions: nail-fold infarcts, chronic leg ulceration, and purpuric rash.

Determine how the joint disease affects the patient's daily activities (e.g., holding a pan, making a cup of tea).

## Osteoarthritis

In the hands in OA look for the following (see Fig. 36.4):
- Heberden's nodes: swelling of the DIP joints.
- Bouchard's nodes: swelling of the PIP joints.
- Subluxation of the first metacarpal: square hand appearance.
- Crepitus of affected joints.
- Hip pain: common in patients with OA.
- Wasting and weakness of the quadriceps and glutei.
- Positive Trendelenburg's sign: this is a downward tilting of the pelvis when the patient stands on the affected leg.
- Joint effusions.
- Loss of function.

The causes of joint pain can be remembered by the mnemonic **SOFTER TISSUE: s**epsis, **o**steoarthritis, **f**ractures, **t**endon/muscle, **e**piphyseal, **r**eferred, **t**umor, **i**schemia, **s**eropositive arthritides, **s**eronegative arthritides, **u**rate, **e**xtra-articular rheumatism (e.g., polymyalgia).

## Gout

Look for the following:

- Asymmetrical swelling of the small joints of the hand and feet.
- Tophi: look especially on the helix of the ear and tendon sheaths.
- Look for associations: hyperlipidemia (xanthalasmata and corneal arcus), hypertension, signs associated with diabetes mellitus.

## Seronegative arthritides
### Ankylosing spondylitis

Ask the patient to sit or stand up. Look for the following:

- Loss of lumbar lordosis and a fixed kyphosis.
- A stooped "question mark" posture.
- Rigid spine.
- Reduced chest expansion.
- Prominent abdomen.

Also examine for complications and extra-articular manifestations:

- Eyes: iritis.
- Cardiovascular system: aortitis (listen for aortic regurgitation and conduction defects).
- Chest: apical fibrosis.
- Neurologic: atlantoaxial dislocation leading to paraplegia or sciatica.

### Reiter's syndrome

This is a triad of urethritis, conjunctivitis, and seronegative arthritis. It follows nonspecific urethritis or occasionally dysentery. Look for the following:

- Large joint mono- or oligoarthritis.
- Iritis.
- Keratoderma blenorrhagica (brown, aseptic abscesses on the soles and palms).
- Mouth ulcers.
- Circinate balanitis.
- Enthesopathy (plantar fasciitis or Achilles tendinitis).
- Aortic regurgitation.

### Psoriatic arthritis

Look for the following:

- Asymmetrical arthropathy.
- Usually involvement of the DIP joints.
- Pitting of the fingernails and onycholysis.
- Thickened nails.

- Psoriatic plaques: look particularly at the elbows, extensor aspects of limbs, scalp, behind the ears, and the navel.
- Other forms of psoriatic arthropathy: arthritis mutilans, a RA-like picture, asymmetrical mono- or oligoarthropathy, ankylosing spondylitis.

## Septic arthritis

This must be recognized and treated promptly because of potential destruction of the joint and widespread infection. It usually presents as a monoarthritis. The affected joint is swollen, painful, hot, and red.

You must also carry out a general examination. In particular, look for the following:

- Eye signs: keratoconjunctivitis sicca, keratitis, episcleritis, scleromalacia perforans, cataracts due to chloroquine or steroids.
- Dry mucous membranes: Sjögren's syndrome.
- Chest signs: pleural effusion, fibrosing alveolitis.
- Neurologic signs: peripheral neuropathy, mononeuritis multiplex, entrapment neuropathy.
- Vasculitic leg ulceration.
- Felty's syndrome: splenomegaly, neutropenia.
- Cardiac signs: pericarditis, myocarditis, conduction defects, and valvular incompetence.
- Secondary amyloidosis.
- Other autoimmune disorders.

## Investigating the patient with joint disease

An algorithm for the investigation of patients with joint disease is provided in Fig. 16.1. The following investigations should be performed:

- Complete blood count: anemia; raised white cell count occasionally in RA, leukopenia and thrombocytopenia in SLE, eosinophilia in PAN, neutropenia in Felty's syndrome.
- Erythrocyte sedimentation rate/C-reactive protein: nonspecific but raised in the presence of inflammation (therefore often high in RA but less so in OA).
- Rheumatoid factor: positive in about 75% of patients with RA. It may also be positive in SLE, mixed connective tissue diseases, scleroderma, Sjögren's syndrome, and viral illnesses.
- Antinuclear antibodies: positive in 30% of patients with RA and in 80% of patients with SLE.

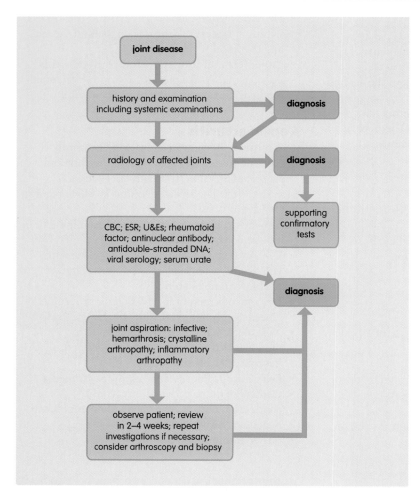

**Fig. 16.1** Algorithm for the investigation of the patient with joint disease. (ESR, erythrocyte sedimentation rate; CBC, complete blood count; U&Es, urea and electrolytes.)

- Anti-double-stranded DNA antibodies: high titers in SLE.
- Other autoantibodies according to clinical suspicion (e.g., anti-Ro and anti-La antibodies in Sjögren's syndrome and anti-Scl70 antibodies in scleroderma).
- Viral serology: if a viral cause for the arthropathy is suspected (e.g., rubella, mumps, infectious mononucleosis, coxsackie virus, and hepatitis B virus).
- Urea and electrolytes: associated renal involvement.
- Liver function tests: liver involvement or drug treatment.
- Creatine phosphokinase: myositis.
- Serum urate: usually high in gout but beware of false positives and false negatives.

Anemia in rheumatoid arthritis may be due to the following:
- Normochromic normocytic anemia of chronic disease.
- Microcytic anemia from chronic blood loss secondary to drug treatment.
- Bone marrow suppression from treatment (e.g., gold or penicillamine).
- Megaloblastic anemia from impaired folate release or pernicious anemia.
- Felty's syndrome.

Joint aspiration should be performed. Examine the following:

- Appearance: purulence indicates infection, frank blood indicates hemarthrosis or traumatic tap.
- Microscopy for bacteria and crystals: monosodium urate indicates gout, calcium pyrophosphate indicates pseudogout.
- White cell count: high in inflammatory arthropathies.
- Culture: gonococci, tubercle bacillus, or fungi when indicated.

A chest x-ray should be performed to look for associated diseases or complications of RA:

- Pleural effusion.
- Diffuse fibrosing alveolitis.
- Rheumatoid nodules or cavities.
- Cricoarytenoid arthritis.
- Obliterative bronchiolitis.
- Rheumatoid pneumoconiosis: Caplan's syndrome.

An x-ray of the affected joints may indicate the following:

- RA: soft tissue thickening, juxta-articular osteoporosis, loss of joint space, bony erosions, subluxation.
- OA: loss of joint space, subchondral sclerosis and cysts, marginal osteophytes.
- Gout: soft tissue swelling and punched-out lesions in juxta-articular bone.
- Ankylosing spondylitis: "bamboo spine" (squaring of the vertebrae and obliteration of sacroiliac joints); also found in Reiter's syndrome and Crohn's disease.

An x-ray of the cervical spine should also be used to look for displacement of the odontoid peg. Finally, arthroscopy allows direct visualization inside the joint space, and can be used for biopsy and the removal of foreign bodies.

In **p**seudogout, crystals are **p**ositively birefringent in plane-polarized light. Remember this by the "Ps." In gout, the crystals are negatively birefringent.

# 17. Skin Rashes

Differential diagnosis
by appearance

## Pigmented lesions

- Freckles (ephelides): flat, brown spots.
- Lentigo: similar to freckles but darker and not affected by sunlight.
- Seborrheic keratosis: benign, beige/brown plaques, 3–20mm in diameter, with a velvety or warty surface.
- Nevus: moles.
- Blue nevus: small, slightly elevated, blue-black lesions.
- Atypical (dysplastic) nevus: over 5mm across, ill-defined, irregular border, irregularly distributed pigmentation with erythema and accentuated skin markings.
- Melanoma: flat or raised pigmented lesion with possibly a recent change in appearance. It has varying colors and typically irregular borders.

## Scaly lesions

- Psoriasis: silvery, scaled, well-demarcated plaques on skin, usually over the extensor surfaces. It can be pustular and involve the nails (nail pitting).
- Dermatitis and eczema: a pruritic, exudative, or lichenified eruption on the face, neck, upper trunk, wrists, and hands, and in the antecubital and popliteal fossae.
- Xerosis: dry skin.
- Lichen simplex chronicus: chronic itching associated with pigmented, lichenified, skin lesions. Lichenified lesions exhibit exaggerated skin lines overlying thickened, well-circumscribed, scaly plaques.
- Tinea corporis: ring-shaped lesion with an advancing scaly border and central clearing or scaly patches with a distinct border.
- Tinea versicolor: pale or hyperpigmented macules, or velvety, tan, pink, whitish, or brown macules that scale with scraping.

- Secondary syphilis.
- Pityriasis rosea: oval, fawn-colored, scaly eruption following the cleavage lines of the trunk ("Christmas tree" pattern). It is commonly preceded by a herald patch.
- Discoid lupus erythematosus: red, asymptomatic, localized plaques, usually on the face and often in a "butterfly" distribution. There is scaling, follicular plugging, atrophy, and telangiectasia of involved areas.
- Exfoliative dermatitis: scaling and erythema over a large area of the body.
- Actinic keratoses: small, pink patches that feel like bits off sandpaper when the finger is drawn over them. They are premalignant.
- Bowen's disease (intraepidermal squamous cell carcinoma): small, well-demarcated, slightly raised, pink-to-red, scaly plaques.
- Extramammary Paget's disease: this resembles chronic eczema and may involve apocrine areas such as the genitals.
- Intertrigo: fissuring, erythema, and sodden epidermis, with superficial denudation in the body folds.

## Vesicular lesions

- Herpes simplex: recurrent, small, grouped vesicles on an erythematous base, especially around the oral and genital areas; often described as "dew drops on a rose petal."
- Herpes zoster: vesicular lesions in a dermatomal distribution.
- Pompholyx: pruritic "tapioca" vesicles or bullae on the palms, soles, and sides of fingers.
- Dermatophytid (allergy or sensitivity to fungi): pruritic, grouped, vesicular lesions involving the sides and flexor aspects of the fingers and palms.
- Dermatitis herpetiformis: pruritic papulovesicular lesions, mainly on the elbows, knees, buttocks,

posterior neck, and scalp. It is associated with gluten-sensitive (i.e., sprue) enteropathy.
- Miliaria (heat rash): superficial, aggregated, small vesicles, papules, or pustules on covered areas of the skin.
- Scabies: pruritic vesicles and pustules especially on the sides of the fingers. Red papules or nodules on the penile glans and shaft are pathognomonic.
- Photosensitivity.

## Weepy or encrusted lesions
- Impetigo: vesiculopustular lesions with thick, golden-crusted exudate associated with group A β-hemolytic streptococci or coagulase-positive *Staphylococcus aureus*, or bullous lesions associated with *S. aureus*.
- Acute-contact allergic dermatitis: erythema and oedema, with pruritus, often followed by vesicles and bullae in an area of contact with a suspected agent. They may later weep, crust, and become infected.
- Any vesicular dermatitis.

## Pustular lesions
Any type of superficial skin infection (bacterial or fungal) can cause pustules.
- Acne vulgaris: the most common skin condition, characterized by open and closed comedones. It varies from purely comedonal to pustular inflammatory acne to cysts to nodules.
- Acne rosacea: erythema and telangiectasia and a tendency to flush easily. May have an acneiform component, or hyperplasia of the soft tissue of the nose (rhinophyma).
- Folliculitis: pustules in the hair follicles.
- Candidiasis: superficial, denuded, beefy-red areas with or without satellite vesicopustules. Whitish, curd-like concretions on the oral and vaginal mucous membranes.
- Miliaria.
- Any vesicular dermatitis.

## Figurate erythema
Figurate erythema lesions look like rings or arcs.
- Urticaria: eruptions of evanescent wheals or hives.
- Erythema multiforme: symmetrical erythematous lesions on the extensor surfaces, palms, soles, or mucous membranes, which may be macular, papular, urticarial, bullous, or purpuric. Target lesions with clear centers and concentric

erythematous rings may be present. This is often associated with drug rashes.
- Erythema migrans: a red expansion around an initial papule with an advancing border, which is usually raised, warm, and red. The center may clear or become indurated, vesicular, or necrotic. This is commonly associated with Lyme disease.
- Cellulitis: a hot, red, diffuse, spreading infection of the skin.
- Erysipelas: edematous, spreading, circumscribed, hot, erythematous area, with or without vesicle or bulla formation, frequently involving the face.
- Erysipeloid: purplish erythema, most often of a finger or the back of the hand, which gradually extends. Caused by *Erysipelothrix insidiosa*, it is often seen in fishermen and meat handlers.

## Bullous lesions
- Impetigo: superficial bacterial infection caused by group A β-hemolytic streptococci or *S. aureus*.
- Pemphigus: relapsing crops of bullae appearing on normal skin, often preceded by mucous membrane bullae, erosions, and ulcerations. There may be superficial detachment of the skin after pressure or trauma (Nikolsky's sign).
- Bullous pemphigoid: tense blisters in flexural areas. They may be preceded by urticarial or edematous lesions.
- Porphyria cutanea tarda.
- Erythema multiforme: "target" lesions, i.e., symmetrically distributed, circular lesions, often with a central blister.
- Toxic epidermal necrolysis: usually secondary to drugs (e.g., sulphonamides, penicillins, and anticonvulsants). This is a severe form of Steven-Johnson syndrome.

## Papular lesions
- Hyperkeratotic: warts, corns, seborrheic keratoses.
- Purple: lichen planus—pruritic, violaceous, flat-topped papules with fine white streaks and a symmetrical distribution, commonly seen along linear scratch marks on the anterior wrists, sacral region, penis, legs, and mucous membranes; drug eruptions; Kaposi's sarcoma—malignant skin lesions with dark plaques or nodules on cutaneous or mucosal surfaces, common in people with human immunodeficiency virus infection.
- Flesh-colored and umbilicated: molluscum contagiosum—a viral infection causing single or

multiple, rounded, dome-shaped, waxy papules, 2–5mm in diameter, which are umbilicated and contain a caseous plug.
- Pearly: basal cell carcinoma—most commonly papules or nodules with a central scab or erosion; intradermal nevi.
- Small, red, and inflammatory: acne, miliaria, candidiasis, intertrigo, scabies, folliculitis.

## Nodular, cystic lesions
- Erythema nodosum: painful red nodules without ulceration on the anterior aspects of the legs; they may regress over weeks to resemble contusions. This is associated with inflammatory bowel disease.
- Furuncle (boils): painful inflammatory swellings of a hair follicle forming an abscess, caused by *S. aureus*.
- Cystic acne.
- Follicular (epidermal) inclusion cyst.

## Photodermatoses
Painful erythema, edema, and vesiculation on sun-exposed surfaces, usually the face, neck, hands, and V of the chest. Causes include drugs (e.g., amiodarone, phenothiazines, sulphonamides, and related drugs), polymorphic light eruption, and systemic lupus erythematosus (SLE).

## Maculopapular lesions
Viral causes and secondary syphilis.

## Erosive lesions
- Any vesicular dermatitis.
- Impetigo.
- Lichen planus.
- Erythema multiforme.
- Oral erosions.
- Psychiatric disorders.

## Ulcerated lesions
- Decubiti: bed sores or pressure sores.
- Herpes simplex.
- Skin cancers.
- Parasitic infections.
- Syphilis: chancre.
- Vasculitis.
- Stasis.
- Arterial disease.

## History in the patient with skin rashes

The following long list of factors should be assessed when taking a history in the patient with skin rashes:
- Rash: onset, duration.
- Aggravating factors: physical or chemical agents; cold (cold urticaria or cryoglobulinemia); heat (worsens seborrheic conditions and superficial skin conditions).
- Precipitants: stress may lead to alopecia or eczema.
- Site of origin: contact dermatitis and pityriasis rosea (herald patch).
- Rate of progression.
- Timing of change in skin lesions, particularly for moles.
- Character: any alteration or progression in lesions.
- Hair and nails.
- Family history: eczema, psoriasis, inherited skin disorders.
- Infective agents: foreign travel (tropical infections), pets (papular urticaria or animal scabies).
- Farm animals: orf (poxvirus), ringworm.
- Occupation.
- Chemical exposure: at home or work, acting as antigens or direct irritants.
- Drugs taken: over-the-counter drugs, steroids may make the rash better (as in dermatitis) or worse (as in acne). How are the drugs being used?
- Foods: nuts and shellfish.
- Laundry detergent or soap.
- Contacts: family and friends.
- Light exposure: herpes simplex, SLE, and vitiligo.
- Hobbies: sportsmen are more prone to viral or fungal infections.
- General state of health and past medical history.
- Patient's explanation for rash.

Systemic symptoms should be assessed and may take the following forms:
- Arthralgias, fever, malaise, fatigue, and weight loss should be considered danger signs and not taken lightly.
- Itching (Fig. 17.1): atopy or urticaria (e.g., scabies, which is worse in bed), eczema, dermatitis herpetiformis, lichen planus, flexural psoriasis.
- Pain: inflammatory conditions, skin tumors.

| Possible causes of generalized and localized itching | |
| --- | --- |
| **Generalized itching** | **Localized itching** |
| • uremia<br>• cholestasis<br>• iron-deficiency anemia<br>• lymphoma<br>• hypo- and hyperthyroidism<br>• pregnancy<br>• carcinoma<br>• multiple sclerosis<br>• syphilis<br>• intestinal parasites<br>• morphine ingestion<br>• allergies, e.g. atopic eczema<br>• diabetes mellitus | • scabies and other mite infestations<br>• contact eczema<br>• dermatitis herpetiformis (associated with celiac disease)<br>• urticaria "nettle rash"<br>• lichen planus<br>• prickly heat<br>• winter itch<br>• aquagenic pruritus<br>• old age |

**Fig. 17.1** Possible causes of generalized and localized itching.

Finally, the mode of spread is significant and may take the form of an annular appearance (e.g., erythema annulare, erythema multiforme, and fungal infections) or irregular spread (e.g., pyoderma gangrenosum or malignancy).

 Drug eruptions may mimic any inflammatory skin condition. They usually start abruptly and are a widespread, symmetrical, erythematous eruption. Constitutional symptoms such as malaise, arthralgia, headache, and fever may be present.

## Examining the patient with skin rashes

Always examine the entire skin and look in the mouth (e.g., with lichen planus, herpes simplex and zoster, and infective exanthemata). Rashes may change with time and become characteristic or diagnostic of common dermatoses, such as the infectious exanthemata. Look at the distribution of lesions:

• If widespread and symmetrical, suspect systemic disease.
• If only areas exposed to the sun are involved, suspect light sensitivity.

• Patterns involving a dermatome distribution suggest herpes zoster.
• Dermatitis involving the hands, face, axillae, ears, and eyelids suggests contact dermatitis.
• Dermatitis involving the axillae, groin, scalp, central chest and back, eyebrows, ears, and beard suggests seborrheic dermatitis.
• Dermatitis involving the popliteal and cubital fossae and the face suggests atopic dermatitis.

In the patient presenting with subcutaneous nodules, think of the following:
  • Rheumatoid nodules.
  • Rheumatic fever.
  • Polyarteritis.
  • Xanthelasmata.
  • Tuberous sclerosis.
  • Neurofibromatosis.
  • Sarcoidosis.
  • Granuloma annulare.

Describe the lesion:
• Bizarrely shaped lesions suggest that the cause is an external agent (e.g., caustic liquid, self-induced injury).
• Fungal infections are characterized by slow growth, a smooth outline, an active edge with a healing center, and asymmetry.

Terms and characteristics of dermatologic lesions are given in Fig. 17.2.

For many skin lesions, multiple diagnoses may be possible. Often these diagnoses do not pose long-term complications, and topical steroids will be the treatment for both. Giving a trial of topical steroids with close follow-up is sometimes the best course of action.

## Investigating the patient with skin rashes

The history and examination may be enough to determine the diagnosis. If the patient is not unwell, it may be possible to examine for skin changes over time to allow for the development of possible characteristic lesions. The following investigations should be performed:

- Blood tests: complete blood count, urea and electrolytes, bacterial and viral titers with immunologic tests for tropical diseases if appropriate, and blood cultures.
- Skin scrapings and nail clippings: fungi.

| Terms and characteristics of dermatological lesions | |
|---|---|
| **Term** | **Characteristics** |
| alopecia | hair loss |
| atrophy | loss of skin thickness |
| blister or bulla | vesicle >1 cm diameter |
| cyst | epithelium-lined cavity containing fluid or semi-solid material |
| erythema | area of reddened skin which blanches with pressure |
| fissure | crack in epidermis |
| indurated | hard and thickened |
| Köebner's phenomenon | skin lesions at sites of external injury |
| lichenification | thickened skin with exaggerated skin markings |
| macule | circumscribed change in the skin color up to 1 cm diameter |
| nodule | solid skin lesion up to 1 cm diameter |
| papule | raised palpable spot up to 1 cm diameter |
| patch | macule >1 cm across |
| plaque | coalesced papules |
| purpura | area of reddened skin caused by hemorrhages which does not blanch with pressure |
| pustule | circumscribed, pus-filled lesion |
| scale | flake of hard skin |
| scar | connective tissue replacement following loss of dermal tissue |
| ulcer | irregularly shaped break in surface continuity of epithelium |
| vesicle | fluid-filled lesion <1 cm diameter |
| wheal | raised, palpable lesion with paler centers |

**Fig. 17.2** Terms and characteristics of dermatologic lesions.

- Examination of the skin under Wood's light.
- Examination of brushings of household pets: mites.
- Culture of fluid-containing lesions.
- Skin biopsy.
- Biopsy of lesions in lymph nodes or other organs.
- Investigations for associated systemic diseases or malignancy.

Drug eruptions may mimic any inflammatory skin condition. They usually start abruptly and are a widespread, symmetrical, erythematous eruption. Constitutional symptoms such as malaise, arthralgia, headache, and fever may be present.

# 18. Loss of Consciousness

Loss of consciousness may be transient (syncope) or ongoing (coma). Many patients are admitted to hospital with "collapse." Patients use the word "collapse" to describe a variety of situations, and it is essential to determine whether or not the patient has actually lost consciousness.

## Differential diagnosis of loss of consciousness

### Syncope ("blackout")
Syncope is caused by a transient loss of consciousness and motor tone due to a reduction in cerebral perfusion. There is spontaneous recovery, and it is often recurrent. Causes and forms of syncope include:
- Vasovagal attack: simple faint.
- Postural hypotension (orthostatic hypotension): may be caused by drugs, alcohol, aging, or hypovolemia.
- Vertebrobasilar insufficiency.
- Cardiac: Stokes-Adams attacks, arrhythmias, hypertrophy obstructive cardiomyopathy (HOCM), aortic stenosis.
- Transient ischemic attacks: posterior cerebral circulation.
- Micturition syncope.
- Cough syncope.
- Carotid sinus syncope: increased carotid sinus sensitivity in the elderly due to atherosclerosis.

### Coma
In coma, the patient remains unconscious and is unarousable. Coma can be caused by the following:
- Vascular: intracranial hemorrhage, cerebral infarction.
- Epilepsy: status epilepticus.
- Shock: anaphylaxis, sepsis, acute blood or fluid loss, cardiogenic, addisonian.
- Drugs overdose: narcotics, barbiturates, benzodiazepines.
- Alcohol: acute intoxication.
- Metabolic: hypoglycemia, hepatic encephalopathy, uremia, porphyria.
- Trauma, particularly closed head injury.
- Infection: meningitis, encephalitis, malaria.
- Respiratory: hypercapnia.
- Electrolyte: hyponatremia, hyper- or hypocalcemia.
- Endocrine: hypopituitarism, hypothyroidism.

## History in the patient with loss of consciousness

When a patient presents in coma, relatives or the PCP should be contacted to gain information regarding previous medical history, prodromal illness, known alcohol or drug abuse, and whether the events leading to the coma were witnessed by anyone.

In syncope, the history should focus on the following details.

### Presyncope
- What was the patient doing at the time?
- Were there any symptoms before the patient lost consciousness?
- In postural hypotension the patient may have stood up suddenly.
- If the patient had just turned his or her head, consider vertebrobasilar insufficiency.
- Prior to an epileptic fit, there is often an aura.
- In arrhythmia, the patient can be aware of palpitations, chest pain, or dyspnea before blacking out.
- In Stokes–Adams attacks there is usually no warning.
- Exertional syncope is seen in aortic stenosis and HOCM.
- Occasionally, cough or micturition may cause syncope.

### The attack itself
- What happened during the episode itself? This is where the history of a witness is vitally important.

- Seizures associated with tongue biting and urinary incontinence indicate epilepsy. (Note that if a patient remains propped upright in other forms of syncope, a secondary seizure may occur).
- In Stokes-Adams attacks the patient is typically seen to go deathly pale with flushing on recovery. The length of time that the patient remained unconscious should be recorded. Note, however, that patients may begin to twitch or have some seizure-like activity during a Stokes-Adams attack secondary to cerebral anorexia. Look for a history of seizures vs. a history of MI, CHF, etc., to help differentiate between these two causes of syncope.

### Postsyncope
- How quickly did the patient recover?
- Was there any injury? Syncope is generally followed by rapid recovery. However, in epilepsy, there is usually postictal sleepiness.
- It is also very important to ask whether patients hurt themselves during the episode. If there is significant injury consider cardiac syncope (lack of warning).

### Risk factors
- Is there a previous history of epilepsy, cardiac disease, cerebrovascular disease, or obstructive airways disease?
- Is the patient a diabetic on insulin?
- Is the patient a health-care worker with access to insulin?
- Is there a history of drug abuse or depression?
- Has there been recent travel to a malarial area?
- Has there been any trauma to the head?

Always try to obtain a history from a witness, even if the patient has regained consciousness.

## Examining the patient with loss of consciousness

The examination should be in three parts, in the order given below:

- How ill is the patient?
- Is there any evidence of the underlying cause?
- Has the patient been injured as a consequence?

Fig. 18.1 summarizes the examination approach.

## How ill is the patient?

In an unconscious patient, the first priority is to establish that there is a patent **airway** and effective **breathing** and **circulation** (**ABC**). A rapid assessment of the Glasgow coma scale should then be made as shown in Fig. 18.2.

Is the patient shocked? Check the blood pressure and pulse.

## Are there any clues as to the underlying cause?

The following signs may indicate the underlying cause:

- Tongue injury or incontinence (urinary or fecal): epilepsy.
- Drop in blood pressure on standing: postural hypotension.
- Dizziness on looking upward: vertebrobasilar insufficiency.
- Rapid or irregular pulse or murmur: cardiac cause.
- Evidence of head injury skull fracture, hematoma, blood or cerebrospinal fluid in ears.
- Needle marks or pinpoint pupils: narcotic overdose.
- Smell of alcohol.
- Meningism: meningitis, subarachnoid hemorrhage.
- Focal neurology: intracranial cause such as hemorrhage or infarction.
- Jaundice: hepatic encephalopathy.
- Trousseau's and Chvostek's signs: hypocalcemia.
- Papilledema, bounding pulse, asterixis and warm peripheries: hypercapnia.
- Tampons in vagina: toxic shock syndrome.
- Carotid bruits: these are found in atherosclerosis and suggest a possible source of emboli in transient ischemic attacks or stroke.

A blood sugar test should be performed urgently in all unconscious patients to exclude hypoglycemia.

**Fig. 18.1** Examining the patient with loss of consciousness. (ABC, airway, breathing, circulation.)

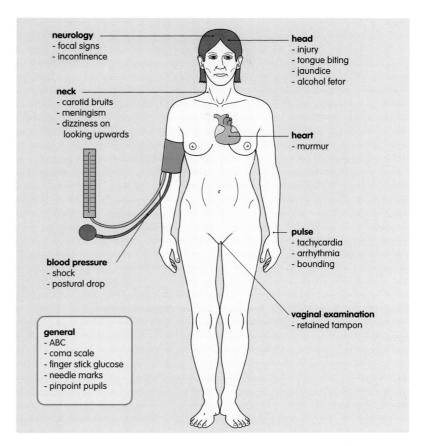

neurology
- focal signs
- incontinence

neck
- carotid bruits
- meningism
- dizziness on looking upwards

blood pressure
- shock
- postural drop

general
- ABC
- coma scale
- finger stick glucose
- needle marks
- pinpoint pupils

head
- injury
- tongue biting
- jaundice
- alcohol fetor

heart
- murmur

pulse
- tachycardia
- arrhythmia
- bounding

vaginal examination
- retained tampon

| The Glasgow coma scale | | |
|---|---|---|
| Category | Response | Score |
| best verbal response | orientated | 5 |
| | confused conversation | 4 |
| | inappropriate speech | 3 |
| | incomprehensible words | 2 |
| | no speech | 1 |
| best motor response | obey commands | 6 |
| | localizes to pain | 5 |
| | withdraws to pain | 4 |
| | flexor posturing | 3 |
| | extensor posturing | 2 |
| | no response | 1 |
| eye opening | spontaneous | 4 |
| | to speech | 3 |
| | to pain | 2 |
| | no eye opening | 1 |

**Fig. 18.2** The Glasgow coma scale, used for assessing loss of consciousness in a patient.

## Has the patient been injured?

If conscious, the patient will be able to describe any injury resulting from the episode. If not, look for bruising or deformities due to fractures. In particular, look for evidence of head injury.

## Investigating the patient with loss of consciousness

Investigation will be guided by findings in the history and clinical examination. The following tests are useful in the different clinical scenarios (Figs 18.3 and 18.4):

- Complete blood count: anemia in severe hemorrhage or hemolysis (malaria); leukocytosis in sepsis.
- Metabolic panel: hypo- or hypernatremia.
- Calcium: hypocalcemia.
- Glucose: hypoglycemia.

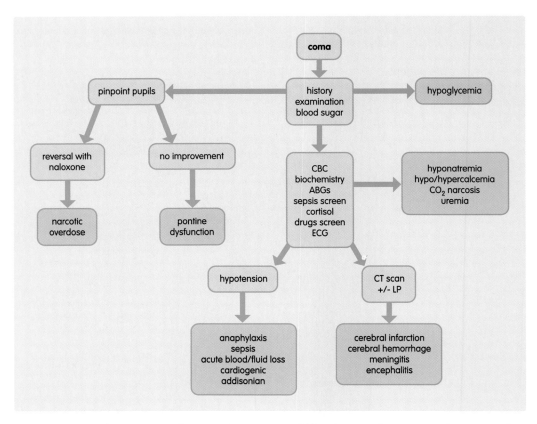

**Fig. 18.3** Diagnosis in the patient with coma. (ABGs, arterial blood gases; CT, computed tomography; ECG, electrocardiogram; CBC, complete blood count; LP, lumbar puncture.)

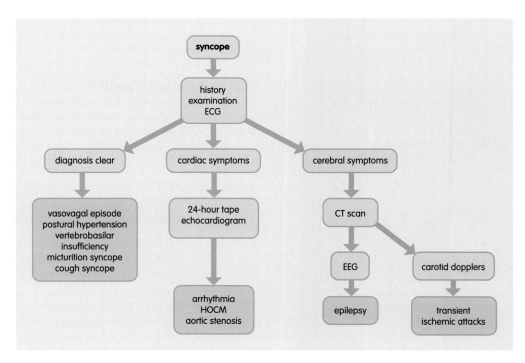

**Fig. 18.4** Diagnosis in the patient with syncope. (CT, computed tomography; ECG, electrocardiogram; EEG, electroencephalogram; HOCM, hypertrophic obstructive cardiomyopathy.)

- Liver function tests: liver failure.
- Thyroid function tests: hypothyroidism.
- Electrocardiogram: arrhythmia, left ventricular hypertrophy in aortic stenosis and HOCM, prolonged QT interval, bundle-branch block/heart block, sinus bradycardia.
- Arterial blood gases: hypercapnia.
- Chest x-ray: pulmonary disease, aspiration pneumonia.
- Drugs screen: urine and blood.
- Tilt table test: helps to determine vasovagal causes of syncope.
- Electroencephalogram: epilepsy (including subclinical status epilepticus), herpes simplex encephalitis.

- Computed tomography head scan: intracranial pathology.
- Carotid Dopplers: carotid atheroma.
- 24-hour/48-hour ambulatory monitoring or Holter monitor 24-hour tape: arrhythmia.
- ECG/echocardiogram: source of emboli, aortic stenosis, HOCM.
- Lumbar puncture: meningitis, subarachnoid hemorrhage.
- Septic screen, including blood cultures and mid-stream urine.

# 19. Confusional States

Confusion can be acute or subacute (delirium) or chronic and progressive (dementia). Confusion is very common, particularly in the elderly, and is often exacerbated by admission to hospital.

> When a patient presents with confusion, try to establish whether it is a longstanding problem which is getting worse or whether it has arisen "out of the blue" by talking to the family or caregivers.

## Differential diagnosis of confusion

### Delirium

Delirium is defined as the acute, decreased ability to maintain or hold concentration/attention with accompanying alterations of perception and mood. It may be caused by the following:

- Infection (almost any!): urinary tract infection, pneumonia, malaria, encephalitis, meningitis.
- Drug intoxication: opiates, anxiolytics, steroids, tricyclics, anticonvulsants, cannabis; in the elderly, anticholinergics can lead to mental status changes.
- Drug withdrawal: benzodiazepines, alcohol.
- Metabolic: liver, kidney, respiratory or cardiac failure, hyper- or hyponatremia, hypoglycemia, hypercalcemia.
- Vitamin deficiency: Wernicke–Korsakoff syndrome (thiamine deficiency).
- Cerebral pathology: abscess, tumor, hemorrhage, infarction, trauma (subdural hematoma).

### Dementia

Among the following, Alzheimer's disease and multi-infarct dementia are the most common causes of dementia:

- Degenerative diseases: Alzheimer's disease, Pick's disease, Huntington's chorea, Creutzfeldt–Jakob disease (CJD), Parkinson's disease, multisystem atrophy.
- Vascular disease: multi-infarct dementia, vasculitis, subdural hematoma.
- Tumor: particularly frontal lobe; can be primary or secondary tumors, or due to paraneoplastic phenomenon.
- Demyelination: multiple sclerosis (MS).
- Infection: human immunodeficiency virus (HIV), syphilis, subacute sclerosing panencephalitis, tuberculosis, meningitis.
- Endocrine: hypothyroidism.
- Vitamin deficiency: vitamin $B_{12}$, folate, thiamine, niacin (pellagra).
- Drugs: sedatives.
- Metabolic: uremia, hepatic failure, or Wilson's disease, following prolonged hypoglycemia or hypoxia.
- Toxic: alcohol, lead, carbon monoxide.
- Normal pressure hydrocephalus.
- Remember that depression can mimic dementia.

> It is important to remember that deaf people are not necessarily confused and that depression can sometimes mimic dementia ("pseudodementia").

## History in the confused patient

The first step is to establish whether the patient has delirium or dementia. A good account from relatives, caregivers, or close friends is almost always the only way of getting a true picture of the pattern of disease. The history should then focus on possible underlying causes.

### Pattern of confusion

Delirium develops over hours or days. It is characterized by clouding of consciousness, which fluctuates in severity, being worse at night with lucid periods in the day. It can be accompanied by poor recent memory, disorientation, and hallucinations. As a result, the patient may be agitated, uncooperative, and sometimes paranoid.

 If delirium develops at around 2 days following hospital admission, consider delirium tremens due to alcohol withdrawal.

Dementia usually has a gradual onset over months or years. It is characterized by a global deterioration in higher cerebral functions, tends to be progressive, and is often exacerbated when the patient is removed from familiar surroundings, such as by admission to hospital. Multi-infarct dementia characteristically progresses in a stepwise fashion.

A more rapid onset is seen in CJD (which presents with dementia, ataxia, and myoclonus) and hydrocephalus. Here, the patient gradually loses memory and intellect and has increasing difficulty in performing even simple tasks around the house. Change in personality may be a prominent feature. Unlike delirium, there is never a change in consciousness level.

## Possible underlying causes

The following should be assessed, as they may reveal an underlying cause:

- Age: dementia becomes increasingly common after the age of 60 years. In younger patients, a thorough search for a treatable underlying cause should be made.
- Symptoms of focal infection (Chapter 6).
- Symptoms of raised intracranial pressure (Chapter 15).
- Risk factors for, or known, vascular disease (Chapter 22).
- Dietary history: vitamin deficiency.
- Alcohol history: while chronic alcohol abuse can cause dementia in its own right, it may also be associated with folate and thiamine deficiency.
- Previous head injury: subdural hematoma.
- Drug history: particular attention should be given to sedatives, anticonvulsants, and steroids.
- Other neurologic symptoms: cerebrovascular disease, MS, cerebral tumor or abscess.

- Previous medical history of any disease may be relevant: longstanding renal disease (uremia), malignancy (cerebral metastases, hypercalcemia, or paraneoplastic syndrome) or diabetes (insulin overdose).
- Family history: Wilson's disease (autosomal recessive); Huntington's chorea (autosomal dominant).

## Examining the confused patient

Since the causes of confusion are so varied, a thorough clinical examination is mandatory. This approach is summarized in Fig. 19.1. Particular attention should be given to the following:

- Consciousness: the level of consciousness should be recorded using the Glasgow coma scale (see Fig. 18.2).
- Mental state: repeated assessments using the same test are useful in determining objectively whether

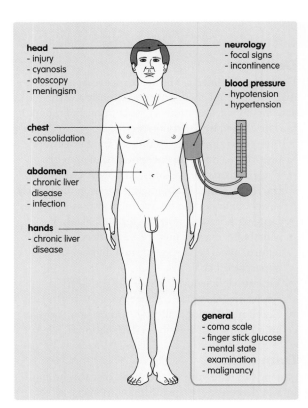

**Fig. 19.1** Examining the confused patient. (BG, stick examination for blood sugar.)

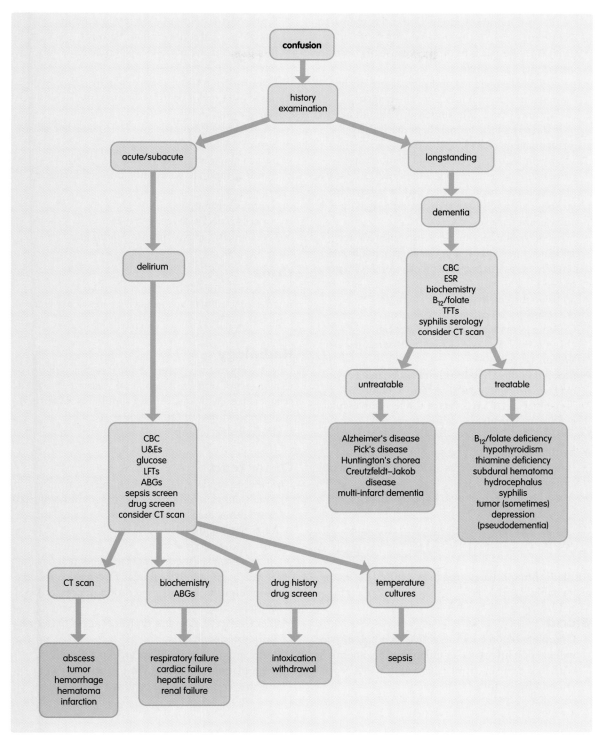

**Fig. 19.2** Algorithm for diagnosing the confused patient. (ABGs, arterial blood gases; CT, computed tomography; ESR, erythrocyte sedimentation rate; CBC, complete blood count; LFTs, liver function tests; TFTs, thyroid function tests; U&Es, urea and electrolytes.)

there is deterioration and its rate and response to treatment.
- Cyanosis: hypoxia is a common cause of confusion in patients in hospital.
- Focal neurologic deficit and the pattern of signs may give important clues as to the diagnosis (Chapters 20 and 22): fundoscopy should be performed looking for papilledema (raised intracranial pressure), optic atrophy (demyelination), or subhyaloid hemorrhages (subarachnoid hemorrhage). Parkinsonism may be present in Parkinson's disease and multisystem atrophy. Myoclonus, extrapyramidal signs, and aphasia are features of CJD.
- Signs of focal infection: look carefully for neck stiffness, consolidation in the chest, abdominal tenderness or otitis media on otoscopy (Chapter 6).
- Signs of chronic liver disease: hepatic encephalopathy can cause confusion. Chronic liver disease may also indicate chronic alcohol abuse or rare disorders such as Wilson's disease.
- Blood pressure: hypotension may be due to overwhelming infection or cardiac failure. Hypertension is a risk factor for cerebrovascular events and can also be caused by raised intracranial pressure.
- Evidence of head injury: subdural hematoma.
- Primary malignancy: this includes breast cancer and melanoma.
- Blood glucose fingerstick: hypoglycemia.

## Investigating the confused patient

An algorithm for diagnosing the confused patient is given in Fig. 19.2.

### Blood
- Complete blood count: reactive blood picture in malignancy, infection, or inflammation; anemia with raised mean corpuscular volume (MCV) in vitamin $B_{12}$ or folate deficiency.

- Erythrocyte sedimentation rate: raised in malignancy, infection, inflammation.
- Metabolic panel: hypo- or hypernatremia and renal failure.
- Liver function tests: abnormal in liver disease, raised γ-glutamyl transferase in excess alcohol consumption.
- Thyroid function tests: low $T_4$ in hypothyroidism.
- Serum calcium: hypocalcemia.
- Serum glucose: hypoglycemia.
- Serum vitamin $B_{12}$ and red blood cell folate: deficiency.
- Syphilis serology.
- Arterial blood gases for hypoxia.
- Drug levels: digoxin, lithium, quinidine.

### Urine
Midstream urine should be obtained for microscopy, culture and sensitivity in urinary tract infection.

### Radiology
Chest x-ray may show pneumonia, cardiac failure, or malignancy. Computed tomography scan or magnetic resonance imaging of the head should be performed to diagnose tumor, infarction, hematoma, hydrocephalus, and abscess.

### Other tests
Consider the following when clinically indicated:
- Thick and thin films: malaria (if patient has visited an endemic area).
- Viral titers and HIV serology.
- Urine: toxicology screen.
- Red cell transketolase for thiamine deficiency.
- Serum copper and ceruloplasmin (reduced) and 24-hour urinary copper excretion (increased): Wilson's disease.
- Electroencephalogram: typical changes of herpes simplex encephalitis.
- Lumbar puncture and cerebrospinal fluid examination: protein, glucose, microscopy, culture, and oligoclonal bands.

# 20. Acute Neurologic Deficit

Focal neurologic deficits are a common cause of presentation to the emergency department. Kit is important to rule out life-threatening causes first; then it is important to maintain supportive care and to expand the differential diagnosis based on the causes. A stroke is a neurologic deficit due to vascular disturbance which develops over minutes (sometimes hours) and persists for at least 24 hours. Identical deficits lasting less than 24 hours are termed transient ischemic attacks (TIAs). Cerebral infarction (embolism or thrombosis) accounts for 80% of strokes; 20% of strokes are caused by intracerebral hemorrhage. Fig. 20.1 outlines the principal types of stroke.

## Differential diagnosis of stroke

The diagnosis is often clear from the history and examination, but the following pathologies can also produce a clinical picture that is identical to stroke and should be considered in atypical presentations:

- Subdural hematoma: elderly, alcoholics.
- Cerebral abscess: consider if patient has bronchiectasis or murmur (infective endocarditis).
- Epilepsy: Todd's paralysis following Jacksonian seizure.
- Hemiplegic migraine: typical features of migraine also present, resolving within 24 hours.
- Demyelination: rare.
- Drugs (e.g., overdose with tricyclic antidepressants: history of depression, younger patients).
- Hypoglycemia.

## History in the stroke patient

The history should focus on three distinct areas. Firstly, does the story fit with the diagnosis of stroke? Secondly, where is the anatomic site of the lesion. Finally, are any risk factors present?

## How has the deficit developed?

The key feature in stroke is that the symptoms develop rapidly over a few minutes or, less commonly, hours, but once the deficit is complete it remains stable and usually improves. Any neurologic deterioration due to vascular disease is in a stepwise fashion. If there is gradual deterioration, consider one of the above differential diagnoses or hydrocephalus secondary to the stroke (edema or blood preventing free drainage of cerebrospinal fluid (CSF)). Improvement can be complete, but there is often some residual deficit.

## Where is the lesion?

Any intracranial artery can be involved in stroke. The symptoms and signs will reflect which artery and therefore which part of the brain has been involved. This is summarized in Fig. 20.2. Remember that the anatomic location of the involved vasculature can help narrow the focus of your studies. For example, a stroke that localizes to the posterior circulation cannot have been caused by carotid artery atherosclerosis. In this case, carotid Doppler studies would not be a first step in elucidation of the stroke's cause.

## Are there any risk factors for stroke?

Fig. 20.3 shows the main risk factors for stroke, which are predominantly the same as for vascular disease elsewhere (Chapter 1).

### Past medical history

A history of TIAs strongly suggests stroke as a possible etiology. In addition, known vascular disease, including coronary artery disease, is a strong predictor of stroke. Patients should be asked about a history of arrhythmias, especially atrial fibrillation. Valvular heart disease (e.g., endocarditis) can increase a patient's risk of stroke as well. A history of hypertension, smoking, diabetes, or hyperlipidemia reveals strong risk factors for the development of vascular disease, including stroke. Drug history can be important, especially if the patient is on an

**Fig. 20.1** Causes of stroke. (PAN, polyarteritis nodosa; SLE, systemic lupus erythematosus.)

| Types of stroke | |
| --- | --- |
| **Cause** | **Aetiology** |
| hemorrhagic | hypertension<br>aneurysm (particularly Charcot-Bouchard microaneurysms; also berry and mycotic aneurysms)<br>arteriovenous malformation<br>tumors<br>bleeding tendency (thrombocytopenia, coagulation defects, anticoagulants)<br>drugs (amphetamines, Ecstasy) |
| infarction | hypertension<br>intracranial arterial atheroma<br>inflammatory vasculopathy (temporal arteritis, SLE, PAN, neurosyphilis)<br>prolonged hypotension (cardiac arrest)<br>prothrombotic hematological disorders (hyperviscosity, antiphospholipid syndrome)<br>drugs (amphetamines, Ecstasy)<br>embolism |
| sources of embolus | carotid or vertebral atheroma<br>cardiac:<br>• atrial fibrillation with left atrial thrombosis<br>• endocarditis<br>• ventricular thrombus due to myocardial infarction or ventricular aneurysm<br>• atrial myxoma<br>paradoxical:<br>• venous thrombus can reach the cerebral circulation via a patent foramen ovale or an atrial septal defect (rare) |

anticoagulation regimen. With warfarin therapy, the dosage may be subtherapeutic (resulting in emboli) or supratherapeutic (resulting in hemorrhage). The social history is important because cocaine can raise blood pressure and cause hemorrhage. A family history of atherosclerosis is also an independent risk factor.

In a pontine stroke, the eyes may be deviated towards the paralyzed side. In a hemispheric lesion, the eyes will deviate away from the paralyzed side.

## Examining the stroke patient

Clinical examination gives information regarding three important areas in the stroke patient. What are the neurologic abnormalities and do they fit with the diagnosis of stroke? Is there any evidence of an underlying cause? Have any complications arisen as a result of the stroke?

Fig. 20.4 summarizes this examination approach.

## Has the patient had a stroke?

A thorough neurologic examination should be performed, including a coma scale. Does the pattern of neurologic deficit fit with disruption of the cerebral vascular supply? (See Fig. 20.2).

Determining the likely site of the lesion helps to focus the search for an underlying cause (e.g., carotid bruits in an anterior or middle cerebral artery stroke).

## Is there any evidence of an underlying cause?

There are many causes and risk factors for stroke. However, pay particular attention to the following:
- Carotid bruits: carotid atheroma.
- Murmurs: endocarditis, valvular disease, atrial septal defect.

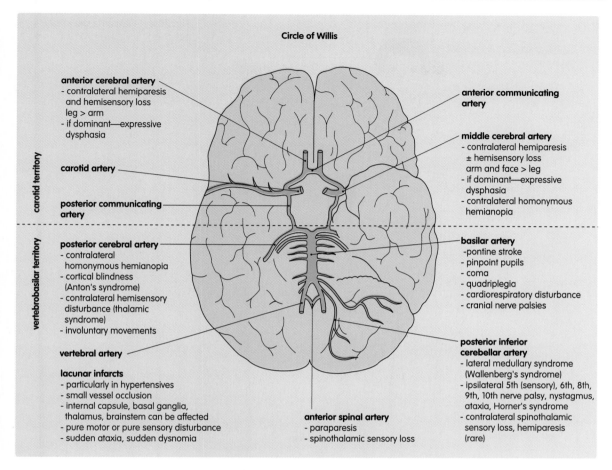

**Circle of Willis**

**anterior cerebral artery**
- contralateral hemiparesis and hemisensory loss leg > arm
- if dominant—expressive dysphasia

**carotid artery**

**posterior communicating artery**

carotid territory

**anterior communicating artery**

**middle cerebral artery**
- contralateral hemiparesis ± hemisensory loss arm and face > leg
- if dominant—expressive dysphasia
- contralateral homonymous hemianopia

**posterior cerebral artery**
- contralateral homonymous hemianopia
- cortical blindness (Anton's syndrome)
- contralateral hemisensory disturbance (thalamic syndrome)
- involuntary movements

vertebrobasilar territory

**vertebral artery**

**lacunar infarcts**
- particularly in hypertensives
- small vessel occlusion
- internal capsule, basal ganglia, thalamus, brainstem can be affected
- pure motor or pure sensory disturbance
- sudden ataxia, sudden dysnomia

**basilar artery**
- pontine stroke
- pinpoint pupils
- coma
- quadriplegia
- cardiorespiratory disturbance
- cranial nerve palsies

**posterior inferior cerebellar artery**
- lateral medullary syndrome (Wallenberg's syndrome)
- ipsilateral 5th (sensory), 6th, 8th, 9th, 10th nerve palsy, nystagmus, ataxia, Horner's syndrome
- contralateral spinothalamic sensory loss, hemiparesis (rare)

**anterior spinal artery**
- paraparesis
- spinothalamic sensory loss

**Fig. 20.2** Symptoms and signs associated with different strokes. Note that hemorrhagic strokes have symptoms and signs determined by the site of the bleed. Patients may also develop headache, loss of consciousness, and vomiting as a result of raised intracranial pressure.

| Risk factors for stoke |
| --- |
| • hypertension |
| • diabetes mellitus |
| • hypercholesterolemia |
| • obesity |
| • alcohol |
| • oral contraceptive pill |
| • established vascular disease (carotid bruit, peripheral vascular disease) |
| • previous stroke or transient ischemic attack |
| • smoking |

**Fig. 20.3** Risk factors for stroke.

- Pulse: atrial fibrillation.
- Blood pressure: hypertension can be the cause or result of stroke; prolonged hypotension can also cause stroke.
- Diminished peripheral pulses: peripheral vascular disease.
- Xanthelasmata, xanthomata: underlying hyperlipidemia.
- Temporal artery tenderness: giant cell arteritis.
- Nicotine-stained fingers from heavy smoking.

## Have any complications developed?

Complications are common following stroke and are related to the size of cerebral damage and the degree of neurological deficit. The more common problems

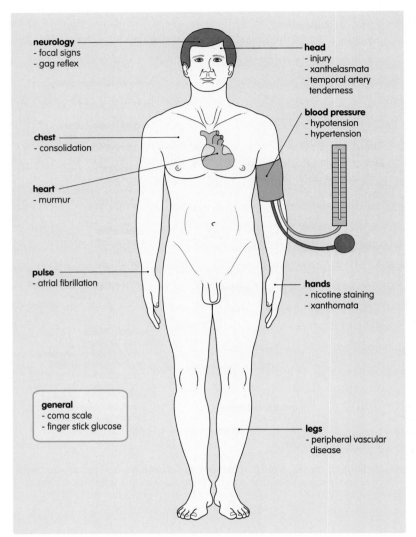

**Fig. 20.4** Examining the stroke patient.

**neurology**
- focal signs
- gag reflex

**head**
- injury
- xanthelasmata
- temporal artery tenderness

**blood pressure**
- hypotension
- hypertension

**chest**
- consolidation

**heart**
- murmur

**pulse**
- atrial fibrillation

**hands**
- nicotine staining
- xanthomata

**general**
- coma scale
- finger stick glucose

**legs**
- peripheral vascular disease

along with prophylactic measures to avoid them are outlined in Fig. 20.5.

## Investigating the stroke patient

The purpose of investigation in these patients is to exclude treatable pathologies and to guide management to prevent further strokes. In atypical presentations, investigation will clearly be important in making the correct diagnosis.

An algorithm for investigating the patient with stroke is given in Fig. 20.6.

The following tests should be performed for all patients:
- Complete blood count: polycythemia may cause a stroke; a reactive picture may indicate inflammation (e.g., temporal arteritis).
- Erythrocyte sedimentation rate: elevated in inflammation, infection, and malignancy.
- Metabolic panel: renal impairment may be due to, or the cause of, hypertension.
- Blood glucose: diabetes and severe hypoglycemia are both associated with stroke.
- Fasting lipids: hypercholesterolemia is an important, treatable, risk factor for stroke.

**Fig. 20.5** Complications of stroke and measures to prevent them.

| Complications of stroke and measures to prevent them | |
|---|---|
| **Complications** | **Prophylactic measures** |
| cerebral edema | particularly in hemorrhagic stroke and usually non-preventable (avoid overenthusiastic rehydration) |
| pressure sores | careful nursing with regular turning |
| pneumonia | patient should be kept nil by mouth until the gag reflex returns to prevent aspiration |
| contractures and spasticity | regular skilled physical therapy |
| malnutrition | feeding via nasogastric tube or, later, gastrostomy |
| depression | provision of adequate social and practical support |
| epilepsy | some institutions are beginning to give prophylactic antiseizure medication to patients who present with stokes involving the parietal lobe of the brain, as a stroke in this area may increase the risk of post-stroke seizure. Treatment may consist of a loading then maintenance dose of phenytoin (Dilantin). |

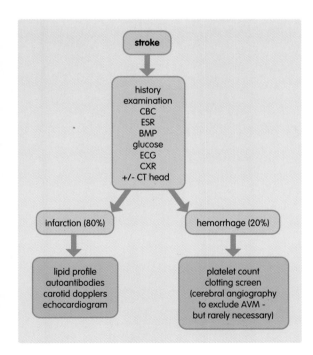

**Fig. 20.6** Algorithm for the investigation of the stroke patient. Note that performing a lumbar puncture in patients with hemorrhagic stroke can precipitate herniation. (AVM, arteriovenous malformation; CT, computed tomography; CXR, chest x-ray; ECG, electrocardiogram; ESR, erythrocyte sedimentation rate; CBC, complete blood count; Gluc, glucose; BMP, basic metabolic panel.)

- Coagulation panel: to exclude coagulopathy or assess degree of anticoagulation (if the patient is receiving warfarin or heparin).
- Electrocardiogram: atrial fibrillation, recent myocardial infarction, ventricular aneurysm.
- Chest x-ray: to exclude malignancy and aspiration.

The following further investigations should be performed where appropriate:
- Syphilis serology: neurosyphilis.
- Blood cultures: infective endocarditis.
- Computed tomography head scan: Note that CT head scan upon arrival at the emergency department is now the standard of care in a patient with neurologic signs. With the increased use of t-PA, it is an absolute necessity to differentiate between ischemic and hemorrhagic strokes before beginning therapy. CT also may be used when cerebellar hemorrhage may be a possibility (urgent surgery is required) and to exclude acute hydrocephalus in patients with continued deterioration.
- MRI is probably the best tool to look for acute ischemia.
- Carotid Dopplers: if bruits or recurrent carotid territory infarction.
- Carotid angiography: carotid territory infarction, in which endarterectomy or angioplasty would be considered.

- Echocardiogram: cardiac source of embolus.
- Autoantibodies: anticardiolipin antibodies (antiphospholipid syndrome) and anti-double-stranded DNA (cerebral lupus), particularly in younger patients.
- 24-hour electrocardiogram monitoring: paroxysmal atrial fibrillation.

## Treatment of acute stroke

Much research has been done over the last several decades surrounding the treatment of acute ischemic stroke. Treatment should first focus on ABCs. Patients with large strokes, increased ICP, or vertebrobasilar ischemia may need to be intubated secondary to respiratory depression or inadequacy.

Monitoring of blood pressure is also important. Since many patients who have strokes also suffer from hypertension, the question of when to treat an increased blood pressure has been researched. It is generally believed that it is best to hold all antihypertensive medications unless the systolic blood pressure is greater than 220mmHg. Any increase in ICP will decrease the MAP within the brain, making the organ dependent on a higher overall BP for perfusion.

Monitoring of ICP in cases of large strokes with much cerebral edema is also important. Measures used to decrease ICP included mechanical hyperventilation and 24 hours of mannitol infusion.

The "hottest" research topic in stroke is the use of thrombolytic therapy. As noted above, it is imperative that hemorrhagic stroke be ruled out prior to treatment. Currently t-PA is given within a 3-hour window (alteplase is the most studied thrombolytic agent). Ongoing research, including using both intravenous and intraarterial thrombolytics, is attempting to increase the temporal window that is available for use of these medications.

# 21. Lymphadenopathy and Splenomegaly

Splenomegaly is often a focus of short case examinations since many of its causes are chronic. Lymphadenopathy may be localized or generalized.

## Differential diagnosis of lymphadenopathy and splenomegaly

### Localized lymphadenopathy
Consider which structures have lymphatic drainage to the nodes affected and examine these carefully for the following:
- Local infection: bacterial (e.g., otitis media, tuberculosis) or viral.
- Metastases: local malignancy.
- Lymphoma: Hodgkin's disease or non-Hodgkin's lymphoma.

### Generalized lymphadenopathy
- Infection: particularly viral (Epstein–Barr virus [EBV], cytomegalovirus [CMV], human immunodeficiency virus [HIV], rubella), but also bacterial (tuberculosis [TB], syphilis, brucellosis) and protozoal (toxoplasmosis).
- Lymphoproliferative: Hodgkin's disease or non-Hodgkin's lymphoma, chronic lymphocytic leukemia, acute lymphoblastic leukemia.
- Connective tissue disorders: systemic lupus erythematosus, rheumatoid arthritis.
- Infiltration: sarcoidosis.
- Drugs: phenytoin ("pseudolymphoma").
- Endocrine: thyrotoxicosis (rare).

### Splenomegaly
In general, different diseases cause different degrees of splenomegaly, as follows.
  Massive splenomegaly is caused by:
- Chronic myeloid leukemia.
- Myelofibrosis.
- Malaria: rarely.
- Kala azar (leishmaniasis, caused by a parasite transmitted by the sand fly): rarely.

Moderate splenomegaly is caused by all of the above plus:
- Portal hypertension.
- Lymphoproliferative disorders (see above).
- Acute leukemias.

Just palpable splenomegaly is caused by all of the above plus:
- Infection: infectious mononucleosis, infectious hepatitis, subacute bacterial endocarditis, TB, brucellosis, schistosomiasis.
- Hemolytic anemias (Chapter 25).
- Immune thrombocytopenias.
- Connective tissue disease: SLE, rheumatoid arthritis.
- Infiltration: amyloid, sarcoid.
- Storage disorders: Gaucher's disease.
- Myeloproliferative disorders: polycythemia rubra vera, essential thrombocythemia.
- Megaloblastic anemias (Chapter 25).

## History in the patient with lymphadenopathy or splenomegaly

It is often not possible to make a diagnosis on the basis of the history in these patients. However, important clues in the history can help to focus the clinical examination and further investigations.

### Localized lymphadenopathy
#### Rate of node enlargement
Lymphadenopathy associated with infection often develops quickly and may be painful. When due to lymphoma or malignancy, the rate of enlargement tends to be slower and can wax and wane in the case of lymphoma.

  Sometimes the lymphadenopathy will not be noticed until it becomes large and causes disfigurement or rubs against clothes. Lymphadenopathy may also result in lymphedema. This is a nonpitting edema caused by blockage of the lymph channels. Lymphedema may be the presenting sign of lymphadenopathy as the increasing size of the lymph nodes cuts off flow of regional lymph channels.

## Symptoms in local structures

Has the patient noticed pain, erythema, or a mass in any of the structures draining into the affected node (e.g., cellulitis in inguinal lymphadenopathy or a breast mass in axillary lymphadenopathy)?

## Systemic symptoms

In lymphoma the patient may experience "B symptoms" (fever, night sweats, weight loss), which indicate a poorer prognosis.

## Generalized lymphadenopathy

A full systemic inquiry is essential in these patients as most of the causes of generalized lymphadenopathy can affect multiple systems. Special attention should be paid to the following:

- Malaise, anorexia and general debility: common but nonspecific.
- "B symptoms": hematologic malignancy.
- Ask about tender lymph nodes after consumption of alcohol (can be seen in Hodgkin's disease).
- Skin rash: rubella, SLE, and sarcoidosis.
- Arthragia and arthropathy: SLE, rheumatoid arthritis, syphilis (Charcot's joints).
- Infectious contacts: rubella, TB, and EBV.
- Risk factors for HIV infection (Chapter 38).
- Drug history: to exclude phenytoin or beryllium as a cause. Also ask about any history of IV drug use.
- Symptoms of thyrotoxicosis: heat intolerance, weight loss, increased appetite, diarrhea, irritability.

## Splenomegaly
### Previous medical history

Is the patient known to have a pre-existing illness that can cause splenomegaly, such as chronic liver disease resulting in portal hypertension, connective tissue disease, thalassemia (hemolysis), Gaucher's disease, or damaged cardiac valves (rheumatic fever or prosthetic valve) with subacute bacterial endocarditis?

### Recent travel abroad or infectious contacts

Consider infectious mononucleosis, TB, schistosomiasis, and malaria.

## Systemic symptoms

Systemic symptoms suggestive of an underlying cause include arthralgia, rash, and "B symptoms" (as above).

## Symptoms of hematologic disturbance

Anemia may be present due to marrow infiltration, chronic disease, hemolysis, vitamin deficiency, or hypersplenism (Chapter 25). Leukopenia causing recurrent infections may result from marrow infiltration, hypersplenism, or infection. Thrombocytopenia may be due to immune platelet destruction, marrow infiltration, or hypersplenism (Chapter 23).

## Examining the patient with lymphadenopathy and splenomegaly

When lymphadenopathy or splenomegaly is present, a full clinical examination of the lymphatic system should be made. The examination should then focus on possible underlying causes. Fig. 21.1 summarizes this examination approach.

## Which lymph nodes are affected? Is there splenomegaly?

Firstly, the extent, sites, sizes, consistency, tenderness, and fixation of enlarged lymph nodes should be documented. Normal reactive nodes are generally less than 1 cm in diameter, feel soft, are not fixed, and can be tender. Lymphomatous nodes are often larger and feel rubbery but are not fixed. Lymph nodes infiltrated by carcinoma feel hard and may be fixed to surrounding tissue. Cervical, occipital, supraclavicular, axillary, and inguinal areas should be palpated carefully.

If splenomegaly is present, the size (in cm) from the left costal margin must be recorded.

It is important to distinguish the left kidney from the spleen when palpating a mass in the left hypochondrium and the differences between the two are commonly asked for in examinations (Fig. 21.2).

## Is there evidence of an underlying cause?

Anemia and purpura may be present as described above. Jaundice may result from chronic liver disease, hemolysis, or infective hepatitis. Cachexia heralds underlying malignancy.

Fig. 21.3 summarizes clinical findings that may point to particular diagnoses. Evidence of chronic liver disease, rheumatoid arthritis, and SLE should also be looked for as described in Chapters 10 and 16. Needle marks may indicate previous exposure to HIV and hepatitis B or C or provide a source of bacteria in infective endocarditis.

### Localized lymphadenopathy

Examine those structures with lymphatic drainage to the affected nodes. Erythema, increased temperature, and tenderness suggest infection, while a hard, nontender mass may indicate malignancy. When there is isolated cervical lymphadenopathy, a formal ear, nose, and throat examination should also be performed since oropharyngeal malignancies commonly metastasize to these nodes.

### Splenomegaly and generalized lymphadenopathy

Where there is both splenomegaly and generalized lymphadenopathy consider lymphoproliferative disorders, infection, connective tissue disease, and sarcoidosis.

## Investigating the patient with lymphadenopathy and splenomegaly

An algorithm for diagnosis of the patient with lymphadenopathy and splenomegaly is given in Fig. 21.4.

### Hematology

- A complete blood count may show anemia, leucopenia, thrombocytopenia, or a combination of these.

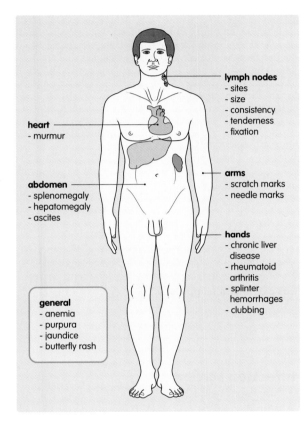

**Fig. 21.1** Examining the patient with lymphadenopathy and splenomegaly.

lymph nodes
- sites
- size
- consistency
- tenderness
- fixation

heart
- murmur

abdomen
- splenomegaly
- hepatomegaly
- ascites

arms
- scratch marks
- needle marks

hands
- chronic liver disease
- rheumatoid arthritis
- splinter hemorrhages
- clubbing

general
- anemia
- purpura
- jaundice
- butterfly rash

| Characteristic clinical features which distinguish between the spleen and left kidney ||
| Spleen | Left kidney |
| --- | --- |
| no palpable upper border | palpable upper border |
| not bimanually palpable (not ballottable) | bimanually palpable (ballottable) |
| notch on medial border | no notch |
| moves inferomedially on inspiration | moves inferiorly on inspiration |
| dull to percussion | resonant to percussion (overlying bowel) |
| occasionally friction rub present | no friction rub |

**Fig. 21.2** Characteristic clinical features which distinguish between the spleen and left kidney.

**Additional clinical features of some conditions presenting with splenomegaly**

| Disease | Clinical features |
|---|---|
| portal hypertension | Caput Medusae, venous hum, ascites |
| infectious mononucleosis | palatal petechiae, tonsillar enlargement, jaundice, tender hepatomegaly, rash |
| bacterial endocarditis | clubbing, splinter hemorrhages, Osler's nodes, Janeway's lesions, Roth's spots, changing murmurs, hematuria, fever |
| sarcoidosis | pulmonary infiltrates, lupus pernio, erythema nodosum, scar infiltration, uveitis, conjunctivitis, arthritis, restrictive cardiomyopathy, peripheral neuropathy, pulmonary infiltrates |
| AA amyloid | hepatomegaly, renal involvement causing nephrotic syndrome (see Chapter 13) |
| Gaucher's disease | adult type: hepatomegaly, pathological fractures, pigmentation<br>childhood type: mental retardation, spasticity |

**Fig. 21.3** Additional clinical features of some conditions presenting with splenomegaly.

- Blood film can provide diagnostic information (Fig. 21.5).
- Erythrocyte sedimentation rate will be elevated in infection, malignancy, and inflammation.
- Bone marrow examination includes aspiration, trephine, and cytogenetic analysis. It is indicated if the blood count or film suggest hematological abnormalities, and it is useful in the diagnosis of leukemias, myeloproliferative disorders, immune thrombocytopenias, and pancytopenia. Occasionally it is helpful in storage diseases, lymphoma, and carcinoma, where there is marrow infiltration.

## Biochemistry
- Liver function tests: transaminases will be abnormal in infective hepatitis and sometimes in EBV and CMV; elevation in alkaline phosphatase and γ-glutamyl transpeptidase will occur when the porta hepatis is obstructed by enlarged lymph nodes; unconjugated hyperbilirubinemia will be present in hemolysis; an elevated lactate dehydrogenase indicates a poor prognosis in lymphoma.
- Serum calcium: raised in malignancy, sarcoidosis, and sometimes lymphoma.
- Serum uric acid: raised when there is rapid cell turnover such as in malignancy.
- Thyroid function tests: thyrotoxicosis.

When asked to palpate a mass in the left upper quadrant, make sure you can distinguish the left kidney from the enlarged spleen.

## Infection screen
- Monospot test: EBV.
- Serology: EBV, CMV, HIV (Chapter 38), rubella, hepatitis, toxoplasmosis, and brucellosis.
- Blood cultures: repeated if infective endocarditis is suspected.
- Sputum culture: TB.

## Autoantibody screen
This is useful in the detection of connective tissue disorders (Chapter 16).

## Imaging
- Chest x-ray: bilateral hilar lymphadenopathy (caused by lymphoma, sarcoidosis, and TB).
- Abdominal ultrasound scan: will confirm the presence of splenomegaly.
- Computed tomography scan of the chest, abdomen, and pelvis: gives clear staging information in malignancy and particularly lymphoma where retroperitoneal

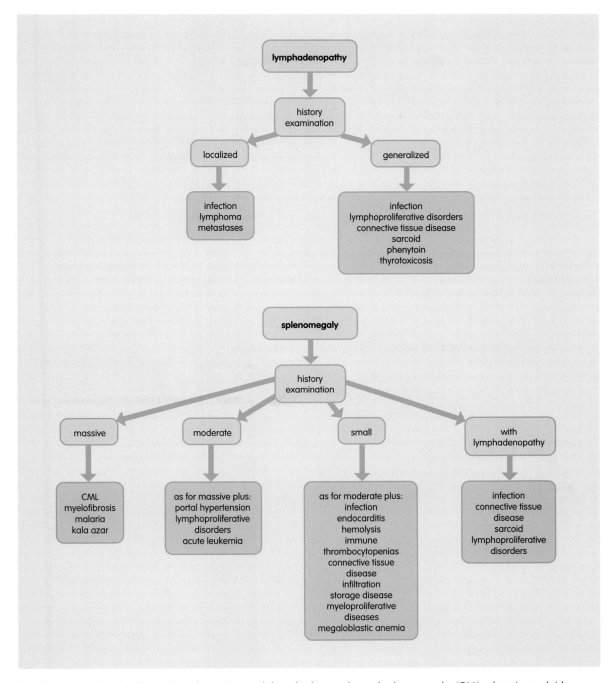

**Fig. 21.4** Algorithm for diagnosis in the patient with lymphadenopathy and splenomegaly. (CML, chronic myeloid leukemia.)

| Blood film abnormalities in conditions presenting with lymphadenopathy and splenomegaly | |
|---|---|
| Disease | Blood film |
| acute leukemia | circulating blasts (Auer rods in AML) |
| chronic lymphocytic leukemia | lymphocytosis, smear cells |
| chronic myeloid leukemia | leukocytosis due to spectrum of myeloid cells |
| myelofibrosis | tear drop poikilocytes, leukoerythroblastic blood film |
| lymphoma | often normal (occasionally mild eosinophilia in Hodgkin's disease) |
| hemolysis | reticulocytosis (polychromasia), micropherocytosis, erythroblasts |
| EBV, infectious hepatitis, toxoplasmosis | atypical lymphocytes |
| malaria (thick and thin films) | parasitemia, thrombocytopenia, hemolysis |

**Fig. 21.5** Blood film abnormalities in conditions presenting with lymphadenopathy and splenomegaly. Many of these disorders may also be associated with a normocytic normochromic anemia. A leukoerythroblastic film will be seen wherever there is heavy bone marrow involvement. Autoimmune hemolytic anemia may also arise in lymphoma and chronic lymphocytic leukemia. (AML, acute myeloid leukemia; EBV, Epstein-Barr virus.)

lymphadenopathy may often be missed by ultrasound scan.

- MRI can evaluate intra-abdominal lymph nodes, look for a primary malignancy, and determine whether masses are cystic.

## Histology
The definitive diagnosis of lymphadenopathy is often made on excision biopsy of an affected node.

A palpable spleen is at least twice its normal size.

# 22. Sensory and Motor Neurologic Deficits

Sensory abnormalities include hyperesthesias (increased pain, touch, or vibration), hypalgesia (decreased sensitivity to painful stimuli), or anesthesia (complete loss of pain, temperature, touch, and vibration sense). Muscle weakness or abnormal sensation can result from disease occurring anywhere along the pathway from the skin or muscle to the brain and back. Such pathologic processes are outlined below.

## Differential diagnosis of sensory and/or motor neurologic deficits

### Muscle
- Drugs: steroids, penicillamine, and procainamide.
- Dystrophy: Duchenne, Becker's, limb girdle, and facioscapulohumeral.
- Endocrine: Cushing's syndrome, thyrotoxicosis, myxedema, and hyperparathyroidism.
- Infection: bacterial (*Clostridium welchii*), viral (influenza), and parasitic (trichinosis).
- Inflammation: polymyositis, dermatomyositis, and sarcoidosis.
- Metabolic: periodic paralyses, McArdle's disease, and mitochondrial myopathy.
- Myotonia: myotonia dystrophica and myotonia congenita (Thomsen's disease).
- Toxin: alcohol.
- Tumor: sarcoma and paraneoplastic syndrome.

### Neuromuscular junction
- Myasthenia gravis.
- Lambert–Eaton syndrome.
- *Clostridium botulinum* infection.

### Peripheral nerves
#### Mononeuropathy
In mononeuropathy, only one peripheral nerve is involved. Consider:
- Trauma.
- Entrapment: carpal tunnel syndrome and meralgia paraesthetica.
- Stretching: ulnar nerve lesion if there is an increased carrying angle at the elbow.
- Tumor: neurofibromatosis.

### Mononeuritis multiplex
In mononeuritis multiplex, two or more individual nerves are affected. The differential diagnosis includes the following:
- Connective tissue disease: polyarteritis nodosa (PAN), systemic lupus erythematosus (SLE), and rheumatoid arthritis (RA).
- Infection: leprosy, herpes zoster, and human immunodeficiency virus (HIV).
- Inflammation: sarcoid.
- Metabolic: diabetes mellitus (DM) and amyloid.
- Tumor: infiltration, paraneoplastic syndrome, and neurofibromatosis.

### Peripheral neuropathy
Peripheral neuropathy is polyneuropathy causing a symmetrical deficit that is most marked distally. The differential diagnosis includes the following:
- Connective tissue disease: PAN, SLE, and RA.
- Drugs: nitrofurantoin, metronidazole, and vincristine.
- Infection: leprosy, HIV, syphilis, and diphtheria.
- Inflammation: Guillain-Barré syndrome.
- Inherited: Charcot-Marie-Tooth disease and Refsum's disease.
- Metabolic: diabetes, renal failure, porphyria, and amyloid.
- Toxins: alcohol and lead.
- Tumor: paraneoplastic syndrome and paraproteinemias.
- Vitamin deficiency: thiamine ($B_1$), niacin ($B_6$), and vitamin $B_{12}$.

### Brachial or lumbar plexus
- Compression: cervical rib.
- Idiopathic: neuralgic amyotrophy.
- Metabolic: DM.
- Trauma: birth injury (Erb's and Klumpke's palsies) and motorbike accidents.
- Tumor: malignant infiltration.

## Spinal nerve root

Spinal nerve roots may be disrupted by the following:

- Infection (e.g., pyogenic meningitis and syphilis).
- Prolapsed intervertebral disc.
- Spinal stenosis.
- Spondylosis.
- Tumor.
- Vertebral fracture dislocation.

## Anterior horn cell

The anterior horn cell may be damaged by the following:

- Motor neuron disease—amyotrophic lateral sclerosis.
- Poliomyelitis.

## The spinal cord

- Degeneration: osteoarthritis.
- Infection: abscess, HIV, tuberculosis (Pott's disease), syphilis.
- Inflammation: multiple sclerosis (MS), sarcoidosis, rheumatoid arthritis (atlantoaxial subluxation).
- Metabolic: Paget's disease.
- Trauma: including radiotherapy and prolapsed intervertebral disc.
- Tumor: metastases, neurofibroma, meningioma, glioma, and ependymoma.
- Vascular: anterior spinal artery occlusion, dissecting aortic aneurysm, arteriovenous malformation, and vasculitis (PAN).
- Vitamin deficiency: subacute combined degeneration of the cord (vitamin $B_{12}$).
- Others: syringomyelia, spina bifida, and motor neuron disease.

## The cerebellum

- Endocrine: hypothyroidism.
- Hereditary: Friedreich's ataxia and ataxia telangiectasia.
- Infection: abscess and postencephalitis miliary TB.
- Inflammation: multiple sclerosis.
- Toxic: alcohol, lead, and phenytoin.
- Trauma: "punch-drunk" syndrome.
- Tumor: metastases, acoustic neuroma, hemangioblastoma (von Hippel–Lindau disease), and paraneoplastic degeneration.
- Vascular: infarction, hematoma, and arteriovenous malformation (AVM).

## The cerebral hemispheres

- Degenerative disease: see Chapter 19.
- Hydrocephalus: primary or secondary.
- Infection: abscess, meningitis, encephalitis, HIV, malaria, rabies, tuberculosis, and syphilis.
- Inflammation: sarcoid, SLE, and MS.
- Metabolic: phenylketonuria and Wilson's disease (basal ganglia).
- Toxic: alcohol, cocaine.
- Trauma.
- Tumor: primary or secondary.
- Vascular: infarction, hemorrhage or hematoma, AVM, and aneurysm.
- Vitamin deficiency: thiamine, niacin, and $B_{12}$.

Other disorders causing cerebral disturbance, such as carbon dioxide narcosis and hepatic encephalopathy, are discussed in Chapters 15, 18, 19, and 20.

Anxiety can often present with bizarre neurologic symptoms.

## History in the patient with sensory and/or motor neurologic deficits

It is often a daunting prospect to be faced with a patient with neurologic symptoms or signs. However, despite the vast number of potential underlying pathologies, a lesion at a particular point in the pathway between brain and muscle or skin will always produce the same clinical signs regardless of the cause. There are five important aspects to consider in the history.

### Onset

Sudden onset usually indicates a vascular problem such as infarction, hemorrhage, or hematoma. Lesions due to trauma, MS, abscess, acute prolapsed disc, and myelitis can also develop rapidly. An insidious onset is more typical of cervical spondylosis, motor neuron disease, neoplasm, myopathy, and syringomyelia.

### Precipitants

Trauma may result in muscular and neurologic deficits. Acute myasthenia can be precipitated by intercurrent illness (particularly infection), or drugs (aminoglycosides or penicillamine). MS may relapse during the puerperium and symptoms may be exacerbated by exertion, hot weather, or after a hot bath.

## Development

Many lesions cause gradually progressive, unremitting disease, including tumor, motor neuron disease, hereditary ataxias, and degenerative brain diseases. Intermittent deficits can be due to transient ischemic attacks, epilepsy, migraine, and myasthenia gravis. MS is characterized by the development of different lesions which are dissociated in time and site. Symptoms and signs due to trauma or vascular events may slowly improve with time or remain static following the initial event.

## Pattern of deficit

Fig. 22.1 summarizes characteristic symptoms and signs which arise as a consequence of a lesion at a specific site. If the neurologic abnormalities do not fit a specific pattern, consider MS, motor neuron disease, or paraneoplastic neuropathy.

## Evidence of cause

The following factors provide evidence of cause:
- Family history: hereditary ataxias, phenylketonuria, neurofibromatosis.
- Drug history, including phenytoin (cerebellar signs), vincristine (peripheral neuropathy), penicillamine (myasthenia).
- Dietary history: intake of vitamins $B_1$, $B_6$ and $B_{12}$.
- Alcohol history.
- Pre-existing illness, such as diabetes, hypertension (cerebrovascular disease), rheumatoid arthritis, or malignancy.
- History of trauma.

## Examining the patient with sensory and/or motor neurologic deficits

When assessing a patient in clinic or hospital, a full neurologic examination should be performed (see Chapter 27). Remember the importance of vital signs, since blood pressure and pulse can help diagnose stroke, arrhythmias, and metabolic disorders. However, in medical school examinations you will only be expected to assess a specific part of the system, such as the eyes, face, legs, arms, or gait. The most common neurologic short cases are peripheral neuropathy (usually due to DM), Parkinson's disease, stroke, and MS, but be prepared for anything!

The clinical examination should aim to answer three questions. Firstly, where is the anatomic site of the lesion or lesions? Secondly, is there anything to suggest the underlying pathologic process? Finally, what disability does the patient have as a consequence of the neurologic deficit?

## Where is the lesion?

The neurologic exam, with particular attention to the cranial nerves, can help localize the lesion. Inspection of the patient's movements on first meeting can lead to the diagnosis—for instance, how the patient is able to move his/her feet or shake hands. From the moment you meet the patient, watch like a hawk. Can the patient lift up the arm? Can the patient let go of your hand (myotonia)? Watch how the patient undresses or gets on to the bed. Any severe deficit will often become apparent before you even lay hands on the patient. Examine the area of interest very carefully.

Fig. 22.1 should help you identify where the anatomic lesion is likely to be on the basis of those neurologic abnormalities present.

## What is the underlying cause?

Once the site of the lesion is identified, think of the differential diagnosis as outlined at the beginning of this chapter. Are there any clues around the patient? Look for diabetic drinks (for peripheral neuropathy or amyotrophy).

If the patient is young, looks well, and is sitting in a wheelchair, MS is the most likely diagnosis. An elderly patient with a hemiparesis is most likely to have had a stroke. Is there a blood pressure chart?

Look at the patient's face for myotonic facies (myotonia dystrophica), Cushing's syndrome (proximal myopathy), or hypothyroidism (myopathy or cerebellar dysfunction). Does the patient have neurofibromatosis (spinal cord or peripheral nerve lesions) or connective tissue disease, such as rheumatoid arthritis (entrapment mononeuropathy,

| Soft of anatomical lesion | Symptoms | Specific signs | Muscle | Reflexes | Sensation |
|---|---|---|---|---|---|
| | | Symptoms and signs associated with different anatomic lesions | | | |
| muscle | weakness (particularly climbing stairs, getting out of chair) pain (inflammation) | myotonia in myotonia dystrophia calf pseudo-hypertrophy and Gowers' sign in Duchenne muscular dystrophy | wasting (usually proximal) tone normal or reduced power reduced | normal reduced or absent in severe muscle disease only plantors downgoing | normal |
| neuromuscular function | diplopia choking on food altered voice proximal limb weakness | fatiguable weakness on looking upwards or counting to 10 | wasting only if severe tone normal power reduction with fatigue | normal | normal |
| peripheral nerve | muscle weakness sensory disturbance can be purely sensory, purely molor, or mixed | mononeuropathy and monoeuritis multiplex—signs in distribution of affected nerves polyneuropathy—signs symmetrical and distal (glove and stocking) | wasting fasciculation reduced tone reduced power | reduced or absent | deficit of all modalities (glove and stocking distribution) |
| brachial or lumbar plexus | muscle weakness sensory disturbance | | wasting fasciculation reduced tone reduced power in distribution affected nerves | | deficit in distribution affected nerves |
| anterior spinal root | muscle weakness | | wasting fasciculation reduced tone reduced power in distribution affected root | reduced or absent | normal |
| posterior spinal root | pain in skin and muscle supplied by that root | | normal | reduced or absent | deficit in distribution affected root |
| anterior horn cell | muscle weakness | | wasting fasciculation reduced tone reduced power in distribution affected nerve | reduced or absent | normal |
| spinal cord | pain at site of lesion worse on coughing, sneezing, at night urinary/bowel disturbance leg weakness sensory disturbance | | at level of lesion: wasting, fasciculation, reduced tone, reduced power below lesion: spasticity, increased tone, reduced power | at level of lesion: reduced or absent below lesion increased, upgoing plantars | below lesion ipsilateral posterior column loss (proprioception, vibration sense) contralateral spinothalamic loss (pain and temperature) |

Fig. 22.1 Symptoms and signs associated with different anatomic lesions.

126

| Symptoms and signs associated with different anatomic lesions | | | | | |
|---|---|---|---|---|---|
| Site of anatomical fusion | Symptoms | Specific signs | Muscle<br>increased tone, reduced power | Reflexes | Sensation<br>loss (pain and temperature) |
| cerebellum | unsteadiness<br>tremor<br>altered speech<br>falls<br>poor coordination | wide-based gait<br>fall to side of lesion<br>intention tremor<br>dysmetria<br>nystagmus<br>staccato speech | reduced tone<br>no wasting<br>normal power | pendular | normal |
| cerebral hemispheres | determined by site of lesion (see Chapters 15, 19, and 20)<br>limb weakness<br>seizure<br>altered speech<br>disturbed higher functions | parietal drift<br>dysphasia<br>dysarthria<br>visual disturbance | increased tone<br>clasp-knife rigidity<br>wasting only if disuse<br>reduced power in pyramidal distribution (flexors stronger than extensors in arms, extensors stronger than flexors in legs) | brisk<br>plantars upgoing | deficit determined by site of lesion |

**Fig. 22.1** *Continued.*

mononeuritis multiplex, or peripheral neuropathy)? Is there a cervical rib?

There are two of most parts of the nervous system, so don't forget to compare one side with the other!

## What disability does the neurologic deficit cause?

The most important thing for the patient is not locating the anatomic site of the lesion but what that lesion prevents the patient from doing.

This is an important part of the examination and is often missed.

Think what tasks the affected part of the body normally performs, and ask the patient to show you how he or she manages, such as doing up buttons (for peripheral neuropathy), brushing hair, or standing out of a chair (for proximal myopathy). Watching the patient walk can give useful information (Fig. 22.2).

## Investigating the patient with sensory and/or motor neurologic deficits

The pathway of investigation is very much determined by findings on the history and clinical examination. The following tests may be useful but each patient will require only those relevant to their presentation:

- Complete blood count and erythrocyte sedimentation rate: reactive picture in inflammation, infection, and neoplasm, and raised mean corpuscular volume in vitamin $B_{12}$ deficiency and alcohol abuse.
- Metabolic panel: raised urea and creatinine in renal failure, potassium high or low in periodic paralyses.
- Serum calcium: raised in hyperparathyroidism.
- Serum glucose: raised in DM.
- Liver function tests: raised γ-glutamyltransferase in alcohol abuse, raised alkaline phosphatase in Paget's disease, and deranged transamines in metastases, infection, and Wilson's disease.
- Thyroid function tests: hyper- or hypothyroidism.

| Abnormalities of gait | |
| --- | --- |
| **Lesion** | **Gait** |
| hemiplegia | foot is plantar flexed; leg is stiff and dragged through a semicircle |
| spastic paraplegia | legs stiff; walk in "scissor fashion" like "walking through mud" |
| proximal myopathy | waddling gait; trunk moves to swing legs forward; difficulty in climbing stairs or standing out of a chair |
| Parkinsonism | stooped posture, hesitation in starting, shuffling, festinant, difficulty in turning, poor arm swing and may freeze |
| cerebellar dysfunction | broad based, ataxic with a tendency to fall to the side of the lesion; unable to walk heel to toe |
| dorsal column disease | stamping; wide based with patient looking at the ground as unable to sense where foot is; clumsy and slaps feet to ground |
| foot drop | stepping; legs lifted high off the ground as no dorsiflexion of the foot |
| musculoskeletal disease | limping; patient avoids weightbearing on affected side due to pain |

**Fig. 22.2** Abnormalities of gait.

- Creatine kinase: markedly raised in muscle inflammation and muscular dystrophies.
- Autoantibodies: RA, SLE, and PAN.
- Serology: HIV, herpes, and syphilis where appropriate.
- Immunoglobulins: paraproteinemias.
- Lumbar puncture: microscopy (infection and malignancy), culture and sensitivity (infection), glucose (reduced in bacterial and tuberculous meningitis), protein (markedly raised in tuberculous meningitis, acoustic neuroma, Guillain–Barré syndrome, Behçet's syndrome, and Froin's syndrome), oligoclonal bands (raised in MS and also in SLE, syphilis, sarcoidosis, and Behçet's syndrome), and xanthochromia (yellow cerebrospinal fluid due to hemoglobin breakdown products) indicating recent subarachnoid hemorrhage.
- Electroencephalogram: may indicate structural cerebral pathology and is characteristic in herpes simplex encephalitis.

- Electromyogram: primary muscle disease (typical changes in myotonia and myasthenia); it also shows denervation but not its cause.
- Nerve conduction studies demonstrate peripheral neuropathies.
- Radiology: plain radiographs may demonstrate degenerative and destructive bone lesions and fractures; computed tomography (CT) scanning and magnetic resonance imaging (MRI) of the brain and spine are extremely useful in diagnosing and localizing central lesions; myelography can be useful in demonstrating compressive cord lesions but this technique has been largely superseded by CT scans and MRI.
- Visual evoked potentials: demonstrate previous retrobulbar neuritis in MS.
- Biopsy: if the diagnosis is in doubt, despite history, examination, and noninvasive procedures. Muscle, nerve, and brain biopsies can be performed to give a definitive histologic diagnosis.

# 23. Bleeding and Bruising

Bruising and bleeding arise when there is abnormal hemostasis. Hemostasis is dependent on normal platelet number and function, an intact coagulation pathway, and normal vessel walls.

## Differential diagnosis of bleeding and bruising

### Platelet abnormalities
Platelets may be reduced in number or function.

#### Thrombocytopenia
- Reduced production: bone marrow failure, drugs (cotrimoxazole), postchemotherapy or postradiotherapy, human immunodeficiency virus (HIV), EBV infection, hepatitis.
- Increased consumption: disseminated intravascular coagulation, thrombotic thrombocytopenic purpura, autoimmune disease, systematic lupus erythematosis (SLE).
- Abnormal distribution: splenic pooling in splenomegaly.
- Dilutional: massive transfusion.

#### Platelet dysfunction
- Hereditary: Glanzmann's thrombasthenia.
- Acquired: aspirin, heparin, uremia.

### Coagulation abnormalities
Coagulopathies may be due to vitamin K deficiency or specific factor deficiency.

#### Factor deficiency
- Hereditary: hemophilia A (factor VIII), hemophilia B (factor IX), von Willebrand's factor.
- Acquired: liver disease.

#### Vitamin K deficiency
Factors II, VII, IX, and X are dependent on vitamin K. Deficiency may be caused by:

- Malabsorption: bowel pathology such as celiac disease or biliary obstruction (vitamin K is fat-soluble).
- Antagonist drugs: coumarins (warfarin).

### Vessel wall abnormalities
Vessel wall abnormalities may be inherited or acquired.

#### Hereditary
Hereditary hemorrhagic telangiectasia.

#### Acquired
- Trauma.
- Physiologic: senile purpura.
- Drugs: corticosteroids.
- Infections: meningococcal septicemia.
- Vitamin deficiency: scurvy (vitamin C).
- Connective tissue disease: pseudoxanthoma elasticum, Ehlers-Danlos syndrome.
- Endocrine: Cushing's syndrome.

## History in the patient with bleeding and bruising

The history should focus on three areas. Firstly, what is the pattern and extent of the bleeding and bruising? Secondly, are there any clues as to the possible underlying cause? Finally, have complications occurred?

### What is the pattern and extent of bleeding and bruising?
As a general rule:
- Platelet abnormalities (low number or dysfunction) cause skin or mucosal purpura and hemorrhage, with prolonged bleeding following trauma or surgery.
- Vessel wall abnormalities cause petechiae and ecchymoses due to bleeding from small vessels,

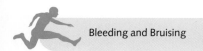

mostly in the skin, but occasionally in mucous membranes.

- Coagulopathies cause hemarthroses, muscle hematomas, postoperative or traumatic bleeding, and mucosal bleeding (von Willebrand's disease).

## What is the underlying cause?

- Bleeding and bruising: "normal" and related to recent trauma or due to an underlying hemostatic abnormality.
- Age: senile purpura seen mostly on the upper limbs.
- Abdominal symptoms: celiac disease, gallstones, liver disease.
- Drug history: aspirin, heparin, warfarin, steroids, previous chemotherapy.
- Family history: hemophilia, hereditary hemorrhagic telangiectasia.
- Symptoms of meningitis: meningococcal sepsis.
- Hyperextensibility of the skin or joints: Ehlers-Danlos syndrome, pseudoxanthoma elasticum.
- Poor diet: scurvy (ecchymoses predominantly on the lower limbs).
- Known acquired immune deficiency syndrome or risk factors for HIV infection.

## Have complications occurred?

- Symptoms of anemia (Chapter 25).
- Symptoms of shock.
- Muscle pain or mass.
- Joint pain or deformity.

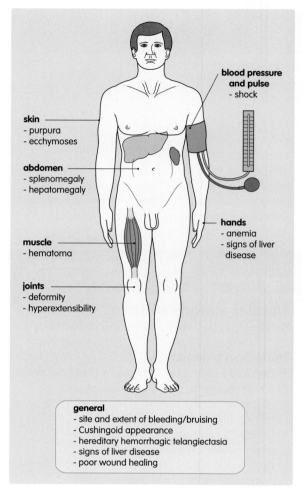

**Fig. 23.1** Examining the patient with bleeding and bruising.

## Examining the patient with bleeding and bruising

The examination should be approached in a similar manner to the history. Fig. 23.1 summarizes the examination approach.

## What is the pattern and extent of bleeding and bruising?

The sites and types of lesions should be documented (see above). "Purpura" includes petechiae (small pinpoint bleeds into the skin) and ecchymoses (small bruises).

## How severe has the bleeding been?

Shock should be looked for urgently in the sick patient by measuring pulse and blood pressure; signs of anemia should also be sought (Chapter 25). Finally, look for joint deformities or a mass in muscle.

## Are there signs suggestive of specific diseases?

- Signs of liver disease (Chapter 10).
- Splenomegaly (whatever cause): platelet pooling.
- Cushingoid appearance: steroid therapy, endocrinopathy.
- Hereditary hemorrhagic telangiectasia: characteristic petechiae on the tongue and lips.
- Meningism (Chapter 15).
- Scurvy: corkscrew hairs with hyperkeratosis of the follicles, perifollicular hemorrhages, gum hypertrophy, poor wound healing.

- Ehlers-Danlos syndrome: hyperextensible skin and joints, "fish-mouth" wounds, pseudotumors over the elbows and knees.
- Pseudoxanthoma elasticum: loose skin in neck, axillae, anticubital fossae and groins, "chicken skin," blue sclera, angioid streaks in the retina, hyperextensible joints.

Thrombocytopenic purpura and vasculitic purpura may look identical, but the lesions in the latter are usually raised and may be tender.

## Investigating the patient with bleeding and bruising

When an abnormality of hemostasis is suspected, a platelet count and simple coagulation assays should be performed. More specific tests to diagnose the underlying cause can then be considered. Fig. 23.2 summarizes the normal coagulation pathway.

An algorithm for investigating the patient with bleeding and bruising is given in Fig. 23.3.

### Platelet count
If thrombocytopenia is present, request a peripheral blood smear (exclude artifactual result due to platelet clumping, look for acute leukemia or disseminated intravascular coagulation) and bone marrow aspirate (increased megakaryocytes in consumptive thrombocytopenia, e.g., idiopathic thrombocytopenic purpura or reduced megakaryocytes in bone marrow failure).

### Prothrombin time
Prothrombin time measures the extrinsic system (VII) and common pathway (X, V, prothrombin, and fibrinogen). It is prolonged in liver disease and warfarin therapy, and is generally expressed as international normalized ratio (INR).

### Activated partial thromboplastin time or kaolin-cephalin clotting time
This measures the intrinsic system (XII, XI, IX, and VIII) and common pathway (X, V, prothrombin, and fibrinogen). It is prolonged in heparin therapy, factor

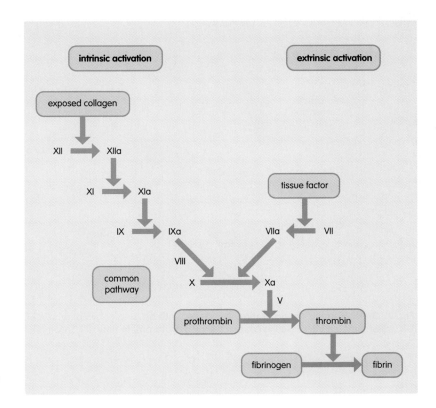

**Fig. 23.2** The normal coagulation pathway.

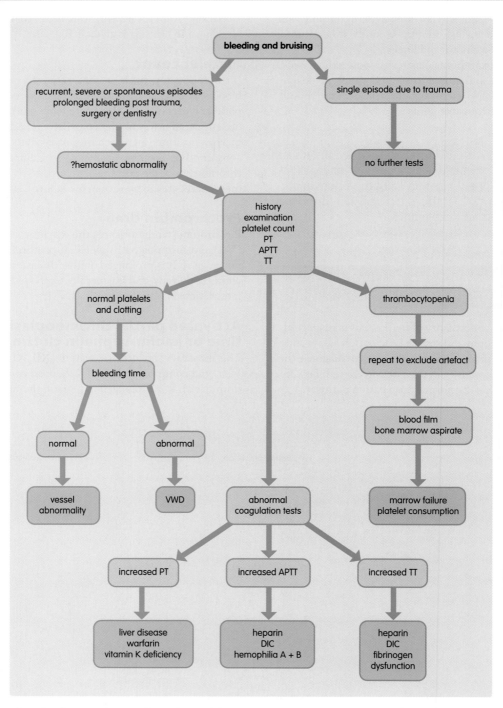

**Fig. 23.3** Algorithm for investigating the patient with bruising or bleeding. (APTT, activated partial thromboplastin time; DIC, disseminated intravascular coagulation; PT, prothrombin time; TT, thrombin time; VWD, von Willebrand's disease.)

deficiency such as factor VIII (hemophilia A) and factor IX (hemophilia B, Christmas disease), and disseminated intravascular coagulation.

### Thrombin time

Thrombin time measures the activity of thrombin and fibrinogen in the common pathway. It is prolonged in fibrinogen deficiency (disseminated intravascular coagulation) or fibrinogen dysfunction. Prolonged thrombin time may also result from heparin therapy (inhibition of thrombin activity).

### Bleeding time (rarely performed)

Bleeding time measures platelet function. It is only performed if platelet count, coagulation screening tests (as above), peripheral blood smear, and bone marrow are normal. It is prolonged in aspirin therapy, uremia, and von Willebrand's disease.

### Fibrin degradation products and D-dimers

Fibrin degradation products and D-dimers will be elevated in disseminated intravascular coagulation.

### Other tests

Other specific tests are also available with hematological advice. These include specific factor assays, von Willebrand's factor, and ristocetin-induced platelet aggregation.

Tests for other diseases given in the differential diagnosis list should be performed as indicated from the history, examination, and basic laboratory tests.

True vertigo is the false perception (illusion) of movement, usually rotational, of a patient of his or her surroundings. This is often accompanied by vomiting, sweating, and pallor. It results from disease in the labyrinth (most common cause), the 8th cranial nerve, or its connections in the brainstem.

Dizziness (i.e., presyncope) or unsteadiness without vertigo can result from a variety of unrelated disorders. Patients often complain of feeling as if they are going to "pass out." They may say that their vision became yellow or that they "saw stars." They do not complain of things spinning. These are discussed in more detail in their appropriate chapters. Dizziness may also be accompanied by sweating and nausea and may be tied to specific movements (i.e., moving from seated to standing). Disorders causing dizziness are discussed in more detail in their appropriate chapters.

When a patient presents with "vertigo" or "dizziness," it is vital to establish whether true vertigo is present or not, as these symptoms result from different pathologies.

## Differential diagnosis in the patient with vertigo or dizziness

### Vertigo
The differential diagnosis in the patient with vertigo includes labyrinth disorders, 8th cranial nerve disease, or brainstem lesions.

### Labyrinth disorders
- Middle ear disease (e.g., otitis media).
- Ménière's disease (triad of vertigo, tinnitus, and sensorineural hearing loss).
- Benign positional vertigo: most commonly caused by free calcium debris within the posterior semicircular canal (canalithiasis).
- Labyrinthitis.
- Traumatic vertigo.
- Perilymphatic fistula.
- Syphilitic labyrinthitis.

### 8th cranial nerve disease
- Vestibular neuronitis.
- Acoustic neuroma.
- Ramsay Hunt syndrome: herpes zoster of the geniculate ganglion.
- Ototoxic drugs: aminoglycosides such as gentamicin.

### Brainstem lesions
- Multiple sclerosis: demyelination.
- Vertebrobasilar ischemia: transient ischemic attack.
- Stroke: lateral medullary syndrome (infraction of interior cerebellar artery).
- Vertebrobasilar insufficiency.
- Migraine.
- Encephalitis.
- Tumor.
- Syringobulbia.
- Alcohol abuse.

Note that vertigo may also be a feature of temporal lobe pathology.

### Dizziness
- Low cardiac output (Chapter 18).
- Hyperventilation, anxiety.
- Anemia.
- Hypoglycemia.
- Pheochromocytoma.
- Postural hypotension due to drugs (e.g., overenthusiastic antihypertensive regimens, antidepressants, tranquilizers).
- Visual disturbance.
- Cerebrovascular disease.

- Fever.
- Psychiatric disturbance—panic attack.

## History in the patient with vertigo

The diagnosis in patients with vertigo is largely made on the history. It is important to elicit the time course of the vertigo and the likely site of the lesion by asking about other auditory and neurological symptoms. Typical features of specific diseases are shown in Fig. 24.1.

## Pattern of vertigo

The following should be established:
- Onset: peripheral lesions generally cause acute severe symptoms; central lesions tend to cause a gradual onset with less severe vertigo. Peripheral lesions also tend to cause nystagmus with a rotary component, whereas central lesions cause nystagmus that lacks rotary movement and is vertical in nature.
- Duration of vertigo.
- Recurrent episodes or a single attack?
- Relation to head position.

### Characteristic features of diseases causing vertigo

| Disease | Cause | Length of vertigo | Aural symptoms | Neurological symptoms | Natural history |
|---|---|---|---|---|---|
| Ménière's disease | excess endolymphatic fluid (hydrops) | 1–8 hours often preceded by sensation of fullness in the ear | fluctuating but progressive deafness tinnitus | none | episodic attacks unilateral at first becomes bilateral in 25% ceases when deafness complete |
| vestibular neuronitis | possibly viral | days to weeks explosive onset | none | none | spontaneously resolves in weeks |
| benign positional vertigo | degeneration of utricular neuroendothelium can follow head injury and vestibular neuronitis | seconds precipitated by changes in head position | none | none | episodic attacks spontaneous resolution over weeks to months |
| perilymphatic fistula | rupture of round window membrane often due to barotrauma can be spontaneous | months to years | deafness and tinnitus | none | often resolves with bed rest can be surgically repaired |
| vertebrobasilar insufficiency | "nipping" of vertebral arteries by osteophytic cervical vertebrae | seconds precipitated by neck extension or rotation | none | dysarthria diplopia visual loss syncope | episodic attacks |
| acoustic neuroma | schwannoma of vestibular nerve | gradual onset progressive | unilateral deafness and tinnitus | 5th and 7th cranial nerve palsies ipsilateral cerebellar signs | symptoms progress until surgical removal |
| central lesions | tumor demyelination vascular migraine | develops gradually unremitting | often spared | usually present and dependent on site of lesion | symptoms progress until underlying cause treated |

Fig. 24.1 Characteristic features of diseases causing vertigo.

- Associated symptoms: dyspnea, tachycardia, and anxiety suggest a panic attack.

## Aural symptoms

The presence of aural symptoms suggests that the lesion is peripheral, involving the labyrinth or 8th cranial nerve:

- Ear pain.
- Ear discharge.
- Deafness (fluctuating or progressive).
- Tinnitus (ringing in the ear[s]).

## Neurologic symptoms

The following symptoms suggest central pathology or acoustic neuroma.

- Facial weakness.
- Dysarthria.
- Dysphagia.
- Diplopia.
- Loss of consciousness.
- Seizures.
- Weakness, altered sensation, poor limb coordination.

## History suggestive of an underlying cause

- Recent viral illness causes vestibular neuronitis.
- Previous head injury may lead to labyrinth concussion, benign positional vertigo.
- Previous otologic surgery.
- Drug history (e.g., aminoglycosides).
- Risk factors for vascular disease: hypertension, high cholesterol, smoking, family history.
- Recent flying or diving (e.g., barotrauma— perilymphatic fistula).

## Examining the patient with vertigo

The clinical examination is often normal. The following specific abnormalities should be looked for carefully:

- Nystagmus: horizontal and away (fast phase) from the side of the lesion. Occasionally, brainstem lesions may also cause vertical nystagmus. Direction of nystagmus is as noted above.
- Romberg's sign: positive if the patient is more unsteady on standing when the eyes are closed compared with when they are open; in vestibular disorders. The patient will tend to fall to the side of the lesion.

- Hallpike's maneuver: the patient is asked to lie down quickly with the head tilted to one side; in benign positional vertigo there will be a latent period of a few seconds followed by nystagmus.
- Focal neurologic signs: if present, these suggest a central lesion, acoustic neuroma, or Ramsay Hunt syndrome. Pay particular attention to assessment of the 8th cranial nerve, gait, and cerebellar signs.
- Eyes: papilledema (tumor with raised intracranial pressure), optic atrophy (demyelination), and ophthalmoplegia (cranial nerve defect, demyelination).
- Ears: otoscopy may reveal otitis media or a herpetic rash. Herpetic lesions may also be found on careful examination of the surrounding skin.
- Lying and standing blood pressures: postural hypotension.

Fig. 24.2 summarizes the examination approach.

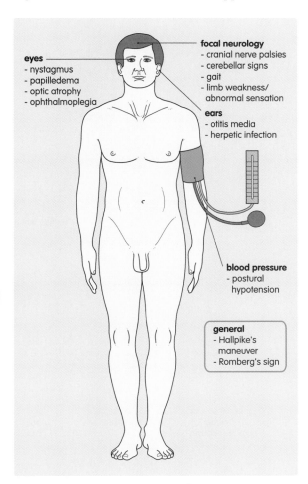

**Fig. 24.2** Examining the patient with vertigo.

## Investigating the patient with vertigo

- Audiometry: to distinguish between conductive and sensorineural deafness.
- Caloric tests: normally, running cold and then warm water into the external auditory meatus causes contralateral and then ipsilateral nystagmus, respectively; where there is pathology in the ipsilateral labyrinth, 8th cranial nerve, or brainstem, this normal response will be reduced or absent.
- Electronystagmography: a more accurate assessment of the presence and type of nystagmus.
- Imaging: high-resolution computed tomography scanning and magnetic resonance imaging are useful tools when a central lesion or acoustic neuroma is suspected.

An algorithm for approaching the diagnosis in the patient with vertigo is given in Fig. 24.3.

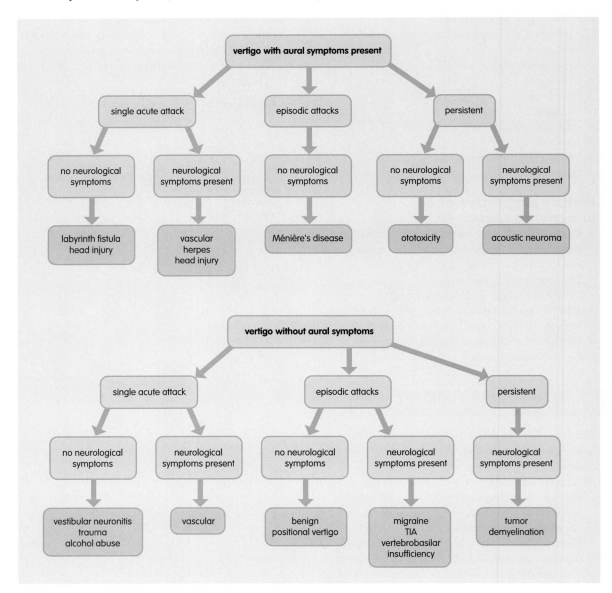

**Fig. 24.3** Algorithm for the diagnosis of a patient with vertigo. (TIA, transient ischemic attack.)

# 25. Anemia

A patient is anemic when the hemoglobin concentration in the blood is less than 13.5g/dL (or hematorcit [Hct] less than 41%) in men and 11.5g/dL (or Hct less than 36%) in women.

## Differential diagnosis of anemia

The size of the red blood cells gives important clues as to the likely underlying abnormality.

### Microcytic red blood cells
Microcytic RBCs have a mean cell volume of less than 80fL; where fL stands for femtoliter (= $10^{-15}$L). Causes include:
- Iron-deficiency anemia (Fig. 25.1).
- Thalassemia.
- Anemia of chronic disease (Fig. 25.2).
- Sideroblastic anemia.
- Lead poisoning.

### Normocytic red blood cells
Normocytic RBCs have a mean cell volume of 80–95fL.
  Causes include:
- Anemia of chronic disease (see Fig. 25.2).
- Hemolysis (Fig. 25.3).
- Acute blood loss.
- Bone marrow hypoplasia.

### Macrocytic red blood cells
Macrocytic RBCs have a mean cell volume of more than 95fL.
  Causes include:
- Megaloblastic anemia: folate deficiency (Fig. 25.4), vitamin $B_{12}$ deficiency (Fig. 25.5).
- Normoblastic anemia: alcohol, liver disease, hypothyroidism, pregnancy, reticulocytosis.
- Several drugs can lead to macrocytosis such as azathioprine, methotrexate, zidovudine, hydroxyurea. In fact, in the case of zidovudine macrocytosis is used as a sign that patients are taking the medication.
- Myelodysplastic syndrome.

## History in the anemic patient

It is important to establish first how symptomatic the anemia is. The history should then focus on whether any complications of anemia are present and whether there are any clues as to the likely underlying diagnosis.

### Symptoms of anemia
When anemia develops over a long time, the hemoglobin can be very low before symptoms occur. Anemia is tolerated less well in the elderly. The following symptoms may present:
- Asymptomatic: particularly if the anemia develops over a long time.
- Lethargy.
- Shortness of breath: most marked on exertion.
- Lightheadedness.
- Palpitations.

### Symptoms of complications
- Symptoms of cardiac failure (Chapters 1 and 2).
- Angina.
- Ischemic claudication.
- Visual disturbance due to retinal hemorrhage: very rare—the anemia must be severe.

### Evidence to suggest underlying cause
- Specific symptoms: menorrhagia, change in bowel habit (including melena or hematochezia), dyspepsia, weight loss, headache. Of note, in adult over 50 years old, microcytic anemia is due to a GI bleed until proved otherwise. It is imperative to ask about dark, malodorous stools and other risk factors for GI bleeding as noted above (e.g., NSAID use).

| Causes of iron-deficiency anemia | |
|---|---|
| **Mechanism** | **Examples** |
| reduced iron intake | poor diet malabsorption (gastrectomy, celiac disease) |
| increased iron utilization | infancy, adolescence, pregnancy |
| abnormal iron loss | chronic bleeding from gastrointestinal tract, uterus, urinary tract |

**Fig. 25.1** Causes of iron-deficiency anemia.

| Causes of anemia of chronic disease | |
|---|---|
| **Mechanism** | **Examples** |
| malignancy | breast, prostate, lung |
| inflammation | rheumatoid arthritis, temporal arteritis |
| chronic infection | tuberculosis, subacute bacterial endocarditis |

**Fig. 25.2** Causes of anemia of chronic disease.

| Causes of hemolytic anemia | | |
|---|---|---|
| | **Mechanism** | **Examples** |
| intrinsic | red blood cell membrane detects enzyme deficiencies | hereditary spherocytosis hereditary elliptocytosis glucose-6-phosphate dehydrogenase deficiency pyruvate kinase deficiency |
| | abnormal hemoglobin | thalassemia sickle cell disease |
| extrinsic | immune | ABO incompatibility (blood transfusion) hemolytic disease of the newborn autoimmune (warm): idiopathic, lymphoma, CLL, SLE, methyldopa autoimmune (cold): idiopathic, lymphoma, mycoplasma, Epstein–Barr virus drugs |
| | non-immune | mechanical heart valves burns malaria microangiopathic (DIC, TTP, pre-eclampsia, Hus) paroxysmal nocturnal hemoglobinuria hepatic or renal disease |

**Fig. 25.3** Causes of hemolytic anemia. (CLL, chronic lymphocytic leukemia; DIC, disseminated intravascular coagulation; SLE, systemic lupus erythematosus; TTP, thrombotic thrombocytopenic purpura.)

| Causes of folate deficiency | |
|---|---|
| **Mechanism** | **Examples** |
| reduced intake | poor diet, e.g., old age, poverty, alcoholics |
| reduced absorption | celiac disease, extensive Crohn's disease, tropical sprue, gastrectomy |
| increased utilization | physiological, e.g., pregnancy, lactation, prematurity increased cell turnover, e.g., malignancy, chronic inflammation, hemolysis, dialysis |
| drugs | trimethoprim, sulphasalazine, anticonvulsants, methotrexate |

**Fig. 25.4** Causes of folate deficiency.

**Fig. 25.5** Causes of vitamin B$_{12}$ deficiency. (TB, tuberculosis; UC, ulcerative colitis.)

| Causes of vitamin B$_{12}$ deficiency | |
| --- | --- |
| **Mechanism** | **Examples** |
| reduced intake | vegans |
| reduced absorption | stomach, e.g. gastrectomy, pernicious anemia<br>small intestine, e.g. Crohn's disease, ileal resection, ileal TB or UC |
| increased utilization | blind loop syndrome (bacterial overgrowth), fish tapeworm (*Diphyllobothrium latum*) |
| abnormal metabolism | transcobalamin II deficiency (autosomal recessive) |
| drugs | nitrous oxide, metformin |

- Pre-existing illness: rheumatoid arthritis, previous abdominal surgery, dialysis.
- Family history: hemolytic anemia.
- Drug history: salicylates (iron deficiency), anticonvulsants (folate deficiency).
- Diet: vegans (vitamin B$_{12}$ deficiency), alcoholics (folate deficiency).
- Pica (craving for specific and often bizarre foods): iron deficiency.
- Pregnancy: folate deficiency.

 Dysphagia plus iron-deficiency anemia: think of Plummer-Vinson or Paterson-Brown-Kelly syndrome (postcricoid esophageal web).

## Examining the anemic patient

### Signs of anemia and its consequences

Fig. 25.6 summarizes the examination approach. The following signs of anemia should be noted:
- Pallor: mucous membranes (mouth and conjunctivae), nails, skin creases.
- Hyperdynamic circulation: tachycardia, collapsing pulse, systolic flow murmur.
- Cardiac failure.
- Retinal hemorrhages.

### Signs of underlying disease

A full general examination should always be performed, including breast examination and rectal examination in iron deficiency. Specific abnormalities include the following:
- Glossitis: megaloblastic anemia, iron deficiency.
- Angular stomatitis: koilonychia, iron deficiency.
- Jaundice: hemolysis, megaloblastic anemia (mild).
- Splenomegaly: hemolysis, megaloblastic anemia (Chapter 21).
- Leg ulcers: sickle cell disease.
- Bone deformities: thalassemia.
- Peripheral neuropathy, optic atrophy, subacute combined degeneration of the cord, and dementia are all neurologic sequelae of vitamin B$_{12}$ deficiency.
- Blue line on the gums (Burton's line), peripheral motor neuropathy, encephalopathy are seen in lead poisoning.

Note the racial origin of the patient as thalassemia is more common in people from South-East Asia and China, while sickle cell anemia is more common among Africans.

## Investigating the anemic patient

### General investigations
#### Complete blood count
- Hemoglobin: anemia.
- Mean corpuscular volume: underlying pathologies.
- White cell count: if low, consider general bone marrow failure; if high, consider infection, inflammation, or malignancy.

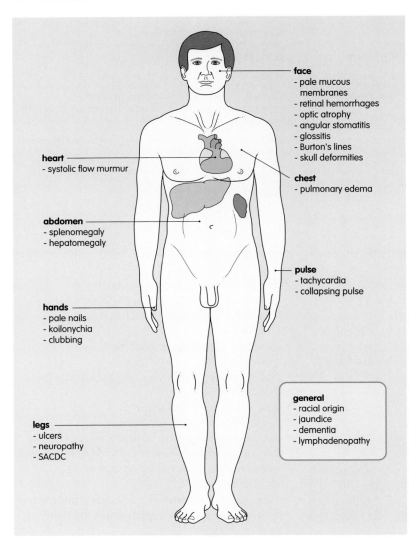

**Fig. 25.6** Examining the anemic patient. (SACDC, subacute combined degeneration of the cord.)

**face**
- pale mucous membranes
- retinal hemorrhages
- optic atrophy
- angular stomatitis
- glossitis
- Burton's lines
- skull deformities

**chest**
- pulmonary edema

**heart**
- systolic flow murmur

**abdomen**
- splenomegaly
- hepatomegaly

**pulse**
- tachycardia
- collapsing pulse

**hands**
- pale nails
- koilonychia
- clubbing

**general**
- racial origin
- jaundice
- dementia
- lymphadenopathy

**legs**
- ulcers
- neuropathy
- SACDC

- Platelet count: if low, consider general bone marrow failure; if high, consider infection, inflammation, or malignancy.

### Erythrocyte sedimentation rate
The erythrocyte sedimentation rate will be raised in infection, inflammation, or malignancy.

### Reticulocyte count
Reticulocytes are young erythrocytes that normally constitute only 0.5–2.0% of circulating RBCs. The reticulocyte count is increased if RBC production is increased and red cells are prematurely released into the circulation. This occurs following hemorrhage, in chronic hemolysis, or with vitamin $B_{12}$, folate, or iron replacement, when there has been a deficiency. This means that macrocytic anemia is normal in some cases (as the body replenishes its circulating RBC volume). Be aware that if the patient does not have macrocytosis after hemorrhage, etc., this may be a sign of inadequate RBC production.

### Peripheral blood smear
The peripheral blood smear can provide diagnostic information, as shown in Fig. 25.7.

### Bone marrow
- Not necessary when the diagnosis is obvious (e.g., iron deficiency).

| Abnormalities on the blood film in anemia | |
|---|---|
| Abnormality | Changes on blood film |
| iron deficiency | hypochromic, microcytic RBCs, target cells, pencil cells, poikilocytosis (variation in RBC shape), anisocytosis (variation in RBC size), often thrombocytosis |
| vitamin $B_{12}$/folate deficiency | oval-shaped macrocytosis, neutrophil nuclei hypersegmented (greater than five lobes), poikilocytosis; white blood cell and platelet count may be low |
| hemolysis | reticulocytosis, microspherocytes, erythroblasts many spherocytes in hereditary spherocytosis elliptocytes in hereditary elliptocytosis |
| thalassemia | hypochromic, microcytic RBCs, basophilic stippling, target cells, reticulocytosis |
| sickle cell disease | sickle cells, target cells features of hyposplenism in adults (Howell–Jolly bodies, Pappenheimer bodies, target cells) |
| anemia of chronic disease | normochromic, normocytic RBCs neutrophilia and thrombocytosis may be present |
| liver disease | macrocytic RBCs, target cells features of iron deficiency and folate deficiency may also be present |

**Fig. 25.7** Abnormalities on the blood film in anemia. (RBCs, red blood cells.)

- Bone marrow aspirate gives information regarding the development of different cell lines, the proportion of these different cell lines, infiltration by abnormal cells (e.g., infiltration with metastatic carcinoma), and the presence of iron stores.
- Bone marrow trephine (core biopsy) provides structural information regarding bone marrow architecture and infiltration.

## Specific investigations

All patients with anemia should have measurement of serum ferritin, vitamin $B_{12}$, and RBC folate, as more than one deficiency can occur at the same time. An algorithm is presented in Fig. 25.8 for the diagnosis of anemia.

### Iron deficiency
- Serum ferritin: low in iron deficiency but raised in iron overload, hemochromatosis and anemia of chronic disease (occasionally).
- Serum iron: low.
- Total iron-binding capacity: increased.
- Menorrhagia or pregnancy: no further investigations are necessary.
- If no menorrhagia or pregnancy: consider upper gastrointestinal endoscopy, rectal examination, and sigmoidoscopy with colonoscopy or barium enema.

- No obvious cause: consider mesenteric angiogram for angiodysplasia.

### Vitamin $B_{12}$ deficiency
- Serum vitamin $B_{12}$: low.
- Bilirubin: mildly raised—intramedullary destruction of abnormal RBCs.
- Lactate dehydrogenase (LDH): elevated—intramedullary destruction of abnormal RBCs.
- Gastric parietal antibodies: positive in 90% of patients with pernicious anemia.
- Intrinsic factor antibodies: positive in approximately 50% of patients with pernicious anemia.
- Schilling test: the patient is given a loading dose of 1000mg vitamin $B_{12}$ intramuscularly, followed by a small oral dose of radioactive vitamin $B_{12}$, and excretion is then measured in the urine; vitamin $B_{12}$ malabsorption is corrected by giving intrinsic factor with labeled vitamin in pernicious anemia, but persists despite the use of intrinsic factor in intestinal disease.
- Endoscopy or barium meal and follow through: may be necessary in underlying intestinal disease.

### Folate deficiency
- RBC folate: more reliable than serum folate.
- Bilirubin: mildly raised—intramedullary destruction of abnormal RBCs.

143

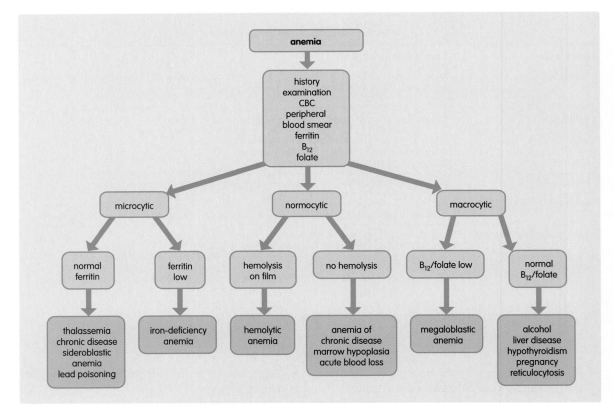

**Fig. 25.8** Algorithm for the diagnosis of anemia. (CBC, complete blood count.)

- LDH: elevated—intramedullary destruction of abnormal RBCs.
- Tests for intestinal malabsorption: including jejunal biopsy, may be necessary when the diagnosis is not clear.

### Hemolysis
- Serum bilirubin: raised and unconjugated.
- Serum haptoglobins: reduced or absent.
- Fecal stercobilinogen: raised.
- Urinary urobilinogen: raised.
- Reticulocyte count: raised.
- Hemoglobin electrophoresis: abnormal in thalassemia and sickle cell disease.
- Coombs' test: positive in autoimmune hemolytic anemias.
- Osmotic fragility: increased if spherocytes are present.

- Enzyme assays: available in specialist centers only for glucose-6-phosphate dehydrogenase and pyruvate kinase deficiencies.
- Ham's test: positive in paroxysmal nocturnal hemoglobinuria.

### Anemia of chronic disease
- Ferritin: high (ferritin is an acute-phase protein).
- Serum iron: low.
- Total iron-binding capacity: low.
- Serum vitamin $B_{12}$: normal.
- RBC folate: normal.

Other investigations should be directed by the clinical scenario. Consider erythrocyte sedimentation rate, C-reactive protein, autoantibody screen, sepsis screen, and search for occult malignancy.

# PART II: HISTORY, EXAMINATION, AND COMMON INVESTIGATIONS

# 26. Taking a History

## General principles— the bedside manner

From the first meeting, patients decide whether or not they think the doctor is trustworthy, based on the doctor's general manner and attitude. Mutual trust is the foundation of the good doctor–patient relationship.

There is no easy recipe for developing a good bedside manner, but courtesy, patience, and letting patients express their ideas, concerns, and expectations are essential ingredients.

Whenever you meet a patient, introduce yourself politely and do not forget relatives or friends who might also be present. Try to put the patient at ease, as visiting the doctor is very stressful for most people, particularly if they think that they have a serious illness. If you cannot speak the same language, try to get an interpreter. If a patient cannot hear you, do not assume they have dementia, but speak louder! Remember that the history is still the most useful tool the clinician has.

The aims of the history are as follows:
- To establish rapport with the patient.
- To obtain an accurate, sequential account of the patient's symptoms and create a differential diagnosis.
- To ask specific questions to focus on the most likely diagnoses.
- To determine risk factors for these possible diagnoses.
- To assess whether complications have occurred on the basis of associated symptoms.
- To put this problem or problems into the context of the patient's life.

We have outlined a standard approach to obtaining the history. However, the important thing is that you develop an approach with which you are comfortable and then practice it again and again. In this way you will not miss things, and you will be able to concentrate more on what the patient is telling you rather than what comes next.

Watch the patient closely, as facial expression and body posture can sometimes tell you more than the words themselves. If you are looking up, the patient will also feel that you are genuinely listening to what he or she is saying. It is important to strike a good balance between recording the history accurately and maintaining eye contact.

As a general principle, start the consultation by asking very open-ended questions, such as "How are you?" or "What symptoms have made you come to the clinic today?" This gives the patient the opportunity to say what he or she wants. Then ask more specific questions to clarify important aspects.

## The history

At the start of every history you should always:
- Document the date, time, and place of consultation. (Remember that the clerking history is a legal document.)
- Record the age, sex, and occupation of the patient.
- Document who referred the patient and whether the patient was seen on an emergency basis.

## Chief complaint

This should be a single sentence that concisely summarizes the main symptom(s) and the length of time they have been present. For example, a 2-hour history of crushing retrosternal chest pain or a 6-month history of alternating constipation and diarrhea with a 4-month history of weight loss of 15 pounds.

Resist the temptation to write the entire history in this section, particularly when there are multiple symptoms.

## History of present illness

Ask when the patient first had this symptom and what has happened since then. Make sure that you establish the following details.

### Onset and offset

Find out whether or not the symptom came on suddenly or gradually, and discover what the patient was doing at the time. For example, chest pain on walking up a hill is likely to be angina, syncope on tilting the head upwards is likely to due to be vertebrobasilar insufficiency, etc.

As for the offset, did the complaint resolve gradually or quickly?

### Duration

Find out whether the complaint is still present. If not, then how long did it last?

### Relieving/exacerbating factors

These are particularly important in describing pain.

### Associated symptoms

Did the patient notice anything else at the time? For example, sweating, clamminess, and vomiting, in association with cardiac chest pain, are usually seen in myocardial infarction rather than angina alone.

### Pattern

Was the symptom a solitary event or a recurrent problem? Did it come on suddenly, and is it gradually settling? Is it getting progressively worse?

Note that patients may often use medical terms to explain what has happened to them, so take time to ask what they actually mean. For example, when the term "vertigo" is used, it might actually mean true vertigo, lightheadedness, or unsteadiness of gait, which have very different underlying etiologies.

It is often useful to list the risk factors for the likely diagnosis at the end of this section.

Also ask about location (if applicable). Ask the patient to point with one finger to where pain or discomfort is. Ask about radiation of pain.

Ask about the quality of the discomfort (especially if pain is involved). Have the patient describe the sensation that he or she is feeling. Is there a cramping discomfort or a burning sensation when the patient performs a specific activity? Tease out exactly what, when, and where the patient is feeling discomfort or pain.

## Past medical history

Ask the patient if he or she has had any previous operations or medical problems. It is prudent to probe a little about each illness and how the diagnosis was made. If applicable, ask for the most recent test results (e.g., the results of a recent HbA1c test, a previous cardiac catheterization, or a recent cholesterol screen). This is done in an attempt to determine the severity of the other medical condition. While knowing that a patient with chest pain has diabetes is good information, it is also important to try to get a feel as to whether or not the diabetes is under good control.

Record the history in chronological order and, when possible, record the year, hospital and attending physician involved (where appropriate) for each episode. Many patients may forget past illnesses, particularly if anxious, and it is worth asking them specifically about diabetes, hypertension, angina or heart disease, rheumatic fever, tuberculosis, epilepsy, asthma, jaundice, stroke, or transient ischemic attacks.

## Review of systems

Patients occasionally focus on one minor symptom while omitting to tell you of another more significant symptom. In fact, this can be a deliberate act, asking the doctor to deal with a simple problem (e.g., sore throat), while deciding whether to ask for help with the real worry such as impotence or chest pain. Performing a quick systems review will prevent you from missing other important diseases. The symptoms to ask about in each system are outlined below.

### General symptoms
#### Fatigue

This is a nonspecific symptom which can accompany many organic as well as psychiatric diseases. Look particularly for evidence of anemia or hypothyroidism.

## Appetite

Anorexia is a feature of many diseases, again organic and psychiatric; increased appetite despite weight loss is seen in hyperthyroidism.

## Weight changes

### Weight loss

Weight loss can be deliberate (dieting) or due to chronic disease. The causes are discussed in detail in Chapter 9.

### Weight gain

Weight gain is seen in pregnancy, hypothyroidism, Cushing's syndrome, polycystic ovarian disease, and "comfort eating" due to anxiety or depression.

## Sweats

Drenching sweats occurring at night are seen in lymphoma, chronic leukemia, and tuberculosis. Sweats at any time of the day are a feature of the menopause.

## Pruritus (itching)

Pruritus can be due to local skin disease or systemic disease as shown in Fig. 26.1.

## Sleep pattern

If there is difficulty in sleeping, ask if the problem is in going to sleep or in waking early. Difficulty in getting off to sleep is often due to worry or anxiety, whereas early morning wakening is a feature of depression.

# Cardiovascular symptoms

## Chest pain

Establish the site, radiation, character, exacerbating and relieving factors, and severity discussed in detail in Chapter 1.

## Dyspnea

Exertional dyspnea can be due to poor left ventricular function, pulmonary edema, arrhythmia, or valvular disease.

Orthopnea is breathlessness while lying flat (pulmonary venous congestion). Note that this symptom can be present in chronic obstructive airways disease, as diaphragmatic respiration is less efficient when the patient is lying flat.

Paroxysmal nocturnal dyspnea is waking during the night due to severe breathlessness (pulmonary edema).

Sudden onset of breathlessness, regardless of body position or exercise, is often due to arrhythmia. See Chapter 2 for more information.

## Syncope

Syncope is the transient loss of consciousness and motor tone, which may be due to arrhythmia, valvular heart disease, postural hypotension, or vertebrobasilar insufficiency (Chapter 18).

## Palpitations

Ask the patient to tap out the rhythm (Chapter 3). Is the beat fast or slow, regular or irregular?

## Ankle swelling

This can be due to right ventricular failure, drugs (e.g., $Ca^{2+}$ channel blockers), or it can be gravitational.

## Calf swelling

This can be due to:

- Deep vein thrombosis: recent travel, immobility or surgery, pregnancy, combined oral contraceptive pill, family history, malignancy.
- Ruptured Baker's cyst: in elderly, secondary to osteoarthritis of the knee.
- Muscle trauma.
- Cellulitis.
- Tumor: sarcoma (rare).

| Causes of pruritus | |
| --- | --- |
| **Cause** | **Examples** |
| skin disease | scabies, eczema, lichen planus, urticaria, dry skin (elderly, hypothyroidism) |
| systemic disease | hepatic (biliary obstruction, pregnancy) malignancy (particularly lymphoma) hematological (polycythemia, iron deficiency) chronic renal failure drugs (sensitivity opiates) endocrine (diabetes mellitus, hyper/ hypothyroidism, carcinoid syndrome) parasitic (trichinosis) neurological (multiple sclerosis) psychogenic |

**Fig. 26.1** Causes of pruritus.

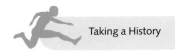

## Claudication

Intermittent claudication due to peripheral vascular disease causes calf, thigh, or buttock pain on exercise. The amount of exercise required to cause pain tends to be consistent although it often deteriorates slowly. It is relieved within a predictable period of time on rest.

Spinal claudication due to spinal stenosis also causes calf, thigh, or buttock pain on exertion, possibly by causing occlusion of the spinal arteries. However, the claudication distance tends to be variable. The pain can also be brought on by prolonged standing and is also often bilateral. The pain improves with rest (though improvement takes longer with ischemic pain) or with lumbar spine flexion (less pain on climbing hills than going downhill).

## Respiratory symptoms

### Dyspnea

See Chapter 2 for more information about dyspnea.

### Cough

Is the cough dry or productive? Is there diurnal variation? (See Chapter 5.)

### Sputum

How much sputum is produced? There is often little sputum in bronchial carcinoma but copious amounts in bronchiectasis. Ask about its color:

- Yellow: infection, acute asthma (due to eosinophils).
- Green: infection.
- Frothy: pulmonary edema.
- Rusty: lobar pneumonia (pneumococcal).
- Blood: see Chapter 5.
- Taste: foul in bronchiectasis and abscess.
- Smell: foul in bronchiectasis.

### Chest pain

Chest pain is usually pleuritic in chest disease (Chapter 1) and is often due to pneumonia, pneumothorax, and pulmonary embolus.

### Wheeze

Patients with airways obstruction sometimes notice an audible expiratory wheeze.

### Hoarse voice

This may be caused, for example, by recurrent laryngeal nerve palsy in bronchial carcinoma.

## Gastrointestinal disease

### Abdominal pain

Establish the site, radiation, character, exacerbating and relieving factors, and severity. This is discussed in detail in Chapter 11.

### Dysphagia

Dysphagia means difficulty in swallowing. Ask about:

- Where do things get stuck? This may give a clue as to the site of the lesion.
- Is there difficulty with solids, fluids or both? Neuromuscular disorders tend to present with dysphagia for fluids at onset, whereas mechanical obstruction results in dysphagia for solids at onset.

The causes of dysphagia are outlined in Fig. 26.2.

### Vomiting

What does the vomitus look like?

- Yellow–green: upper gastrointestinal (GI) contents plus bile.
- Brown (feculent): lower small bowel contents.
- Bright-red blood: active upper GI bleeding (Chapter 7).
- "Coffee grounds": old upper GI bleeding.

How "violent" was the vomiting? Projectile vomiting indicates pyloric stenosis, most commonly seen in infants, but may arise as a consequence of duodenal ulceration in adults.

### Indigestion

"Heartburn" or "dyspepsia" is due to reflux of the gastric contents into the esophagus.

### Bowel habit

Has there been a change? Ask about diarrhea and constipation, or the presence of one alternating with the other. For more about this, see Chapter 8.

### Rectal bleeding

Is the bleeding with or without mucus? The causes of rectal bleeding are summarized in Fig. 26.3. Anal and rectal lesions result in fresh blood on the outside of the stool, on the paper on wiping, or in the pan. Higher lesions result in blood intermixed with the stool.

Ask if the patient has passed any black or very malodorous stools. As with all other symptoms noted above and below, it is very important to determine on how many occasions the symptoms have occurred. Does the patient have blood in the stool once a week

**Fig. 26.2** Causes of dysphagia.

| Causes of dysphagia | |
| --- | --- |
| **Disorder** | **Examples** |
| oropharyngeal lesions | stomatitis, pharyngitis, lymphoma |
| intrinsic esophageal and gastric lesions | peptic stricture<br>carcinoma of esophagus or gastric fundus<br>foreign body<br>esophageal web (Paterson–Brown–Kelly or Plummer–Vinson syndrome)<br>infection (*Candida albicans*)<br>pharyngeal pouch<br>Schatzki's ring (esophagogastric junction in hiatus hernia) leiomyoma of esophageal muscle |
| extrinsic esophageal compression | goiter with retrosternal extension<br>intrathoracic tumors (lymphoma, bronchial carcinoma)<br>enlarged left atrium |
| neuromuscular disorders | achalasia<br>scleroderma<br>diffuse esophageal spasm<br>diabetes mellitus<br>myasthenia gravis<br>myotonia dystrophica<br>bulbar or pseudobulbar palsy<br>diphtheria |
| psychological | globus hystericus |

| Causes of rectal bleeding |
| --- |
| • hemorrhoids<br>• anal fissure<br>• carcinoma (anus, rectum, or colon)<br>• polyps<br>• diverticulitis (including Meckel's diverticulum) but not diverticulosis<br>• colitis (infective, ulcerative, Crohn's, ischemic)<br>• angiodysplasia |

**Fig. 26.3** Causes of rectal bleeding.

or every day? Has the patient seen blood with every bowel movement for a week? Is the patient now feeling tired and short of breath? Determining the frequency of symptoms can help paint a better picture of the illness.

## Tenesmus

Tenesmus is the painful desire to defecate when there is no stool in the rectum. This is due to a lesion in the lumen or wall of the rectum mimicking feces.

# Genitourinary symptoms
## Dysuria

This is discomfort during or after micturition due to urinary tract infection or recent urethral instrumentation (catheter or cystoscope).

## Urine

What does the urine look like?
- Cloudy: infection, precipitated urates or phosphates.
- Frothy: proteinuria.
- Orange: very concentrated urine, bilirubin, rifampicin.
- Red: hematuria, hemoglobinuria, myoglobinuria, rifampicin.
- Black: "blackwater fever" due to *Plasmodium falciparum*.
- Dark on standing: porphyria.

See Chapter 13 for the causes of hematuria and proteinuria.

### Frequency

Increased frequency of micturition can be due to:
- Bladder irritation: infection, stones, tumor.
- Outflow obstruction: prostatic hypertrophy, urethral stricture.
- Neurologic: multiple sclerosis.

*Note:* In polyuria there is an increased volume of urine as well as frequency of micturition.

### Nocturia

This can be due to any of the causes of polyuria (see Chapter 12) and increased frequency.

### Hesitancy

Hesitancy, followed by a poor stream with terminal dribbling, is suggestive of prostatic enlargement.

### Groin pain

This can be associated with renal disease (Chapter 11).

### Incontinence

This can be either urge incontinence (e.g., detrusor instability) or stress incontinence (e.g., weak pelvic musculature following childbirth).

### Menstruation

Determine the pattern of the normal cycle. Then ask about flow (heavy or light), intermenstrual bleeding, postcoital bleeding, or dysmenorrhea.

### Discharge

Vaginal or penile discharge can indicate infection.

## Neurologic symptoms
### Headache

See Chapter 15.

### Dizziness

This can also be unsteadiness (Chapters 18 and 22).

### Limb weakness and sensory loss

These are covered in detail in Chapter 22.

### Syncope

See Chapter 18.

### Disturbed vision

Vision can be affected by lesions of the optic pathway or of the nerves controlling eye movements (3rd, 4th, 6th), or conjugate gaze.

### Disturbed hearing

Ask about deafness, tinnitus, and vertigo (Chapter 24).

### Disturbed smell

Anosmia can result from head injury, nasal polyps, following viral upper respiratory tract infections or frontal lobe tumors.

### Altered speech

There are three types of disordered speech:
- Dysarthria: difficulty in articulating speech, but language content is completely normal.
- Dysphonia: difficulty in voice production.
- Dysphasia: difficulty in understanding or expressing language; caused by lesions affecting the dominant cerebral hemisphere (usually the left).

Fig. 26.4 shows the characteristic speech abnormalities that result from lesions at specific anatomic sites.

## Metabolic and endocrine symptoms

Most symptoms will have been described in previous chapters. In particular, look for a history suggestive of hyper- or hypothyroidism (Fig. 26.5) and diabetes mellitus (Fig. 26.6).

## Musculoskeletal symptoms
### Weakness

This is covered in detail in Chapter 20.

### Pain

Pain can arise in the muscles (Chapter 20), joints (Chapter 16), or bones (Fig. 26.7).

### Stiffness

Stiffness, particularly after inactivity (e.g., early morning stiffness), is a feature of inflammation.

### Joint swelling

This can be caused by infection, inflammation, blood (hemarthrosis), or crystal deposition.

### Disability

How do the symptoms affect lifestyle? This is extremely important in patients with rheumatologic diseases.

| Causes and features of abnormalities of speech arising from lesions at specific anatomical sites | | |
|---|---|---|
| Site of lesion | Causes | Features of speech |
| **dysarthria** | | |
| mouth | ulcers, macroglossia | slurred |
| lower cranial nerve lesions (9th to 12th) | bulbar palsy (stroke, poliomyelitis, motor neuron disease, syringobulbia, malignancy) | nasal quality, slurred associated features such as dysphagia |
| upper cranial nerve lesions (9th to 12th) | pseudobulbar palsy (stroke, motor neuron disease, multiple sclerosis) | spastic speech like "Donald duck" associated features like dysphagia and emotional lability |
| cerebellum | multiple sclerosis, stoke, tumor, hereditary ataxias, alcohol, hypothyroldism | scanning "staccato" speech flow is broken syllables explosive |
| extrapyramidal | parkinsonism | difficulty initiating speech monotonous and slightly slurred |
| toxic | acute alcohol intoxication | slurred |
| **dysphonia** | | |
| neuromuscular junction | myasthenia gravis | weak nasal speech deteriorates on repetition |
| vocal cord disease | tumor, viral laryngitis, tuberculosis syphilis | weak volume, husky quality |
| vocal cord paralysis | recurrent laryngeal nerve palsy (mediastinal carcinoma, intrathoracic surgery or trauma, aortic aneurysm) | weak volume, husky quality |
| **dysphasia** | | |
| Broca's area (inferior frontal gyrus) | infarction, bleeding, space-occupying lesion | expressive dysphasia comprehension intact difficulty in finding appropriate words and so speech non-fluent |
| Wernicke's area (superior temporal gyrus) | infarction, bleeding, space-occupying lesion | receptive dysphasia fluent speech but words are disorganized or unintelligible comprehension impaired |
| frontotemporoparietal lesion | infarction (left middle cerebral artery), bleeding, space-occupying lesion | global dysphasia marked receptive and expressive dysphasia |
| posterior part of superior temporal/inferior parietal lobe | infarction bleeding, space-occupying lesion and raised intracranial pressure, dementia | nominal aphasla unable to name specific objects other aspects of speech preserved |

**Fig. 26.4** Causes and features of abnormalities of speech arising from lesions at specific anatomic sites.

| Differences in the history between hyperthyroidism and hypothyroidism | | |
|---|---|---|
| Symptom | Hyperthyroidism | Hypothyroidism |
| temperature intolerance | heat | cold |
| weight | decreased | increased |
| appetite | increased | decreased |
| bowel habit | diarrhea | constipation |
| psychiatric | anxiety, irritability | poor memory, depression |
| menstruation | oligomenorrhea | menorrhagia |
| other | palpitations, sweating, eye changes, pretibial myxoedema, acropachy | dry skin, brittle hair, arthralgia, myalgia |

**Fig. 26.5** Differences in the history between hyperthyroidism and hypothyroidism.

153

| Symptoms of diabetes mellitus | |
|---|---|
| Mechanism | Symptoms |
| due to hyperglycemia | polyuria<br>polydipsia<br>fatigue<br>blurred vision<br>recurrent infections, e.g. *Candida*<br>weight loss (type I) |
| due to complications | peripheral neuropathy<br>retinopathy<br>vascular disease |

**Fig. 26.6** Symptoms of diabetes mellitus.

| Causes of bone pain | |
|---|---|
| Cause | Example |
| tumor | primary tumor (benign or malignant), metastases |
| infection | osteomyelitis (*Staphylococcus, Hemophilus influenzae, Salmonella,* tuberculosis) |
| fracture | traumatic, pathological |
| metabolic | Paget's disease, osteomalacia |

**Fig. 26.7** Causes of bone pain.

## Skin symptoms
### Rash
The distribution may be very helpful in determining the diagnosis (Chapter 17).

### Pruritus
For the causes of pruritus, see Fig. 26.1.

### Cause
Has there been any recent change in detergents, soap, shampoo, etc.?

## Hematologic symptoms
These can be summarized as follows:
- Symptoms of anemia: low hemoglobin (Chapter 25).
- Recurrent infections: low white cell count.
- Bleeding or bruising: low platelets (Chapter 23). Ask the patient if he or she has noticed any bruises for which they do not recall the cause.

## Medications

Record which drugs the patient is taking and at what dose. Ask if there have been any recent changes in medication. Has the patient had any adverse reactions (e.g., rash, facial swelling, or bronchospasm) to drugs or anesthetics in the past? If so, record exactly what that reaction was, as it may have not been a true allergy (e.g., thrush with broad-spectrum antibiotics).

## Family history

Do any diseases run in the patient's family? Record illnesses in close relatives, including age of death where relevant. Drawing a family tree can be helpful in some patients.

In some conditions, such as adult polycystic disease, the family history should be more detailed as family members may need to be screened and considered for genetic counseling.

## Social history

The importance of this part of the history is to establish how the illness affects the patient's life and how they are coping at home. Ask about:
- Who is at home? If the patient has a partner, is the partner fit and well?
- Does the patient have dependent children? Who is looking after them at the moment?
- What is the home like? If the patient is elderly, is there a caregiver?
- If the patient is disabled, have appropriate modifications been made?
- Does the patient need help with daily tasks, such as washing, dressing, feeding, cleaning, or shopping?

- Is there a nearby relative who helps, or does the patient have meals-on-wheels, home help, or a visiting nurse?
- In a diabetic patient with retinopathy, can he or she see to draw up the insulin and monitor blood sugar? If not, who does it for the patient?
- What is the patient's occupation? Details of past and present occupation can be important (e.g., industrial lung disease).
- Is the patient still able to work despite the current problem?
- Some diagnoses can be particularly important in relation to work, such as truck drivers and epilepsy.
- Does the patient smoke? Smoking is a significant cause of many diseases.
- Alcohol past and present. Record as drinks per week (Fig. 26.8).
- Does the patient use "recreational" drugs? These have health, social, and financial implications.
- Has the patient recently been abroad? The patient

may have been exposed to different infectious agents.
- Does the patient have pets (particularly budgerigars, pigeons, and parrots)?
- Sexual history is not appropriate in every history but may be important (e.g., for hepatitis or HIV).

**units of alcohol**

1 drink = 1 glass of (5OZ) = 1 pint of beer (12OZ) = 1 measure of a short (1.5OZ)

**Fig. 26.8** Drinks of alcohol.

At the end of the history ask two questions:
- "Is there anything else you are worried about or want to tell me?" It is possible that the patient may now feel ready to tell you about their main concern.
- "Is there anything that you are worried this might be?" There is often visible relief when this question is asked and it enables you to address the patient's real feelings about his or her illness.

# 27. Examination of the Patient

When it comes to examining patients, practice really does make perfect. Attendings will be able to tell whether you have examined many patients or not within the first 2 or 3 minutes of seeing you in action! Therefore, take every opportunity you have to rehearse your technique. The more you do it, the more comfortable you will be with the patient; you will use the right words to get the patient to do what you need and, as in history taking, you will stop worrying about what comes next and start thinking about which physical signs are absent or present.

## First things first

There are three essential things you must do whenever you see a patient:

- Introduce yourself, shake hands, and tell the patient what you are going to do (e.g., "Hello Mr Bloggs, my name is Dr.—and I would like to examine your chest").
- Ask the patient to move into the position required for the system you are looking at, expose the area concerned, and then make sure that the patient is comfortable.
- From the moment you first see the patient, try to decide whether the patient looks well or ill. There is plenty of time for you to gain a lot of information while an examiner introduces you to the patient and while the patient undresses and gets on to the examining table. Can the patient walk? Can the patient undo buttons? Is the patient breathless or in pain? Can the patient see? Is the patient deaf? Are there any handy clues around the bed (diabetic drinks, wheelchair, nebulizer, catheter)? Taking time to do this has several advantages: it helps you with the diagnosis, it helps to prioritize your approach as a practicing clinician, and it calms your nerves in clinical examinations.

You will probably find that all clinical teachers will show you a slightly different format for examination technique. The important thing is to develop an approach that you are comfortable with and then keep practicing it until it becomes second nature.

In examinations you will almost always be asked to examine a particular system: "Examine the patient's chest," "What do you notice about the patient's face?" This chapter describes the technique for each system and how to interpret the clinical signs you will find. When, as a doctor, you see a patient, you will need to be able to examine the whole patient and focus your attention on relevant areas.

## Vital signs

The vital signs should always be taken first before the rest of the physical exam of a stable patient.

### Temperature
Fever can accompany numerous infectious, inflammatory, and malignant diseases. If it is associated with an acute infection, the patient often looks flushed, sweaty, and unwell. A swinging fever may be a feature of lymphoma and is known as Pel-Ebstein fever. A fever that recurs every few days is seen in malaria (see Chapter 6).

Hypothermia is a particular problem of the elderly, alcoholics, and patients with dementia. A patient becomes hypothermic when the core temperature falls below 35°C. The causes are summarized in Fig. 27.1

### Blood pressure
- Level: hypertension is a risk factor for vascular disease.
- Lying and standing: postural hypotension.
- Right and left: left may be lower than right in aortic dissection.
- Narrow pulse pressure: aortic stenosis.
- Pulsus paradoxus: exaggerated fall in pulse pressure during inspiration, resulting in a faint or

**Causes of hypothermia**

| Cause | Examples |
|---|---|
| exposure | at home in patients who are immobile on treks or after prolonged water immersion in the young |
| infection | septicemia from any cause |
| endocrine | hypothyroidism, hypopituitarism |
| toxic | alcohol abuse, drug overdose |
| drugs | hypnotics, e.g. benzodiazepines |
| stroke | failure of thermoregulation |

**Fig. 27.1** Causes of hypothermia.

absent pulse in inspiration; caused by severe asthma or cardiac tamponade.

## Pulse

Tachycardia (>100 beats per minute) can indicate stress on the body, e.g., infection, fever, hyperparathyroidism, pain, anxiety. Bradycardia (<60 beats per minute) can signal heart failure, arrhythmias, drug therapy, etc.

## Respiratory rate

Respiratory rate is normally around 14–18 breaths per minute. Decreased rate can indicate excessive sedation, tiring under respiratory distress, central neurologic damage, or neuromuscular disease. Increased respirations are a sign of respiratory distress, anxiety, pain, etc.

## General inspection

It is medical etiquette that all clinical examinations are performed from the right hand side of the patient. The most important thing is to decide is how well or ill the patient is, as described above. Other specific abnormalities should then be looked for.

## Cyanosis

This is a bluish discoloration which is seen when the concentration of reduced (deoxygenated) hemoglobin in the blood rises above 5g/dL. Central cyanosis is seen best in the tongue and lips. It is caused by underlying respiratory or cardiovascular disease. Peripheral cyanosis can be due to either central cyanosis or reduced peripheral circulation, as poorly perfused peripheral tissue will take up oxygen more readily. Reduced peripheral circulation is seen in shock, cold weather, and vascular abnormalities. Cyanosis is seen rarely in anemia but occurs more readily in polycythemia.

## Jaundice

Jaundice is the yellow discoloration of the skin, sclera, and mucous membranes due to serum bilirubin concentrations greater than 30μmol or 2mg/dl, which becomes more obvious at concentrations greater than 50μmol or 3mg/dl. Jaundice can be due to increased bilirubin production, abnormal bilirubin metabolism in the liver, or reduced bilirubin excretion (Chapter 10). Causes of increased conjugated hyperbilirubinemia are genetic (Dubin-Johnson syndrome, Rotor syndrome), biliary obstruction, hepatocellular damage, and intrahepatic cholestasis.

Yellow skin (particularly palms and soles) with normal sclera can be due to carotenemia (excessive consumption of carrots or hypothyroidism). Note that the first place that jaundice can be observed is the frenulum of the tongue.

## Pallor

Generalized pallor can be racial, inherited (albinism), or due to anemia, shock, myxedema, or hypopituitarism. Localized pallor is seen in disruption of the arterial supply, as in Raynaud's phenomenon.

## Hydration

Signs of dehydration include dry mucous membranes, tachycardia, postural hypotension, decreased skin turgor, and altered consciousness level if severe. If the patient is in hospital, hydration status should be monitored more accurately using weight, fluid balance charts, and central venous pressure (if very ill).

Overhydration can sometimes result from the overenthusiastic administration of intravenous fluids, particularly in the elderly. Clinical signs include raised jugulovenous pressure (JVP), pulmonary edema, and peripheral edema.

## Pigmentation

Generalized pigmentation is usually of racial origin but may also arise in hemochromatosis (grayish-bronze), occupational exposure (slate-gray appearance with argyria in silver workers), and with some drugs (slate-gray with amiodarone).

Localized pigmentation is seen in Addison's disease (brown lesions in the buccal mucosa, skin creases, and sites of pressure, e.g., beneath the bra strap), Peutz–Jeghers syndrome (brown lesions around the lips), and neurofibromatosis (*café-au-lait* patches). Obese patients can also have increased local pigmentation, especially in their skin folds.

Localized areas of depigmentation, particularly affecting the back of the hand and neck, are seen in vitiligo, an autoimmune disease of the skin affecting melanocytes. It may be associated with other autoimmune diseases.

## Breast examination

Breast examination should be performed in women who have symptoms of breast disease or when an underlying malignancy is suspected. Do not forget that breast tissue extends into the axillae. It is not always appropriate to examine the breasts, and male students (and doctors) should have a female chaperone when possible.

## Lymphadenopathy

Examine all lymph node sites (Fig. 27.2). Always examine the cervical lymph nodes standing behind the patient. The causes for generalized and localized lymphadenopathy are discussed in Chapter 21. If

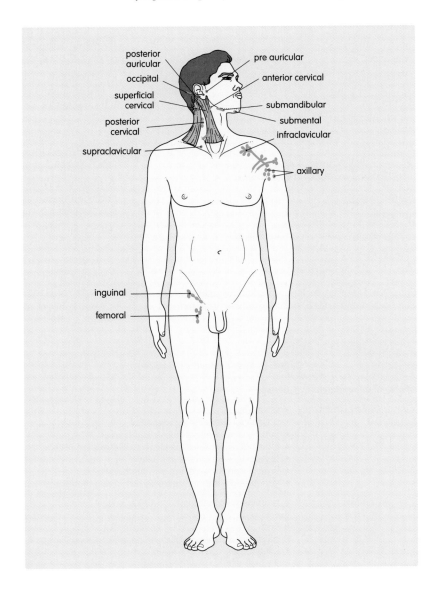

**Fig. 27.2** Examination of lymph node sites.

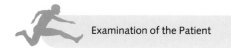

lymphadenopathy is present, pay special attention to examination of the spleen and liver.

## The face and body habitus

When looking at the face and body habitus consider the diagnosis listed in Fig. 27.3.

Whenever you see a lower motor neuron lesion of the facial nerve, look around the ear for a herpes zoster rash (Ramsay Hunt syndrome).

## The neck

When examining the neck, be on the lookout for a thyroid mass or lymphadenopathy. However, do not forget the salivary glands, branchial cyst, pharyngeal pouch, cervical rib, carotid body tumor, and cystic hygroma. Causes of lymphadenopathy are described in Chapter 21. Fig. 27.4 lists the causes of thyroid enlargement.

First, look very carefully at the neck, lifting the hair out of the way if necessary. Look for obvious masses, scars, skin changes, or deformity. If there is a mass in the region of the thyroid gland, ask the patient to take a sip of water into the mouth and then swallow. A goiter will move upward on swallowing. Also ask the patient to open the mouth and then watch as the patient protrudes the tongue forward. A thyroglossal cyst will move upward. If a mass is present, determine the properties shown in Fig. 27.5.

Bruits may be audible in the thyroid gland (thyrotoxicosis) or carotid artery (atheroma). If you find a thyroid mass, you should then assess thyroid status as shown in Fig. 27.6.

| Disease causing typical abnormalities of the face and body habitus | |
|---|---|
| **Disease** | **Examples** |
| endocrine | hypothyroidism, hyperthyroidism, acromegaly, Cushings syndrome |
| metabolic | Paget's disease |
| neuromuscular | Parkinson's disease, myotonia dystrophica, facial nerve palsy, Horner's syndrome |
| connective tissue | SLE, scleroderma, Marfan's syndrome |
| hereditary | Turner's syndrome, Klinefelter's syndrome, achondroplasia |
| cardiovascular | mitral facies |
| physiologic | chloasma of pregnancy |
| hematologic | thalassemia |
| infection | congenital syphilis |

**Fig. 27.3** Diseases causing typical abnormalities of the face and body habitus. (SLE, systemic lupus erythematosus.)

| Causes of thyroid gland enlargement | |
|---|---|
| **Form of enlargement** | **Causes** |
| diffuse enlargement (goiter) | • idiopathic<br>• physiologic—puberty, pregnancy<br>• autoimmune—Hashimoto's and Graves' diseases<br>• iodine deficiency—endemic, e.g., Derbyshire neck<br>• thyroiditis—de Quervain's (viral), Riedel's (autoimmune)<br>• drugs—carbimazole, lithium, sulphonylureas<br>• genetic—dyshormonogenesis (Pendred's syndrorne) |
| solitary nodule | • prominent nodule in multinodular goiter<br>• adenoma<br>• cyst<br>• carcinoma (papillary, follicular, anaplastic, medullary)<br>• lymphoma |

**Fig. 27.4** Causes of thyroid gland enlargement.

Always palpate the neck from behind the patient with the neck slightly flexed to relax the sternocleidomastoid muscles.

If you find no abnormality in the neck, examine the jugulovenous pressure, listen to the carotid artery for bruits, and re-examine for cervical rib.

**Features of any mass**

- site
- shape
- size including upper, lower and lateral limits
- consistency
- tenderness
- fluctuance
- fixation to underlying or overlying structures
- transillumination (where appropriate)
- local lymph node involvement
- bruit

**Fig. 27.5** Features to determine for any mass.

## The hands and associated structures

The hands can provide a wealth of information for the alert clinician. When you are asked to examine the hands, consider the normal structures present and examine them in turn. Where appropriate, go on to examine the functional use of the hand (e.g., undoing a button or picking up a pen). This is particularly important in neurologic abnormalities and destructive arthritides (e.g., rheumatoid arthritis).

### Hands

- Blue: peripheral cyanosis.
- Pallor: anemia (skin creases) and Raynaud's phenomenon.
- Pigmentation: Addison's disease (skin creases).
- Depigmentation: vitiligo.
- Palmar erythema (Fig. 27.7).

### Nails

- Koilonychia: spoon-shaped nails seen in iron deficiency.
- Leukonychia: white nails due to hypoalbuminemia (Fig. 27.8).
- Clubbing: an increase in angle between nail-plate and fold to over 180°. The causes are shown in Fig. 27.9.
- Splinter hemorrhages: terminal lesions usually due to trauma, proximal lesions found in subacute bacterial endocarditis (SBE), and vasculitis.

| Examination of thyroid status | | |
|---|---|---|
| | **Hyperthyroidism** | **Hypothyroidism** |
| mood | irritability, anxiety | depression, slowness |
| weight | thinness | overweight |
| hands | fine tremor, palmar erythema, sweaty palms, acropachy | puffiness, anemia, Tinel's sign (carpal tunnel syndrome) |
| pulse | tachycardia, atrial fibrillation | bradycardia |
| face | lid lag, lid retraction, exophthalmos, ophthalmoplegia, chemosis | loss of outer third of eyebrow, puffy eyes, "toad-like" facies, xanthelasmata |
| skin | pretibial myxedema (shins) | dry, thin hair |
| neuromuscular | proximal myopathy | delayed ankle jerks, cerebellar signs |

**Fig. 27.6** Examination of thyroid status.

| Causes of palmar erythema | |
|---|---|
| Cause | Example |
| physiologic | pregnancy<br>puberty<br>familial |
| pathologic | chronic liver disease<br>rheumatoid arthritis<br>thyrotoxicosis<br>oral contraceptive pill<br>polycythemia |

**Fig. 27.7** Causes of palmar erythema.

| Causes of hypoalbuminemia | |
|---|---|
| Causes | Examples |
| reduced intake | malnutrition |
| reduced synthesis | liver disease |
| increased utilization | chronic illness |
| increased loss | nephrotic syndrome (kidneys)<br>protein-losing enteropathy (gut)<br>severe burns (skin) |

**Fig. 27.8** Causes of hypoalbuminemia.

- Quincke's sign: capillary pulsation in the nail-bed due to aortic regurgitation.
- Beau's lines: horizontal grooves in the nails caused by temporary arrest of nail growth due to acute severe illness.
- Onycholysis: separation of the nail from the nail-bed due to psoriasis, trauma, fungal infections, and hyperthyroidism.
- Yellow nails: yellow nail syndrome with lymphatic hypoplasia (peripheral edema and pleural effusions).
- Half-and-half nails where the proximal nail is white and the distal nail is brown or red due to chronic renal failure.

## Tendons
- Xanthomata: hypercholesterolemia.
- Dupuytren's contractures (thickening of the palmar fascia): associated with alcoholic liver disease, epileptics treated with phenytoin, vibrating tools, and familial and idiopathic causes.

| Causes of clubbing | |
|---|---|
| Causes | Examples |
| respiratory | tumor: bronchial carcinoma, mesothelioma<br>chronic suppuration: abscess, bronchiectasis, empyema<br>fibrosis: from any cause<br>vascular: arteriovenous malformation |
| cardiovascular | congenital cyanotic heart disease<br>subacute bacterial endocarditis<br>atrial myxoma |
| gastrointestinal | inflammatory bowel disease<br>lymphoma<br>cirrhosis |
| endocrine | thyrotoxicosis (acropachy) |
| familial | autosomal dominant |

**Fig. 27.9** Causes of clubbing.

## Joints
- Destructive arthropathy: RA, psoriasis, gout.
- Heberden's nodes: osteophytes of the distal interphalangeal joints.
- Bouchard's nodes: osteophytes of the proximal interphalangeal joints.

## Muscles
- Localized wasting: ulnar or median nerve lesions.
- Generalized wasting: $T_1$ lesion (brachial plexus, root) or RA.
- Myotonia: failure to relax after voluntary contraction seen in myotonia dystrophica.

## Other signs
- Sclerodactyly (tightening of the skin causing tapering of the fingers): look also for calcinosis, Raynaud's phenomenon, esophageal dysmotility (ask the patient about difficulty on swallowing), and telangiectasia—hence **CREST** syndrome (where the **S** stands for sclerodactyly).
- Spade hands: acromegaly.
- Asterixis: a coarse flapping tremor seen when the hand is oustretched with the wrist extended and fingers apart. It is caused by metabolic encephalopathy (e.g., liver failure, carbon dioxide retention, uremia).

When examining the hands always look at the elbows for a psoriatic rash, rheumatoid nodules, or gouty tophi.

## The cardiovascular system

### General inspection
- Does the patient look well or ill?
- Is the patient lying flat?
- Is the patient cachectic (cardiac cachexia)?
- Does the patient have Marfan's syndrome (aortic regurgitation, mitral regurgitation) or Down's syndrome (atrial septal defect)?

### Position
Help the patient to adopt a comfortable position at 45° with the chest exposed. In women cover the chest until ready to examine the precordium.

### Hands
- Clubbing: SBE and congenital cyanotic heart disease.
- Cyanosis: peripheral vasoconstriction, pulmonary edema, and right-to-left shunt.
- Splinter hemorrhages: SBE.
- Janeway's lesions: nontender macules in the palms due to SBE.
- Osler's nodes: painful nodules on the pulps of the fingers due to SBE.
- Quincke's sign: aortic regurgitation.
- Xanthomata: hypercholesterolemia—vascular disease.

### Radial pulse
- Rate: normally between 60 and 100 beats per minute (see Chapter 3).
- Rhythm: regular or irregular (Chapter 3).
- Radioradial delay: dissecting thoracic aortic aneurysm.
- Radiofemoral delay: coarctation of the aorta.
- Character: best determined by palpation of a larger artery (e.g., brachial or carotid arteries).

### Blood pressure
- Level: hypertension is a risk factor for vascular disease.
- Lying and standing: postural hypotension.

- Right and left: left may be lower than right in aortic dissection.
- Wide pulse pressure: in the elderly and aortic regurgitation.
- Narrow pulse pressure: aortic stenosis.
- Pulsus paradoxus: exaggerated fall in pulse pressure during inspiration resulting in a faint or absent pulse in inspiration; caused by severe asthma or cardiac tamponade.

### Brachial and carotid artery
- Character: collapsing (Fig. 27.10), slow-rising (aortic stenosis), bisferiens (mixed aortic valve disease), alternans (severe left ventricular failure), and jerky (hypertrophic obstructive cardiomyopathy).
- Corrigan's sign: prominent carotid pulsation due to aortic regurgitation.

When looking at the JVP, concentrate on the a and v waves. These are the easiest and most reliable to detect.

When assessing JVP, the patient should be at 45° with their head rested on a pillow (this relaxes the sternocleidomastoid muscles). Pulsation should be up to 3cm above the sternal angle (8cm above right atrium). Differences between JVP and carotid pulsation in normal subjects are shown in Fig. 27.11. JVP acts as a manometer for right atrial pressure and

| Causes of a collapsing pulse | |
|---|---|
| Causes | Examples |
| physiologic | elderly<br>pregnancy<br>exercise |
| pathologic | aortic regurgitation<br>patent ductus arteriosus<br>fever<br>thyrotoxicosis<br>anemia<br>arteriovenous shunts |

**Fig. 27.10** Causes of a collapsing pulse.

**Fig. 27.11** Differences between jugulovenous pulsation (JVP) and carotid pulsation.

| Differences between JVP and carotid pulsation | | |
|---|---|---|
| Feature | Carotid pulsation | JVP |
| palpable | yes | no |
| number of visible peaks | one | two |
| occlusion by gentle pressure | no | yes (fills from above) |
| sitting upright | no change | height falls |
| lying flat | no change | height rises |
| gentle pressure on liver | no change | height rises (hepatojugular reflex) |
| deep inspiration | no change | height falls |

| Causes of a raised JVP |
|---|
| • right ventricular failure |
| • volume overload (overenthusiastic intravenous fluids) |
| • superior vena caval obstruction (JVP is nonpulsatile) |
| • tricuspid valve disease (stenosis and regurgitation) |
| • pericardial effusion |
| • constrictive pericarditis |

**Fig. 27.12** Causes of a raised jugulovenous pressure (JVP).

is raised when right atrial pressure is raised (Fig. 27.12). Abnormalities in the waveform result from specific underlying pathologies (Fig. 27.13).

## Face

- Central cyanosis: pulmonary edema and right-to-left shunt.
- Anemia: possible high output cardiac failure.
- Malar flush: pulmonary hypertension due to mitral valve disease.
- Jaundice: hemolysis due to mechanical valves.
- Xanthelasmata: hypercholesterolemia (vascular disease).
- Teeth: source in bacterial endocarditis.
- Mouth: high-arched palate in Marfan's syndrome.
- De Musset's sign: head nodding due to aortic regurgitation.
- Roth's spots in the retina: bacterial endocarditis.

## Precordium

Look for scars and deformities, including:

- Sternotomy scar: arterial bypass grafts and valve replacements.
- Mitral valvotomy scar under the left breast: always look for it as it indicates a previously closed mitral valvotomy.
- Skeletal deformities—can cause an ejection systolic flow murmur.

## Point of maximal impulse

The point of maximal impulse (PMI) should be at the mid-clavicular line in the fifth left intercostal space.

- Lateral displacement: left or severe right ventricular dilatation.
- Impalpable: obesity, pleural effusion, pericardial effusion, chronic obstructive airways disease, and dextrocardia (palpable on the right!).
- Tapping: mitral stenosis (palpable first heart sound).
- Heaving: pressure overload in aortic stenosis or hypertension.
- Thrusting: volume overload in aortic regurgitation, pulmonary regurgitation (ventricle usually markedly displaced); diffuse: left ventricular dilatation, double impulse: left ventricular aneurysm (uncommon).

## Palpation

Parasternal heave is caused by the enlargement or hypertrophy of the left atrium or right ventricle.

A thrill is a palpable murmur and indicates significant valve disease; it can be systolic or diastolic. Palpate in all valve areas (Fig. 27.14).

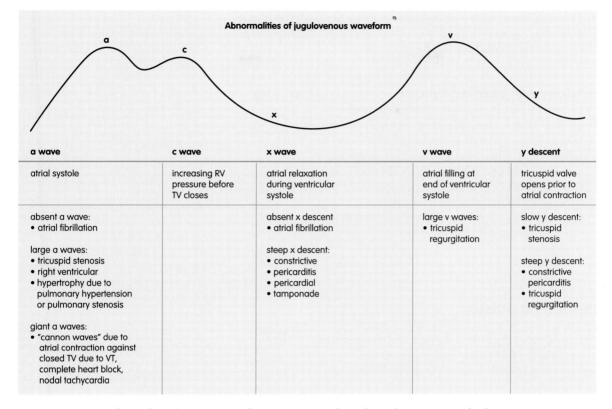

**Abnormalities of jugulovenous waveform**

| a wave | c wave | x wave | v wave | y descent |
|---|---|---|---|---|
| atrial systole | increasing RV pressure before TV closes | atrial relaxation during ventricular systole | atrial filling at end of ventricular systole | tricuspid valve opens prior to atrial contraction |
| absent a wave:<br>• atrial fibrillation<br><br>large a waves:<br>• tricuspid stenosis<br>• right ventricular<br>• hypertrophy due to pulmonary hypertension or pulmonary stenosis<br><br>giant a waves:<br>• "cannon waves" due to atrial contraction against closed TV due to VT, complete heart block, nodal tachycardia | | absent x descent<br>• atrial fibrillation<br><br>steep x descent:<br>• constrictive<br>• pericarditis<br>• pericardial<br>• tamponade | large v waves:<br>• tricuspid regurgitation | slow y descent:<br>• tricuspid stenosis<br><br>steep y descent:<br>• constrictive pericarditis<br>• tricuspid regurgitation |

**Fig. 27.13** Abnormalities of jugulovenous waveform. (VT, ventricular tachycardia; TV, tricupsid valve.)

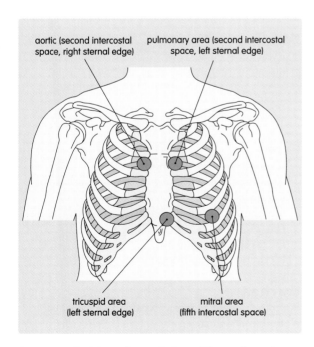

aortic (second intercostal space, right sternal edge)

pulmonary area (second intercostal space, left sternal edge)

tricuspid area (left sternal edge)

mitral area (fifth intercostal space)

**Fig. 27.14** Positions of auscultation of the cardiac valves.

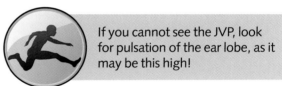

If you cannot see the JVP, look for pulsation of the ear lobe, as it may be this high!

## Auscultation
- Listen in all four areas with the bell and diaphragm (see Fig. 27.14).
- Roll the patient to the left hand side to listen with the bell at the axilla for mitral stenosis.
- Sit the patient forward to listen with the diaphragm at the left sternal edge in expiration for aortic regurgitation.
- Listen to the first and second sounds, then for third and fourth sounds.
- Are there any murmurs? (See Chapter 4.)
- Listen for additional sounds including opening snap, ejection click, pericardial knock or rub, and mechanical valves.

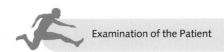

- Time any abnormalities against the carotid pulsation.
- Listen to the carotid arteries for bruits (atheroma) or radiation of aortic stenotic murmur.

### Evidence of cardiac failure

- Examine lung bases for pulmonary edema and pleural effusions indicating left ventricular failure.
- Sacral edema occurs in right ventricular failure. Remember to check for this if you are examining a patient who has been lying in bed. The sacral area will be most dependent in this position; therefore, the edema will accumulate there.
- Hepatomegaly occurs in right ventricular failure; it will be pulsatile if there is tricuspid regurgitation.
- Pitting edema occurs in right ventricular failure and is almost always bilateral.

### Peripheral pulses

Pulses in the legs may be diminished in peripheral vascular disease. Systolic and diastolic murmurs may be heard in the femoral arteries due to aortic regurgitation (pistol shots and Duroziez's sign).

 There are four main features of Horner's syndrome. Remember that everything "gets smaller."

## The respiratory system

### General inspection

- Does the patient look well or ill? Is the patient alert?
- Cachexia: underlying malignancy.
- Sputum cup: examine.
- Nebulizer: bronchospasm.
- Distress: breathless at rest and moving around in the bed.
- Voice: hoarse in bronchial carcinoma (recurrent laryngeal nerve palsy).
- Lymphadenopathy: supraclavicular, cervical, and axillary.
- Respiratory rate: normally around 14–18 breaths per minute.

### Position

Help the patient to adopt a comfortable position at 45° with the chest exposed. In women cover the chest until you are ready to examine it.

### Hands

- Clubbing: malignancy, fibrosis, and chronic suppuration.
- Cyanosis: peripheral vasoconstriction and respiratory failure.
- Wasting of small muscles: infiltration of $T_1$ by bronchial neoplasm.
- Nicotine-stained fingers: increased likelihood of malignancy and obstructive airways disease.
- Asterixis: carbon dioxide retention.
- Hypertrophic pulmonary osteoarthropathy: swelling and pain, particularly in wrists or ankles, due to bronchial carcinoma (particularly squamous cell).

### Pulse

- Tachycardia: severe respiratory disease (e.g., acute asthma or pneumonia).
- Bounding: carbon dioxide retention.
- Atrial fibrillation: malignancy and pneumonia.

### Blood pressure

Pulsus paradoxus is seen in severe acute asthma.

### JVP

- Right ventricular failure: chronic respiratory disease with pulmonary hypertension.
- Superior vena caval obstruction: bronchial carcinoma.
- Large a waves: cor pulmonale.

### Face

- Central cyanosis: respiratory failure.
- Anemia: chronic respiratory disease, particularly malignancy.
- Horner's syndrome: bronchial malignancy (Fig. 27.15).
- Fine tremor: β-agonists.
- Plethoric facies: polycythemia.

### Trachea

Warn the patient before you palpate the trachea! Note the following:
- Tracheal deviation (Fig. 27.16).
- Feel for tracheal tug in acute respiratory distress.

| Features of Horner's syndrome |
|---|
| **Ipsilateral**<br>• partial ptosis<br>• enophthalmos<br>• pupillary constriction<br>• reduced sweating |

**Fig. 27.15** Features of Horner's syndrome. These result from interruption of the sympathetic innervation of the eye.

| Causes of tracheal deviation | |
|---|---|
| **Towards lesion** | **Away from lesion** |
| collapse | tension pneumothorax |
| apical fibrosis | massive pleural effusion |
| pneumonectomy | large mass (e.g. thyroid) |

**Fig. 27.16** Causes of tracheal deviation.

- The distance from the cricoid cartilage to the suprasternal notch should be three to four finger breadths—this distance reduces in hyperinflation.
- Check the position of the apex beat to confirm mediastinal shift.

## Inspection

Perform inspection, palpation, percussion, and auscultation on the front of the chest first. Then sit the patient forward, palpate for lymphadenopathy, and then repeat the examination on the back of the chest. Typical patterns of respiratory abnormalities are shown in Fig. 27.17.

On inspecting the chest assess the following:
- Respiration: use of accessory muscles (respiratory distress).
- Recession: intercostal and subcostal (respiratory distress).
- Scars: including previous surgery and chest drains.
- Deformity: in particular Harrison's sulci (indrawn costal margins) and pectus carinatum due to severe childhood asthma; barrel chest is seen in long-standing airways obstruction due to hyperinflation.
- Radiotherapy: markings or skin changes indicate previous treatment for underlying malignancy.

## Expansion
- Ask the patient to take a deep breath in and out and watch closely.
- Place your hand firmly on the chest laterally with fingers apart and thumbs lifted off the chest wall touching each other.
- The lungs should expand by at least 5 cm on deep inspiration.
- Any significant pulmonary disease will reduce expansion.

- In unilateral disease, the affected side will move less than the other.
- Note any chest wall tenderness, which is usually caused by musculoskeletal abnormalities.

## Vocal fremitus
Ask the patient to say "99" and palpate with the ulnar border of the hand. Increased vocal fremitus indicates consolidation (sometimes fibrosis and above pleural effusion); decreased indicates pleural effusion or collapse.

## Percussion
Compare one side with the other and remember the axillae. The following signs are important:
- Hyperresonant: pneumothorax.
- Dull: solid organ (liver or heart), consolidation, collapse, pleural thickening, peripheral tumors, and fibrosis.
- Stony dull: pleural effusion.

## Auscultation
- Vesicular breath sounds: these are normal.
- Bronchial breathing: consolidation (sometimes fibrosis and above pleural effusion).
- Wheeze: airways obstruction (polyphonic or generalized), lung cancer (monophonic or localized), and cardiac failure.
- Fine crackles: pulmonary fibrosis.
- Medium crackles: cardiac failure.
- Coarse crackles: infection.
- Absent breath sounds: pleural effusion.
- Pleural rub: pleural irritation due to pneumonia or pulmonary embolus.
- Click: during systole this is occasionally heard in pneumothorax (Hamman's sign).
- Whispering pectoriloquy: consolidation (sometimes fibrosis and above pleural effusion).

**Findings on clinical examination of common respiratory diseases**

| Pathology | General signs | Tracheal deviation | Palpation | Percussion note | Breath sounds | Causes |
|---|---|---|---|---|---|---|
| pneumothorax | tachycardia and hypotension in tension pneumothorax | away from affected side if tension | reduced expansion, reduced VF | normal or hyperresonant | reduced or absent | spontaneous (particularly tall healthy males and Marfan's syndrome), trauma, airways obstruction, cystic fibrosis, pulmonary abscess |
| consolidation | fever, tachycardia | none | reduced expansion, increased VF | dull | bronchial breathing, inspiratory crepitations | pneumococcus, Hemophilus influenzae, Staphylococcus aureus, Klebsiella, Pseudomonas, Mycoplasma, Legionella, influenza type A, Aspergillus |
| pleural effusion | | away from affected side if large | reduced expansion, reduced VF | stony dull | absent | if any of the 3 criteria below are met, the fluid is an exudate:<br>• pleural fluid protein/serum protein ration >0.5<br>• pleural fluid LDH/serum LDH ratio >0.6<br>• pleural LDH $>2/3$ the upper limits of normal of the serum LDH<br>transudate:<br>  cardiac failure, liver failure, nephrotic syndrome, Meigs' syndrome, myxedema<br>exudate:<br>  malignancy, pneumonia, pulmonary embolus, rheumatoid arthritis, SLE, subphrenic abscess, pancreatitis, trauma, Dressler's syndrome |
| collapse | | towards affected side | reduced expansion, reduced VF | dull | reduced or absent | foreign body or mucus plugs (asthma, aspergillosis) within the bronchial lumen, bronchial carcinoma arising from the bronchus itself, extrinsic compression by enlarged lymph nodes (malignancy, tuberculosis) |
| fibrosis | clubbing | towards affected side if apical disease | reduced expansion, increased VF | normal or dull | fine inspiratory crepitations | cryptogenic fibrosing alveolitis, sarcoidosis, drugs (amiodarone, bleomycin), radiation, inhalation of dusts (asbestos, coal), extrinsic allergic alveolitis, ankylosing spondylitis, rheumatoid arthritis, systemic sclerosis, tuberculosis |
| bronchiectasis | clubbing, purulent sputum | normal | normal or reduced expansion, normal or increased VF | normal or dull | coarse inspiratory crepitations, occasional polyphonic wheeze | congenital (cystic fibrosis, Kartagener's syndrome, hypogammoglobulinemia), idiopathic, bronchial obstruction (foreign body, carcinoma, lymphadenopathy), infection (childhood measles or whooping cough, tuberculosis, aspergillosis, postpneumonia) |
| bronchospasm | hyperexpanded chest, tremor, Harrison's sulci, pectus excavatum | normal | reduced expansion, normal VF | normal, hyperresonant over bullae, reduced liver dullness | polyphonic wheeze, crackles in chronic obstructive airways disease | asthma, chronic bronchitis, emphysema (cardiac failure—"cardiac asthma") |

**Fig. 27.17** Findings on clinical examination of common respiratory diseases. (VF, vocal fremitus.)

## Other signs

- The liver may be palpable if it is pushed down by hyperexpanded lungs (ptosis), enlarged due to right ventricular failure, or if there are metastases from a bronchial carcinoma.
- Pitting edema indicates right ventricular failure.
- Peak flow should be assessed if available.

The upper border of the liver is normally at the sixth rib in the right midclavicular line. If the percussion note remains resonant below this, the lungs are hyperinflated.

- Bullae (blisters): porphyria cutanea tarda due to alcoholic liver disease.

## Arms

- Scratch marks: obstructive jaundice (particularly primary biliary cirrhosis) and lymphoma.
- Muscle wasting: proximal myopathy due to alcohol, steroid excess, or underlying malignancy (paraneoplastic).
- Bruising: hepatic impairment.

Always look at the patient's face when palpating the abdomen—it will often tell you a lot!

## The abdomen

### General inspection

- Appearance: does the patient look well or ill?
- Pain.
- Patient's position: think of peritonism if very still, appendicitis (psoas irritation) if right knee flexed, and renal colic if rolling around in agony.
- Cachexia: chronic disease, particularly malignancy.
- Drowsy: encephalopathy (hepatic or uremia).
- Hydration.

### Position

Ask the patient if he or she is comfortable lying flat. If so, help the patient to do this with the head on one pillow and arms relaxed by the sides. Expose from below the breasts (in women) or the nipples (in men) down to the symphysis pubis.

### Hands

- Clubbing: cirrhosis, inflammatory bowel disease and gastrointestinal lymphoma.
- Leukonychia: liver failure, nephrotic syndrome, protein-losing enteropathy.
- Koilonychia: chronic iron deficiency, consider occult neoplasm particularly in the stomach and caecum.
- Palmar erythema: cirrhosis.
- Asterixis: hepatic encephalopathy and uremia.
- Dupuytren's contracture: alcoholic liver disease.
- Half-and-half nails: renal failure.

### Face

- Jaundice: prehepatic, hepatic, or posthepatic (Chapter 10).
- Anemia: from any cause (Chapter 25).
- Xanthelasmata: hypercholesterolemia (primary biliary cirrhosis or nephrotic syndrome).
- Kayser-Fleischer rings: Wilson's disease (best seen by slit-lamp examination).

### Mouth

- Hydration.
- Glossitis: iron deficiency and megaloblastic anemia.
- Pigmentation: Addison's disease and Peutz-Jeghers syndrome.
- Telangiectasia: hereditary hemorrhagic telangiectasia (Osler-Weber-Rendu syndrome).
- Crohn's disease: lip swelling and mucosal ulceration.
- Gingival hypertrophy (Fig. 27.18).

### Neck

Look for left supraclavicular lymphadenopathy—caused by metastasis from underlying gastrointestinal carcinoma (Virchow's node or Troisier's sign).

### Trunk

Spider nevi arise in the distribution of the superior vena cava—five or more suggest underlying chronic liver disease, pregnancy, or hyperthyroidism.

Gynecomastia and sexual hair loss indicates chronic liver disease.

**Causes of gingival hypertrophy**

| Cause | Examples |
|---|---|
| acute myeloid leukemia | monocytic, myelomonocytic |
| drugs | cyclosporin, phenytoin, nifedipine |
| infection | gingivitis |
| scurvy | see p. 130 |
| physiologic | pregnancy |

**Fig. 27.18** Causes of gingival hypertrophy.

**Causes of generalized abdominal swelling**

| Cause | Etiology |
|---|---|
| fluid | ascites |
| feces | constipation |
| fetus | pregnancy |
| flatus | bowel obstruction |
| fat | obesity |
| fibroids | and any other tumor or organomegaly |

**Fig. 27.19** Causes of generalized abdominal swelling.

**Causes of hepatomegaly**

| Cause | Examples |
|---|---|
| cirrhosis | any cause, particularly primary biliary cirrhosis and hemochromatosis |
| tumor | benign, malignant, primary (hepatocellular carcinoma), and metastases |
| venous congestion | right ventricular failure, Budd–Chiari syndrome, tricuspid stenosis |
| infection | viral hepatitis, abscess, syphilis, Well's disease, hydatid disease |
| cysts | polycystic disease |
| hematologic | lymphoproliferative disease, myeloproliferative disease |
| metabolic | storage diseases, amyloidosis |
| inflammatory | sarcoidosis |

**Fig. 27.20** Causes of hepatomegaly. Remember the "Cs" for common causes: **c**irrhosis, **c**arcinoma, and **c**ardiac failure. Note that the liver may appear large in the absence of true hepatomegaly when it is pushed down by a hyperinflated lung (as in acute asthma or chronic obstructive airways disease) and when a Riedel's lobe is present (normal anatomical variation of the right hepatic lobe).

## Inspection

Ask the patient to breathe in and then out—watch carefully for the following:

- Scars: previous surgery or trauma. Be on the lookout for laparoscopy scars that are not as obvious.
- Distention (Fig. 27.19).
- Obvious mass: including movement with respiration.
- Bruising: Cullen's (paraumbilical) and Grey Turner's (flanks) signs in acute pancreatitis.
- Dilated veins: inferior vena cava (venous flow is upwards).
- Caput Medusae: portal hypertension (venous flow is away from the umbilicus).
- Pulsation: abdominal aortic aneurysm.
- Striae: pregnancy or Cushing's syndrome.
- Node: umbilical nodule (Sister Mary Joseph's nodule) is a metastasis from intra-abdominal malignancy.
- Peristalsis: if visible this indicates an obstruction, though it may be normal in a thin or elderly patient.

## Palpation

Before you touch the patient, ask if he or she is tender anywhere and start palpation away from that area. Feel gently in each of the four quadrants, noting tenderness or masses. Then feel more deeply in each quadrant to determine the characteristics of any mass found (see Fig. 27.5).

If a mass is present, consider what structures normally lie at that site and what disease processes might affect that structure (Chapter 11). Next, palpate for hepatomegaly and splenomegaly, starting in the right iliac fossa. Examine for renal masses by bimanual palpation. If hepatomegaly or splenomegaly is present, comment on consistency and size in centimeters (not finger breadths) beneath the costal margin. The causes of hepatomegaly are shown in Fig. 27.20; the causes of splenomegaly are discussed in detail in Chapter 21.

Do not forget the distinguishing features of the spleen and kidney (see Fig. 21.2); the causes of a renal mass are summarized in Fig. 27.21.

Finally, palpate for abdominal aortic aneurysm and examine the groin for lymphadenopathy and hernias.

## Percussion

Always percuss from resonance to dullness. Use percussion to determine the size of the liver and spleen starting at the chest, moving inferiorly. Percuss over any masses to determine their consistency. Always assess for ascites by looking for a fluid thrill and shifting dullness. Fig. 27.22 summarizes the causes of ascites.

| Causes of unilateral and bilateral palpable kidneys | |
| --- | --- |
| Type | Cause |
| unilateral | tumor (hypernephroma, nephroblastoma) hydronephrosis, pyonephrosis hypertrophy of single functioning kidney, perinephric abscess or hematoma, polycystic disease (only one kidney palpable) |
| bilateral | polycystic kidneys (autosomal dominant in adults, autosomal recessive in children) amyloidosis bilateral hydronephrosis |

**Fig. 27.21** Causes of unilateral and bilateral palpable kidneys.

| Causes of ascites | |
| --- | --- |
| Type | Cause |
| transudate (portal hypertension) serum-ascites albumin gradient >1.1 | cardiac failure liver failure nephrotic syndrome Meigs' syndrome myxedema constrictive pericarditis (rare) |
| exudate (capillary permeability abnormality) serum-ascites albumin gradient <1.1 | intra-abdominal malignancy cirrhosis with portal hypertension infection (tuberculosis, perforation, spontaneous) pancreatitis Budd–Chiari syndrome lymphatic obstruction (chylous) |

**Fig. 27.22** Causes of ascites.

## Auscultation

- Bowel sounds may be normal, increased, or decreased: increased in bowel obstruction (high-pitched and tinkling) and absent in the ileus (functional motor paralysis of the bowel) due to any cause (Fig. 27.23).
- Arterial bruits: may be heard over stenosed vessels such as renal arteries.
- Venous hum in the epigastrium: portal hypertension.
- Friction rubs: may rarely be heard over the liver (infarction, tumor, or gonococcal perihepatitis) or spleen (infarction).
- The "scratch test" can be used to estimate liver and spleen size. By placing the stethoscope over the liver, then lightly scratching the skin above the liver, you can find the margins because of differences in sound.
- Succussion splash: pyloric stenosis.

## Other signs

- Look at the legs for pitting edema (Fig. 27.24).
- When seeing patients as a practicing clinician, always consider whether examination of genitalia or regal examinations are appropriate. In some circumstances they are essential, such as rectal bleeding, iron deficiency, or change in bowel habit.
- If there is hepatosplenomegaly, go on to examine all lymph node sites, bearing in mind lymphoproliferative disorders, sarcoidosis, and viruses such as Epstein-Barr virus.

| Causes of ileus |
| --- |
| • following intra-abdominal surgery where the gut has been handled |
| • peritonitis |
| • pancreatitis |
| • hypokalemia |
| • uremia |
| • diabetic ketoacidosis |
| • intra-abdominal hemorrhage |
| • retroperitoneal hematoma |
| • retroperitoneal trauma, e.g. surgery for aortic aneurysm |
| • anticholinergic drugs |

**Fig. 27.23** Causes of ileus.

| Causes of lower limb edema | |
|---|---|
| **Cause** | **Examples** |
| pitting | unilateral:<br>    deep venous thrombosis<br>    unilateral compression of veins (nodes,<br>      tumor)<br>bilateral:<br>    right ventricular failure<br>    tricuspid stenosis<br>    constrictive pericarditis<br>    hepatic failure<br>    nephrotic syndrome<br>    protein-losing enteropathy<br>    inferior vena cava obstruction<br>      (thrombosis, nodes, tumor)<br>    immobility<br>    kwashiorkor |
| lymphatic<br>(non-pitting) | obstruction by nodes, tumor or infection<br>    (filariasis)<br>congenital hypoplasia (Milroy's disease)<br>myxedema |

**Fig. 27.24** Causes of lower limb edema.

## The nervous system

Although it is true that neuroanatomy is complicated and many different diseases can affect each part, the end result is a limited repertoire of patterns of signs. The best approach is to identify which signs are present using a well-rehearsed technique and consider where the lesion is likely to be. You can then think of which diseases affect that part of the nervous system and look for additional evidence to support the diagnosis.

Chapter 22 has discussed in detail the clinical signs and common diseases associated with different parts of the nervous system. This section covers a practical approach to the examination technique itself. It is particularly important to practice this routine over and over again as it is the most difficult to perform competently and will be all the more impressive if you can do it well!

### General inspection
- Appearance: does the patient look well or ill?
- Level of consciousness: is the patient conscious or unconscious?

- Age: a young patient is more likely to have multiple sclerosis or an inherited disease; an elderly patient is more likely to have had a stroke.
- General clues: is there a wheelchair (the problem also affects the legs) or diabetic drinks (peripheral neuropathy or stroke)?
- Posture: how is the patient sitting? Is the patient leaning towards one side (hemiparesis)? Is there a tremor at rest (parkinsonism)?
- Speech: when the patient speaks does the speech sound normal? (See Fig. 26.4.)

## Cranial nerves
Features and examinations of the cranial nerves include the following.

### 1st cranial nerve (olfactory)
- Sensory only.
- This is not routinely tested, but ask if the patient has noticed anything abnormal about the sense of smell.
- Sense of smell can be tested using bottles containing essences, though this test is rarely performed. (Note: Ammonia should not be used because it also stimulates the trigeminal nerve).
- Anosmia can result from head injury (fracture of the cribriform plate), upper respiratory tract infection, tumor (olfactory groove meningioma or glioma), or Kallmann's syndrome (anosmia with hypogonadotrophic hypogonadism).

### 2nd cranial nerve (optic)
- Sensory only.
- Visual acuity: ask the patient to read some print or Snellen's chart (with glasses if normally worn). Test each eye separately. Any lesion from the cornea, lens, retina, optic nerve, optic chiasm, optic radiation, or occipital cortex can result in reduced acuity.
- Visual fields: test each eye individually. Make sure your eyes are on the same level as the patient's. Move your fingers from beyond your visual field inwards and ask the patient to tell you when they can see them. Check each quadrant. Use a red hat pin to determine the blind spot. Typical field defects are shown in Fig. 27.25. Vision can be formally assessed using perimetry.

| Visual field defects | | |
|---|---|---|
| **Defect** | **Site of lesion** | **Causes** |
| tunnel vision | retina | glaucoma, retinitis pigmentosa, laser therapy for diabetic retinopathy |
| enlarged blind spot | optic nerve | papilledema (due to any cause) |
| central scotoma | macular, optic nerve | optic atrophy, optic neuritis, retinal disease affecting macula |
| monocular visual loss | eye, optic nerve | optic nerve infarction, optic neuritis, optic atrophy, extensive retinal disease |
| bitemporal hemianopia | optic chiasm | pituitary tumor, craniopharyngioma, sella meningioma |
| quadrantic hemianopia | temporal lobe (superior) parietal lobe (inferior) | stroke, tumor |
| homonymous hemianopia | occipital cortex, optic tract | stroke, tumor |

**Fig. 27.25** Visual field defects.

- Fundoscopy: common abnormalities on fundoscopy are papilloedema (Fig. 27.26), optic atrophy (Fig. 27.27), diabetic retinopathy (Fig. 27.28), hypertensive retinopathy, and retinitis pigmentosa. Retinitis pigmentosa is associated with Refsum's disease, hereditary ataxias, abetalipoproteinemias, Laurence-Moon-Biedl syndrome, and mitochondrial cytopathies.

### 3rd, 4th, and 6th cranial nerves
- Control the eye's movements.
- Ask the patient to follow your finger with both eyes and tell you if he or she "sees double."
- Look for nystagmus and failure of eye movements.
- Assess conjugate gaze by asking the patient to look at your hand and then to a finger on your other hand, and then from one to the other as quickly as possible. If there is an internuclear ophthalmoplegia (a lesion in the medial longitudinal fasciculus) there will be slow movement in the adducting eye and nystagmus in the abducting eye. Internuclear ophthalmoplegia is usually caused by multiple sclerosis but may occasionally result from vascular lesions.
- Diplopia in all directions of gaze may result from myasthenia gravis or disease in the surrounding tissue of eye, such as Graves' disease, tumor, or orbital cellulitis.

| Cause of papilledema | |
|---|---|
| **Cause** | **Examples** |
| raised intracranial pressure | tumor, abscess, hydrocephalus, hematoma, benign intracranial hypertension, cerebral edema (trauma) |
| venous occlusion | central retinal vein thrombosis, cavernous sinus thrombosis |
| malignant hypertension | grade IV hypertensive retinopathy |
| acute optic neuritis | multiple sclerosis, sarcoidosis |
| metabolic | hypercapnia, hypoparathyroidism |
| hematologic (rare) | severe anemia, acute leukemia |

**Fig. 27.26** Causes of papilledema.

### 3rd cranial nerve (oculomotor)
- Motor supply to levator palpebrae superioris, all orbital muscles except the superior oblique and lateral rectus muscles, and parasympathetic tone to pupillary reflex.
- Controls pupillary reflexes, in addition to the 2nd cranial nerve. Test the reaction to light and accommodation.
- Lesion of this nerve results in ptosis and a dilated pupil with no reaction to light or accommodation.

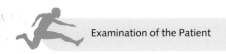 

| Causes of optic atrophy | |
|---|---|
| **Cause** | **Examples** |
| pressure on optic nerve | tumor, glaucoma, aneurysm, Paget's disease |
| demyelination | multiple sclerosis |
| vascular | central retinal artery occlusion |
| metabolic | diabetes mellitus, vitamin B$_{12}$ deficiency |
| toxins | methyl alcohol, tobacco, lead, quinine |
| trauma | including surgery |
| consecutive | due to extensive retinal disease such as choroidoretinitis |
| hereditary prolonged papilledema | Friedreich's ataxia, Leber's optic atrophy |

**Fig. 27.27** Causes of optic atrophy.

| Stages of diabetic retinopathy | |
|---|---|
| **Stage** | **Features** |
| background | dot hemorrhages (microaneurysms), blot hemorrhages, hard exudates |
| preproliferative | all of the above, plus soft exudates (cotton wool spots), flame hemorrhages, venous beading and loops |
| proliferative | all of the above, plus new vessel formation on retina or iris (rubeosis iridis), retinal detachment, preretinal or vitreous hemorrhage, glaucoma (with rubeosis iridis) |
| maculopathy | hard exudates at maculae (sometimes form rings) |

**Fig. 27.28** Stages of diabetic retinopathy. Note that cataracts are also more common in diabetes, and that retinopathy may have been treated by laser photocoagulation (burns around the periphery of the retina, destroying ischemic tissue and thus reducing the drive for new vessel formation).

The eye looks "down and out" at rest and is unable to look upward or inward.

- Causes of 3rd cranial nerve lesions are infarction, posterior communicating artery aneurysm, mononeuritis multiplex, demyelination, tumor, and neurosyphilis.

 Patients with a fourth cranial nerve palsy have difficulty with vision when walking downstairs or reading a book.

### 4th cranial nerve (trochlear)
- Motor supply to the superior oblique muscle.
- Patient may have the head tilted away from the lesion.
- Diplopia on looking down and away from the lesion with one image at an angle to the other.
- 4th cranial nerve lesions are usually associated with 3rd cranial nerve lesions and have a similar etiology.

### 6th cranial nerve (abducens)
- Motor supply to the lateral rectus.
- There is diplopia on abduction of the affected eye with two images side by side.

- 6th cranial nerve lesions are caused by mononeuritis multiplex, demyelination, tumor, infarction, thiamine deficiency (Wernicke's encephalopathy), raised intracranial pressure (false localizing sign), and neurosyphilis.

### 5th cranial nerve (trigeminal)
- Sensation to the face (ophthalmic, maxillary, and mandibular branches).
- Motor supply to the muscles of mastication (temporalis, masseter, and pterygoid muscles).
- Test sensation in the distribution of each division comparing one side with the other.
- Remember the corneal reflex, which requires intact motor function of the 3rd cranial nerve for blinking.
- Ask the patient to clench the teeth.
- Ask the patient to hold the mouth open while you try to push it shut.
- Test jaw jerk, which is increased in pseudobulbar palsy and reduced or absent in bulbar palsy.
- The causes of 5th cranial nerve lesions are shown in Fig. 27.29.

**Fig. 27.29** Causes of a trigeminal nerve lesion.

| Causes of a trigeminal nerve lesion | |
|---|---|
| **Cause** | **Examples** |
| brainstem | tumor, infarction, demyelination, syringobulbia |
| cerebellopontine angle | acoustic neuroma, meningioma |
| petrous temporal bone | trauma, tumor, middle ear disease, herpes zoster |
| cavemous sinus | tumor, thrombosis, aneurysm of internal carotid artery |
| peripheral | meningeal tuberculosis, syphilis, lymphoma, carcinoma, sarcoid |

| Causes of facial nerve palsies | |
|---|---|
| **Cause** | **Examples** |
| upper motor neuron central | stroke, tumor |
| lower motor neuron<br>pons<br>cerebellopontine angle<br>petrous temporal bone<br>middle ear disease<br>peripheral | stroke, tumor, demyelination, motor neuron disease<br>acoustic neuroma, meningioma<br>Bell's palsy, herpes zoster<br>infection, tumor<br>trauma, parotid disease, mononeuritis multiplex, sarcoid |

**Fig. 27.30** Causes of facial nerve palsies.

## 7th cranial nerve (facial)
- Sensation of taste from the floor of the mouth, the soft palate, and anterior two-thirds of the tongue.
- Motor supply to the muscles of facial expression and the stapedius muscle.
- Parasympathetic supply to the salivary and lacrimal glands.
- Ask the patient to wrinkle the forehead, screw the eyes tightly shut, show the teeth, and blow the cheeks out.
- In lower motor neuron lesions all the muscles are affected.
- In upper motor neuron lesions the upper half of the face and emotional expressions are spared (e.g., normal eye closure and wrinkling of the forehead).
- Taste is not usually examined formally, but ask if the patient has noticed any recent change.
- Fig. 27.30 summarizes the causes of facial nerve palsies.

## 8th cranial nerve (vestibulocochlear)
- Sensory from the utricle, saccule, and semicircular canals (vestibular), and from the organ of Corti (cochlea).

- Ask if the patient has noticed any difficulty with hearing.
- Rub your fingers in front of each of the patient's ears and ask if he or she can hear it.
- Rinne's test: place a vibrating tuning fork on the mastoid process and then at the external auditory meatus—the test is positive if the sound is louder when the fork is held at the external auditory meatus (i.e., air conduction) than when placed on the mastoid process (i.e., bone conduction). This is normal. An abnormal test (Rinne negative) indicates conductive deafness.
- Weber's test: place a vibrating tuning fork at the center of the forehead; the sound will be heard towards the normal ear in sensorineural deafness or towards the affected ear in conductive deafness.
- The causes of vestibular disease are shown in Fig. 24.1.
- The causes of conductive and sensorineural deafness are described in Fig. 27.31.

## 9th and 10th cranial nerves
- Look at palatal movement (ask the patient to say "Aah").

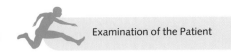
| Causes of deafness | |
|---|---|
| Cause | Examples |
| conductive | wax, foreign body, otitis externa, injury to tympanic membrane, otitis media, otosclerosis, middle ear tumor (e.g. cholesteatoma) |
| sensorineural | presbycusis (due to old age), noise induced, drugs (aminoglycosides, aspirin overdose), infection (meningitis, syphilis, measles), congenital (maternal rubella, cytomegalovirus, toxoplasmosis), Ménière's disease, acoustic neuroma, trauma, Paget's disease |

**Fig. 27.31** Causes of deafness. (CMV, cytomegalovirus.)

| Causes of glossopharyngeal, vagus, and accessory nerve palsies | |
|---|---|
| Cause | Examples |
| central (brainstem) | tumor, infarction, syringobulbia, motor neuron disease |
| peripheral | tumor or aneurysm near the jugular foramen, trauma of skull base, Guillain–Barré syndrome, poliomyelitis |

**Fig. 27.32** Causes of glossopharyngeal, vagus, and accessory nerve palsies.

- No palatal elevation on the affected side, with the uvula pulled towards the normal side.
- Check the gag reflex (9th, sensory; 10th, motor).
- Fig. 27. 32 summarizes diseases affecting these nerves.

### 9th cranial nerve (glossopharyngeal)
- Sensory to pharynx and carotid sinus and taste to the posterior third of the tongue.
- Motor supply to the stylopharyngeus muscle.
- Parasympathetic to the parotid gland.

### 10th cranial nerve (vagus)
- Sensory to the larynx.
- Motor supply to the cricothyroid and the muscles of the pharynx and larynx.
- Parasympathetic to the bronchi, heart, and gastrointestinal tract.

### 11th cranial nerve (accessory)
- Cranial root provides the motor supply to some muscles of the soft palate and larynx.
- Spinal root provides the motor supply to the trapezius and sternocleidomastoid muscles.
- Ask the patient to shrug the shoulders and test against resistance.
- Ask the patient to turn his or her head to each side and test against resistance.

### 12th cranial nerve (hypoglossal)
- Provides the motor supply to the styloglossus, hyoglossus, and all intrinsic muscles of the tongue.
- Ask the patient to open the mouth. Look for wasting and fasciculation, indicating a lower motor neuron lesion of the tongue.
- Then ask the patient to protrude the tongue. If there is a unilateral lesion the tongue will deviate toward the side of the lesion.
- Upper motor neuron lesions are due to stroke, tumor, or motor neuron disease.
- Lower motor neuron lesions are due to diseases in the posterior fossa, skull base, and the neck, including tumor, motor neuron disease, syringobulbia, trauma, and poliomyelitis.

## The upper limbs
### Inspection
- Wasting: lower motor neuron lesion, muscle disease, and disuse.
- Fasciculation: lower motor neuron lesion.
- Scars: particularly from surgery.
- Deformity: may cause mononeuropathy by entrapment, and contractures may be the result of neurologic disease.
- Tremor (Fig. 27.33).

**Fig. 27.33** Causes of tremor.

| | Causes of tremor | |
|---|---|---|
| **Type** | **Features** | **Causes** |
| resting | seen when patients relaxed with hands at rest | parkinsonism |
| postural | seen when hands held outstretched | benign essential tremor anxiety thyrotoxicosis β₂-agonists |
| intention | seen when patients try to touch examiner's finger with their own finger | cerebellar disease |

## Pronator drift
- Ask the patient to hold his or her arms outstretched with the palms facing upward.
- Marked weakness due to any cause will become immediately apparent.
- Ask the patient to keep the arms still and close the eyes.
- If there is an upper motor neuron lesion (affecting the parietal lobe), the arm will drift downward and the palms will turn downward.

## Tone
Reduced tone is a feature of a lower motor neuron lesion or cerebellar lesion. Tone may be increased throughout a movement, when it is called "lead pipe" rigidity (as in parkinsonism) or more pronounced at the beginning of a movement, so-called "clasp knife" rigidity (as with an upper motor neuron lesion).

## Strength
All muscle groups should be tested and scored (Fig. 27.34). You will need to learn the spinal root for each movement (Fig. 27.35). Remember to compare muscle power of one side to the other for each group.

## When assessing coordination
Ask the patient to alternately touch their nose and your finger. In cerebellar disease there will be an intention tremor and past pointing, i.e., the patient overshoots the examining clinician's finger consistently towards the side of the lesion. Ask the patient to tap one palm with alternating sides of the other hand as quickly as possible (demonstrate to the patient what you would like him or her to do). In cerebellar disease this will be slow, poorly

| | Grading muscle power |
|---|---|
| **Grade** | **Features** |
| 0 | no movement at all |
| 1 | flicker of movement only |
| 2 | movement only when gravity excluded |
| 3 | movement against gravity only |
| 4 | movement against gravity and some additional resistance |
| 5 | normal power |

**Fig. 27.34** Grading muscle power.

coordinated, and the action of the moving hand has a high amplitude—this is dysdiadochokinesis.

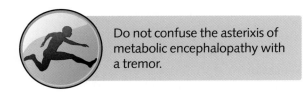

Do not confuse the asterixis of metabolic encephalopathy with a tremor.

## Reflexes
Practice as often as you can. Learn the spinal root of each reflex—these are clinically useful as well as helpful in examinations! (Fig. 27.36). Reflexes can be reduced, normal or increased. They will be reduced or absent in lower motor neuron lesions, sensory neuropathy, and severe muscle disease (disruption of reflex arc), and will be exaggerated in upper motor neuron lesions.

177

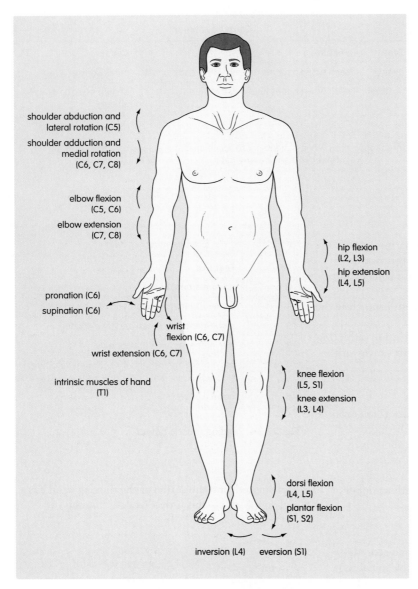

**Fig. 27.35** Roots for each muscle group movement.

shoulder abduction and lateral rotation (C5)

shoulder adduction and medial rotation (C6, C7, C8)

elbow flexion (C5, C6)

elbow extension (C7, C8)

pronation (C6)

supination (C6)

wrist flexion (C6, C7)

wrist extension (C6, C7)

intrinsic muscles of hand (T1)

hip flexion (L2, L3)

hip extension (L4, L5)

knee flexion (L5, S1)

knee extension (L3, L4)

dorsi flexion (L4, L5)

plantar flexion (S1, S2)

inversion (L4)     eversion (S1)

## Sensation

Test each dermatome (Fig. 27.37) for the sensation of light touch, pinprick, and temperature. Then, starting distally, check vibration and joint position sense. Remember the different pathways these senses take (Fig. 27.38).

## The lower limbs

### Inspection

- Wasting: lower motor neuron lesion, muscle disease, and disuse.
- Fasciculation: lower motor neuron lesion.
- Scars: particularly from surgery.

- Deformity: may cause mononeuropathy by entrapment, and contractures may be the result of neurologic disease.
- Pes cavus: Charcot-Marie-Tooth disease.
- Catheter: neurogenic urinary incontinence.
- Walking aids: wheelchair and stick indicating degree of disability.

S2, 3, 4 feels your bottom on the floor!

**Fig. 27.36** Eliciting reflexes. (A) Upper limb tendon reflexes. (B) A simple way to remember root values of reflexes. (C) Testing ankle jerk with reinforcement. (D) The normal response is a downgoing hallux. In an upper motor neuron lesion, the hallux dorsiflexes and other toes fan out (the Babinski response).

**Fig. 27.37** Dermatome testing.

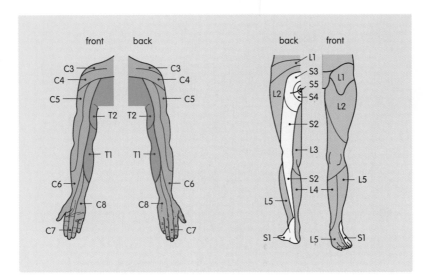

## Gait

- Ask the patient to walk for 2–3 yards, turn and walk back, then walk heel to toe (cerebellar ataxia), and finally stand on toes and on heels (any muscle weakness will now manifest itself).
- Make sure you walk with the patient so you can catch them if they fall.
- An immense amount of information can be gained by careful study of these aspects of gait (see Fig. 22.2).
- Have the patient attempt to walk on the heels, toes, and heel-to-toe to test gait and strength at the same time.

## Tone

Reduced tone is a feature of a lower motor neuron lesion or cerebellar lesion. Tone may be increased in an upper motor neuron lesion or parkinsonism. Test for clonus, signifying an upper motor neuron lesion.

## Strength

All muscle groups should be tested and scored (see Fig. 27.34). Learn the roots for each movement (see Fig. 27.35). Remember to compare muscle power of one side to the other for each group.

## Coordination

Ask the patient to gently run the heel of one leg down the shin of the other. In cerebellar disease this will be slow and clumsy.

## Reflexes

Learn the root value of each reflex (see Fig. 27.36). Reflexes will be reduced or absent in lower motor neuron lesions, sensory neuropathy, and severe muscle disease, and will be exaggerated in upper motor neuron lesions. Check plantar response, which is normally downgoing but will be upgoing in upper motor neuron lesions.

## Sensation

Test each dermatome (see Fig. 27.37) for sensation of light touch, pinprick, and temperature. Then, starting distally, check vibration and joint position sense. Check specifically for peripheral neurology— "stocking" distribution.

The sensory pathways are shown in Fig. 27.38.

## The joints

### Examination

Diseases affecting the musculoskeletal system and how to distinguish between different disease processes on clinical examination have been discussed in detail in Chapter 16. However, remember the following broad components to the examination of joints.

### General

- Does the patient look well or ill?
- Anemia: chronic disease, blood loss (peptic ulcer due to non-steroidal use), bone marrow

**Fig. 27.38A** Anatomy of sensory pathways within the spinal cord.

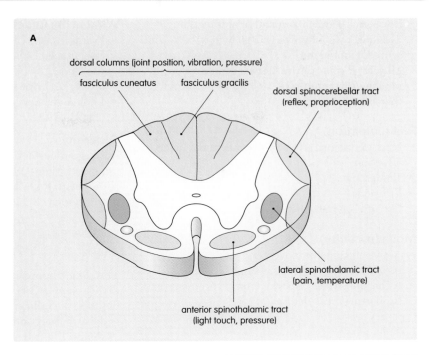

**Fig. 27.38B** Tests for different sensory modalities.

| Sensory pathways | | | |
|---|---|---|---|
| Sensation | Tested using | Pathway | Level of decussation |
| pain | pin | lateral spinothalamic tract | at level of sensory root within one spinal segment |
| temperature | tuning fork for cold | lateral spinothalamic tract | at level of sensory root within one spinal segment |
| light touch | cotton wool | anterior spinothalamic tract | at level of sensory root within several spinal segments |
| vibration | tuning fork | posterior columns (fasciculus gracilis and fasciculus cuneatus) | medulla oblongata |
| joint position sense | move fixed joints | posterior columns (fasciculus gracilis and fasciculus cuneatus) | medulla oblongata |
| two-point discrimination | orange stick | posterior columns (fasciculus gracilis and fasciculus cuneatus) | medulla oblongata |

suppression (immunosuppressive therapy), hemolysis (autoimmune associated with systemic lupus erythematosus), and hypersplenism (Felty's syndrome in RA).
- Face: scleroderma, systemic lupus erythematosus, cushingoid facies (long-term steroid therapy).

- Stooped: ankylosing spondylitis and osteoporosis.

## Look (inspection)
- Deformity.
- Scars: previous surgery.

- Erythema: acute inflammation or infection.
- Swelling: osteophytes, synovial hypertrophy, and acute inflammation.
- Muscle wasting: disuse, nerve entrapment, mononeuritis multiplex, or long-term steroid therapy.

## Feel (palpation)

- Increased temperature: acute inflammation or infection.
- Tenderness.
- Effusions.
- Crepitus on movement.

## Move (mobility)

- Active and passive movement.
- Is pain associated with movement?
- Is the joint stable? Are there intact ligaments and supporting musculature?

---

### Problems of long-term steroid therapy

- Cushing's syndrome (thin skin with easy bruising, moon-like facies, central obesity)
- proximal myopathy
- osteoporosis
- psychosis
- edema (sodium retention)
- hypertension
- diabetes mellitus
- avascular necrosis of femoral head
- peptic ulceration

**Fig. 27.39** Problems of long-term steroid therapy.

## What is the underlying cause?

- Psoriatic rash.
- Subcutaneous rheumatoid nodules: particularly at the elbow.
- Gouty tophi: on the pinna and elbow.
- Look for evidence of long-term steroid treatment (Fig. 27.39).

## Disability

It is very important to get an impression of how limiting the joint problem is. For example, in a patient with RA, ask the patient to undo some buttons or write their name with a pen.

## The skin

The clinical approach to skin rashes has been discussed in detail in Chapter 17. Remember to describe the following:

- Distribution: this can be diagnostic in itself.
- Shape.
- Size.
- Color.
- Consistency.
- Temperature.
- Tenderness.
- Margins.
- Relation to the surface: raised, flat, or ulcerated.
- Fixation to underlying structures.

Fig. 27.40 summarizes skin disorders associated with underlying systemic disease.

### Skin disorders associated with underlying systemic disease

| Disease | Skin manifestation |
|---|---|
| diabetes mellitus | necrobiosis lipoidica diabeticorum, granuloma annulare, acanthosis nigricans |
| sarcoidosis | lupus pernio, scar infiltration, erythema nodosum |
| malignancy | dermatomyositis, acanthosis nigricans, necrolytic migratory erythema (glucagonoma), erythema gyratum repens (usually bronchial carcinoma), thrombophlebitis migrans (pancreatic carcinoma) |
| liver disease | spider nevi, palmar erythema, leukonychia, porphyria cutanea tarda |
| renal disease | uremic frost (rare), pale yellow pigmentation, half-and-half nails |
| hyperlipidemia | xanthelasmata, tendon xanthomata, eruptive xanthomata |
| neurofibromatosis | *café-au-lait* patches, axillary freckling, neurofibromas, plexiform neuromas |

**Fig. 27.40** Skin disorders associated with underlying systemic disease.

# 28. Medical Record of History and Physical Examination (H&P)

The doctor's "H&P" is a written summary of the patient's history and examination. It is a legal document and should be precise, complete, and legible. Avoid using abbreviations—although the meaning may be obvious to you, they may be interpreted very differently in a different specialty or hospital.

At the end of the H&P, the salient points should be emphasized in a summary statement. You should then compile a "problem list." This is often forgotten by students and junior doctors alike, but it is invaluable in planning appropriate investigations and management. You can compile a plan that states the problems based on a problem list or in an organ/system approach, followed by the tests and other strategies that will be performed. In some patients it will not be appropriate, or even possible, to take a full history and perform a full clinical examination (e.g., in an emergency situation). We have outlined a clinical example.

As a student it is good practice to be very thorough as it helps you to learn the relevant questions and to avoid missing anything important. However, with practice, you will learn to tailor carefully the clinical approach to each patient based on their individual, and often very different, needs.

## Checklist example

| | |
|---|---|
| Date: | 1 January 2000 |
| Time: | 0720 |
| Name: | John Doe |
| Place: | A&E |
| Age: | 47 |
| Sex: | Male |
| Occupation: | Truck driver |
| Referred by: | 999 call |

### Presenting chief complaint (CPC)
4 hour crushing retrosternal chest pain

### History of presenting illness (HPI)
JD, a 47-year-old white male with known CAD, presents to the ED with 4 hours crushing 9/10 retrosternal chest pain, radiating to neck and both arms; gradual onset over 5–10 mins.
Duration: persistent since onset.

### Relieving/exacerbating factors
Sublingual nitroglycerine provided no relief, although it normally relieves pain in mins; no other relieving/exacerbating factors.

### Associated symptoms
nausea, vomiting (×2), sweating, dizzy.

### Relevant previous history
1986: myocardial infarction, full recovery
1997: exertional chest tightness and dyspnea initially controlled on atenolol
Dec. 2003: symptoms worse, exercise tolerance 200 yards on flat, limited by chest pain, no rest pain, no orthopnea or PND

### Risk factors
| | |
|---|---|
| Hypertension | —no. |
| Smoking | —20 cigarettes per day from 16 years. |
| FH | —father died of "heart attack" at 52 years. |
| Diabetes | —no. |
| Cholesterol | —never checked. |
| Ischemic heart disease | —angina, previous MI. |

### Past medical history (PMH)
1963: appendectomy.
1972: duodenal ulcer (no symptoms since).
1989: gout (quiescent on treatment).
NO diabetes, hypertension, rheumatic heart disease, tuberculosis, epilepsy, asthma, jaundice, cerebrovascular disease.

### Surgical history
1963: appendectomy

### Review of systems (ROS)
*General*
Fatigue lately, appetite unchanged, weight stable, no sweats or pruritus, sleeping well.

*CVS*
As above.

*RS*
Dyspnea on exertion, particularly uphill, but not limiting. No cough/sputum/wheeze

*GIT*
No current indigestion. No symptoms like previous duodenal ulcer. No vomiting, dysphagia, abdominal pain.

*GUS*
No change in bowel habit, no rectal bleeding. No urinary symptoms.

*NS*
No headache or syncope. No dizziness, limb weakness, or sensory loss. No disturbed vision, hearing, smell, or speech.

*MS*
No painful gout for 5 years. No joint pain, stiffness, or swelling. No disability.

*Skin*
No rash, pruritus, or bruising.

**Drug history**
Atenolol          100mg once daily.
Allopurinol       300mg HS.
Sublingual nitroglycerine as required.
Not taking aspirin.
Allergies: penicillin: skin rash.

**Family history (FH)**
Father died of "heart attack" at age 52.
Mother died of "old age" at 76.

**SH (social history)**
Lives with wife, who is fit and well.
Owns house.
Completely independent.
Smoking 20 cigs/day for many years.
Alcohol: 24 units per week.
Sexual history: not appropriate.
Overseas travel: not appropriate.
Pets: not appropriate.
Occupation: heavy goods truck driver.

**Physical examination (PE)**
*Vital signs:* T 37.5°C, HR 104, BP 110/70, RR 15
*General:* unwell, sweaty, clammy, no cyanosis/jaundice.
Cigarette-stained fingers.
No arcus, xanthomas, or xanthelasma

*CVS*
Pulse: 104bpm regular, normal character.
BP: 110/70mmHg (right), 112/74mmHg (left).
JVP: normal.
No precordial scars or chest deformities.
PMI displaced to anterior axillary line 6th intercostal space.
No parasternal heave or thrills.
Auscultation: Heart sounds normal, but soft pansystolic murmur at apex radiating to axilla and ejection systolic murmur in aortic area with no radiation.

hs ——————————————————— PSM at apex
    1        2        3

hs ——————————————————— ESM in
    1        2        3     aortic area

Peripheral pulses: absent right popliteal to dorsalis pedis.
No sacral or ankle edema.

*RS*
Trachea central.
Respiratory rate 15/min, no respiratory distress.
Expansion symmetrical and normal.
Vocal fremitus normal.
Percussion note normal.
Breath sounds vesicular throughout, no added sounds.

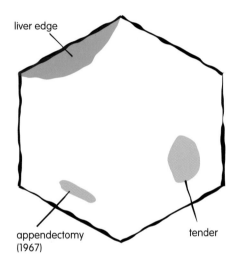

*Abdomen*
No scars, veins, or distention.
Palpation: soft, but tender LIF (left iliac fossa).
Percussion note normal.
Auscultation bowel sounds normal.
Genitalia not examined.
Rectal examination: not performed.

*NS*
Higher function normal.
Cranial nerves:
I: normal.
II: PERRLA (pupils equal in reaction to light and accommodation), normal fundi and visual fields.
III, IV, VI: no diplopia/nystagmus.
V, VII, VIII, IX, X, XI, XII: normal.
Upper and lower limbs: power, tone, coordination, sensation all normal.

| *Reflexes* | | *Right* | *Left* |
|---|---|---|---|
| | Biceps | ++ | ++ |
| | Supinator | ++ | ++ |
| | Triceps | ++ | ++ |
| | Knee | ++ | ++ |
| | Ankle | + | + |
| | Plantar | ↓ | ↓ |

*Joints and skin*
Normal.

**Assessment**
47-year-old male smoker, with a family history and previous history of ischemic heart disease, presents with a 4-month history of increasing exertional chest pain and a 4-hour history of persistent, severe pain at rest which is unrelieved by sublingual nitroglycerin and associated with nausea, vomiting, and sweating. On examination he has a resting tachycardia and evidence of left ventricular dilatation with a displaced apex beat and possible secondary mitral regurgitation. The most likely diagnosis is acute myocardial infarction.

**Plan**
Attending physicians and senior residents vary in how they want the plan presented, either systems-based or problem-based. As a student, it is often helpful to use both. See below.

*I. CVS*
Chest pain—given the slight elevation in cardiac enzymes, classic history of angina, known previous CAD, and ECG changes, the most likely diagnosis is NSTEMI.
- have instituted emergent PTCA, will determine pathology of lesion and whether stent will be placed.
- will continue Gp. IIb/IIIa inhibitor for post-catheterization.
- will maintain beta blocker and will add statin, ACE inhibitor, and daily aspirin therapy. Will add clopidogrel therapy for 3–12 months if stent was placed.
- have SL nitroglycerine at bedside and educate patient to report any additional chest pain.
- fractionated heparin injections (Lovenox injections) until patient is ambulatory.
- will refer patient for cardiac rehabilitation, smoking cessation counseling, and dietary counseling.

*II. Respiratory*

No acute pathology, will have incentive spirometry to bedside with education.

*III. Metabolic*

Will continue allopurinol while patient is in hospital.

*IV. Disposition*

Patient will be considered for discharge if he remains free of chest pain for 24 hours and no complications of MI exist. He will follow up with outpatient cardiology and cardiac rehabilitation.

# 29. Common Investigations

By the time it comes to organizing investigations, the good clinician will already have a fairly clear idea of what he or she is likely to find. The investigation plan should be well structured, starting with simple noninvasive tests designed to answer specific questions. Remember two important rules:

- Do not request a test if you do not know why you are doing it. There is nothing worse than getting an abnormal result and wondering whether it is important or not!
- If a test is worth requesting, always make sure you see the result—it may be the clue you need.

If you are given a study to comment on, always describe what the investigation is, the patient's name, and the date it was performed. This is a good habit to get into, as the name will usually tell you what sex the patient is and possibly their ethnic background, which may be useful. As a practicing clinician, it is also important as patients' results occasionally find their way into the wrong set of notes.

## The cardiovascular system

### Cardiac enzymess

The enzymes released by necrotic myocardium following myocardial infarction (MI) include troponin T and troponin I, creatinine kinase (CK), aspartate aminotransferase (AST), and troponins. Each enzyme is released and reaches a peak level at different times and can help to determine when the infarct occurred. Unfortunately these enzymes are also present in other tissues and are not specific (Fig. 29.1). Isoenzymes of CK (CK-MB) and troponin can be measured and are more indicative of acute MI. Note that some emergency departments now use myoglobin as a cardiac marker. Levels of this marker rise more quickly than other cardiac enzymes, peaking at 6–7 hours, whereas troponin and CK peak at 18–24 hours.

## Electrocardiogram

The 12-lead electrocardiogram (ECG) is an assessment of the electrical activity of the heart. Twelve electrodes are attached to the patient, as shown in Fig. 29.2, giving 12 different "views" of the heart (Fig. 29.3). Diagnostic information is obtained by considering the different components of the ECG.

### Rate

Divide 300 by the number of large squares between two QRS complexes to give the number of beats per minute (each large square represents 0.2 seconds). Normal rate is 60–100 beats per minute. Causes of sinus tachycardia and bradycardia are shown in Fig. 29.4.

### Rhythm

Are the QRS complexes regular? Is each QRS preceded by a p wave (Chapter 3)?

#### Tachycardia

In sinus tachycardia a P wave precedes each QRS complex and the rhythm is regular. If there are no P waves and the rhythm is irregular, consider atrial fibrillation, atrial flutter with variable block, and frequent ectopic beats.

If no P waves are present and the rhythm is regular, consider atrial tachycardia, atrial flutter with 2:1 block, and ventricular tachycardia.

#### Bradycardia

If P waves are small or absent, check for hyperkalemia. In sinus bradycardia P waves are present and the rhythm is regular.

In first-degree heart block, P waves are present with a regular rhythm, but the PR interval is prolonged.

In second-degree heart block two or more P waves are present between each QRS (2:1 or 3:1 heart block). In Mobitz I (second-degree heart block) the

| Tissues containing cardiac enzymes and the differential diagnosis of raised levels | | | | |
| --- | --- | --- | --- | --- |
| | Creatinine kinase | Aspartate aminotransferase | Lactate dehydrogenase | Troponin |
| tisses found in | cardiac muscle<br>skeletal muscle<br>smooth muscle<br>brain | cardiac muscle<br>skeletal muscle<br>liver<br>kidney<br>red blood cells | cardiac muscle<br>skeletal muscle<br>liver<br>kidney<br>brain<br>red blood cells | cardiospecific |
| raised levels in | MI<br>muscle trauma<br>postintramuscular<br>   injection<br>muscular dystrophy<br>hypothyroidism<br>   following surgery<br>severe head injury | MI<br>hepatitis<br>cirrhosis<br>malignant hepatic<br>   infiltration<br>muscle disease<br>   following surgery<br>severe hemolytic anemia | MI<br>megaloblastic anemia<br>lymphoma<br>acute leukemia<br>malignancy<br>muscle disease<br>pulmonary embolus<br>hepatitis<br>renal infarction | MI<br>myocarditis<br>acute RV overload<br>   (as in large PE) |

**Fig. 29.1** Tissues containing "cardiac enzymes" and the differential diagnosis of raised levels. (MI, myocardial infarction; RV, right ventricle; PE, pulmonary embolus.)

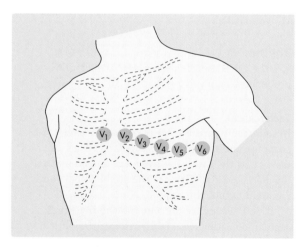

**Fig. 29.2** The position of the anterior electrodes for a 12-lead electrocardiogram.

PR interval gradually lengthens until one P wave is not conducted. In Mobitz II, the PR interval is constant with dropped beats.

In third-degree heart block, P waves are present but are completely independent of QRS complexes, creating an irregular rhythm (see Chapter 30—cardiovascular disease).

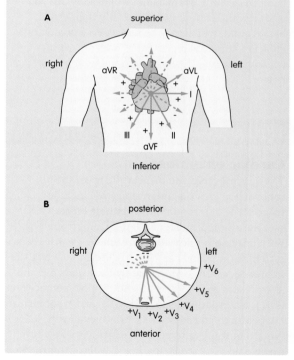

**Fig. 29.3** The 12 different views of the heart given by a 12-lead electrocardiogram. (A) Superior perspective. (B) Posterior perspective.

188

| Causes of sinus tachycardia and sinus bradycardia | |
| --- | --- |
| **Sinus tachycardia** | **Sinus bradycardia** |
| anxiety | physical fitness |
| exercise | sinoatrial node disease |
| anemia | hypothermia |
| shock | hypothyroidism |
| fever | cholestatic jaundice |
| pregnancy | raised intracranial pressure |
| thyrotoxicosis | postmyocardial infarction |
| pulmonary embolus | drugs, e.g. β-blockers |
| cardiac failure | |
| drugs, e.g. β-agonists | |

**Fig. 29.4** Causes of sinus tachycardia and sinus bradycardia.

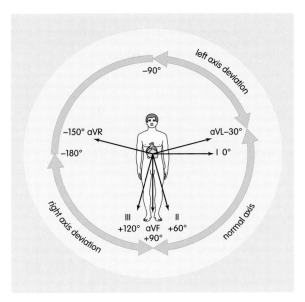

**Fig. 29.5** Axis determination on ECG.

Check whether the complexes are regular by marking five QRS complexes on a piece of paper. Move it along by one complex, and your marks should coincide exactly.

## Axis

The axis is the average direction of spread of electrical activity through the ventricles. The normal axis lies between −30° and +90° (Fig. 29.5). Look at leads I, II, and III. If the axis in normal, all three will have a predominantly upwards or positive deflection (i.e., R > S). If lead I is negative (with the others positive), there is right axis deviation. If lead II is negative (with I positive and III negative), there is left axis deviation.

## P wave

The P wave represents electrical activity of the right and left atria.

It is tall in P pulmonale (i.e., >2.5mm), which is caused by hypertrophy of the right atrium, as in tricuspid stenosis or pulmonary hypertension. The P wave is bifid (like an "m") in P mitrale, which is caused by hypertrophy of the left atrium as in mitral stenosis.

## PR interval

The PR interval represents the time for electrical activity to pass from the sinoatrial node to the atrioventricular (AV) node—it should be 0.12–0.2 seconds (3–5 small squares).

It is prolonged in heart block (see above) and shortened in Wolff-Parkinson-White and Lown-Ganong-Levine syndrome due to accessory pathways connecting the atria and ventricles. In Wolff-Parkinson-White syndrome there is also a slurred upstroke of the R wave, which is called a delta wave.

## QRS complex

The QRS complex represents ventricular depolarization; it should last less than 0.12 seconds (3 small squares).

It is broad if depolarization has spread through an abnormal route, either due to disruption of the pathway, as in bundle branch block, or because it has started somewhere other than the AV node, as in ventricular ectopic beats or ventricular tachycardia.

Q waves result from depolarization of the septum and should be less than 0.04 seconds (1 small square) and less than 2 small squares deep. Abnormally wide and deep Q waves are permanent features of MI.

The height of the R wave in $V_5$ and $V_6$ should be less than 25mm. The R wave may be abnormally tall in left ventricular hypertrophy (Fig. 29.6); the QRS complexes may be abnormally small in pericardial effusion.

**Features of left ventricular hypertrophy**

- S wave in $V_1$ and R wave in $V_5$ or $V_6 \geq 35\,mm$
- R wave in $V_{5-6} > 27\,mm$
- S wave in $V_{1-3} > 30\,mm$
- ST depression in I, aVl, $V_{4-6}$
- T wave inversion in I, aVl, $V_{4-6}$
- left axis deviation

**Fig. 29.6** Features of left ventricular hypertrophy.

### ST segment

The ST segment should not be greater than 1 mm above or below the isoelectric line. (Causes of ST elevation are shown on p. 7, fig. 1.3.) ST depression is an indication of myocardial ischemia.

### T wave

The T wave represents ventricular repolarization and should be less than 10 mm in height. Peaked T waves are seen in acute MI and hyperkalemia. Small, flattened T waves may be seen in hypokalemia. Inverted T waves are a feature of myocardial ischemia, infarction, and digitalis effect (reverse tick sign—downsloping of the ST segment).

### QT interval

The QT interval is the time from ventricular depolarization (start of QRS) to complete ventricular repolarization (end of T wave). It should be less than 0.44 seconds (which is 2 large squares). The QT interval varies inversely with heart rate (e.g., shortens in tachycardia). It can be corrected for rate by calculating $QT/_{R-R}$.

The QT interval is increased in hypocalcemia, hypomagnesemia, drugs (amiodarone, beta blockers, tricyclics), or severe myocardial disease.

### U wave

The U wave is often a normal variant but is more prominent in hypokalemia.

### Exercise electrocardiogram

The resting ECG is taken. The patient then performs exercise until symptoms develop or the protocol is complete. Regular pulse, blood pressure, and ECGs are recorded. Evidence of myocardial ischemia (ST depression and T wave inversion) and rate induced arrhythmias are looked for.

The test is useful for the following:
- Assessment of severity of ischemic heart disease.
- Prognosis following MI.
- Exercise-induced palpitations.
- Diagnosis of atypical chest pain—is it angina or not?

## 24-hour electrocardiogram

The 24-hour ECG records cardiac rhythm over a 24-hour period while the patient continues with their normal daily activities. It will detect transient arrhythmias and is useful in the investigation of episodic syncope, palpitations, dizziness, and dyspnea.

## Chest x-ray

Chest x-ray (CXR) can give much information regarding both the underlying diagnosis, as well as subsequent complications. This information is summarized in Fig. 29.7. Further related details are shown for mitral valve disease in Fig. 29.8 and for pulmonary edema in Fig. 29.9.

## Echocardiography

Echocardiography is an ultrasound technique that can be performed via a transthoracic or transesophageal approach. It gives structural information of the heart.

To make a definite diagnosis of left ventricular hypertrophy, voltage criteria in addition to repolarization abnormalities must be present.

Color Doppler can be used to look at blood flow and pressure gradients across valves. Echocardiography is useful in the diagnosis of the following:
- Pericardium: effusion.
- Myocardium: left ventricular hypertrophy, left ventricular dysfunction, cardiomyopathies.
- Endocardium: atrial myxoma, vegetations, thrombus.
- Valves: stenosis and regurgitation with estimation of pressure across valves.
- Congenital heart disease: including atrial and ventricular septal defects.
- Aorta: aneurysm.

**Underlying diagnoses and complications in the cardiovascular system detectable on chest X-ray**

| Region | Diagnosis | X-ray findings |
| --- | --- | --- |
| pericardium | tuberculosis or constrictive pericarditis | calcification |
| myocardium | effusion<br>left ventricular dilatation<br>right ventricular dilatation<br>left atrium<br>left ventricular aneurysm | globular cardiomegaly<br>cardiomegaly with left ventricle displaced inferolaterally<br>cardiomegaly with PMI elevated<br>double right heart border; splaying of carina<br>calcified mural thrombus |
| endocardium | rheumatic heart disease | calcification |
| valves | valve replacement<br>mitral valve disease<br>atheroma | sternal wires; metallic valves; surgical clips<br>Fig. 29.8<br>calcification |
| aorta | coarctation<br>dissection | rib notching<br>widened mediastinum |
| lungs | pulmonary edema | Fig. 29.9 |

**Fig. 29.7** Underlying diagnoses and complications in the cardiovascular system detectable on chest x-ray.

**Chest x-ray features of mitral stenosis**

- calcified mitral valve
- dilated left atrium (makes the left heart border look straight)
- splayed carina with elevation of left main bronchus
- prominent pulmonary arteries indicating pulmonary hypertension
- pulmonary edema may be present

**Fig. 29.8** Chest x-ray features of mitral stenosis.

**Chest x-ray features of pulmonary edema**

- upper lobe veins dilatation
- Kerley B lines
- bat's wing shadowing (perihilar edema)
- fluid in the horizontal fissure
- pleural effusion (usually bilateral but can be unilateral)

**Fig. 29.9** Chest x-ray features of pulmonary edema.

## Thallium perfusion scan

Thallium perfusion scan monitors cardiac uptake of radioactive thallium. Areas with a poor coronary blood supply are identified as "cold spots." This test can be used in patients unable to use a treadmill, such as those with osteoarthritis affecting the lower limbs.

## Cardiac catheterization

The right side of the heart is catheterized via the femoral vein (usually the right). The left side of the heart and coronary arteries are catheterized via the femoral artery. It provides the following information:
- Pressure in different chambers of the heart and the great vessels.
- Pressure gradient across the valves.
- Anatomy of the coronary arteries: following injection of radiopaque dye.
- Assessment of blood flow: valvular regurgitation or across septal defects.
- Oxygen concentrations: in different heart chambers in assessment of shunts.

Therapeutic measures include:
- Angioplasty (Fig. 29.10).
- Valvotomy.
- Arterial stent insertion.

## The respiratory system

### Chest x-ray

You should develop your own routine for looking at a CXR so as not to miss important features, particularly when there is a glaring abnormality that immediately demands attention. This should include

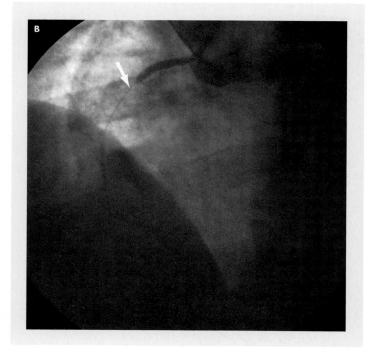

**Fig. 29.10** Percutaneous transluminal coronary angioplasty (PTCA) of the right coronary artery. **A**, The right coronary artery is occluded proximally. **B**, A guide wire is introduced into the artery. **C**, A balloon is inflated over the site of the obstruction, and a stent is deployed. **D**, The whole artery is patent at the end of the procedure.

**Fig. 29.10** *Continued.*

the trachea, mediastinum (nodes, vessels), cardiac outline, diaphragms (including the costo- and cardiophrenic angles), lung fields themselves, bones, and soft tissues. The radiologic findings for common respiratory diseases are outlined in Fig. 29.11.

Always look at a chest x-ray in a systematic way as outlined in this section. Never comment on heart size unless the film is a posterior—anterior (PA) projection.

If you cannot see any abnormality, look specifically at the apices for a small pneumothorax or cervical rib, behind the heart for a hiatus hernia (air-fluid level), at the soft tissues for unilateral mastectomy, and below the diaphragms for free gas.

## Spirometry

Measurements of airflow rates and forced vital capacity are obtained using a spirometer. The patient breathes in to maximum inspiration and then exhales into the spirometer as quickly and for as long as possible. The volume expelled is plotted against time.

The $FEV_1$ (forced expiratory volume in 1 second) is the volume exhaled in the first second of the test. The FVC (forced vital capacity) is the total volume exhaled. Both measurements are related to age, sex, and height, and nomograms are used to provide

| Radiologic findings associated with common respiratory diseases | |
| --- | --- |
| **Abnormality** | **Radiologic findings** |
| airways obstruction (asthma, emphysema, chronic bronchitis) | lungs hyperexpanded with flat hemidiaphragms allowing visualization of anterior aspects of sixth ribs; apical bullae may be seen in emphysema; look specifically for pneumothorax which may complicate bronchospasm or for evidence of infection which may have caused it |
| pneumonia | hazy opacification, often limited to one lobe or segment but may be diffuse; bronchi remain patent and may form air bronchograms; sometimes associated with collapse or pleural effusion |
| pulmonary embolus | often no abnormality, elevated hemidiaphragm, local oligemia, wedge atelectasis, and pleural effusions may be seen |
| tumor | localized opacification; look for small rounded opacifications or hilar lymphadenopathy suggesting metastases |
| pleural effusion | dense opacity in the lower zone with edges curved upwards (meniscus); hemidiaphragm and heart border not visible; mediastinum may shift if effusion massive; look for causes of effusion such as tumor; need at least 500 ml of fluid before detectable on chest x-ray |
| fibrosis | diffuse "ground glass" nodular or reticular may progress to honeycomb lung if severe; mediastinum may shift towards disease due to loss of lung volume |
| pneumothorax | increased translucency due to absence of vascular shadowing and visible visceral pleura; mediastinum will shift only if pneumothorax massive or under tension; look for underlying pathology such as airways obstruction |
| tuberculosis | apical mass with hilar lymphadenopathy with or without pleural effusion; may become calcified; apical fibrosis and military mottling indicate postprimary disease |
| bronchiectasis | may be normal; thickened bronchi may be visible as tramline or ring shadows; look for dextrocardia (Kartagener's syndrome) |
| pulmonary edema | see Fig. 29.9 |

**Fig. 29.11** Radiologic findings associated with common respiratory diseases.

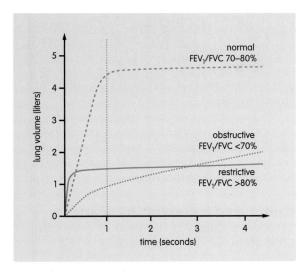

**Fig. 29.12** Spirometry in normal patients, and those with obstructive and restrictive pulmonary defects.

predicted or "normal" parameters. The $FEV_1$ is expressed as a percentage of the FVC and is 70–80% in normal subjects.

Where there is obstruction to airflow, as in bronchospasm due to chronic bronchitis, the $FEV_1$ is very much reduced. Although the total lung volume is increased, the FVC will also be slightly reduced due to air trapping as the small airways collapse. However, the reduction in $FEV_1$ is much greater than that for FVC and the $FEV_1/FVC$ ratio is reduced (Fig. 29.12).

A repeat test should be performed after the administration of bronchodilators to determine if there is a reversible element present.

Restrictive defects due to pulmonary fibrosis are characterized by reduced lung volumes and reduced FVC. The $FEV_1$ will be normal or slightly reduced. The $FEV_1/FVC$ ratio is therefore normal or increased (see Fig. 29.12).

## Diffusion factor

Diffusion factor (DLCO) is a measurement of the diffusing capacity of a low concentration of carbon monoxide. The diffusion is across the alveolar-capillary membrane (i.e., movement from the alveolus to the blood) and is dependent on three conditions:

- An adequate blood supply to the areas of lung ventilated, i.e., ventilation–perfusion (V/Q) matching.

- Efficient diffusion across the alveolar-capillary membrane.
- Adequate amounts of normal hemoglobin.

DLCO should be corrected for the hemoglobin concentration. If it remains abnormal, it indicates that the pathology present has disrupted diffusion.

DLCO will be low when any of the three above steps are affected, as in emphysema, pulmonary fibrosis (from any cause), and *Pneumocystis carinii* pneumonia in patients with acquired immunodeficiency syndrome. It will be raised in polycythemia, left-to-right shunts, and pulmonary hemorrhage.

## Arterial blood gases

The partial pressures of oxygen and carbon dioxide in the blood are dependent on the following factors:
- Neuromuscular control of ventilation.
- Patent airways for ventilation.
- Diffusion across the alveolar-capillary membrane.
- Pulmonary capillary blood flow matching the areas of ventilation.

When looking at blood gas results, remember these three handy tips:
- If the $pCO_2$ is high the problem is poor ventilation.
- If the $pCO_2$ is high, look at the $HCO_3^-$. If there is chronic carbon dioxide retention, it will be high due to renal compensation. Giving oxygen to these patients can be disastrous as they rely on hypoxic drive to maintain respiration.
- Administration of oxygen to hypoxic patients will improve or correct the $pO_2$ in all cases except right-to-left shunt.

Oxygen is carried in the blood in an easily reversible combination with hemoglobin. Carotid and aortic body chemoreceptors detect low partial pressures of oxygen $pO_2$.

Carbon dioxide is carried in the blood mainly as bicarbonate (reaction catalyzed by carbonic anhydrase principally in the red blood cells [RBCs]) but is also bound to protein or dissolved. It therefore has a profound effect on the acid–base balance. Increased levels are detected by central chemoreceptors (increasing hydrogen ions) and peripheral chemoreceptors (increasing partial pressure of carbon dioxide [$pCO_2$] and falling pH).

Arterial blood is sampled from a peripheral artery (usually the radial artery). The $pO_2$, $pCO_2$, pH, bicarbonate ($HCO_3^-$), and oxygen saturations can be measured. The $pO_2$ will be low if atmospheric oxygen is low (e.g. at high altitude), if ventilation is poor (see below), if diffusion is reduced (interstitial lung disease), if there is a V/Q mismatch (pulmonary embolus [PE]), or if there is a right-to-left shunt (ventricular septal defect with Eisenmenger's phenomenon).

The $pCO_2$ will be high if ventilation is inadequate. This may be due to reduced central drive (sedative drugs, cerebral trauma), neuromuscular disease (Guillain-Barré syndrome, myasthenia gravis), thoracic wall abnormalities (kyphoscoliosis, ankylosing spondylitis) or airways obstruction (chronic bronchitis).

The $pCO_2$ will be low in hyperventilation due to anxiety or panic.

## Respiratory failure

Respiratory failure is defined by a $pO_2$ of less than 60mmHg and can be subdivided according to the $pCO_2$.

In type I respiratory failure there is a low $pO_2$ with normal $pCO_2$. This can be caused by lung disease (pneumonia, pulmonary fibrosis, pulmonary edema), V/Q mismatch (PE), or right-to-left shunts.

If the $pO_2$ is very low, ventilation will increase and the $pCO_2$ may also be low.

In type II respiratory failure there is a low $pO_2$ with high $pCO_2$. This results from inadequate ventilation (see above).

## Ventilation–perfusion scan

Technetium-99m-($^{99m}$Tc)-labeled albumin is injected intravenously and detected in the lungs by a gamma camera—this is the perfusion scan. Areas not perfused are identified as "cold spots."

Pulmonary ventilation is demonstrated by the inhalation of xenon-133 ($^{133}$Xe), which is also detected by a gamma camera.

In PE an area of well-ventilated lung is deprived of its blood supply. This will create a discrepancy ("mismatch") in the V/Q scans which is diagnostic of PE. Where a V/Q scan is not possible, a pulmonary angiogram should be considered. In other pulmonary diseases, such as pneumonia, both ventilation and perfusion are reduced. This results in a nonspecific "matched" defect.

V/Q scans are reported in most centers as showing a high, intermediate, or low probability of PE. When the probability is intermediate or low, careful clinical re-evaluation and further investigations are usually required.

## Computed tomography scan

Most lung pathology can be detected by a standard CXR. However, computed tomography (CT) scanning provides more detailed information regarding the mediastinum and pleura and is particularly valuable in two scenarios:
- Demonstration and staging of bronchogenic carcinoma.
- Demonstration of pulmonary disease not detectable by CXR (e.g., industrial lung disease, lymphangitis carcinomatosis, sarcoidosis).

## Bronchoscopy

Fiberoptic bronchoscopy is performed under local anesthetic and allows direct visualization of the bronchial tree. It is important in the diagnosis and sometimes treatment of pulmonary disease.

Central tumors can be visualized and biopsied. Transbronchial biopsy of the lung will provide diagnostic tissue in interstitial lung disease.

Bronchoalveolar lavage is important in the diagnosis of some infections (tuberculosis, P. carinii), peripheral tumors, and some unusual diseases (e.g., histiocytosis X).

Laser therapy can obliterate small endobronchial tumors and palliate large symptomatic tumors that have not responded to other therapeutic modalities.

## Lung biopsy

Biopsy may be necessary in the diagnosis of tumors, interstitial lung disease, and infections when other techniques have failed to provide adequate information. The tissue can be obtained by transthoracic needle biopsy under ultrasound or CT guidance, mediastinoscopy, mediastinotomy, thoracoscopy, and open biopsy at thoracotomy.

## The gastrointestinal system

### Serum amylase

Amylase breaks down starch to glycogen and maltose. It is found at highest concentrations in saliva and pancreatic juice and is excreted in the urine. It is used as an indicator of acute pancreatitis where levels may be very high (i.e., greater than five times normal upper limit). However, serum amylase may also be elevated in the conditions listed in Fig. 29.13.

### Plain abdominal x-ray

Plain x-rays are of limited use in gastrointestinal (GI) disease. Fig. 29.14 shows radiologic changes that may be found in specific diseases.

### Ultrasound scan, CT scan, and magnetic resonance imaging

These are useful in defining intra-abdominal anatomical abnormalities and pathologies such as

fluid (ascites, abscess), tumor and stones (biliary, urinary tract). Ultrasound is cheaper, more accessible and is often used as the first-line investigation. CT and magnetic resonance imaging (MRI) are particularly helpful in examining the deeper structures that are not always adequately visualized on ultrasound, which include the pancreas and retroperitoneum.

### Barium swallow

The progress of swallowed barium is recorded. This procedure is used in the investigation of dysphagia. It should be performed prior to endoscopy in these patients to demonstrate esophageal anatomy and prevent perforation by the endoscope. It will demonstrate anatomic lesions in the esophagus, including strictures, carcinoma, web, or pharyngeal pouch, and motility abnormalities such as achalasia.

### Double contrast upper GI series

Barium is taken with effervescent tablets, producing a double-contrast image of the stomach and proximal duodenum. This will demonstrate anatomic abnormalities including ulcers and polyps. However, most patients with gastric pathology will need a histologic diagnosis and endoscopy with the option of biopsy is the investigation of choice.

### Small bowel contrast studies

Barium can be introduced into the small bowel in two ways—in a small bowel follow-through, barium is swallowed and its journey to the terminal ileum is

| Causes of a raised serum amylase |
|---|
| • acute pancreatitis |
| • perforated peptic ulcer |
| • ruptured ectopic pregnancy |
| • acute cholecystitis |
| • diabetic ketoacidosis |
| • severe glomerular disease |
| • myocardial infarction |
| • mumps |
| • salivary calculi |

**Fig. 29.13** Causes of a raised serum amylase.

| Radiologic abdominal abnormalities associated with gastrointestinal diseases | |
|---|---|
| **Diagnosis** | **Radiologic abnormality** |
| intestinal obstruction | proximal bowel distension; absent bowel gas distally; air—fluid levels on the erect film |
| perforation of a viscus | subdiaphragmatic free gas on the erect film |
| sigmoid volvulus | grossly distended loop of sigmoid colon often extending from the pelvis to the xiphisternum (looks like a coffee bean) |
| acute pancreatitis | "sentinel loop" of dilated adynamic small bowel "ground glass" appearance if ascites present |
| chronic pancreotitis | pancreatic calcification |
| calculi | 90% of urinary tract stones and 10% of gallstones are radiopaque |
| abdominal aortic aneurysm | calcified aneurysmal abdominal aorta |

**Fig. 29.14** Radiologic abdominal abnormalities associated with gastrointestinal diseases.

recorded; and in a small bowel enema, barium is delivered to the distal duodenum via a nasojejunal tube. It is useful in the diagnosis of small bowel polyposis, Crohn's disease, and malignancies, such as lymphoma.

## Barium enema

A double-contrast picture of the colon and terminal ileum is produced by introducing barium and air into the rectum. The rectum is poorly visualized and should be examined by sigmoidoscopy. Typical abnormalities will be seen in polyps, malignancy, ulcerative colitis, and Crohn's disease.

## Endoscopy

Various "scopes" are now available, enabling direct visualization of the whole GI tract, with the exception of the third part of the duodenum to the terminal ileum (Fig. 29.15).

As well as visualizing pathology, biopsies can be taken for histological diagnosis. Contrast can also be injected into the pancreatic and biliary tree (endoscopic retrograde cholangiopancreatogram [ERCP]).

Endoscopy is also important in treatment for the following reasons:

- Strictures can be dilated.
- Stents and prosthetic tubes can be placed through malignant lesions causing obstruction (esophagus, urinary tract, ampulla of Vater).
- Varices can be injected with sclerosing agents.
- Polyps can be removed.
- Bleeding lesions can be cauterized.

| "Scopes" used to examine the gastrointestinal tract | |
|---|---|
| **"Scope"** | **Bowel visualized** |
| esophagogastroscope | esophagus, stomach, first two parts of duodenum |
| colonoscope | rectum, entire colon, terminal ileum |
| flexible sigmoidoscope | rectum, descending colon |
| rigid sigmoidoscope | rectum, lower sigmoid colon |
| proctoscope | anus, lower rectum |

**Fig. 29.15** "Scopes" used to examine the gastrointestinal tract.

## The urinary system

### Urine

Urine should be collected by taking a midstream specimen which minimizes contamination by skin commensals.

The urine should have a dipstick test, which gives an indication of urinary pH, specific gravity, protein, glucose, ketones, and blood. Causes of proteinuria and hematuria are discussed in detail in Chapter 13. Glycosuria is usually due to high plasma glucose concentration (diabetes mellitus) though it may rarely be due to renal glycosuria, an autosomal dominant condition characterized by a reduction in tubular glucose reabsorption.

Heavy ketonuria is a feature of diabetic ketoacidosis, although ketones will become present in the urine on fasting for several hours.

Microscopy is performed to determine the number of RBCs and white blood cells (WBCs) and the presence of bacteria or casts. A urinary tract abnormality is likely to be present if there is more than 2 RBC or 5 WBCs per high-powered field, RBC or WBC casts, or a large number of bacteria (>1 × $10^5$/mL). The urine can be cultured to confirm a urinary tract infection and to determine sensitivities to available antibiotics. If tuberculosis is suspected, three early morning specimens should be examined.

### Urea and creatinine

Urea is produced by the liver from amino acids, while creatinine is a product of tissue breakdown; both are excreted by the kidneys. Levels of both in the plasma are dependent on a balance between production and excretion.

In renal failure, urea and creatinine will be raised proportionally. In an upper GI bleed, urea will be raised but creatinine remains normal (high protein intake—blood absorbed by the small intestine). The urea:creatinine ratio is also raised in dehydration and tetracycline administration. A low ratio occurs in chronic liver disease, low-protein diet, and hemodialysis. Creatinine may also be low in those with reduced muscle bulk.

### Plain x-ray

A plain x-ray (KUB film) is most useful in the diagnosis of renal stones, of which 90% are radiopaque. It also demonstrates renal size, shape, and position.

## Renal ultrasound

Renal ultrasound is good at detecting renal size, cysts, stones, tumors, and urinary outflow obstruction (hydronephrosis), but gives little information regarding the pelvicalyceal system and is a poor predictor of renal artery stenosis. It provides no information about renal function.

## Intravenous urography

Renally excreted contrast is injected intravenously and a series of x-rays are taken at specific time intervals. Information regarding anatomy and excretion are gained by following the movement of contrast from the renal parenchyma, through the pelvicalyceal system, to the ureters and bladder. It detects renal scarring due to chronic parenchymal disease, pelvicalyceal pathology, the location of calculi and is a good predictive indicator of renal artery stenosis.

## CT scan

CT scan provides detailed anatomical information. It is important in staging malignancy and the examination of regions poorly visualized by other techniques, such as the retroperitoneal and perinephric areas.

## Radioisotope studies

Renal scintigraphy can provide information about gross renal anatomy, obstruction, the relative contribution of each kidney to overall renal function, and features suggestive of renal artery stenosis. Its accuracy is increased by the coadministration of captopril—the "captopril renogram."

## Renal angiography

Contrast is injected directly into the renal arteries via a catheter introduced into the femoral artery. This is the gold standard test for the diagnosis of renovascular disease.

## Cystoscopy

Cystoscopy allows the direct visualization of the bladder mucosa. It is useful in the diagnosis and sometimes treatment of bladder carcinoma.

 A slightly elevated creatinine may indicate significant renal impairment.

## Renal biopsy

Renal biopsy is performed transcutaneously under ultrasound guidance. It is particularly useful in the assessment of rapidly deteriorating renal function, nephrotic syndrome, and assessment of transplanted kidneys. It may be complicated by significant hematuria, pain, and, in the long term, arteriovenous malformation. Biopsy material should be evaluated by light microscopy, electron microscopy, and immunofluorescence.

# The nervous system

Tests useful in the diagnosis of neurologic disease have been described in Chapter 22.

# Metabolic and endocrine disorders

## Diabetes mellitus

Diabetes mellitus (DM) is characterized by chronic hyperglycemia. It can be primary, as in type 1 (IDDM—insulin-dependent DM) and type 2 (NIDDM—non-insulin-dependent DM), or secondary to pancreatic disease (chronic pancreatitis, hemochromatosis, cystic fibrosis), endocrine disease (Cushing's syndrome, acromegaly), pregnancy, or drugs (steroids, thiazide diuretics).

### Diagnosis

Diagnostic criteria for diabetes mellitus include:
- Fasting blood glucose >126 mg/dl.
- On two separate occasions, random blood glucose >200 mg/dl.
- Oral glucose tolerance test >200 mg/dl 2 hours after ingestion of 75 g oral glucose.

### Monitoring response to diet or treatment

Glycated hemoglobin (HBA1c) gives a measurement of overall glycemic control over the previous 2–3 months. Fructosamine gives a measurement of overall glycemic control over the previous 1–3 weeks.

### Hypothalamus-pituitary-adrenal axis

Fig. 29.16 summarizes the normal control of cortisol. Excess circulating cortisol causes the clinical picture

**Fig. 29.16** Hypothalamus–pituitary–adrenal axis. (ACTH, adrenocorticotrophic hormone; CRH, corticotrophin-releasing hormone.)

of Cushing's syndrome. It may result from increased release of adrenocorticotrophic hormone (ACTH) from an anterior pituitary adenoma (Cushing's disease), ectopic ACTH from a bronchogenic carcinoma or carcinoid tumor, excess cortisol production by an adrenal adenoma or carcinoma, or by the oral administration of corticosteroids. Pseudo-Cushing's syndrome may arise in alcohol abuse and endogenous depression.

Reduced circulating cortisol results from reduced pituitary ACTH production (tumor, infarction, prolonged corticosteroid therapy), or reduced adrenal cortisol production (autoimmune Addison's disease, tuberculosis, metastases, amyloidosis, Waterhouse-Friderichsen syndrome).

Tests useful for determining the site of the lesion in cortisol excess and deficiency are given in Fig. 29.17.

### Plasma cortisol

Plasma cortisol will vary throughout the day in normal individuals and should be measured at 9 AM and 11 PM. Normal circadian rhythm will be lost and levels raised in Cushing's syndrome. Very low or absent cortisol levels at a time of suspected

| Investigations in abnormalities of the hypothalamus-pituitary-adrenal axis | | | | | |
|---|---|---|---|---|---|
| | Cushing's disease | Ectopic ACTH production | Adrenal hyperproductiion of cortisol | Pituitary hypoproduction of ACTH | Adrenal hypoproduction of cortisol |
| causes | pituitary adenoma | bronchial carcinoma, carcinoid tumor | adenoma, carcinoma | tumor, infarction, corticosteroids | Addison's disease, amyloid, TB, metastases. Waterhouse—Friderichsen syndrome |
| plasma cortisol | high | high | high | low | low |
| plasma ACTH | high | very high | very low | low | high |
| urinary free cortisol | high | high | high | low | low |
| overnight dexamethasone suppression test | no suppression | no suppression | no suppression | not applicable | not applicable |
| high-dose dexamethasone suppression test | suppression | no suppression | no suppression | not applicable | not applicable |
| short ACTH test | not applicable | not applicable | not applicable | no stimulation | no stimulation |
| long ACTH test | not applicable | not applicable | not applicable | stimulation | no stimulation |

**Fig. 29.17** Investigations in abnormalities of the hypothalamus–pituitary–adrenal axis. (ACTH, adrenocorticotrophic hormone.)

Addisonian crisis confirms hypoproduction of cortisol.

## Tests for cortisol excess
### Urinary cortisol
A 24-hour estimation of urinary free cortisol is a better predictor of Cushing's syndrome than plasma cortisol.

### Plasma ACTH
This is very high in ectopic ACTH production, moderately raised in Cushing's syndrome (pituitary adenoma), and very low in adrenal adenoma or carcinoma.

### Overnight dexamethasone suppression test
Here, 2mg oral dexamethasone is taken at 11 pm; plasma cortisol is measured at 9 am the next morning. In normal patients, ACTH and cortisol production will be suppressed by negative feedback, and plasma levels of cortisol will be <5µg/dl (140nmol/L).

In all cases of Cushing's syndrome suppression will not occur. In patients with Cushing's disease the feedback mechanism is less sensitive than normal as ACTH levels are chronically elevated. Ectopic ACTH production has no feedback mechanism; ACTH is always suppressed in those with an adrenal cause.

### High-dose dexamethasone suppression test
Plasma cortisol is measured; 2mg oral dexamethasone is taken every 6 hours for 2 days. After 48 hours from the first dose, plasma cortisol is remeasured. In normal individuals the plasma cortisol should be suppressed to at least half its initial value. This dose of dexamethasone should overcome the less sensitive feedback mechanism in Cushing's disease but will not cause suppression in ectopic ACTH production and adrenal hyperfunction.

## Tests for cortisol deficiency
### Short ACTH stimulation test
Plasma cortisol is measured (>170nmol/L normally) and 0.25mg cosyntropin (synthetic ACTH, which has the same biologic action as ACTH) is given intramuscularly or intravenously. Plasma cortisol is remeasured after 60 minutes. In normal patients, cortisol will rise by a minimum of 190nmol/L to at least 580nmol/L. The response will be poor in any case of cortisol hypoproduction.

### Long ACTH stimulation test
Here, 1mg ACTH is given by intramuscular injection daily for 3 days. Adrenal glands suppressed by the prolonged admistration of corticosteroids show a response to this level of stimulation. No response will be seen in adrenal hypofunction.

## The hypothalamus–pituitary–thyroid axis
Fig. 29.18 summarizes the normal control of thyroid hormones. Thyroid status can now be easily assessed by the measurement of thyroid-stimulating hormone (TSH), total thyoxine ($T_4$) and total tri-iodothyronine ($T_3$) (Fig. 29.19). Around 99% of circulating $T_4$ and $T_3$ is bound to protein (mostly thyroxine-binding globulin—TBG). It is the free $T_4$ and $T_3$ that is physiologically active and can be measured separately.

The TRH stimulation test, which used to be important in the diagnosis of hyperthyroidism, is now almost never necessary.

## Calcium metabolism
Calcium homoeostasis is dependent on the normal availability of calcium and vitamin D and normal functioning of the parathyroid glands, kidneys, and gut (Fig. 29.20).

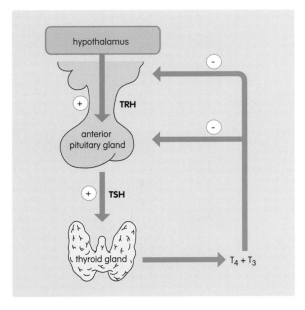

Fig. 29.18 Hypothalamus–pituitary–thyroid axis. (TRH, thyrotropin-releasing hormone; TSH, thyroid-stimulating hormone.)

| Biochemical abnormalities in thyroid disease | | | | | |
|---|---|---|---|---|---|
| | **Primary thyrotoxicosis** | **Secondary thyrotoxicosis** | **Primary hypothyroidism** | **Secondary hypothyroidism** | **Sick euthyroid syndrome** |
| causes | thyroiditis, toxic adenoma, multinodular goiter, carcinoma, amiodarone | pituitary adenoma | thyroiditis, iodine deficiency, dyshormonogenesis, antithyroid drugs, postirradiation/$^{131}$I therapy | hypopituitarism, isolated TSH deficiency | acute severe illness |
| TSH | low | high | high | low | normal or low |
| total or free $T_4$ and $T_3$ | $T_3$ high (first) then $T_4$ high | $T_3$ high (first) then $T_4$ high | $T_4$ low (first) then $T_3$ low | $T_4$ low (first) then $T_3$ low | $T_4$ and $T_3$ low |

**Fig. 29.19** Biochemical abnormalities in thyroid disease. ($T_3$, tri-iodothyronine; $T_4$, thyroxine; TSH, thyroid-stimulating hormone.)

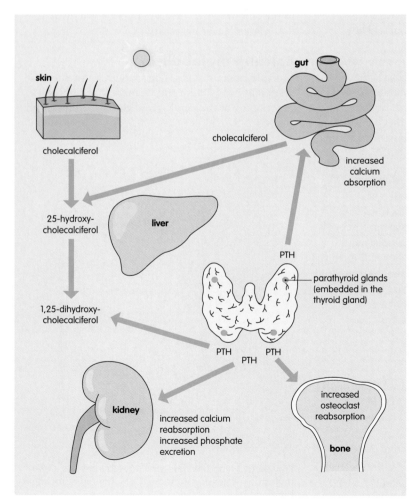

**Fig. 29.20** Calcium homeostasis. (PTH, parathyroid hormone.)

## Plasma calcium

Total plasma calcium is measured and should be adjusted for albumin concentration (half is protein-bound, but it is the unbound that is physiologically active). The most accurate measurement is in the fasted patient with a sample taken without a cuff. Causes of hypercalcemia and hypocalcemia are shown in Figs 29.21 and 29.22.

## Phosphate

Phosphate levels are dependent on a balance between release from bone by osteoclastic activity, and renal tubular reabsorption. Parathyroid hormone (PTH) increases phosphate release from bone but reduces renal reabsorption, with the overall effect of lowering phosphate concentrations.

Hyperphosphatemia occurs in renal disease and hypoparathyroidism.

Hypophosphatemia occurs as a result of hyperparathyroidism, reduced intake due to dietary deficiency or long-term parenteral feeding, and increased phosphate loss as in renal tubular acidosis.

> Calcium and phosphate levels vary in the same direction (i.e., all higher or all lower) in all diseases with the exception of hypo- and hyperparathyroidism, and renal failure.

| Causes of hypercalcemia | |
|---|---|
| **Mechanism** | **Example** |
| increased calcium intake | milk—alkali syndrome |
| increased vitamin D intake | self-administered, iatrogenic |
| increased activity of vitamin D | sarcoidosis, lymphoma Addison's disease |
| increased production of PTH | primary hyperparathyroidism (adenoma, hyperplasia, carcinoma), tertiary hyperparathyroidism (hyperplasia) |
| production of PTH-related peptide | squamous carcinoma, renal cell carcinoma |
| increased osteoclastic activity | osteolytic metastases, multiple myeloma |
| increased bone turnover | hyperthyroidism |
| increased renal tubular calcium reabsorption | familial hypocalciuric hypercalcemia (autosomal dominant) |

**Fig. 29.21** Causes of hypercalcemia. (PTH, parathyroid hormone.)

| Causes of hypocalcemia | |
|---|---|
| **Mechanism** | **Example** |
| reduced calcium intake | dietary deficiency, malabsorption |
| reduced vitamin D intake/production | dietary deficiency, malabsorption, reduced sunlight exposure |
| reduced activation of vitamin D | renal disease, liver disease |
| increased inactivation of vitamin D | enzyme induction by anticonvulsants |
| reduced production of PTH | surgical removal of parathyroid glands, autoimmune, congenital (DiGeorge syndrome) |
| resistance to PTH | pseudohypoparathyroidism |
| hypoalbuminemia | shock |

**Fig. 29.22** Causes of hypocalcemia. (PTH, parathyroid hormone.)

## Urinary calcium

Hypercalciuria will occur whenever there is hypercalcemia if glomerular function is normal or if the renal tubules "leak" calcium (idiopathic hypercalciuria).

## Alkaline phosphatase

Alkaline phosphatase is found in osteoblasts, liver, and the placenta. Isoenzymes can be measured to determine the origin of high levels. Alkaline phosphatase concentrations will be increased in bone disease if there is an increase in the number or activity of osteoblasts, as in Paget's disease, osteomalacia, metastases, healing fractures, and hyperparathyroidism.

## Parathyroid hormone

PTH concentrations can be measured by radioimmunoassay. They are elevated in hyperparathyroidism and pseudohypoparathyroidism, and low or undetectable in primary hypoparathyroidism.

The overall patterns of abnormalities in these investigations are typical, as shown in Fig. 29.23.

## Musculoskeletal and skin disease

Muscle disease is investigated by measuring muscle enzymes, electromyography, and muscle biopsy, as described in Chapter 22. The investigation of joint and connective tissue diseases is described in Chapter 16, and characteristic findings on investigation of skin pathology are discussed in Chapter 17.

## Hematologic disorders

## Complete blood count

### Hemoglobin

Normal values for hemoglobin are 13.5–17.5g/dL in men and 11.5–15.5g/dL in women. Anemia is present when the hemoglobin level falls below these values. The causes and investigation of anemia are described in Chapter 25.

In polycythemia, hemoglobin levels are above the normal range. It may be true where the total RBC volume is increased, or relative where the total RBC volume is normal but the plasma volume is decreased (Fig. 29.24).

### Mean corpuscular volume

Normal values for mean corpuscular volume are 80–100 fL. The causes of a raised and low mean corpuscular volume are described in Chapter 25.

### Reticulocytes

Reticulocytes normally comprise 0.5–2% of the RBCs; they are immature RBCs that still contain ribosomal RNA. They are demonstrated by supravital staining with methylene blue. They are present in the

| Pattern of biochemical abnormalities in bone disease | | | | |
|---|---|---|---|---|
| Disease | Calcium | Phosphate | Alkaline phosphatase | PTH |
| osteoporosis | N | N | N | N |
| osteomalacia | ↓ | ↓ | ↑ | N or ↑ |
| Paget's disease | N | N | ↑↑ | N |
| metastases | ↑ | ↑ | ↑ | PTH-rp may be ↑ |
| renal failure | ↓ | ↑ | N or ↑ | N or ↑ |
| primary hypoparathyroidism | ↑ | ↓ | N (slightly ↑) | ↑ |
| primary hypoparathyroidism | ↓ | ↑ | N | ↓ |
| pseudo-hypoparathyroidism | ↓ | ↑ | N | ↑ |

**Fig. 29.23** Pattern of biochemical abnormalities in bone disease. (N, normal; PTH-rp, parathyroid hormone resorption.)

**Fig. 29.24** Causes of polycythemia.

| Causes of polycythemia | | |
|---|---|---|
| **Primary polycythemia (myeloproliferative disorder)** | **Secondary polycythemia (↑erythropoietin production)** | **Relative (↓ plasma volume)** |
| polycythemia rubra vera | chronic hypoxia: pulmonary disease, cyanotic heart disease, high altitudes, obesity (pickwickian syndrome), methemoglobinemia inappropriate erythropoietin: renal disease, cerebellar hemangioblastoma, hepatocellular carcinoma, uterine myomata, pheochromocytama | stress polycythemia dehydration plasma loss (burns) |

| Causes of abnormalities of the white cell count | | | |
|---|---|---|---|
| **White cell** | **Normal value (× 10$^9$/L)** | **Increased** | **Decreased** |
| neutrophils | 2.5–7.5 | bacterial infections, uremia, inflammation, malignancy, steroids, acute hemorrhage, myeloproliferative disorders | bone marrow failure, hypersplenism, infections (HIV, typhoid), racial, drugs (phenytoin, tolbutamide), connective tissue disease (SLE, rheumatoid arthritis) |
| lymphocytes | 1.5–3.5 | infections (viral, TB, brucellosis), CLL, ALL, non-Hodgkin's lymphoma, thyrotoxicosis | bone marrow failure, HIV, drugs (cytotoxics) |
| monocytes | 0.2–0.8 | infection (TB, brucellosis), inflammation (UC, Crohn's disease), connective tissue disease (SLE, rheumatoid arthritis), AML, malignancy | bone marrow failure |
| eosinophils | 0.04–0.44 | allergy (urticaria, drugs), parasite infection (filariasis, amoebiasis), skin disease (psoriasis, dematilis herpetiformis), polyarteritis nodosa, Hodgkin's disease, pulmonary eosinophilia, eosinophilic leukemia | bone marrow failure |
| basophilis | 0.01–0.1 | infection (varicella), hypothyroidism, myeloproliferative disorders | bone marrow failure |

**Fig. 29.25** Causes of abnormalities of the white cell count. (ALL, acute lymphoblastic leukemia; AML, acute myeloid leukemia; CLL, chronic lymphocytic leukemia; HIV, human immunodeficiency virus; SLE, systemic lupus erythematosus; TB, tuberculosis; UC, ulcerative colitis.)

peripheral blood for up to 2 days after leaving the bone marrow before they become mature RBCs. The number of reticulocytes present in the peripheral blood will increase when the bone marrow is producing large numbers of RBCs. This is seen 2–3 days after acute blood loss and in hemolysis.

## Total white cell count

The normal range for total white cell count is $4.0–11.0 × 10^9$/L. The total count comprises neutrophils, lymphocytes, monocytes, eosinophils, and basophils (Fig. 29.25).

| Causes of thrombocytosis | |
|---|---|
| primary | essential thrombocythemia |
| secondary | inflammation<br>malignancy<br>chronic infection<br>postsplenectomy<br>hemorrhage<br>surgery or trauma |

**Fig. 29.26** Causes of thrombocytosis.

## Platelet count

The normal range for platelet count is $150-400 \times 10^9$/L. The causes of thrombocytopenia are discussed in Chapter 23, and the causes of thrombocytosis are shown in Fig. 29.26.

## Erythrocyte sedimentation rate

The erythrocyte sedimentation rate (ESR) is a measure of the rate of RBC sedimentation over 1 hour. The normal range varies between laboratories, increases with age, and is higher in women. It is a nonspecific indicator of inflammation, infection, and malignancy.

A "reactive" blood picture consists of a normochromic normocytic anemia, neutrophilia, thrombocytosis and raised erythrocyte sedimentation rate. It suggests underlying inflammation, infection or malignancy.

## Bone marrow examination

Aspirate and trephine are usually taken from the posterior iliac crest under local anesthesia (aspirate may also be obtained from the sternum). A smear of bone marrow cells is made from the aspirate, allowing a detailed examination of the proportion and differentiation of different cell lines in the bone marrow. Infiltration by other cells (carcinoma) and iron reserves can also be assessed. Cytogenetic analysis of the aspirate may give diagnostic and prognostic information. The trephine consists of a core of bone containing marrow cells, is important in determining marrow cellularity and infiltration.

## Coagulation assessment

Coagulation is assessed by measurement of the prothrombin time, activated partial thromboplastin time, thrombin time, and bleeding time (Chapter 23).

## Computed tomography scan

Deep intra-abdominal and mediastinal lymphadenopathy are well demonstrated on CT scans and often missed on other imaging techniques such as ultrasound. CT scans are useful in the staging of hematologic malignancies such as lymphoma.

# PART III: DISEASES AND DISORDERS

# 30. The Cardiovascular System

## Coronary heart disease

Coronary heart disease (CHD) is the result of an imbalance between myocardial oxygen supply and demand. The term covers a group of clinical syndromes that includes angina pectoris, acute myocardial infarction (MI), and sudden death. The most common underlying pathology is atherosclerosis of the coronary arteries. More rarely, CHD can result from coronary artery spasm, embolis, coronary ostial stenosis, aortic stenosis, hypertrophic obstructive cardiomyopathy, arrhythmias causing decreased coronary perfusion pressures, and anemia.

Ischemia may also occur with normal coronary arteries and is then termed syndrome X. It is thought to be due to abnormalities of small coronary vessels, resulting in a reduction of coronary flow reserve.

The incidence of CHD shows large geographic variations, ranging from a mortality rate below 100 in 100,000 in Japan to 600 in 100,000 in Finland and Northern Ireland. The incidence appears to be declining in Western Europe, although there has been a noticeable increase in CHD mortality rates in several Eastern European countries. In England and Wales, 1 in 6 men aged 40–44 years have some evidence of CHD; at 55–59 years, this rises to 1 in 3, showing the increase in prevalence with age.

Current measures of the prevalence of CHD in the U.S. (although thought to be underestimates) show that the risk increases in men from 7% at ages 40–49 to 22% at ages 70–79. In women the incidence is 5% at 40–49 years and 14% at ages 70–79.

### Risk factors for coronary heart disease

A number of predictors have been found to be associated with an increased likelihood of developing CHD and are called risk factors (Fig. 30.1).

The complete list of possible risk factors for CHD is extremely long and includes environmental factors as well as personal characteristics. Not all these factors will ultimately be shown to be truly causal. For example, obesity may act as a risk factor because it is associated with raised serum cholesterol, hypertension, and decreased glucose tolerance.

### Age

Mortality from CHD rises steeply with increasing age. This may be due to the accumulative effects of raised serum total cholesterol, hypertension, cigarette smoking, and other factors over time.

### Sex

The rate in young men is about six times higher than in women of the same age, although this difference diminishes with increasing age. Premenopausal women are thought to be protected by their hormonal status, and this protection diminishes progressively during and after menopause.

### Family history

The effect of family history appears to be independent of other major risk factors if first-degree relatives below the age of 50 years are affected. Although high levels of serum total cholesterol may cluster in families, only a very small proportion of these are associated with genetically conditioned familial hypercholesterolemia.

### Cigarette smoking

The risk of developing coronary artery disease is directly proportional to the number of cigarettes smoked. The rate of CHD in current smokers is about three times that of those who have never smoked. Giving up smoking leads to an initial rapid decrease in the risk of developing CHD, followed by a more gradual decline in risk, so that the risk of CHD is almost the same as a nonsmoker after about 10 years.

### Blood lipids

The risk of CHD increases as serum total cholesterol and low-density lipoprotein (LDL) cholesterol

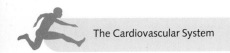

| Major risk factors for coronary artery disease | |
|---|---|
| **Type** | **Risk factors** |
| fixed | age<br>male sex<br>positive family history<br>race |
| modifiable | cigarette smoking<br>hyperlipidemia<br>hypertension<br>diabetes mellitus<br>left ventricular hypertrophy |

**Fig. 30.1** Major risk factors for coronary artery disease.

increase. High-density lipoprotein (HDL) cholesterol is "protective" for CHD, and the risk of IHD decreases as HDL increases. Triglycerides are also positively related to CHD risk, although, when the relationship of CHD to other blood lipids is taken into account, the independent contribution of triglycerides to CHD is very small.

### Hypertension
Both systolic and diastolic hypertension are associated with the risk of developing IHD, as well as hypertensive heart disease, stroke, and renal failure. Treatment of hypertension with drugs reduces the incidence of cardiac events by about 16% overall, with a greater benefit obtained in the elderly.

### Diabetes mellitus
In countries where CHD is prevalent, diabetes mellitus (DM) is associated with an approximately two-fold increase in the risk of a major CHD event. The role of asymptomatic hyperglycemia is uncertain.

### Race
The prevalence of CHD in South Asians in the U.S. is high compared with their family members remaining in the Indian subcontinent. The explanation is only partly accounted for by a low HDL cholesterol and a higher prevalence of DM and glucose intolerance.

### Obesity
Overweight individuals have twice the risk of a major CHD event. This is probably mediated through increased blood pressure levels, total cholesterol,

insulin resistance, and with decreased HDL and physical activity.

### Psychosocial factors
Although stress and other strong emotional responses can precipitate major CHD events in individuals with severe atherosclerosis, it remains to be shown whether stress plays a role in the pathogenesis of coronary artery disease in the absence of other standard risk factors. People from lower socioeconomic classes are at an increased risk for CHD. In addition, patients who were small for gestational age (SGA) have an increased risk of CHD. The risk associated with SGA decreases with increasing birth weight.

Combining risk factors is a more accurate way of predicting those at risk from CHD than relying on any one individual risk factor. Many models and scoring systems have been devised incorporating the different risk factors so that those at high risk may be targeted for preventative treatment. This should be accompanied by population-based measures to reduce the risk of CHD.

## Pathology
Atherosclerosis is a slowly progressive focal proliferation of connective tissue within the intima, which begins early in life. It is linked to high lipid levels, although the principal constituent of atherosclerotic plaques is collagen synthethized by smooth muscle cells.

The initial process consists of endothelial dysfunction in association with a high circulating cholesterol, inflammation, shear forces, and chemical irritants from tobacco smoke. Macrophages enter the arterial wall between endothelial cells. The accumulation of lipid-laden macrophages in the subendothelial zone leads to the formation of fatty streaks. Toxic products released from the macrophages lead to the adhesion of platelets and results in smooth muscle cell proliferation and thrombus formation. This then becomes organized, leading to the development of an atherosclerotic plaque surrounded by a fibrotic cap. Progressive enlargement of these lesions leads to segmental narrowing of the lumen, which, when sufficient to be flow limiting on exercise, causes stable exertion-associated angina. Atherosclerotic plaques are liable to rupture, resulting in sudden thrombosis, which is responsible for the acute manifestations of IHD. Factors associated with plaque disruption and consequent thrombosis include a large lipid core, a high monocyte density, and low smooth muscle cell density.

The onset or worsening of angina is due predominantly to intraplaque thrombosis leading to rapid plaque growth. Extension of thrombus into the lumen results in unstable angina or non-Q-wave MI.

## Investigations

### Electrocardiogram

A normal electrocardiogram (ECG) does not exclude a diagnosis of angina. During attacks, there may be ST segment depression or symmetrical T wave inversion. T wave inversion in leads $V_{1-3}$ often indicates a critical left anterior descending coronary artery (LAD) stenosis. The ECG may show signs of an old MI or left ventricular hypertrophy.

### Exercise electrocardiogram

The exercise ECG is a useful indicator of exercise performance and is an independent indicator of prognosis. The test is most useful in patients with known CHD risk factors and an indeterminate clinical history. It is contraindicated in unstable angina, recent (within 7 days) MI, severe aortic stenosis, severe pulmonary hypertension, and significant rhythm disturbances. Relative contraindications include infirmity and ataxia.

The test is usually regarded as positive if there is more than 1 mm of J point depression, the junction of the ST segment and the T wave. If the pretest probability of angina is high, the number of false positives is low. Causes of false positive tests include hyperventilation, digoxin and other antiarrhythmic agents, hypokalemia, hypertension, valvular heart disease, left ventricular hypertrophy, and pre-excitation syndromes. The test should be terminated if there is a fall in blood pressure, ventricular tachycardia, or if the patient becomes pale, indicating peripheral circulatory collapse. Relative contraindications for termination include ST segment depression of more than 4 mm, incoordination, or paroxysmal rhythm disturbances other than ventricular tachycardias (VTs).

### Echocardiography

This can be used to assess ventricular function and localize areas of ventricular wall involvement. In patients with angina but no evidence of infarction, the echocardiogram may be normal. With diffuse ischemic changes, left ventricular function may be globally impaired. Exercise or pharmacological stress echocardiography may be used to detect areas of "hibernating" myocardium. These are areas that show reduced function on exercise, due to decreased blood flow secondary to decreased coronary flow reserve, but which show improved function at rest.

### Nuclear imaging

This technique may be used to assess myocardial structure and function. A radioactive isotope (e.g., thallium) is injected during exercise and an image is taken soon after. The isotope is taken up by healthy myocardium, whereas areas of infarction show up as "cold spots."

Repeat images are taken at rest to obtain a redistribution image. The disappearance of the cold spot implies ischemia provoked by exertion and reversed by rest; a fixed cold spot indicates infarction. It is a useful technique when the exercise test is equivocal or contraindicated, or to indicate the clinical significance of angiographically equivocal stenoses.

### Coronary angiography and cardiac catheterization

This is a technique for radiographically visualizing the coronary arteries, and measuring intracardiac pressures, blood oxygen saturation in different cardiac chambers, and cardiac output. The test is usually used to determine the exact coronary anatomy and is used to decide on further management, i.e., medical therapy, coronary angioplasty, or coronary artery bypass surgery. It is usually indicated for patients with:

- Angina resistant to medical treatment.
- Strongly positive exercise tests indicating a poor prognosis.
- Non-ST elevation MI
- Unstable angina.
- Persisting angina after MI.

More rarely, coronary angiography is used as a diagnostic test when other noninvasive tests have not been helpful and symptoms persist.

The mortality from the procedure is about 1 in 1000. Complications include:

- Hemorrhage at the site of arterial puncture and retroperitoneal hemorrhage (patients can lose enough blood in this location to become anemic.

There may be no physical findings, but the patient may complain of some pain. Diagnose with ultrasound or CT).

- Emboli into arteries resulting in MI.
- Stroke.
- Arrhythmias.
- Coronary artery dissection.
- Infection.

## Treatment
### General measures
It is important to explain the condition to the patient, emphasizing that the prognosis is generally good and that treatment can alleviate symptoms. The diagnosis can lead to severe emotional upset, and patients should be encouraged to return for discussion. Noncoronary causes for angina (e.g., valvular heart disease, calcific aortic stenosis, intermittent tachycardias, hyperthyroidism, or anemia) should be sought and treated appropriately.

Risk factors should be evaluated and steps taken to correct them. All patients should be advised to stop smoking and should lose weight if overweight. Dietary control of hyperlipidemia should be considered if total cholesterol is above 4.8mmol/L.

Factors precipitating angina (e.g., cold weather or emotion) should be avoided, although exercise within the patient's limits should be encouraged to promote the formation of a collateral cardiac circulation.

### Drugs
All patients should be prescribed aspirin 81–325mg daily as this lowers the incidence of subsequent MI and death. If cholesterol is more than 4.8mmol/L after diet or if LDL is more than 100mg/dl, patients with CHD and/or diabetes will also benefit from HMG-CoA reductase inhibitors (statins) to lower cholesterol. During an acute attack the patient should be advised to stop any precipitating factors such as exercise and to take sublingual nitroglycerin (NTG); the acute attack usually subsides within 5 minutes. Patients may also be advised to take sublingual NTG prophylactically before exertion.

When angina occurs frequently, regular prophylactic therapy should be advised. This consists of β-adrenoreceptor blockers, nitrates, calcium antagonists, and potassium channel openers.

### β-blockers
These act by reducing sympathetic tone, depressing myocardial contractility (negatively inotropic), and reducing the heart rate (negatively chronotropic). In addition to these effects (which reduce the oxygen demand), β-blockers may also increase the perfusion of the ischemic area because the decrease in heart rate increases the duration of diastole and hence the time available for coronary blood flow.

Typical β-blockers include atenolol 50–100mg daily, or metoprolol 25–50mg 3 times/day if a shorter half-life is required. Heart rate with beta blocker therapy should be 50–60bpm, if blood pressure tolerates this level. Contraindications include asthma, peripheral vascular disease with skin ulceration, and second and third -degree heart block.

### Nitrates
Nitrates cause peripheral vasodilatation, especially in the veins. This reduces venous return and the ventricular volume is decreased. Reduction in the distension of the heart wall decreases oxygen demand, resulting in relief of pain. Sublingual GTN acts for about 30 minutes. Nitrates work by conversion to nitric oxide, a free radical, which activates guanylate cyclase. This results in an increase in intracellular cyclic GMP in the smooth muscle; by stimulating calcium binding processes the free calcium available to trigger muscle contraction is reduced.

Longer-acting nitrates are more stable and can be effective for several hours. Isosorbide dinitrate (ISDN) is rapidly metabolized by the liver to the mononitrate, which is the main active metabolite. Isosorbide mononitrate (ISMN) may avoid the variable absorption and unpredictable first-pass metabolism of the dinitrate.

Typical doses include ISMN 10–60mg b.i.d. or slow release ISMN 60–120mg q.d. Adverse effects are normally due to arterial dilatation and include headaches, flushing, hypotension, and, rarely, fainting.

Patients may also benefit from a transdermal nitroglyerine patch. The patch needs to be worn for only 12 hours/day to avoid drug tolerance.

### Calcium channel blockers
Calcium antagonists have direct actions on the heart but they relieve angina mainly by causing peripheral arteriolar dilatation and afterload reduction. They

are especially useful if there is some degree of coronary artery spasm. The dihydropyridines such as nifedipine can cause reflex tachycardia and should not generally be used without a β-blocker. Typical doses are slow-release nifedipine 10–30mg b.i.d. Diltiazem has slight negative inotropic and chronotropic effects, and the patient should be closely monitored if on concomitant β-blockers for the development of heart block. Verapamil is the drug of choice if β-blockers are contraindicated (e.g., in patients with asthma or patients who have supraventricular tachycardias in addition to angina). They are contraindicated in heart block and heart failure. Side effects include constipation.

Side effects with the dihydropyridines include headache, flushing, dizziness, and gravitational edema.

## Angiotensin-converting enzyme inhibitors (ACE-Is)

These medications work to decrease afterload and blood pressure. They are also very beneficial in diabetic patients who have microalbuminemia. Currently they are not first-line choices to treat angina because their benefit in this setting is still under investigation. However, they are still very beneficial because of their proven efficacy in patients with prior MI.

Possible side effects include hyperkalemia and a chronic dry cough in some patients.

## Antiplatelet medications

The mere fact that one of the most important medications given during an acute MI is aspirin should tell you how important antiplatelet medication is to decrease mortality rates. New medications that inhibit platelets in ways different from aspirin have recently been shown to be beneficial in keeping stents and arteries open.

Clopidogrel, an adenylate cyclase inhibitor, is now the standard of care, particularly for patients receiving a stent during catheterization (see below). The medication is prescribed for a period ranging from three months to life-long in order to decrease the restenosis rate.

GIIb/IIIa inhibitors affect platelet aggregation. Recent data have shown their usefulness in patients who will undergo catheterization and stenting within 24 hours of their administration. As more research is done on these medications, they may be used in other settings.

## Potassium channel activators

This is a new class of drug with arterial and venous vasodilating properties. They may be useful in patients refractory to treatment with other antianginal agents. The only licensed drug (in Europe, not U.S.) in this group at present is nicorandil 10–30mg b.i.d.

Side effects include headache, flushing, nausea, vomiting, and dizziness.

## Unstable angina

Angina which occurs with increasing frequency and severity, even at rest, is termed unstable. Patients should be admitted to hospital to facilitate rapid adjustments to drug therapy. Antianginal therapy should be added and titrated to control symptoms, and the patient should be on bed rest. Aspirin reduces the incidence of death and MI.

Intravenous NTG is useful for patients who do not become free of chest pain with oral treatment, and intravenous heparin or high-dose, low-molecular-weight heparin is used to reduce the incidence of occlusive coronary thrombosis and MI. If the patient still does become free of chest pain, it may be appropriate to proceed to coronary angiography with a view to urgent PCI or coronary artery bypass surgery.

## Percutaneous coronary intervention (PCI)

Patients should be sent for emergent PCI if two of the following indications are present:
- ECG changes consistent with ischemia (ST segment elevations or depressions, T wave inversions, new LBBB).
- Clinical history consistent with ischemic chest pain.
- Elevation of blood troponin I, CK-MB.

It is important to know that, if ECG changes and angina are present, PCI is indicated. Cardiac markers may not be present because they take time to rise, and patients benefit from reperfusion as soon as possible. In addition, three or more cardiac risk factors, prior documented 50% stenotic lesion, and age >65 years are independent factors in considering a patient for emergent PCI.

PCI is a similar technique to diagnostic angiography except that a fine wire is passed through the obstructing lesion, followed by a small catheter with a nonelastic balloon near its tip. The balloon is inflated to a pressure of several atmospheres to dilate the lesion and hence relieve the obstruction. After the obstruction is relieved, a stent is frequently placed. This procedure involves the insertion of a metal tube mounted on the balloon and inflated over the stenosis. If there are no complications, the patient is mobilized the next day and allowed home. The technique is used on selected patients, ideally with a discrete stenosis of a major vessel, including lesions of bypass grafts. One exception is stenosis of the left main stem as occlusion during attempted angioplasty is likely to be catastrophic.

The procedure may be carried out in multiple vessels, and repeat procedures can be undertaken. Complications occur in about 5% of cases, usually resulting from acute occlusion at the lesion within a few hours following the procedure. This may be due to spasm, thrombosis, or dissection of the artery. About 3% of patients will require urgent coronary artery bypass surgery and/or will sustain a MI. The mortality is less than 1%.

About one-third of lesions will restenose within the first 6 months. This can be dealt with by repeat PCI, although a substantial proportion will eventually require coronary artery bypass surgery. Some lesions are now amenable to coronary artery "stenting," which involves the insertion of a metal tube mounted on the balloon and inflated over the stenosis. Recent changes include post-catheterization treatment (with antiplatelet therapy) and new stents coated with drugs that prevent thrombosis or emit very low-dose radiation to reduce the acute closure of the blood vessel.

## Surgical management

Surgery should be considered in patients whose symptoms persist despite optimal medical management. The most common operation involves harvesting the saphenous vein from the leg and bypassing the coronary obstruction by suturing the vein between the aorta and the coronary artery distal to the obstruction. The internal mammary artery may also be used as a conduit and has a lower occlusion rate than vein grafts. The overall mortality with surgery is about 2%, and certain factors confer a reduced risk or mortality compared to medical treatment (Fig. 30.2).

The main determinants of risk are increasing age, the degree of ventricular damage, the extent and diffuseness of coronary artery disease, and gender, with females at higher risk. Seventy per cent of patients obtain total relief, and 20% have improved

| Patient factors associated with reduction in mortality with surgery |
| --- |
| • left main stem stenosis<br>• triple vessel coronary artery disease<br>• two vessel disease with proximal LAD disease<br>• benefit is greater in those with left ventricular impairment |

**Fig. 30.2** Factors associated with reduction in mortality with coronary artery bypass surgery compared to medical management of patients with coronary artery disease. (LAD, left anterior descending coronary artery.)

symptoms, although pain returns to 50% in 5 years.

All patients should be given aspirin 81–325 mg daily and treated with an HMG-CoA reductase inhibitor if total cholesterol is greater than 4.8 mmol/L or LDL is greater than 100 mg/dl.

## Prognosis

The mortality of patients with some evidence of CHD in the general population is less than 1% per year. In those with definite angina who are treated with aspirin, the risk of a major coronary heart disease event is about 3% per year. Mortality increases with multivessel disease and with left ventricular dysfunction. It is highest in those with left main stem stenosis, where the mortality is over 10% per year. In unstable angina the annual mortality is up to 40% per year.

Poor prognostic factors include pain lasting for more than 48 hours, heart failure, an enlarged heart, persistent ST/T changes in the ECG, and a long past history of CHD.

## ST-elevation myocardial infarction (STEMI)

Myocardial infarction (MI) affects 5 in 1000 of the general population per year in the U.S. and is the most common cause of mortality in the Western world. Ninety per cent of transmural MIs are caused by an occlusive intracoronary thrombus overlying an ulcerated or fissured stenotic plaque. Underlying most cases is a dynamic interaction between severe coronary atherosclerosis, an acute atheromatous plaque change, superimposed thrombosis, platelet activation, and vasospasm. The microscopic changes

**Fig. 30.3** Changes induced by acute myocardial infarction.

| | Changes induced by acute myocardial infarction | |
|---|---|---|
| Time after onset of symptoms | Macroscopic changes | Microscopic changes |
| up to 18 hours | none | none |
| 24–48 hours | pale edematous muscle | edema, acute inflammatory cell infiltration, necrosis of myocytes |
| 3–4 days | yellow rubbery center with hemorrhagic border | obvious necrosis and inflammation, early granulation tissue |
| 3–6 weeks | silvery scar becoming rough and while | dense fibrosis |

of acute MI follow a predictable sequence (Fig. 30.3).

The overall fatality rate from acute MI in community studies is 50% in the first month. About half these deaths occur within the first 2 hours, while in-patient mortality is about 20%. After the first 6 months the annual mortality, with appropriate prophylactic treatment, is about 2%.

Adverse risk factors in patients admitted to hospital with acute MI are:
- Older age.
- Previous medical history (diabetes, previous MI).
- Indicators of a large infarct size, including the site of infarction (anterior versus inferior).
- Low initial blood pressure.
- The presence of pulmonary congestion.
- The extent of ischemia as expressed by ST elevation with or without depression on the ECG.

## Diagnosis

The diagnosis of acute MI is based on two or three out of the following: history, ECG changes, and enzyme changes.

## Cardiac markers

Cardiac markers are intracellular enzymes which leak out of infarcted myocardium into the bloodstream (Fig. 30.4):
- Creatinine kinase (CK) peaks within 24 hours. It is a cardiac enzyme that is also produced by skeletal muscle and brain. The myocardial-bound isoenzyme fraction of CK—i.e., CKMB—should be requested which is specific for heart muscle

damage. The site of the infarct is related to the serum level of enzyme.
- Aspartate aminotransferase (AST) peaks at 24–48 hours. It is also released by damaged red blood cells (RBCs), kidney, liver and lungs.
- Lactate dehydrogenase (LDH) peaks at 3–4 days. The predominant isoenzyme released with cardiac necrosis is ∝-hydroxybutarate dehydrogenase (HBD). LDH is also released from the liver, skeletal muscle, and RBCs.
- Troponin T and I is a regulatory protein with high specificity for cardiac injury. It is released within 2 hours of myocardial infarction. Troponin measurement is now the cardiac marker test of choice in almost all institutions in the U.S.
- Myoglobin is a small heme molecule that is quickly leaked from damaged tissue due to its small size. It is currently used in some EDs to help diagnose MI because it can be detected much faster than the other cardiac markers (peak release is approximately 1 hour after injury). However, because its half life in the blood is under 10 minutes and because it lacks cardiac specificity, it has yet to widely replace CK-MB and troponin I as the prime markers of cardiac injury. It is not yet widely available as a diagnostic tool.

## Electrocardiogram

The earliest ECG changes or "hyperacute" changes consist of tall, pointed, upright T waves, followed by elevation of the ST segment. This is shortly followed by T wave inversion, the R wave voltage decreases, and Q waves develop. After weeks or months the T

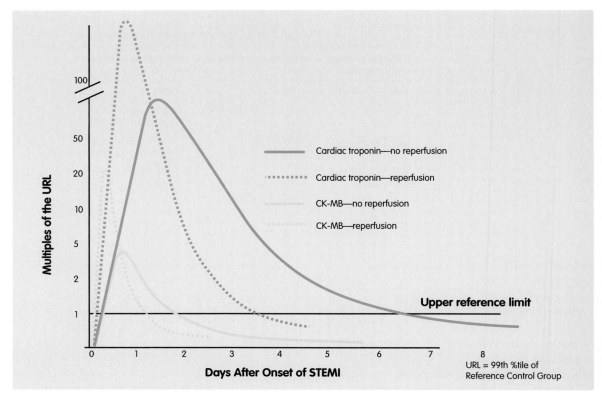

**Fig. 30.4** The pattern of serum enzymes after acute myocardial infarction. (AST, aspartate aminotransferase; CK, creatinine kinase; LDH, lactate dehydrogenase.)

**Fig. 30.5** Progressive ECG changes in myocardial infarction.

wave may become upright again but the Q waves remain (Fig. 30.5).

The site of the infarction may also be deduced from the affected leads on the ECG.

- Inferior MI involves leads II, III, and aVF.
- Anterior MI: affects the precordial leads.
- Anteroseptal MI: affects leads $V_{1-3}$.
- Lateral MI: affects leads I and aVF.
- Posterior MI; there is a tall R wave in leads $V_1$ and $V_2$ with ST segment depression and upright T waves.

There may also be "reciprocal" ECG changes with ST segment depression in leads opposite to the site of infarction. The absence of Q waves in a proven infarct denotes a subendocardial or "non-Q-wave" infarct and is represented by T wave inversion in any lead.

Other investigations to help with management include:

- A complete blood count (CBC) to exclude anemia.
- Metabolic panel to exclude electrolyte abnormalities.
- A chest x-ray (CXR) to exclude aortic dissection, to look for signs of heart failure, and to assess changes in cardiac size.

## Management
### Emergency care

The main aims are to prevent or treat cardiac arrest, and to relieve pain—the patient should ideally be managed on a coronary care unit and an intravenous cannula should be inserted for emergency medicines.

Intravenous opiates, such as diamorphine, 2.5–10mg IV, are given for pain relief. This relieves pain not only for humane reasons but alleviates sympathetic activation associated with the pain which causes vasoconstriction and increases the work of the heart. Side effects include nausea and vomiting, hypotension with bradycardia, and respiratory depression. Antiemetics should be administered concurrently with opiates (e.g., metoclopramide, 10mg IV; cyclizine, 50mg IV; or prochlorperazine, 12.5mg IV). If respiratory depression occurs, intravenous naloxone, which is a specific opioid antagonist, should be given. High-dose oxygen should be given via a face-mask or nasal cannula, especially to those who are breathless or who have any features of heart failure or shock.

Anxiety is a natural response to the pain and to the circumstances surrounding a heart attack. Reassurance of patients and those closely associated with them is therefore of great importance.

### Early care
The aims are to initiate reperfusion therapy, limit infarct size, prevent infarct extension, and treat life-threatening arrhythmias.

### Thrombolytic treatment
Within 12 hours of the onset of pain, treatment with thrombolysis should be given for patients with ST elevation or bundle branch block. This prevents 30 deaths in 1000 patients treated within 6 hours, or 20 deaths if treated between 7 and 12 hours. The benefit from aspirin is additive so that 50 lives are saved in 1000 patients treated.

The largest benefit is seen for those at highest risk:
- The elderly.
- Those with presenting systolic blood pressure of below 100 mmHg.
- Those with anterior infarction.
- Those treated soonest after the onset of thrombolysis.

Contraindications to thrombolytic therapy are given in Fig. 30.6.

Alteplase (rt-PA) is the best thrombolytic agent. Although much more expensive than streptokinase, alteplase was associated with a 1% reduction in mortality in a comparison study of the two drugs. Since the greatest benefit with thrombolysis was seen within the first 2 hours, prompt treatment is necessary. New tools such as thrombolytic predictive instruments (TPIs) help to calculate patient prognosis and to give recommendations for treatment on the ECG. In one study, this tool helped patients achieve thrombolytic therapy for inferior MI more often and sooner.

Streptokinase is the most frequently used fibrinolytic agent in the U.K., but it increases the patient's antistreptokinase antibody level. These antibodies reduce the effectiveness of a repeat dose and increase the risk of an anaphylactic reaction. It should therefore not be readministered in the period between 5 days and a minimum of 2 years following initial treatment. Frequently used thrombolytic regimens are given in Fig. 30.7.

### PCI
PCI with or without stent placement has now become the standard of care for treatment of acute

| Contraindications to thrombolytic therapy | |
|---|---|
| contraindications | stroke<br>major surgery, trauma, or head injury within 3 weeks<br>gastrointestinal bleed within the last week<br>known bleeding disorder<br>dissecting aneurysm |
| relative contraindications | transient ischemic attack in the preceding 6 months<br>warfarin therapy<br>pregnancy<br>non-compressible punctures<br>traumatic resuscitation<br>refractory hypertension (SBP > 180mmHg)<br>recent retinal laser treatment |

**Fig. 30.6** Contraindications to thrombolytic therapy. (SBP, systolic blood pressure.)

217

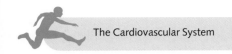

| Frequently used thrombolytic regimens | | |
|---|---|---|
| **Drug** | **Initial treatment** | **Heparin treatment** |
| streptokinase | 1.5 million units i.v. over 30–60 minutes | none |
| anistreplase | 30 units i.v. over 3–5 minutes | none |
| alteplase (rtPA) | 15mg i.v. bolus 0.75mg/kg i.v. over 30 minutes 0.5mg/kg i.v. over 60 minutes total dosage not to exceed 100mg | i.v. for 48 hours determined by the APTT |

**Fig. 30.7** Frequently used thrombolytic regimens. (APTT, activated partial thromboplastin time.)

MI. A recent study showed that it is more beneficial to transfer the patient emergently to a center at which catheterization is available than to give thrombolytic agents despite the increased time from presentation to treatment. Studies have shown that PCI gives patency of the infarct-related artery in 91% of patients at 3 months compared with 68% for thrombolytic therapy. In addition, PCI was associated with fewer adverse events in hospital than thrombolysis. Additional studies have shown that PCI is associated with overall mortality benefits.

It is important to note that only 20% of U.S. hospitals have catheterization capabilities, and benefits of PCI over thrombolysis may be erased by the additional time needed to transfer a patient from one institution to another. Remember: if a patient cannot be catheterized in the first two hours because of delays, thrombolysis should be performed.

If the first ECG does not show diagnostic changes, despite a strong history, then frequent or continuous ECG recordings should be obtained.

## Prophylactic therapy in the acute phase
### Aspirin
Aspirin therapy, 325mg, should be prescribed early. This leads to a 29% reduction in deaths or 24 lives saved in 1000 treated. Contraindications include:
- Known hypersensitivity.
- Bleeding peptic ulcer.
- Blood dyscrasias.
- Severe hepatic disease.

| Treatment regimens for angiotensin-converting enzyme inhibitors | | |
|---|---|---|
| **Drug** | **Initial dose** | **Target dose** |
| enalapril | 2.5mg | 20mg q day |
| lisinopril | 2.5mg | 10mg q day |
| captopril | 6.25mg | 50mg tid |
| ramipril | 2.5mg | 5mg bid |
| trandolapril | 0.5mg | 4mg q day |

**Fig. 30.8** Treatment regimens for angiotensin-converting enzyme inhibitors.

### β-blockers
The intravenous adminstration of β-blockers in the acute phase potentially limits infarct size, reduces the risk of fatal arrhythmias, and relieves pain. There is a 15% reduction in mortality at 1 week. It is particularly appropriate when the patient has tachycardia (in the absence of heart failure), relative hypertension, or pain unresponsive to opioids. Do not give beta blockers to patients with acute heart failure; their negative inotropic and chronotropic effects will worsen the symptoms.

### Angiotensin-converting enzyme inhibitors
Angiotensin-converting enzyme (ACE) inhibitors are of definite value in patients with clinical symptoms or signs of heart failure, or impaired left ventricular function echocardiographically. Opinions differ as to the best time to initiate treatment—whether acutely or after a few days. The benefits appear to be a class effect, and doses should be titrated to the target dose (Fig. 30.8).

## Complications of myocardial infarction
A summary of the complications that may occur in MI is given in Fig. 30.9.

| Complications of myocardial infarction | | |
|---|---|---|
| **Complication** | **Interval** | **Mechanism** |
| sudden death | usually within hours | often ventricular fibrillation |
| arrhythmias | first few days | — |
| persistent pain | 12 hours to a few days | progressive myocardial necrosis (extension of MI) |
| angina | immediate or delayed (weeks) | ischemia of non-infarcted muscle |
| cardiac failure | variable | ventricular dysfunction following muscle necrosis; arrhythmias |
| mitral incompetence | first few days | papillary muscle dysfunction, necrosis or rupture |
| pericarditis | 2–4 days | transmural infarct with inflammation of the pericardium |
| cardiac rupture and ventricular septal defects | 3–5 days | weakening of wall following muscle necrosis and acute inflammation |
| mural thrombus | one week or more | abnormal endothelial surface following infarction |
| ventricular aneurysm | 4 weeks or more | stretching of newly formed collagenous scar tissue |
| Dressler's syndrome | weeks to months | autoimmune |
| pulmonary emboli | 1 week or more | deep venous thrombosis in lower limbs |
| late ventricular arrhythmias | — | — |

**Fig. 30.9** Complications of myocardial infarction.

| The Killip classification | |
|---|---|
| **Class** | **Features** |
| 1 | no crepitations or third heart sound |
| 2 | crepitations over less than 50% of lung fields or third heart sound |
| 3 | crepitations over 50% of the lung fields |
| 4 | shock |

**Fig. 30.10** The Killip classification.

## Pump failure and shock

Left ventricular failure (LVF) during the acute phase of MI is associated with a poor prognosis. Repeated examination of the heart and lungs for signs of incipient heart failure should be practiced in all patients (Fig. 30.10). Patients with LV dysfunction should be considered for treatment with eplerenone (an aldosterone receptor blocker) because it improves survival rates.

General measures include monitoring for arrhythmias, and checking for electrolyte abnormalities and for the diagnosis of concomitant conditions such as valvular dysfunction or pulmonary disease.

Chest x-rays and echocardiography for assessing ventricular function, mitral regurgitation, and ventricular septal defects may be of help.

The management of heart failure is described on pp 227–229. Cardiogenic shock is defined as a systolic blood pressure less than 90mmHg in association with signs of circulatory deterioration expressed as peripheral vasoconstriction, low urinary output (<2.0mL/hour), and mental confusion and dulling.

Other causes of hypotension should be excluded such as hypovolemia, vasovagal reactions, electrolyte disturbance, drugs, or arrhythmias. Ventricular function should be evaluated by echocardiography, and hemodynamics measured with a balloon flotation catheter. Inotropic agents are of value. Low-dose dopamine (2.5µg/kg/min) may be given to improve renal function, and additional administration of dobutamine (5–10µg/kg/min) should be considered. Correction of acidosis is important.

Emergency PCI or surgery should be considered.

## Cardiac rupture and mitral regurgitation

Free wall rupture, if acute, is usually fatal within minutes. If subacute, there is hemodynamic deterioration with hypotension and signs of cardiac tamponade. Immediate surgery should be considered.

Ventricular septal defect (VSD) occurs in 1–2% of all infarctions, appearing early after MI. Without surgery the mortality is 54% within the first week and 92% within the first year. It should be suspected if there is clinical deterioration and a loud holosystolic murmur. Treatment is by surgical closure of the defect and bypass grafts as necessary. Predictors of poor postoperative outcome are:

- Cardiogenic shock.
- Posterior location.
- Right ventricular dysfunction.
- Age.
- Long delay between septal rupture and surgery.

### Mitral regurgitation

The incidence of moderately severe or severe mitral regurgitation is about 4% and the mortality without surgery is high at about 24%. Valve replacement is the procedure of choice in papillary muscle dysfunction and rupture.

### Arrhythmias and conduction disturbances

These are extremely common in the early period following MI. Often, however, the arrhythmias are not hazardous in themselves but are a manifestation of a serious underlying disorder, such as continuing ischemia, vagal overactivity, or electrolyte disturbance that requires attention. Arrhythmias are also discussed on pages 221–224.

### Ventricular arrhythmias

Ventricular arrhythmias may present as ventricular ectopics, VT, or ventricular fibrillation.

Ventricular ectopics are almost universal on the first day and require no treatment if the patient is asymptomatic.

Short episodes of VT may be well tolerated and require no treatment. More prolonged episodes may cause hypotension and heart failure. Amiodarone is becoming the drug of first choice (superseding lidocaine). Direct current (DC) cardioversion may be required if hemodynamically significant VT persists.

If ventricular fibrillation occurs, immediate defibrillation should be performed.

### Supraventricular arrhythmias

Atrial fibrillation complicates 15–20% of MIs and is often associated with severe left ventricular damage and heart failure; it is usually self limiting. If the heart rate is fast, digoxin is effective in slowing the rate, but amiodarone may be more efficacious in terminating the arrhythmia.

Other supraventricular arrhythmias are rare but are also usually self limiting. They may respond to carotid sinus massage. Beta blockers may be effective and DC shock should be employed if the arrhythmia is poorly tolerated.

### Sinus bradycardia and heart block

Sinus bradycardia is common in the first hour, especially in inferior MI, and usually responds to atropine in 300-μg boluses titrated against response. The administration of unnecessarily large doses of atropine should be avoided.

Atrioventricular (AV) block is common in inferior MI and may respond to atropine, though some patients will need a permanent pacemaker. However, it may take up to 14 days before normal conduction is restored.

Heart block with anterior MI is ominous because it indicates a large infarct. The development of left bundle branch block or bifasicular block may presage complete heart block and is an indication for temporary pacemaker insertion. If complete heart block does occur and persists, a permanent pacemaker will be needed.

## Management of the later inpatient course
### General management

Patients should be on bed rest for the first 24 hours. If uncomplicated, the patient can then sit out of bed, use a commode, and undertake self care and self feeding. Ambulation can be started the next day up to about 200m on the flat, and the exercise is gradually built up to climbing stairs within a few days.

### Deep venous thrombosis and pulmonary embolism

Deep venous thrombosis (DVT) and pulmonary embolism (PE) may be prevented by subcutaneous heparin when in bed. If they do occur, the patient should be treated initially with intravenous heparin, followed by oral anticoagulation for 3–6 months. Patients are usually started on subcutaneous heparin, 5000μ 2 times/day, or a low-molecular-weight heparin (e.g., enoxaparin subcutaneously 20mg once daily) after admission to the coronary care unit.

### Intraventricular thrombus and systemic emboli

This may be confirmed on echocardiography and treated with intravenous heparin followed by oral anticoagulation for 6 months.

### Pericarditis

This may occur within the first few days, causing pain that is sharp in nature and varies with posture and respiration. The diagnosis can be confirmed by a pericardial rub. If troublesome it may be treated with high-dose aspirin, non-steroidal anti-inflammatory drugs (NSAIDs), or steroids.

> Remember the causes of pericarditis by the mnemonic **CARDIAC RIND**: **C**ollagen vascular disease, **A**ortic aneurysm, **R**adiation, **D**rugs (e.g. hydralazine), **I**nfections, **A**cute renal failure, **C**ardiac infarction, **R**heumatic fever, **I**njury, **N**eoplasms, and **D**ressler's syndrome.

### Late ventricular arrhythmias

When arrhythmias occur late in the course of MI, they are liable to recur and are associated with a high risk of death. If it is probable that the arrhythmia is induced by ischemia, revascularization should be considered. If this is unlikely, antiarrhythmic agents, e.g., β-blockers and amiodarone, and electrophysiologically guided treatment may be given. In some cases an implantable defibrillator is indicated.

## Rehabilitation

Rehabilitation is aimed at restoring the patient to as full a life as possible, and must take into account physical, physiological, and socio-economic factors. The process should start as soon as possible after hospital admission and should be continued in the succeeding weeks and months. Depression and denial are common. Lifestyle advice should be individualized and include advice on diet, exercise, and stopping smoking.

## Secondary prevention
### Smoking

Observational studies show that those who stop smoking have a mortality in the succeeding years of less than half that of those who continue to smoke. It is potentially the most effective of all the secondary prevention measures. All smokers should be counseled to stop smoking. Nicotine replacement therapy may be of value.

### Diet

A weight-reducing diet should be prescribed to the overweight. Eating fatty fish at least twice a week may reduce the risk of reinfarction and death.

### Antiplatelet treatment

Aspirin, 81–325 mg daily, reduces the risk of reinfarction and death by 25%. There is no clear benefit of oral anticoagulation over antiplatelet therapy, although it may be considered for patients with left ventricular aneurysm, atrial fibrillation, or echocardiographically proven left ventricular thrombus.

For those patients receiving a stent during catheterization, clopidogrel has been shown to be beneficial to prevent closure of the stent. Currently the trend is to place patients on this medication for at least 3 months after stenting. However, more and more patients are taking clopidogrel indefinitely.

### β-blockers

β-blockers reduce the risk of mortality and reinfarction by 20–25%. About 25% of patients have contraindications to β-blockers because of uncontrolled heart failure, respiratory disease, or other conditions.

### Calcium antagonists

Verapamil may prevent reinfarction and death and should be considered in patients in whom β-blockers are contraindicated because of airways obstruction.

### Angiotensin-converting enzyme inhibitors

Provided there are no contraindications, ACE inhibitors are of potential benefit to all those after MI. However, patients at low risk gain only marginal benefit and they are often reserved for people with clinical signs of heart failure, people with low ejection fraction on echocardiography, or people with anterior MI.

### Lipid-lowering agents

There are clear benefits from treatment with HMG-CoA reductase inhibitors, or statins, if LDL cholesterol is above 75 mg/dL after dietary measures have been tried. The risk of subsequent major coronary heart disease events is lowered by about

30%. All subgroups of patients appear to benefit from treatment.

## Arrhythmias

Arrhythmias are usually secondary to CHD, particularly after MI. Ventricular ectopic beats are extremely common in the first 24 hours following an MI, but any arrhythmia including conduction disturbances may occur.

Other causes include drugs, cardiomyopathy, myocarditis, thyroid dysfunction, and electrolyte disturbances.

### Clinical features
Arrhythmias may present with palpitations (Chapter 3), dizziness, angina, shortness of breath (Chapter 2), syncope, cardiac arrest, or sudden death; they may also be symptomless. The history should focus on symptoms and possible underlying etiologies.

### Investigations
An ECG with a long rhythm strip will allow diagnosis of the arrhythmia, if present at the time of the test. For infrequent symptoms, 24-hour Holter monitoring (with a diary of events) may catch and record the rhythm disturbance. Other routine investigations should include CBC, U&Es, calcium, magnesium, thyroid function tests (TFTs), and a CXR. An echocardiogram should be considered if an underlying cause is not evident, to look for cardiomyopathy or valve disease.

Finally, electrophysiologic studies may reveal an arrhythmogenic focus, and response to treatment may be assessed, but this is only available in specialized centers.

### Supraventricular arrhythmias
#### Sinus tachycardia
There is usually an underlying cause, which should be treated on its own merits. Also see Fig. 3.1.

### Atrial fibrillation
This is an irregular, chaotic atrial rhythm at a rate of 300–600 beats per minute (bpm). It is transmitted to the ventricles via the AV node at different intervals, leading to an irregular heart rate, dependent on the speed of conduction and refractoriness down the AV node. The incidence rises with age and is over 10% in the very elderly.

Common causes include:
- CHD.
- Mitral valve disease.
- Hyperthyroidism.
- Hypertension.
- Cardiomyopathy.
- Pericarditis.
- Pneumonia.
- Bronchial carcinoma.
- Atrial myxoma.
- Endocarditis.
- Infiltrative diseases of the heart (e.g., sarcoidosis).
- Alcohol.
- Electrolyte abnormalities.

Clinically, there is an irregularly irregular pulse and the apical rate is greater than the rate at the radial artery. The first heart sound is of variable intensity.

The ECG shows absent P waves and irregular narrow complex QRS complexes (unless there is associated bundle branch block).

#### Treatment
The ventricular rate can usually be controlled with digoxin. If not, a β-blocker or diltiazem can be added if left ventricular function is good. Other classes of drugs may sometimes be required. Patients should be anticoagulated to reduce the risk of emboli. If the patient has contraindications to warfarin, aspirin should be considered.

If the atrial fibrillation is of recent onset, DC cardioversion or intravenous amiodarone to restore sinus rhythm may be attempted. If after more than 2 days the patient should be "warfarinized" for at least 1 month before cardioversion. If this is unsuccessful, the aim is control of the ventricular rate.

If the atrial fibrillation is paroxysmal, drugs such as amiodarone or sotalol may maintain the patient in sinus rhythm.

### Atrial flutter
This is due to circus movement of continuous atrial depolarization. As the AV node cannot conduct that fast, it is usually transmitted with a degree of block.

The causes and treatment are similar to those for atrial fibrillation.

The ECG shows a "sawtooth" appearance to the baseline at 300bpm due to flutter or F waves (Fig. 30.11). The ventricular rate is usually divisible into this, e.g., 150bpm in 2:1 block, or 100bpm in 3:1 block.

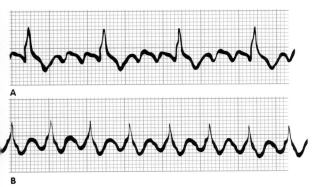

**Fig. 30.11** ECG of atrial flutter. (A) Atrial flutter with 4:1 block. (B) Atrial flutter with 2:1 block.

**Fig. 30.12** ECG of ventricular tachycardia.

## Paroxysmal supraventricular tachycardias

This is normally due to the presence of a second pathway between the atria and ventricles. An impulse is conducted normally through one AV connection and is then reconducted retrogradely up the other, causing a premature atrial contraction. This is then conducted down the first AV connection. On each occasion, the ventricle also depolarizes, giving rise to a fast ventricular rate. The refractory period for an accessory pathway may be shorter than the AV node, leading to ventricular rates exceeding 200 bpm.

### Management

Initially, try vagal stimulation, which can be achieved in the following ways:
- Valsalva maneuver: ask the patient to blow against resistance for about 15 seconds, as if straining at stool. The tachycardia usually terminates in the relaxation (parasympathetic) phase.
- Carotid sinus massage: massage of the carotid artery at the level of the thyroid cartilage.
- Diving reflex: the patient holds his breath while the face is wetted with cold water.
- Vomiting: this may be induced if the patient gives a clear history of termination by vomiting.
- Eye pressure: this should not now be done as it may cause retinal detachment.

 If the heart rate is 150 bpm, always consider atrial flutter with 2:1 block as the diagnosis (Fig. 30.12B).

### Drug treatment

Intravenous adenosine is the treatment of choice. Digitalization or intravenous β-blockers may also be effective. Intravenous verapamil may be useful for patients without MI or valvular disease. If the arrhythmia is poorly tolerated, synchronized DC shock usually provides rapid relief.

Metabolic panel should be checked for hypokalemia and corrected.

If the patient is already on digoxin, the levels should be checked to exclude toxicity.

## Ventricular tachycardia

This is defined as three or more consecutive ventricular extrasystoles with a rate greater than 120 bpm (Fig. 30.12).

### Treatment

If there is circulatory collapse, the patient should be treated with synchronized DC cardioversion. If conscious, the patient will require a brief anesthetic. Electrolyte abnormalities should be corrected.

Drug treatment is also used for prophylaxis of recurrent attacks. The most common setting is after MI; lidocaine is the preferred therapy for emergency use. Other options include amiodarone or procainamide.

## Torsade de pointes ("twisting of the points")

This is a special form of VT, which tends to occur in the presence of a long QT interval. It may progress to ventricular fibrillation and is often refractory to treatment, which is with intravenous magnesium sulphate. Antiarrhythmics may further prolong the QT interval and worsen the condition. Overdrive pacing may be effective.

**Fig. 30.13** ECG of ventricular fibrillation. Coordinated activity of the ventricles ceases. The ECG shows irregular waves of no defined shape. In this trace there are short periods suggestive of ventricular flutter.

Before carotid sinus massage:
- Always check that there are two carotid pulses.
- Never massage both carotids at the same time.

Listen for carotid bruits first—don't massage if one is present as it may cause a cerebral embolus.

**Fig. 30.14** ECG of first-degree heart block.

A favorite exam question is how to distinguish VT from SVT with aberrant conduction. The following features suggest VT:
- Fusion or capture beats (these are pathognomonic).
- Different QRS morphology to that in sinus rhythm.
- QRS duration >0.14 seconds with RBBB configuration or >0.16 seconds with LBBB configuration.
- QRS axis: left axis deviation with RBBB morphology, or extreme left axis deviation (northwest axis) with LBBB morphology.
- Concordance in the chest leads (all complexes have similar polarities).

### Ventricular fibrillation
This is an emergency and requires immediate DC cardioversion with cardiopulmonary resuscitation (Fig. 30.13).

### Bradycardias
#### Sinus bradycardia
For notes on sinus bradycardia, see Fig. 3.2.

#### Heart block
All negatively chronotropic drugs should be stopped. If the patient is symptomatic, atropine can be tried. If this fails, consider temporary pacing. If the patient remains symptomatic or has second or third-degree block, permanent pacing may be required.

#### Sick sinus syndrome
This is due to dysfunction of the sinus node and can lead to periods of sinus bradycardia with periods of asystole, and tachycardia. Atrial pacing is the treatment of choice if there is no AV conduction defect. Otherwise dual chamber pacing (atria and ventricles) is the treatment of choice.

#### First-degree heart block
The ECG shows a long PR interval (more than 0.2 seconds) (Fig. 30.14).

### Second-degree heart block
In Wenckebach (Mobitz type I) heart block there is progressive widening of the PR interval, culminating in non-conduction through the AV node. The cycle then continues (Fig. 30.15).

Mobitz type II heart block is intermittent failure of AV conduction (Fig. 30.16).

**Fig. 30.15** ECG of Wenckebach heart block.

**Fig. 30.16** ECG of Mobitz type II heart block showing two p waves for each QRS complex (i.e., 2:1 block).

**Fig. 30.17** ECG of complete heart block.

In complete heart block, work out the atrial rate and the ventricular rate separately by marking them on a piece of paper. They should both be regular but at different rates.

### Third-degree or complete heart block

Here, there is dissociation between the atria and ventricles (Fig. 30.17).

## Antiarrhythmic drugs

Traditionally, antiarrhythmics are classified according to their effects on the action potential (Vaughn Williams classification; Fig. 30.18). However, this is now of less clinical relevance than a classification based on the site of action in the heart—supraventricular, ventricular, and both. Some examples of antiarrhythmic drugs are given below.

| The Vaughn Williams classification of antiarrhythmic drugs | |
|---|---|
| **Class** | **Features** |
| Ia, b, c | membrane stabilizing drugs (e.g. quinidine, lidocaine and flecainide, respectively) |
| II | β-blockers |
| III | amiodarone, bretylium, sotalol |
| IV | calcium channel blockers (excluding dihydropyridines, e.g. nifedipine) |

**Fig. 30.18** The Vaughn Williams classification of antiarrhythmic drugs.

### Supraventricular arrhythmias
#### Adenosine

Adenosine is used for terminating paroxysmal supraventricular tachycardia (SVT). The half-life is 8–10 seconds but is longer if the patient is on dipyridamole. It can cause flushing and bronchospasm.

## Verapamil

Verapamil should not be used for wide complex tachycardias unless a supraventricular origin has been established beyond doubt. It should not be used with β-blockers.

## Supraventricular and ventricular arrhythmias
### Amiodarone

Amiodarone is the drug of first choice. It can be used orally or intravenously for rapid effect. The half-life is several weeks. It may therefore take some weeks to achieve steady-state plasma concentration.

Side effects include hypo- and hyperthyroidism and liver dysfunction. TFTs and liver function tests (LFTs) should therefore be checked at baseline and every 6 months. It may also cause pneumonitis, corneal microdeposits (which are reversible on stopping treatment), and photosensitivity.

### β-blockers

Beta blockers act mainly by attenuating the effects of the sympathetic nervous system on automaticity and conductivity within the heart.

### Disopyramide

Disopyramide may be used intravenously to control arrhythmias after MI. It is negatively inotropic and has antimuscarinic side effects.

### Flecainide

Flecainide is useful for symptomatic ventricular arrhythmias and paroxysmal atrial fibrillation. It has been shown to increase mortality in patients treated for asymptomatic ventricular ectopics after MI, and is therefore contraindicated in patients with CHD.

### Procainamide

Procainamide is used for ventricular arrhythmias and paroxysmal atrial fibrillation. It can cause a syndrome resembling systemic lupus erythematosus (SLE) with prolonged use.

### Propafenone and quinidine

Propafenone and quinidine are also useful for ventricular and some supraventricular arrhythmias.

## Ventricular arrhythmias
### Bretylium

Bretylium is only used as an antiarrhythmic drug in resuscitation. It can cause severe hypotension, nausea, and vomiting.

| \multicolumn{2}{c}{The New York Heart Association classification of heart failure} | |
|---|---|
| Class | Features |
| I | symptoms only with maximal unaccustomed exertion |
| II | symptoms with minimal unaccustomed exertion |
| III | symptoms with activities of daily living |
| IV | symptoms at rest |

Fig. 30.19 The New York Heart Association classification of heart failure.

### Lidocaine

Lidocaine is used commonly for VT after an MI, but it can only be given intravenously. The dose should be decreased with cardiac or liver failure to avoid convulsions, depression of the central nervous system, or depression of the cardiovascular system.

### Mexiletine

Mexiletine has a similar action to lidocaine. It is negatively inotropic.

## Heart failure

Heart failure occurs when the heart is unable to maintain sufficient cardiac output to meet the demands of the body, despite the presence of normal filling pressures. The incidence rises with age and is present in over 1% of the over-65s. It is classified by its severity (Fig. 30.19). The mortality in severe heart failure is about 50% at 1 year.

## Causes of heart failure
### High output failure

The heart maintains a normal or increased cardiac output in the face of grossly elevated requirements. It is then unable to meet these requirements. Conditions causing this include:

- Thyrotoxicosis.
- Nephritis.
- Anemia.
- AV shunts.
- Beriberi.
- Fever.
- Paget's disease.
- Pregnancy.

## True heart failure

True heart failure is due primarily to an abnormality of the heart, when the cardiac output at rest is low or normal, but low on exercise. Causes include the following:

- Myocardial disease: ischemia and infarction; structure (e.g., hypertrophic obstructive cardiomyopathy, hypertension); fibrosis (e.g., infections, immunologic reactions, small vessel disease); others (e.g., thyroid disease, beriberi, amyloidosis, sarcoidosis, heavy metals, alcohol).
- Drugs (e.g., antiarrhythmics, calcium antagonists, β-blockers).
- Arrhythmias (e.g., atrial fibrillation).
- Volume overload (e.g., aortic and mitral regurgitation).
- Outflow obstruction (e.g., aortic stenosis).
- Restricted filling (e.g., constrictive pericarditis or tamponade, restrictive cardiomyopathy).

## Clinical features

### Left heart failure

Symptoms include:

- Exertional dyspnea.
- Orthopnea.
- Paroxysmal nocturnal dyspnea.
- Fatigue.
- Wheeze.
- Cough.
- Hemoptysis.

Signs include:

- Tachypnea.
- Tachycardia.
- Pulsus alternans (alternating large and small pulse pressures).
- Peripheral cyanosis.
- Cardiomegaly.
- A third heart sound.
- Functional mitral regurgitation secondary to dilatation of the mitral annulus.
- Basal crepitations.
- Pleural effusions.

### Right heart failure

This may occur secondary to chronic lung disease, multiple pulmonary emboli, pulmonary hypertension, right-sided valve disease, left-to-right shunts, or isolated right ventricular cardiomyopathy. It is most commonly secondary to LVF, in which case the term congestive heart failure is used.

Symptoms include:

- Fatigue.
- Nausea.
- Wasting.
- Swollen ankles.
- Abdominal discomfort.
- Anorexia.
- Breathlessness.

The signs include:

- A raised jugulovenous pressure (JVP).
- Smooth hepatomegaly.
- Liver tenderness.
- Pitting edema.
- Ascites.
- Functional tricuspid regurgitation.
- Tachycardia.
- Right ventricular third heart sound.

## Investigations

The cause for the heart failure must always be sought as heart failure itself is an inadequate diagnosis. After the history and examination, investigations include the following:

- CBC: anemia.
- Metabolic panel (e.g., for hypokalemia with diuretics).
- LFTs: liver congestion.
- Echocardiography: left ventricular function and valves.
- TFTs.
- Cardiac enzymes: if acute onset, to exclude MI.
- ECG: CAD, arrhythmias, and left ventricular hypertrophy.
- CXR: cardiomegaly, alveolar edema, bat's wings shadowing, prominent upper lobe vessels, Kerley B lines, pleural effusions.

Other investigations to consider are:

- Exercise testing: functional severity and prognosis.
- Cardiac catheterization.
- Nuclear techniques: ejection fraction, cardiac function, prognosis.

## Management

The aims of management are to relieve symptoms and to improve the prognosis. The cause of the heart failure should be sought and treated appropriately (e.g., valve lesions). Exacerbating factors such as anemia and hypertension should be treated. Check the patient's drugs as some may cause fluid retention (e.g., nonsteroidal anti-inflammatory drugs [NSAIDs]). Patients should be advised to maintain an optimal weight, avoid excessive salt intake and large amounts of alcohol, and stop smoking.

## Drug treatment

Diuretics relieve the symptoms of heart failure, and ACE inhibitors improve symptoms and prognosis. They reduce the risk of MI and increase survival. Treatment is best planned as a stepped care plan.

### Step 1

If the heart failure is mild, start a thiazide diuretic (e.g., HCTZ 2.5mg q.d.). Many patients are started on a loop diuretic from the outset (e.g., furuosemide 20–40mg daily). Diuretics increase the excretion of sodium and water, and, by reducing the circulatory volume, they decrease the preload and edema. Loop diuretics have a thiazide-like action on the early distal tubule but more importantly they inhibit sodium and chloride reabsorption in the thick ascending loop of Henle. This segment has a high capacity for absorbing sodium and chloride, and so drugs which act on this site produce a diuresis that is much greater than that of other diuretics. Side effects include hyperglycemia, hyperuricemia, hypotension, and hypokalemia.

### Step 2

An ACE inhibitor should be commenced at the same time if there are no contraindications. The dose should be increased to the maximum tolerated dose (see Fig. 30.8). As the name suggests, ACE inhibitors inhibit the conversion of angiotensin I to angiotensin II. To avoid dangerous hyperkalemia, any potassium-sparing diuretic should be omitted from the diuretic regimen before introducing an ACE inhibitor, changing to the loop diuretic alone. Potassium supplements should be discontinued.

Profound first-dose hypotension may occur when ACE inhibitors are introduced to patients with heart failure who are already on a high dose of a loop diuretic (e.g., furosemide 80mg q.d. or higher). Temporary withdrawal of the loop diuretic reduces the risk but may cause severe rebound pulmonary edema. The ACE inhibitor should therefore be started at a very low dosage with the patient recumbent and under close medical supervision, and with facilities to treat profound hypotension.

Patients with severe heart failure should start ACE inhibitors in hospital. Initiation in hospital is

### Recommendation for inpatient initiation of ACE inhibitors

- furosemide 80mg o.d. or more
- hypovolemia (check for diarrhea and vomiting)
- hyponatremia (plasma sodium <130mmol/L)
- systolic blood pressure <90mmHg
- unstable heart failure
- renal impairment: plasma creatinine >150mmol/L
- high-dose vasodilator therapy
- age 70 years or more

Fig. 30.20 Recommendations for inpatient initiation of angiotensin-converting enzyme (ACE) inhibitors. ACE inhibitors are contraindicated in people with known or suspected bilateral renal artery stenosis, in aortic stenosis, or outflow tract obstruction, pregnancy, and porphyria. Common side effects include a dry cough, hypotension, dizziness, and headache.

also recommended for patients with mild to moderate heart failure and the conditions given in Fig. 30.20.

### Alternative step 2

The contributions of venodilators such as long-acting nitroglycerine, which will reduce preload, and arterial dilators such as hydralazine, which will reduce afterload, have been shown to be of prognostic benefit in people with heart failure but are inferior to ACE inhibitors in this respect. They may be prescribed to patients in whom ACE inhibitors are contraindicated. The combination of hydralazine and isosorbide dinitrate has been found to be beneficial in black patients. Aldosterone receptor blockade with spironolactone (25mg orally once daily) has been shown to improve mortality rates in class III–IV CHF. Renal function and serum potassium should be monitored carefully after initiating treatment with spironolactone.

### Step 3

This next stage is to increase the dose of loop diuretic. For patients with intractable heart failure, very high doses of furosemide may be needed—up to 1g per day.

### Step 4

The addition of digoxin for its inotropic effect has been shown to reduce hospital admissions and symptoms, although not mortality. It is of particular benefit in patients with atrial fibrillation. It should be used with caution in the elderly, who are particularly susceptible to digoxin toxicity.

Common toxic effects are anorexia, nausea, and vomiting. Digoxin may also cause almost any supraventricular or ventricular arrhythmia and heart block. These unwanted effects depend both on the plasma digoxin concentration and on the sensitivity of the conducting system or myocardium, which is often increased in heart disease.

Hypokalemia predisposes to toxicity, and serum potassium should be monitored. Renal function is the most important determinant of digoxin dosage. Typical maintenance doses are 125–250mg daily although lower doses may be needed if there is renal impairment. Toxicity can often be managed by discontinuing therapy and correcting hypokalemia if appropriate. Digoxin-specific antibody fragments are available for the reversal of life-threatening overdosage.

## Step 5

Traditionally, beta blockers are contraindicated in patients with heart failure because of their negative inotropic effect. However, carvedilol, which is a beta blocker with additional arteriolar vasodilating action, may be of benefit if heart failure is severe.

## Step 6

If heart failure is intractable, the addition of metolazone, a powerful thiazide diuretic, produces a profound diuresis, acting synergistically with loop diuretics.

Angiotensin II antagonists are being increasingly used in patients with heart failure. They should be considered if there are contraindications to ACE inhibitors.

## Other drug options

Other drug options to consider are phosphodiesterase inhibitors such as enoximone and milrinone, which increase myocardial contraction and are vasodilators. Sustained hemodynamic benefit has been shown after administration but as yet there is no conclusive evidence of any beneficial effect on survival.

Bed rest may promote diuresis. Prophylaxis for DVT should be given with subcutaneous heparin. It may sometimes help giving frusemide intravenously, either as a slow bolus or continuous intravenous infusion. As a last resort, β-adrenergic agonists, dopamine and dobutamine produce a positive inotropic effect but must be given intravenously. They may be useful for acute exacerbations of heart failure but may induce inotrope dependence, making it difficult to wean the patient off them.

For patients with severe heart failure, heart transplantation should be considered. This can dramatically improve the quality of life; 5-year survival is over 70%.

## Acute heart failure

This is an emergency characterized by acute breathlessness, wheezing, anxiety, and sweating. There may be pink frothy sputum, as well as signs of pulmonary edema. If severe, the management (listed below) should begin before investigations are performed:

- Sit the patient upright.
- Give high-concentration oxygen unless there is coexisting chronic hypercapnia due to long-standing respiratory failure. It may even be necessary to ventilate the patient.
- Give intravenous furosemide or bumetanide. These cause an immediate vasodilatation, as well as their more delayed diuresis.
- Give 5mg intravenous morphine slowly unless there is liver failure of chronic obstructive pulmonary disease. This causes sedation, relieves dyspnea, and causes vasodilatation. It should be given with an antiemetic.
- Give intravenous venodilators (e.g., nitrates, nitroglycerine) if systolic blood pressure is greater than 100mmHg. This will reduce preload.
- Load the patient with digoxin, orally or intravenously, to slow the heart rate if the patient is in fast atrial fibrillation. Other arrhythmias should be treated appropriately. This can be done with an esmolol or diltiazem IV drip.
- Consider giving intravenous aminophylline 5mg/kg intravenously over 10 minutes. This is positively inotropic and causes vasodilatation and bronchodilation. It is usually reserved only for those patients with bronchospasm.
- Intravenous inotropic agents may be of value if there is hypotension. If signs of renal hypoperfusion are present, dopamine is recommended intravenously at 2.5–5µg/kg/min. If pulmonary congestion is dominant, dobutamine is preferred at 2.5µg/kg/min, increasing gradually to 10µg/kg/min if needed.

## Hypertension

The prevalence of hypertension differs depending on blood pressure cut-off points, age, sex, and race. It increases with age and is more common in men, and African-Americans. It is estimated that 27% of the population in the U.S. has hypertension. Unfortunately, only 23% of these patients achieve blood pressure control with medications. It is important, therefore, not only to treat patients but also to ensure appropriate follow-up and compliance. The risk of morbidity and mortality rises continuously with increasing blood pressure, and marginal risk is greater at higher blood pressures. Similarly, the lower the blood pressure achieved with treatment, the lower the risk of complications of hypertension. However, the benefit of lowering diastolic blood pressure to below 90mmHg is minimal in uncomplicated hypertension in young or middle-aged patients.

Definitions of hypertension differ, but whatever the blood pressure thresholds used, the mean of several blood pressure measurements should be taken over time, as an isolated reading predicts cardiovascular risk very poorly. Blood pressure should be taken sitting or lying after 2–3 minutes rest. The bladder cuff should cover at least 80% of the arm circumference; otherwise, in obese patients artificially high readings are observed. The dial or mercury column should fall at 2mm per second, i.e., slowly, and be read to the nearest 2mm. The diastolic pressure is recorded at the disappearance of sounds, i.e., phase V. The new JNC-7 guidelines define normal blood pressure as less than 120/80mmHg, prehypertension as 120–139/80–89mmHg, hypertension I as 140–159/90–99mmHg, and hypertension II as >160/100mmHg. In patients with DM or renal disease, the target blood pressure is 130/80mmHg.

## Etiology

In over 90% of people, the diagnosis of hypertension is idiopathic ("essential"), i.e., no cause can be found. Genetic influences on blood pressure regulation have been suggested by family studies. A number of environmental factors are also associated with the developments of hypertension. These include obesity, alcohol, dietary sodium intake, dietary potassium, and smoking.

Vegetarians have less hypertension than meat eaters, although it is difficult to know whether the blood pressure differences are due to diet *per se* or other causes. It is not clear whether psychological factors play a significant part in long-term blood pressure regulation, though there is no doubt that

emotional factors can induce pronounced but transient variations in blood pressure.

### Obesity

There is a continuous linear relationship between excess body fat and blood pressure levels.

### Alcohol

Increasing alcohol consumption is related to higher blood pressure levels, and the effects are additive to those of obesity.

### Dietary sodium intake

Salt intake has a small effect on population blood pressure levels. Salt restriction may reduce systolic blood pressure by 3–5mmHg in hypertensives and is most clear-cut in older subjects and those with more severe hypertension.

### Dietary potassium

Dietary sodium and potassium intake are generally inversely related. Dietary potassium may have a blood pressure-lowering effect, and estimates of dietary sodium/potassium ratios are more strongly associated with blood pressure levels than either of the cations independently.

### Smoking

This leads to an acute elevation in blood pressure, which subsides within 15 minutes of finishing a cigarette. Regular smokers actually have slightly lower blood pressures than nonsmokers, although the small potential benefit is greatly outweighed by the increased cardiovascular risk.

## Secondary hypertension

A definite underlying cause for hypertension is more common in younger people and should be looked for specifically in people under 35:

- Renal disease: chronic glomerulonephritis, chronic pyelonephritis, renal artery stenosis, polycystic kidney disease, and polyarteritis nodosa. Although it only accounts for 1% of all hypertension, the diagnosis of renal artery stenosis is important as it is the most common curable cause.
- Endocrine disease: Cushing's and Conn's syndromes, pheochromocytoma, acromegaly, and hypercalcemia.
- Pregnancy-induced hypertension and pre-eclampsia: associated with edema and proteinuria.
- Coarctation of the aorta.

**Fig. 30.21** Clinical evaluation of the patient with hypertension. Look for the "five Cs."

| Clinical evaluation of the patient with hypertension | |
|---|---|
| causes of hypertension | drugs causing hypertension? paroxysmal features? (pheochromocytoma) present, past or family history of renal disease? general appearance? (Cushing's syndrome) radiofemoral delay? (coarctation) kidney(s) palpable? (polycystic, hydronephrosis, neoplasm) abdominal or loin bruit? (renal artery stenosis) |
| contributory factors | overweight? alcohol intake? |
| complications | cerebrovascular disease left ventricular hypertrophy or cardiac failure ischemic heart disease fundal hemorrhages and exudates (accelerated phase) |
| contraindications to drugs | gout, diabetes (thiazides) asthma, heart block (β-blockers) heart failure, heart block (verapamil) |
| cardiovascular risk | assessment of other cardiovascular risk factors |

- Drugs: estrogen-containing oral contraceptive pill, NSAIDs, steroids, sympathomimetics in cold cures, carbenoxolone, and liquorice.

## History

Patients with hypertension are usually asymptomatic. The history should concentrate on environmental predisposing factors, associated cardiovascular risk factors, and the symptoms of underlying secondary causes. For example, patients with pheochromocytoma may have symptoms of panic, headache, sweating, nausea, tremor, and pallor. Accelerated hypertension may lead to symptoms secondary to heart failure, renal failure, headaches, nausea and vomiting, visual impairment, or seizures.

## Examination

The clinical approach to the patient with hypertension is summarized in Fig. 30.21. Apart from the blood pressure itself, the examination should focus on complications of hypertension or underlying secondary causes. The patient should be examined for left ventricular hypertrophy (displaced apex beat), coarctation of the aorta (difference in blood pressure in the arms, weak femoral pulses, radiofemoral delay), renal bruits for possible underlying renal artery stenosis, and palpable kidneys, e.g. in polycystic kidney disease. There may

| The Keith–Wagener classification of retinopathy | |
|---|---|
| **Grade** | **Features** |
| I | arterial narrowing and increased tortuosity |
| II | arteriovenous nipping |
| III | hemorrhages and soft exudates |
| IV | grades I–III and papilledema |

**Fig. 30.22** The Keith–Wagener classification of retinopathy.

be retinopathy, classified by the Keith–Wagener changes (Fig. 30.22).

## Investigation policy

The minimum tests include urinalysis and serum biochemistry for evidence of renal disease and ECG for evidence of left ventricular hypertrophy or ischemia.

Consideration should also be given to the following:

- CXR: cardiac size and signs of heart failure.
- Serum lipids: cardiovascular risk.
- Echocardiography: left ventricular hypertrophy and left ventricular function.

231

Further invesigations are warranted in young patients, in whom a secondary cause is more likely, in patients with rapidly rising blood pressure or severe hypertension, in patients with hypertension resistant to treatment, and in patients with deranged metabolic panel. These investigations include urinary vanillylmandelic acids for pheochromocytoma and an intravenous urogram (IVU) for evidence of renal artery stenosis. If this is abnormal, renal arteriography is indicated.

Further investigations depend on clinical suspicion (e.g., aortography for coarctation of the aorta).

## Management of hypertension

For secondary hypertension, treatment of the underlying condition may sometimes be indicated (e.g., treatment of an underlying endocrine condition or surgical correction of aortic coarctation). In renovascular hypertension, drug treatment may effectively control blood pressure. It is therefore reasonable to consider angioplasty or surgery only for young patients, who are more likely to have fibromuscular hyperplasia compared to atherosclerosis, patients with severe hypertension, or patients whose blood pressure is difficult to control medically. Surgery may also be indicated where progressive renal failure in a hypertensive patient is due either to bilateral renal artery stenosis or stenosis of an artery to a single kidney.

An algorithm of the decision-making process in patients with hypertension is given in Fig. 30.23. The aim is to reduce blood pressure to below 160/90 mmHg, although getting blood pressure as close as possible to 120/80mmHg is ideal, especially for patients with diabetes and other cardiovascular risk factors.

### Accelerated hypertension

Malignant hypertension or very severe hypertension (diastolic blood pressure over 140mmHg) requires urgent treatment in hospital. Treatment is normally given orally with beta blockers or calcium antagonists to reduce diastolic blood pressure to 100–110mmHg within the first 24 hours. Over the next few days, further antihypertensives should be given to lower blood pressure further. If there are signs of malignant hypertension (i.e., altered mental status, renal failure, papilledema), IV nitroprusside labetelol should be instituted. Diastolic blood pressure should be lowered to 100–105mmHg (or 25% in total, whichever is lower) over 2–6 hours.

Very rapid falls in blood pressure should be avoided because the reduction in cerebral perfusion may lead to cerebral infarction, blindness, worsening renal function, and myocardial ischemia. Parenteral antihypertensive drugs are rarely required.

In moderate-to-severe hypertension (i.e., diastolic blood pressure over 110mmHg) or in patients with vascular complications, drugs are best added stepwise until control has been achieved. An attempt can then be made to "step down" treatment under supervision. Monotherapy controls blood pressure in only 30–50% of patients, and most patients therefore need two or more drugs. In uncomplicated mild hypertension, drugs may be substituted rather than added.

A good stepped care plan is given in Fig. 30.24.

### Drug treatment
#### Thiazides

Thiazides lower blood pressure mainly by lowering body sodium stores. Initially blood pressure falls because of a decrease in blood volume, venous return, and cardiac output. Gradually the cardiac output returns to normal but the hypotensive effect remains because the peripheral resistance decreases. Side effects include impaired glucose tolerance and gout. Low doses (bendrofluazide, 2.5mg) cause little biochemical disturbance without loss of the antihypertensive effect. Higher doses are never needed, nor usually are potassium supplements. Thiazides are better tolerated in women than men and are more effective in the elderly.

#### Potassium-sparing diuretics

Potassium-sparing diuretics may be used for the prophylaxis or treatment of diuretic-induced hypokalemia (Fig. 30.25).

#### β-blockers

Beta blockers initially produce a fall in blood pressure by decreasing cardiac output. With continued treatment the cardiac output returns to normal but the blood pressure remains low because the peripheral resistance is "reset" at a lower level.

Side effects include negative inotropism, provocation of asthma, decreased libido and heart block. Less serious side effects include cold hands and fatigue. Beta blockers are more effective in young patients and less effective in black patients.

#### Calcium antagonists

Calcium antagonists work in different ways. The dihydropyridines (e.g., nifedipine) may cause a reflex

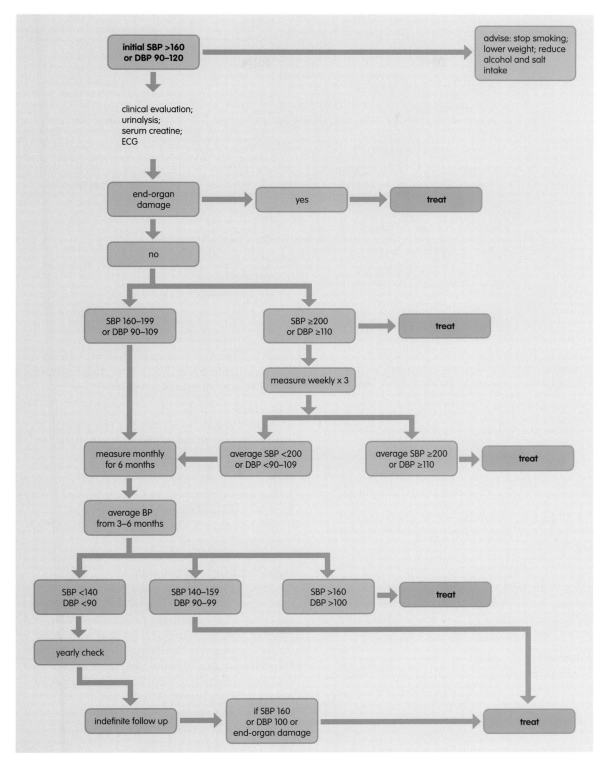

**Fig. 30.23** Algorithm for making decisions in systolic and diastolic hypertension. (BP, blood pressure; DBP, diastolic blood pressure; SBP, systolic blood pressure.)

| Stepped care plan for management of hypertension | |
|---|---|
| Step | Measures |
| 0 | non-drug treatment: weight reduction, alcohol reduction, moderate salt restriction, stop smoking |
| 1 | women, and men over 60 years—HCTZ 12.5–25mg<br>men under 60 years—HCTZ 12.5–25mg or β-blocker, e.g. atenolol 50mg |
| 2 | HCTZ 12.5–25mg + atenolol 50mg |
| 3 | add ACE inhibitor, e.g. enalapril 2.5–40mg (alternatives: dihydropyridine calcium antagonist, e.g. amlodipine 5–10mg o.d., selective α-blocker, e.g. doxazosin 1–8mg o.d., angiotensin II antagonist, e.g. losartan 50–100mg o.d.) |
| 4* | substitute furosemide 40–80mg for thiazide<br>exclude non-compliance, drug interactions, secondary hypertension<br>consider referral for detailed investigation |
| 5* | non-urgent: try other step 3 drugs<br>urgent: minoxidil (men only–causes hirsuitism) |

Fig. 30.24 Stepped care plan for the management of hypertension. *Steps 4 and 5 require detailed investigation and intensive biochemical monitoring, best performed in a specialist clinic. Drugs may also be chosen with concomitant conditions in mind. For example, β-blockers and calcium antagonists may be used early for patients with angina; ACE inhibitors are a sensible first choice in DM because they may delay the progression of nephropathy.

| Indications for use of a potassium-sparing diuretic for prophylaxis or treatment of diuretic-induced hypokalemia |
|---|
| • digoxin treatment<br>• chronic liver disease<br>• history of arrhythmia or antiarrhythmic treatment<br>• severe or unstable angina<br>• Conn's syndrome and other states of mineralocorticoid excess<br>• severe hypokalemia, i.e. serum potassium <3.0mmol/L |

Fig. 30.25 Indications for use of a potassium-sparing diuretic for prophylaxis or treatment of diuretic-induced hypokalemia.

tachycardia, flushing, headache, edema, and indigestion. The edema does not respond to diuretics.

Verapamil cannot be used with a β-blocker. It may cause constipation.

### Minoxidil

Minoxidil is a potent vasodilator and decreases peripheral resistance. It may cause a reflex tachycardia, which can be prevented by combination with a β-blocker. It may also cause fluid retention, which is prevented by combination with a diuretic.

### ACE inhibitors

ACE inhibitors are well tolerated and more effective in younger patients. They cause a persistent dry cough in 20% of women and 10% of men. Renal function should be checked before starting treatment and when dose titration is complete.

### α-blockers

α-blockers reduce both arteriolar and venous resistance and maintain a high cardiac output.

### Methyldopa

Methyldopa stimulates $\alpha_2$-receptors in the medulla and reduces sympathetic outflow. In 20% of patients it causes a positive Coombs' test and, rarely, hemolytic anaemia. Drug-induced hepatitis with fever may also occur.

### Hypertension in pregnancy

Good blood pressure control in pregnancy is important—oral methyldopa is safe. Beta blockers are effective and safe in the third trimester but may cause intrauterine growth retardation when used earlier in pregnancy. Hydralazine may also be used. Hypertension may indicate pre-eclampsia, and consultation with an obstetrician/gynecologist is essential. This is especially important if the hypertension is of new onset, the patient is beyond 20 weeks, and proteinuria is also present. Also remember that pre-eclampsia can be superimposed on existing hypertension. A worsening of hypertension beyond 20 weeks of pregnancy should merit urinalysis in every patient.

| Age and hypertension—factors associated with advancing age |
|---|
| • greater likelihood of hypertension (>50%) |
| • greater damage when hypertensive |
| • disatolic threshold for treatment 90mmHg |
| • as much or more benefit from treatment |
| • no increase in treatment side effects |
| • elderly should be offered treatment unless suffering other life-shortening illness |
| • erect pressures should be measured |

Fig. 30.26 Age and hypertension—factors associated with advancing age.

## Age and hypertension

Factors relating to hypertension associated with advancing age are summarized in Fig. 30.26.

## Follow-up

Of patients, 25–50% default or discontinue treatment, so an effective follow-up system is needed. When the blood pressure is satisfactorily controlled, it should be checked once every 3 months. More frequent checks are needed during dose titration if the control is borderline, if compliance is a problem, or if the treatment regimen is complex. On routine visits, the blood pressure and weight should be measured, and the patient should be asked about side effects. The urine should be checked for protein and glucose yearly.

Apart from this, routine re-examination or investigation is unnecessary and should be performed only if there is a special indication (e.g., variable or borderline blood pressure control) or at the onset of new symptoms.

## Prognosis

Patients with untreated malignant hypertension have a 90% mortality in 1 year, and treatment is therefore life-saving. The risk of hypertension in other cases depends on the level of blood pressure, the presence of complications, e.g. cardiac or renal failure, and the presence of other cardiovascular risk factor (e.g., male sex, smoking, diabetes, and older age). Those at highest risk gain most benefit from treatment.

# Valvular heart disease

## Mitral stenosis

The cause of mitral stenosis is usually rheumatic fever although only about half of all patients give a positive history. It is four times more common than mitral regurgitation, and is more common in women than men.

Progressive stenosis of the mitral valve, via thickening of the cusps and fusion of the commissures, results in a pressure gradient between the left atrium and the left ventricle. As the stenosis worsens, ventricular filling becomes impaired, and this is compounded by fibrosis of the subvalvar apparatus, leading to left atrial dilatation and hypertrophy. Left atrial dilatation predisposes the patient to atrial fibrillation and thrombosis. Pulmonary congestion may ensue, and an increase in pulmonary artery pressure may lead to right heart failure.

### Management

Anticoagulation is indicated in patients with atrial fibrillation, although some would anticoagulate all patients with mitral stenosis. The risk of emboli is greater with a large left atrium or left atrial appendage.

Pulmonary congestion is treated with diuretics, and digoxin is used to control the ventricular rate in atrial fibrillation. It may be necessary to add in other rate-controlling drugs such as β-blockers or verapamil.

If symptoms persist, the patient should be considered for mitral valvotomy or valve replacement. If the valve is not calcified and the leaflets are pliable, balloon valvuloplasty may be attempted.

All patients should receive antibiotic prophylaxis before dental and surgical procedures to avoid subacute bacterial endocarditis.

## Mitral regurgitation

The incidence of mitral regurgitation is equal in men and women. It is usually secondary to rheumatic fever, floppy prolapsing mitral valve leaflets, papillary muscle dysfunction, rupture after an inferior MI or cardiomyopathy, or secondary to ventricular dilatation or dysfunction. Less common causes include congenital malformations, which may be associated with an ostium primum atrial septal defect, infective endocarditis, rupture of the chordae tendineae, cardiomyopathy, rheumatoid arthritis, or left atrial tumor interfering with mitral valve closure.

The circulatory changes depend on the speed of onset and severity of mitral regurgitation. Acute regurgitation may lead to acute pulmonary edema, whereas chronic regurgitation allows for compensatory left ventricular and atrial dilatation (also see page 22).

## Management

Diuretics are used for pulmonary congestion, and vasodilators are helpful in acute regurgitation. Digoxin and anticoagulants are given to patients in atrial fibrillation. Antibiotic prophylaxis is needed prior to dental and surgical procedures.

Mitral valve replacement is indicated if symptoms are severe and uncontrolled by medical treatment, or if pulmonary hypertension develops. Good results are achieved if left ventricular function is preserved, and early referral may allow repair of the valve rather than replacement.

## Mitral valve prolapse

This is due to prolapse of the mitral valve leaflets into the left atrium during ventricular systole. It may affect up to 15% of the population and is three times commoner in women. Pathologically, there is an increase in the zona spongiosa of the valve leaflets.

### Clinical signs and symptoms

It is often asymptomatic and found incidentally. An apical midsystolic click is heard, associated with a late systolic murmur if the valve is regurgitant. It may be associated with palpitations and atypical chest pains, although the latter is more common in people aware of their condition. Systemic emboli and syncope are rare.

### Investigations
#### Electrocardiography

The ECG may show inferolateral ST/T segment changes. Arrhythmias may be confirmed by Holter monitoring. The commonest rhythm disturbance is ventricular extrasystoles.

#### Echocardiography

Echocardiography is diagnostic.

## Management

Patients should receive endocarditis prophylaxis. Treatment is only indicated for complications (e.g., antiarrhythmic drugs for significant rhythm disturbances or anticoagulants for emboli).

## Aortic stenosis

The most common cause of aortic stenosis is a calcified bicuspid valve, and this is more common in men. In younger patients the cause may be congenital or due to rheumatic fever, but in older patients it may be due to senile degenerative calcification, which is more common in women. Aortic stenosis tends to progress gradually, causing obstruction to the left ventricular outflow with resultant hypertrophy. Typical symptoms of aortic stenosis include angina, syncope, and dyspnea. Ventricular dilatation and heart failure are late complications. Conduction defects may result from calcification extending into the ventricular system (also see p. 233).

## Management

Valve replacement is indicated for severe stenosis because of the risk of sudden death, or for symptomatic aortic stenosis. Drugs do not alter the progression of the disease though diuretics and digoxin can be given for heart failure.

## Aortic regurgitation

The more common causes include cusp malformation (e.g., bicuspid valve) and cusp erosion (e.g., infective endocarditis). (Also see p. 244.)

Other causes include:
- Cusp distortion (e.g., senile calcification and rheumatic fever).
- Loss of support (e.g., VSD).
- Aortic wall disease due to inflammation (e.g., syphilis).
- Ankylosing spondylitis.
- Reiter's syndrome.
- Psoriatic arthropathy.
- Aortic wall disease due to dilatation (e.g., hypertension with or without dissection). Chronic regurgitation causes left ventricular dilatation and hypertrophy.

## Management

Valve replacement is indicated for symptomatic patients. In the meantime, diuretics and digoxin may be given to control symptoms of heart failure. The prognosis is good while ventricular function is good but death usually occurs within 2–3 years after the onset of ventricular failure.

## Tricuspid regurgitation

This may be functional secondary to right heart failure, commonly as a result of pulmonary hypertension. It may also be rheumatic in association with mitral valve disease, or due to endocarditis in drug addicts.

## Miscellaneous cardiovascular conditions

## Congenital heart disease
### Ventricular septal defect

VSD is the most common congenital heart lesion, accounting for about one-third of all malformations. Blood moves from the high pressure left ventricle to the right ventricle. If the defect is large, pulmonary flow increases leading to obliterative pulmonary vascular changes and an increase in pulmonary vascular resistance. The pulmonary arterial pressure may then equal the systemic pressure reducing or reversing the shunt, and central cyanosis may develop (Eisenmenger's syndrome).

### Clinical features

A small defect (maladie de Roger) may cause no symptoms but there is a loud pansystolic murmur at the left sternal edge; it may close spontaneously. Larger VSDs produce dyspnea and fatigue, and the pulse volume may be decreased. The apex beat is prominent due to left ventricular hypertrophy, and there may be a left parasternal heave if there is right ventricular hypertrophy (RVH) with pulmonary hypertension. There is a thrill at the left sternal edge as well as a pansystolic murmur in the same place. A mitral diastolic flow murmur implies a large shunt.

### Investigation

*Electrocardiography*   There may be no changes in small VSDs. There may be features of right and left ventricular hypertrophy.

*Chest x-ray*   This may be normal in small VSDs. Prominent pulmonary arteries are present in pulmonary hypertension. There may be left atrial and ventricular enlargement.

*Echocardiography*   This is diagnostic if the defect can be imaged. Doppler studies identify abnormal flow across the septum.

*Cardiac catheterization*   There is a step-up in oxygen saturation at the right ventricular level due to shunting of oxygenated blood from the left ventricle to the right ventricle. Left ventricular angiography produces opacification of the right ventricle through the defect.

### Management

Antibiotic prophylaxis should be advised to prevent endocarditis. Moderate and large defects should be closed surgically to prevent pulmonary hypertension and Eisenmenger's syndrome.

## Atrial septal defect

Atrial septal defect (ASD) accounts for 10% of congenital heart defects and is more common in women than men. There are two types: ostium secundum (the more common type) and ostium primum. The communication between the atria allows for left-to-right atrial shunting. Atrial arrhythmias are common. In ostium primum defects, there may be involvement of the mitral and tricuspid valves producing regurgitation.

### Clinical features

Most patients are asymptomatic; a few have dyspnea and weakness. The patient may have palpitations secondary to atrial arrhythmias, and right heart failure may develop later in life. Auscultation reveals wide, fixed splitting of the second heart sound. The increased right heart output gives rise to a pulmonary systolic flow murmur. There may be a tricuspid diastolic flow murmur with large defects. There may be a left ventricular heave of RVH.

### Investigations

*Electrocardiography*   There may be evidence of atrial arrhythmia (e.g., atrial fibrillation). In ostium secundum defects there is right bundle branch block (RBBB), right axis deviation and RVH. In ostium primum defects, there is RBBB, left axis deviation, and RVH.

*Chest x-ray*   Pulmonary arteries are prominent and the lung fields are plethoric. The right atrium and ventricles are enlarged.

*Echocardiography*   This shows dilatation of the right-sided cardiac chambers. Doppler studies allow visualization of the left-to-right shunt across the atrial septum.

*Cardiac catheterization*    There is a step-up in oxygen saturation at the right atrial level due to shunting of oxygenated blood from the left atrium to the right atrium. The catheter can be directed across the defect into the left atrium.

### Management
The defect should be closed surgically if the pulmonary/systemic flow ratio is greater than 2:1.

## Patent ductus arteriosus
Patent ductus arteriosus (PDA) accounts for about 10% of congenital heart defects and is more common in women. The ductus arteriosus connects the pulmonary artery to the descending aorta but it should close off at birth. The condition is sometimes associated with maternal rubella. Because the aortic pressure is higher than the pulmonary artery pressure throughout the cardiac cycle, the PDA produces continuous shunting from the aorta to the pulmonary artery, leading to increased pulmonary venous return to the left heart and an increased left ventricular volume load.

### Clinical features
There are usually no symptoms. Large defects lead to left ventricular failure with dyspnea. The pulse is collapsing. There may be left ventricular hypertrophy. There is a continuous "machinery" murmur with systolic accentuation loudest in the first or second left intercostal space.

### Investigations

*Electrocardiography*    This is normal or shows features of left atrial and left ventricular hypertrophy.

*Chest x-ray*    The aorta and pulmonary arteries are prominent. The lung fields are plethoric.

*Echocardiography*    There is dilatation of the left-sided cardiac chambers. Doppler studies identify the abnormal flow across the ductus.

*Cardiac catheterization*    There is a step-up in oxygen saturation at pulmonary artery level. The catheter can sometimes be passed across the ductus into the descending aorta.

### Management
Indomethacin given within the first few days of birth may stimulate duct closure by inhibiting prostaglandin synthesis. If this fails, the duct can be ligated surgically or with an umbrella occlusion device. Antibiotic prophylaxis is advised.

## Pulmonary stenosis
This accounts for about 7% of defects. It may be valvar or subvalvar (infundibular).

### Clinical features
If very severe there is peripheral cyanosis. There is a pulmonary systolic thrill and murmur, louder on inspiration. The second heart sound is widely split due to a delayed $P_2$. There may be signs of right heart failure. In severe stenosis, the pulse volume is small and $P_2$ is soft or absent.

### Investigations
*Electrocardiography*    Electrocardiography may exhibit features of right atrial hypertrophy (P pulmonale) and RVH.

*Chest x-ray*    There may be poststenotic dilatation of the pulmonary artery and pulmonary oligemia.

*Echocardiography*    This will confirm the diagnosis if adequate views are obtainable. Doppler studies can be used to measure the gradient across the valve.

### Management
For severe pulmonary stenosis, balloon valvuloplasty or valvotomy is indicated.

## Coarctation of the aorta
This accounts for 5–7% of congenital heart defects. It is twice as common in men, and is associated with Turner's syndrome, Marfan's syndrome and berry aneurysms. There is a narrowing of the aorta at or just distal to the ductus arteriosus; the vast majority are distal to the origin of the left subclavian artery. The condition is a cause of secondary hypertension. It encourages the formation of a collateral arterial circulation involving the intercostal arteries. In 80% of patients there is an associated bicuspid aortic valve.

### Clinical features
The condition is often asymptomatic. When present, symptoms include headache, intermittent claudication, stroke, and endocarditis. On examination the femoral pulses are weak or absent, and there is radiofemoral delay. The upper limbs may

be hypertensive or have unequal blood pressure, and the lower limbs have a low pressure. There may be features of LVH. There is a mid- or late systolic murmur over the upper praecordium or back due to turbulent flow through the coarctation. Collateral murmurs may be heard over the scapulae and there may be an aortic systolic murmur of an associated bicuspid valve.

### Investigation
*Electrocardiography*   There may be LVH.

*Chest x-ray*   Tortuous and dilated collaterals may erode the undersurface of the ribs to produce "rib notching." There is a double aortic knuckle due to stenosis and poststenotic dilatation. There may be cardiomegaly.

*Aortography*   This confirms the diagnosis.

### Management
Antibiotic prophylaxis should be advised. Treatment is by surgical resection.

## Tetralogy of Fallot
This represents 6–10% of cases of congenital heart disease. The four features comprising the tetrad are as follows:
- VSD.
- Right ventricular outflow obstruction (pulmonary stenosis—infundibular or valvar).
- The aorta is positioned over the ventricular septum ("overriding aorta").
- RVH.

Because there is right ventricular outflow obstruction, the shunt through the VSD is from right to left. This results in central cyanosis.

### Clinical features
Children may present with deep cyanosis and syncope. Squatting helps to decrease the right-to-left shunt by increasing systemic resistance. Signs include cyanosis and finger clubbing. There is a parasternal heave and systolic murmur in the pulmonary area (second left intercostal space), P$_2$ is soft or absent, and there may be growth retardation.

### Investigation
*Electrocardiography*   Features of right atrial and ventricular hypertrophy are present.

*Chest x-ray*   The heart is boot-shaped ("coeur en sabot"). The pulmonary artery is small and the lung fields are oligemic.

*Echocardiography*   This can be diagnostic, but it may be necessary to proceed to cardiac catheterization studies to confirm the diagnosis.

### Management
This is by total surgical correction. There are palliative procedures for the very young as holding measures (e.g., the Blalock shunt, which is anastamosis of a subclavian artery to a pulmonary artery to increase pulmonary blood flow).

## Cardiomyopathy
Cardiomyopathy is a disorder of heart muscle. They are classified into three types as hypertrophic, dilated, and restrictive. Fig. 30.27 gives a classification.

### Hypertrophic cardiomyopathy
Hypertrophic cardiomyopathy (HCM) follows an autosomal dominant inheritance although half of all cases occur sporadically. There is asymmetrical left ventricular hypertrophy, which leads to symptoms of dyspnea, angina, palpitations, and syncope. On examination there is a jerky pulse, the apex beat has a double impulse, there may be third and fourth heart sounds, and there is a late systolic murmur best heard at the left sternal edge. There may also be associated mitral regurgitation.

HCM may be complicated by atrial fibrillation, systemic emboli, heart failure, and sudden death, the risk of which is probably increased by strenuous exercise.

### Investigation
*Electrocardiography*   Electrocardiography shows left ventricular hypertrophy, and sometimes left bundle-branch block.

*Echocardiography*   Echocardiography shows asymmetrical septal hypertrophy and systolic anterior movement of the mitral valve.

*24-hour ECG monitoring*   This may identify silent arrhythmias.

*Cardiac catheterization*   This shows a small left ventricular cavity with obliteration in systole. There is a systolic gradient within the ventricle.

### Management
Beta blockers help with symptoms and are useful for angina or dysrhythmias. Some treat dysrhythmias prophylactically with amiodarone. The patient should be anticoagulated if there is atrial fibrillation.

### 239

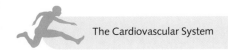
| Causes of cardiomyopathy | |
|---|---|
| **Cause** | **Examples** |
| toxic | alcohol, cyclophosphamide, corticosteroids, lithium, phenothiazines |
| metabolic | thiamine deficiency, pellagra, obesity, porphyria, uremia |
| endocrine | thyrotoxicosis, acromegaly, myxedema, Cushing's disease, diabetes mellitus |
| collagen diseases | SLE, PAN |
| infiltrative | amyloidosis, hemochromatosis, neoplastic, sarcoidosis, mucopolysaccharidosis, Whipple's disease |
| infective | viral, rickettsial, mycobacterial |
| genetic | hypertrophic cardiomyopathy, muscular dystrophies |
| fibroplastic | endomyocardial fibrosis, Loeffler's endomyocardial disease, carcinoid |
| miscellaneous | ischemic heart disease, postpartum |

**Fig. 30.27** Causes of cardiomyopathy. (PAN, polyarteritis nodosa; SLE, systemic lupus erythematosus.)

If medical treatment is ineffective, the patient should be considered for septal myectomy or myotomy or cardiac transplantation. A new treatment option is the use of alcohol to decrease the septal hypertrophy. In this procedure, pure EtOH is injected selectively into small septal arterioles, causing local tissue destruction.

### Dilated (congestive) cardiomyopathy

The ventricles are dilated and contract poorly. Clinically, there are usually signs of right and left heart failure, cardiomegaly, and atrial fibrillation with emboli. More dangerous arrhythmias and conduction defects occur.

There are a number of possible heterogeneous causes, which include infiltrative disorders, collagen diseases, infective, toxic, metabolic, and genetic conditions. Echocardiography shows a globally hypokinetc and dilated heart. Coronary arteriography is usually normal.

### Management

Heart failure should be treated in the usual manner with diuretics, beta blockers, and ACE inhibitors and aldosterone receptor blockers. All patients with markedly reduced ejection fraction should be considered for implantable defibrillators. Any underlying condition is treated as appropriate. Some prescribe anticoagulants to reduce the risk of emboli. The mortality rate is 40% at 2 years. Patients should be considered for cardiac transplantation.

### Restrictive cardiomyopathy

This is due to endomyocardial stiffening and includes fiboplastic and infiltrative conditions in Fig. 30.28. The most common cause in the U.S. is idiopathic amyloidosis. Infiltrative diseases such as sarcoidosis and amyloidosis are other causes. The presentation of right heart failure (elevated JVP, peripheral edema, dyspnea) is similar to that of constrictive pericarditis. Since constrictive pericarditis can be treated with surgery, a distinction should be made between the two.

## Pericarditis

Symptoms of pericarditis include a sharp retrosternal pain relieved by sitting forward. It may radiate to the left arm, or inferiorly. It is worse on lying down, with inspiration and coughing. There may be a "scratchy" friction rub on examination.

The causes of pericarditis are given in Fig. 30.28.

### Investigations

In addition to ECG and CXR (below), the following investigations should be performed:
- Blood and sputum culture for bacteria.
- Viral titers and viral culture from throat swabs and stools.
- Autoantibodies if there is evidence of connective tissue disease.
- ESR, CRP.
- Blood cultures, urea, creatinine, and electrolytes.

| Causes of pericarditis |
| :-- |
| • idiopathic |
| • infections—viral (e.g., coxsackie virus B), bacterial (e.g., *Mycobacterium*), parasitic |
| • neoplastic (e.g., breast, lung, lymphoma) |
| • connective tissue disease (e.g., SLE, RA) |
| • uremia |
| • myocardial infarction |
| • Dressler's syndrome following myocardial infarction or cardiac surgery |
| • radiotherapy |
| • trauma |
| • hypothyroidism |

**Fig. 30.28** Causes of pericarditis. (RA, rheumatoid arthritis; SLE, systemic lupus erythematosus.)

- PPD if TB is suspected (e.g., immigrant population, known exposure).
- TFTs.

### Electrocardiography
This shows concave upward ST segments; T wave inversion may also occur.

### Chest x-ray
This is usually normal. If there is an associated pericardial effusion, the heart appears large and globular.

### Management
The underlying cause is treated. NSAIDs (e.g., indomethacin, 25–50mg 6–8 hourly, or aspirin, 600mg 6 hourly) relieve pain. Occasionally, oral prednisone with a short taper needs to be used to decrease inflammation.

Clinical features of an associated pericardial effusion include signs of left and right heart failure. Pericardial tamponade means that the intrapericardial pressure increases, with reduced cardiac filling and hypotension. Clinically there is tachycardia, pulsus paradoxus, Kussmaul's sign (the JVP increases on inspiration), and muffled heart sounds. The CXR shows a globular heart. The ECG may show a changing axis and low amplitude QRS complexes. Echocardiography is diagnostic. Management is by pericardiocentesis.

### Constrictive pericarditis
This is usually idiopathic or secondary to tuberculosis, although it may follow any cause of pericarditis. The heart is encased within a nonexpansile pericardium. Clinically the signs are of right heart failure with ascites, hepatomegaly, and a raised JVP. There may be pulsus paradoxus, hypotension, and auscultation reveals a pericardial "knock" due to an abrupt end to ventricular filling. The CXR may show pericardial calcification. Management is by pericardiectomy if constriction is severe.

## Infective endocarditis
Infective endocarditis is an illness caused by microbial infection of the cardiac valves or endocardium. It follows invasion of the bloodstream by micro-organisms from the mouth, gastrointestinal and genitourinary tracts, respiratory tract, or the skin. Platelets adhere to endothelial breaks and form "vegetations," which are then colonized by circulating bacteria. Common sites of infection are bicuspid aortic valves and mitral valves with prolapse and regurgitation.

Prosthetic valve endocarditis is becoming increasingly important and may occur early postoperatively or late; 50% of patients have no previously known valve disease. In this group, endocarditis tends to follow a more acute course.

*Streptococcus viridans* is the most common pathogen; others include *Strep. fecalis*, *Staphylococcus aureus*, and *Staph. epidermidis*, especially in drug addicts.

### Clinical features
The diagnosis of endocarditis requires the combination of many different sources of information. The evidence combines the physical exam, radiology, blood tests, and many clinical symptoms. Duke's critieria for the diagnosis of infectious endocarditis are the gold standard.

Definite infectious endocarditis is demonstrated by culturing organisms from heart vegetation or histology, showing vegetation or intracardiac abscess.

The Duke system requires (1) two major criteria, (2) one major and three minor criteria, or (3) five minor criteria.

Major criteria include:
1. Positive blood cultures (all 3 or 3 of 4), separated by time and location, that grow typial endocarditis organisms.
2. New regurgitant murmur.
3. Positive echocardiogram, showing vegetation. TEE is preferred.

Minor criteria include:
1. Predisposing factors (valve damage, prosthetic valves, IV drug use).
2. Evidence of emboli and other vascular phenomena (e.g., Janeway lesions, retinal hemorrhages).
3. Immunologic phenomena (e.g., Osler's nodes, Roth spots).
4. Microbiologic evidence not included above (i.e., infection with Staphylococcus aureus, single positive blood culture, or serologies positive for typical infectious endocarditis organisms).
5. Echocardiographic (minor criteria eliminated).

The diagnosis should be suspected in a patient with fever and changing heart murmurs. The clinical features are:
- Infection: malaise and lassitude, sweats, myalgia, arthralgia, weight loss, finger clubbing, anemia, and splenomegaly. Fever is often low grade.
- Heart disease: listen for murmurs. In tricuspid endocarditis the patient may be murmur free. The patient may present with embolic pneumonia, pleurisy or hemoptysis, or later with a raised venous pressure, jaundice and a pulsating liver.
- Embolism: this is the most common cause of death in endocarditis. Most emboli are sterile but large fungal mycelia may embolize.
- Immunologic phenomena: examples include vasculitic skin lesions, splinter hemorrhages, Roth spots in the retina, and Osler's nodes.
- Urine: this is normal in uncomplicated endocarditis. There may be mild proteinuria resulting from fever, or hematuria as a result of embolism with infarction.

## Investigations
Numerous sets of blood cultures from different sites at different times are the essential investigation. A positive culture confirms the diagnosis. Other investigations are only supportive.

### Erythrocyte sedimentation rate and white cell count
The erythrocyte sedimentation rate (ESR) and white cell count are usually raised. There is a normochromic normocytic anemia.

### Chest x-ray
A CXR with right-sided endocarditis may show multiple shadows due to an embolic pneumonia with infarction.

### Electrocardiography
The ECG may show changes of MI due to coronary embolism, or conduction defect due to the development of an aortic root abscess.

### Echocardiography
Echocardiography may show vegetations or paravalvular abscess formation. A negative echo does not exclude the diagnosis of endocarditis.

## Management
Treatment should be started after blood has been taken for culture, but before obtaining confirmation of a positive culture, because valve destruction can occur rapidly and vegetations may grow and embolize.

### Prophylaxis
Prophylactic antibiotics should be given before dental procedures for patients with heart valve lesions, septal defects, patent ductus, or prosthetic valves. For dental procedures under local or no anesthesia, oral amoxycillin 3g is given 1 hour before the procedure.

Patients who are penicillin-allergic or who have received more than a single dose of penicillin in the previous month are given oral clindamycin, 600mg, or azithromycin, 1g, 1 hour before the procedure. For procedures under general anesthesia, intravenous amoxycillin 1g is given at induction, followed by oral amoxicillin, 500mg, 6 hours later.

Patients at special risk (e.g., those with prosthetic valves or who have had endocarditis) are given 1g intravenous amoxycillin and 120mg intravenous gentamicin at induction, followed by 500mg oral amoxycillin 6 hours later.

Patients who are penicillin-allergic are given 1g vancomycin over 100 minutes, then 120mg intravenous gentamicin at induction. The regimen for patients with upper respiratory tract infection is the same as for dental procedures.

For patients undergoing genitourinary or gastrointestinal procedures, the regimen includes ampicillin (2g IV or IM) plus gentamicin (1.5mg/kg up to a maximum dose of 120mg) 30 minutes before procedure, followed by amoxicillin (1g orally, IM, or IV) 8 hours later. Penicillin-allergic patients should receive the same dose of gentamicin plus vancomycin (1g IV) 1 hour before the procedure.

### Treatment
Treatment will depend on the organism being cultured and its sensitivities. Culture-negative

endocarditis should be treated empirically with broad-coverage antibiotics. Patients with aggressive disease that is unresponsive to treatment may have fungal endcocarditis and will need antifungal coverage.

Patients with endocarditis caused by penicillin-sensitive streptococci (e.g., *Strep. viridans*) are given intravenous benzylpenicillin (or vancomycin if penicillin-allergic) plus low-dose gentamicin (i.e., 60–80mg twice daily). Treatment is for 4 weeks. Gentamicin is stopped after 2 weeks if the organism is fully sensitive to penicillin. Oral amoxycillin may be substituted for benzylpenicillin after 2 weeks.

For patients with endocarditis caused by streptococci with reduced sensitivity to penicillin (e.g. *Strep. fecalis*), intravenous benzylpenicillin (or vancomycin) plus low-dose gentamicin is given for 4 weeks. If the organism is *Staph. aureus*, intravenous flucloxacillin plus either gentamicin or fusidic acid (or vancomycin alone if penicillin allergic) is given for at least 4 weeks. The gentamicin may be stopped after 2 weeks.

### Surgery
This is needed for hemodynamic complications with acute severe valvular regurgitation, for valve obstruction by vegetations, for intractable heart failure, for cardiac abscess formation, and for resistant infections.

### Culture-negative endocarditis
Possible causes of culture-negative endocarditis are given in Fig. 30.29.

## Acute rheumatic fever
Acute rheumatic fever is a multisystem disease following a group A, β-hemolytic, streptococcal infection. The multisystem involvement reflects the generalized vasculitic process of the underlying pathology of the disease. It usually affects children of 5–15 years of age, but no age or race is immune. Risk factors include crowding and low socioeconomic status.

The diagnosis of acute rheumatic fever is based on clinical findings. The presence of two major or one major and two minor criteria indicates a high probability of rheumatic fever (Fig. 30.31). Evidence of a preceding streptococcal infection greatly strengthens the possibility of rheumatic fever.

**Possible causes of endocarditis in the event of negative culture**

- *Coxiella burnetii* (Q fever)
- fungi, e.g. aspergillus, histoplasma
- partially treated bacterial endocarditis
- polyarteritis nodosa or SLE
- atrial myxoma
- non-bacterial endocarditis associated with carcinoma

**Fig. 30.30** Possible causes of endocarditis in the event of negative culture (SLE, systemic lupus erythematous).

**Revised Jones' criteria for guidance in the diagnosis of rheumatic fever**

| major criteria | polyarthritis carditis chorea erythema marginatum subcutaneous nodules |
|---|---|
| minor criteria | fever arthralgia previous rheumatic fever or rheumatic heart disease raised acute phase reactants (ESR, CRP, WCC) prolonged PR interval in ECG |

**Fig. 30.31** Revised Jones' criteria for guidance in the diagnosis of rheumatic fever. For a diagnosis of rheumatic fever there must also be supporting evidence of preceding streptococcal infection, i.e. increased antistreptolysin O (ASOT) or other streptococcal antibodies, positive throat culture for group A *Streptococcus*, or recent scarlet fever. (CRP, C reactive protein; ESR, erythrocyte sedimentation rate; WCC, white cell count.)

### Notes on Jones' criteria for rheumatic fever
#### Carditis (40–50%)
There may be myocarditis (tachypnea, dyspnea, pulmonary edema), endocarditis (listen regularly for transient murmurs—the mitral valve is most commonly affected), or pericarditis (friction rub, effusion). It may be asymptomatic or result in death in the acute stage, and it can lead to heart failure and chronic valvular heart disease.

#### Arthritis (80%)
This is the most common major criterion and usually presents as migratory joint pain affecting larger joints. The onset is sudden with signs of

inflammation and limitation of movement. Symptoms last for 3–6 weeks.

### Chorea (10%)
There is a latent period of 2–6 months. Symptoms last for about 6 months. It is more common in girls. Movements are involuntary, involving mainly the face and limbs and may be unilateral. It is associated with emotional lability.

### Erythema marginatum (<5%)
This is a painless rash appearing as large, pink macules, that spread quickly to give a serpiginous edge with a fading center.

### Subcutaneous nodules (rare)
These are round, firm, and painless, ranging from 0.5–2cm. They are mobile and occur mainly over bony prominences.

### Fever
This is usually low grade.

### Management
This is bed rest for 2 weeks. Painful joints immobilized. Anti-inflammatory drugs relieve the pain and swelling of joints and possibly the later development of valvular heart disease. Treatment is usually for 12 weeks, or longer for severe carditis.

Aspirin, 80–100mg/kg/day, or corticosteroids in severe carditis are the drugs of choice. Diazepam is given to control choreiform movements. Intramuscular penicillin G is given in the acute stages, and is followed by oral penicillin for 5 years in those patients without carditis, and probably indefinitely for those with cardiac involvement.

## Atrial myxoma
These are rare, benign, primary tumors usually in the left atrium, which are twice as common in women as in men. They present with vague symptoms (e.g., fever, weight loss, general malaise, atrial fibrillation, left atrial obstruction, or systemic emboli). Auscultation may reveal a "tumor plop." They are diagnosed by echocardiography, and treatment is by surgical excision.

## Asthma

### Diagnosis

Asthma is a disease of the airways characterized by an increased responsiveness of the tracheobronchial tree to many different stimuli. It is manifested by paroxysms of shortness of breath, cough, and wheezing. These symptoms may resolve spontaneously or be relieved by treatment.

Asthma is episodic with acute exacerbations interspersed by symptom-free periods. Typically, most attacks are short (minutes to hours), and clinically the patient appears to recover completely after an attack.

In more severe asthma, patients can experience some degree of airway obstruction daily with accompanying symptoms.

### Incidence

Asthma is very common and occurs in about 5% of the population in most Western countries. Bronchial asthma occurs at all ages but peaks in childhood and is more common in boys. However, in adult asthma, the sex ratio is about equal by the age of 30 years.

### Etiology

It is helpful to classify asthma by the main factors associated with acute episodes, i.e., into allergic asthma and intrinsic asthma.

Allergic asthma is often associated with a personal or family history of allergy such as hay fever, urticaria, and eczema. There may also be increased levels of immunoglobulin (Ig) E in the serum and a positive response to provocation tests (e.g., methacholine challenge.)

Intrinsic (or idiosyncratic) asthma is a term used to define those patients presenting with no personal or family history of allergy, with negative skin tests, and with normal serum levels of IgE. Many develop typical symptoms following an upper respiratory infection, which, after several days, leads to paroxysms of wheezing and shortness of breath that can last for months.

In general, asthma that occurs in childhood or early adult life tends to have a strong allergic component, whereas asthma that develops late tends to be nonallergic.

Despite this, many patients do not fit into either category but fall into a group with a mixture of allergic and nonallergic features.

### Pathophysiology

Many theories have been proposed to explain the increased airway reactivity of asthma, but the basic mechanism remains unknown.

The most popular hypothesis is that of airway inflammation. This is based on the observation that increased numbers of mast cells, epithelial cells, neutrophils, eosinophils, and lymphocytes have been found in the bronchoalveolar lavage fluid of patients with asthma. Along with these cellular components of inflammation a variety of inflammatory mediators such as histamine, bradykinin, the leukotrienes C, D, and E, and platelet-activating factor; prostaglandins $E_2$ and $F_2\alpha$ have also been found.

The clinical features of asthma probably derive from an interaction between the normally resident and infiltrating inflammatory cells in the airways and the surface epithelium. These produce an intense immediate inflammatory reaction involving bronchoconstriction, vascular congestion, and edema formation—the pathologic hallmarks of asthma. Leukotrienes, in addition to evoking contraction of airway smooth muscle and mucosal edema, may also account for other typical features of asthma, such as increased mucus production and impaired mucociliary transport.

A number of factors interact with normal airway responsiveness and provoke acute episodes and include the following:

- Allergens (e.g., house dust, mites, and animal dander).

- Drugs (e.g., β-blockers).
- The environment (e.g., climatic conditions, cold air, and air pollution).
- Occupations (e.g., exposure to industrial chemicals, drugs, metals, dusts).
- Infections (e.g., viral and bacterial).
- Exercise.
- Emotion.

## Clinical features of asthma

The symptoms of asthma consist of a triad of shortness of breath, cough, and wheezing. In its most typical form, asthma is an episodic disease, and all three symptoms coexist.

At the onset of an attack, patients experience a sense of constriction in the chest, often with a nonproductive cough. Respiration becomes audibly harsh, wheezing in both phases of respiration becomes prominent, expiration becomes prolonged, and patients frequently have both tachypnea and tachycardia. If the attack is severe or prolonged, there may be a loss of breath sounds, and wheezing becomes either very high-pitched or inaudible. Accessory muscles of respiration can be seen, and pulsus paradoxus often develops.

Less typically, a patient with asthma may present with intermittent episodes of nonproductive cough or shortness of breath on exertion. These patients often have a normal physical examination but may wheeze after repeated forced exhalations or may show evidence of airways obstruction with spirometry. Occasionally a provocation test may be required to make the diagnosis of airway hyperresponsiveness.

## Confirming the diagnosis of asthma

Diagnosing asthma is usually not difficult, especially if the patient is seen during an acute attack. In addition, the history of episodic symptoms and a history of eczema, hay fever, or urticaria is valuable. Nocturnal symptoms (e.g., awakening short of breath or wheezing), are very common features.

### Investigations

The diagnosis of asthma is established by demonstrating reversible airways obstruction. Reversibility is traditionally defined as a 15% or greater increase in the forced expiratory volume in 1 second ($FEV_1$) following two puffs of a $\beta_2$-agonist.

Once the diagnosis is confirmed, peak expiratory flow rates (PEFRs) at home or the $FEV_1$ in the clinic can be used to monitor the course of the illness and the effectiveness of therapy. Sputum and blood eosinophilia and measurement of serum IgE levels may be helpful but are not specific for asthma. Similarly, a chest x-ray (CXR) showing hyperinflation is not diagnostic of asthma.

### Differential diagnosis

In a small minority of patients the diagnosis can cause some difficulty, and the following differential diagnoses for wheezing and shortness of breath should be considered:

- Upper airway obstruction: tumor, vocal cord paralysis, or laryngeal edema.
- Endobronchial disease (e.g., foreign body aspiration, neoplasm, bronchial stenosis).
- Left ventricular failure.
- Carcinoid tumors.
- Recurrent pulmonary emboli.
- Chronic bronchitis (COPD).
- Eosinophilic pneumonias.
- Systemic vasculitis with pulmonary involvement.

## Management of asthma

The elimination of the causative agent from the environment of an allergic asthmatic is the most successful means available for treating this condition.

The treatments available for asthma can be divided into two general categories:

- Drugs that inhibit smooth muscle contraction (e.g., $\beta_2$-agonists, methylxanthines or theophylline derivatives, anticholinergics).
- Drugs that prevent or reverse inflammation (e.g., corticoidsteroids, mast cell-stabilizing agents, and leukotriene antagonists).

In clinical practice the two most common settings in which patients require treatment are emergency treatment of acute severe asthma and chronic therapy.

### Chronic therapy

Patients should be divided into categories depending on disease severity. Although firm distinctions do not exist among these groups, treatment guidelines are based on the severity of symptoms.

## Mild
- Symptoms occur only with heavy exercise.
- 1 or 2 nocturnal awakenings per month.
- Lung function does not deteriorate over the course of the day.

## Moderate
Symptoms occur with mild exercise.

1 or 2 nocturnal awakenings per week.

$FEV_1 = 60$–70% of predicted with symptoms worse upon awakening.

## Severe
Symptoms occur with minimal exercise.

Nocturnal symptoms more than twice per week.

$FEV_1 < 60$% of predicted.

Therapy is aimed at achieving a stable, asymptomatic state with the best pulmonary function possible. The first step is to educate patients to function as partners in their management. The severity of the illness needs to be assessed and monitored with objective measures of lung function. Asthma triggers should be avoided or controlled, and plans should be made for both chronic management and treatment of exacerbations. Regular follow-up care is mandatory.

Drug therapy should be kept as simple as possible and infrequent symptoms require only the use of an inhaled $\beta_2$-agonist on an as-needed basis.

When features such as nocturnal wakenings and worsening daytime symptoms develop, inhaled steroids or mast cell-stabilizing inhalers should be added. If symptoms do not improve, the dose of inhaled steroids can be increased. Severe asthma can be treated with long-acting inhaled $\beta_2$ agonists, and antimuscarinic agents, (e.g., ipratropium). Note, however, that theophylline is not commonly used because of the need to check blood levels on a regular basis. Also note that ipratroprium is not used frequently for asthma but remains popular in the treatment of COPD.

Some patients with severe recurrent symptoms need oral steroids in a single daily dose. Once control is reached and sustained for several weeks, a step-down reduction in therapy should be undertaken, beginning with the most toxic drug, to find the minimal amount of treatment needed to keep the patient well. The PEFR should be monitored and treatment adjusted accordingly, particularly when corroborated by the patient's symptoms. This stepped–care management of chronic adult asthma is illustrated in Fig. 31.1.

## Emergency treatment
Emergency treatment of acute asthma is one of the most common emergencies seen in ordinary medical practice, and its life-threatening nature can be underestimated by the less experienced.

Features indicating severe airway obstruction include the presence of pulsus paradoxus, the use of accessory muscles, and marked hyperinflation of the thorax with absent breath sounds. Failure of these signs to remit promptly after aggressive therapy requires objective monitoring of the patient using measurements of arterial blood gases (ABGs) and the PEFR or $FEV_1$.

A checklist for the assessment and treatment of these patients is shown in Fig. 31.2.

Generally, there is a direct correlation between the severity of the obstruction with which the patient presents and the time it takes to resolve it. When the PEFR falls by more than 20% of its previous value, if the magnitude of the pulsus paradoxus is increasing, and if serial measures of ABGs show that the partial pressure of carbon dioxide ($pCO_2$) is within the normal range or elevated, then the patient should be monitored in an intensive care setting and may need assisted ventilation.

# Chronic bronchitis and emphysema

## Definitions
### Chronic bronchitis
Chronic bronchitis is a condition associated with excessive mucus production sufficient to cause cough with expectoration for at least 3 months of the year for more than 2 consecutive years.

Simple chronic bronchitis is characterized by mucoid sputum production, while chronic mucopurulent bronchitis is identified by persistent or recurrent purulent sputum in the absence of localized suppurative diseases such as bronchiectasis.

### Emphysema
Emphysema is defined as the permanent, abnormal distention of the air spaces distal to the terminal bronchiole with destruction of alveolar septa.

### Chronic obstructive pulmonary disease
Chronic obstructive pulmonary disease (COPD) is defined as a condition in which there is chronic

| Stepped-care plan for the management of chronic asthma | |
| --- | --- |
| **Step** | **Measures** |
| 1 | inhaled short-acting $\beta_2$-stimulant as required (up to once daily) |
| 2 | add regular inhaled preventive therapy<br>either regular standard-dose inhaled corticosteroid<br>or regular cromoglycate of nedocromil (but change to inhaled corticosteroid if control not achieved) |
| 3 | add high-dose inhaled corticosteroids<br>or long-acting inhaled $\beta_2$-stimulant (e.g., salmeferol)<br>or trial of regular cromoglycote or nedoctomil if not tried at step 2 |
| 4 | high-dose inhaled corticosteroids plus regular bronchodilators<br>plus sequential therapeutic trial of one or more of the following:<br>• Inhaled long-acting $\beta_2$-stimulant<br>• inhaled ipratropium<br>• modified-release oral $\beta_2$-stimulant<br>• high-dose inhaled bronchodilators<br>• cromoglycate or nedocromil |
| 5 | add regular corticosteroid tablets (prednisone) (note these patients should normally be referred to an asthma clinic) |
| stepping down | review treatment every 3–6 months<br>if control achieved stepwise reduction may be possible<br>if treatment started recently at step 4 or 5 (or contained corticosteroid tablets) reduction may take place after short interval<br>for other patients a 1–3 month or longer period of stability needed before slow stepwise reduction attempted |

**Fig. 31.1** Stepped-care plan for the management of chronic asthma. Treatment is started at the step most appropriate to initial severity, and a "rescue" course of prednisone can be given at any time and with any step to cover an exacerbation. Move up the step ladder if relief bronchodilators are needed frequently or night-time symptoms occur. Check compliance and inhaler technique, and consider the use of spacer devices.

obstruction to airflow due to chronic bronchitis with or without emphysema. Although the degree of obstruction may be less when the patient is free from respiratory infection and may improve somewhat with bronchodilators, significant obstruction is always present in these patients.

## Pathophysiology

The hallmark of chronic bronchitis is hypertrophy of the mucus-producing glands found in the submucosa of large cartilaginous airways. Quantitation of this anatomic change is based on the ratio of the thickness of the submucosal glands to that of the bronchial wall. In lungs from patients with COPD studied at post-mortem there is goblet cell hyperplasia, mucosal and submucosal inflammatory cells, edema, peribronchial fibrosis, intraluminal mucus plugs, and increased smooth muscle in small airways.

Inflammation in chronic bronchitis occurs at the alveolar epithelium and differs from the predominantly eosinophilic inflammation of asthma by the predominance of neutrophils and the peribronchiolar location of fibrotic changes.

Emphysema is classified according to the pattern of involvement of the gas-exchanging units (acini) of the lung distal to the terminal bronchiole. With centriacinar emphysema, the distention and destruction are mainly limited to the respiratory bronchioles with relatively less change peripherally in the acinus. Because of the large functional reserve in the lung, many units must be involved in order for overall dysfunction to be detectable. Panacinar emphysema involves both the central and peripheral

| Assessment and treatment of acute severe asthma | |
|---|---|
| **Tasks to consider** | **Comment** |
| assessment | clinical features indicating severity:<br>• patient unable to speak sentences<br>• respiratory rate >25/min<br>• heart rate >110/min<br>• peak flow <40% predicted (or <200mL)<br>• inspiratory fall in systolic BP >10mmHg<br>life-threatening features:<br>• silent chest on auscultation<br>• cyanosis<br>• bradycardia<br>• exhaustion or confusion<br>ABG:<br>• respiratory failure [$pO_2 < 60mmHg$]<br>• normal or high $pCO_2$<br>• low pH |
| immediate treatment | oxygen at high concentration<br>high doses of inhaled $\beta_2$-agonists (e.g. salbutamol 5mg via nebulizer)<br>high doses of systemic steroids (prednisolone 30–60mg or hydrocortisone 200mg i.v.)<br>intravenous bronchodilators for very severe disease |
| criteria for hospital admission | any life-threatening features<br>any features of severe attack persisting after initial treatment<br>peak flow still <40% predicted or 200mL 30 minutes after nebulizer<br>recent worsening of daytime or nocturnal symptoms over days or weeks<br>poor social circumstances |
| indications for intensive care | respiratory failure despite 60% oxygen<br>hypercapnia [$pCO_2 > 50mmHg$]<br>onset of exhaustion<br>confusion or drowsiness<br>unconscious patient<br>respiratory arrest |
| further investigation in hospital | CXR for pneumothorax, consolidation, or pulmonary edema<br>U&Es and serum creatinine<br>CBC<br>ECG in order patients |
| duration of hospital admission | until symptoms and lung function stable<br>peak flow >75% predicted or best level<br><25% diurnal variability in peak flow<br>no nocturnal symptoms |
| treatment changes before discharge | inhaled steroids started 48 hours before discharge<br>nebulizers replaced by inhalers 24–48 hours before<br>inhaler technique should be checked |
| drugs on discharge from hospital | all patients should be discharged taking:<br>• oral steroids for 1–3 weeks<br>• an inhaled anti-inflammatory drug (usually a steroid)<br>• inhaled or nebulized $\beta_2$-agonists<br>• long-acting $\beta_2$-agonist, or inhaled ipratropium if needed |

**Fig. 31.2** Checklist for the emergency assessment and treatment of asthma. (ABG, arterial blood gases; BP, blood pressue; CXR, chest X-ray; ECG, electrocardiogram; CBC, complete blood count; $pCO_2$, partial pressure of carbon dioxide; $pO_2$, partial pressure of oxygen; U&Es, urea and electrolytes.)

portions of the acinus, which results, if the process is extensive, in a reduction of the alveolar–capillary gas exchange surface and loss of elastic recoil properties.

When emphysema is severe, it may be difficult to distinguish between the two types because, most often, they coexist in the same lung.

## Etiology of chronic bronchitis and emphysema
### Cigarette smoking
Cigarette smoking is the most commonly identified factor associated with both chronic bronchitis during life and extent of emphysema at post-mortem. Prolonged cigarette smoking impairs ciliary movement, inhibits function of alveolar macrophages, and leads to hypertrophy and hyperplasia of mucus-secreting glands. It is probable that smoke also inhibits antiproteases and causes polymorphonuclear leukocytes to release proteolytic enzymes acutely. Inhaled cigarette smoke can produce an acute increase in airways resistance due to vagally mediated, smooth-muscle constriction.

### Air pollution
Air pollution with sulphur dioxide and particulate matter is associated with exacerbations of chronic bronchitis, and the incidence and mortality rates for chronic bronchitis and emphysema is probably higher in heavily industrialized urban areas.

### Occupation
Occupations exposing workers to inorganic or organic dusts, or to noxious gases, result in a higher prevalence of chronic bronchitis among employees.

### Acute respiratory infections
These have been implicated as one of the major factors associated with both the etiology and progression of COPD.

### Familial and genetic factors
Familial aggregation of chronic bronchitis has been well demonstrated. $\alpha_1$-Antitrypsin ($\alpha_1$AT) deficiency is a recognized genetic cause of emphysema. Either decreased or absent serum levels of the protease inhibitor $\alpha_1$AT are found in some patients with early-onset emphysema. Most members of the normal population have two M genes, designated as protease inhibitor type MM, but those with defective (Z and S) genes who are homozygous ZZ or SS have markedly decreased serum levels of $\alpha_1$AT and

develop severe panacinar emphysema in their 20s and 30s.

## Clinical features of COPD
The clinical presentation of COPD varies in severity from simple chronic bronchitis without disability to patients with severe disability and chronic respiratory failure. In clinical practice it is common to encounter patients with fully developed COPD and, even though most patients will have features of both chronic bronchitis and emphysema, it is useful to categorize patients as having predominant features of one or other. The clinical features of emphysema and chronic bronchitis are summarized in Fig. 31.3. It is important to remember, however, that most patients have a combination of features of both emphysema and chronic bronchitis.

## Management of COPD
The management of patients with COPD is based on knowledge of the degree of obstruction, the extent of disability, and the reversibility of the patient's illness.

The extent of the airways obstruction and the potential to reverse this is key as there is a chance that treatment may be effective in improving the overall disability.

Emphysema, however, is an irreversible process and so the prevention of its progression and the avoidance of acute infections are the main approach to management.

### Investigations
History, physical examination, and CXR should be supplemented by tests of lung function performed during a chronic stable period. Complete spirometry, lung volumes, transfer of carbon monoxide, and ABGs should be measured. Also, reversibility should be assessed by spirometry and lung volumes after the administration of bronchodilators.

## Treatment of COPD
Treatment strategies for COPD are varied, and a multidisciplinary approach to the patient is often required. A treatment plan should consider the following:
- Stopping cigarette smoking.
- Education of the patient about the disease.
- Relief of bronchospasm.
- Chest physical therapy.
- Treatment of acute exacerbations.

| | Clinical feature | Emphysema | Chronic bronchitis |
|---|---|---|---|
| history and examination | dyspnea | constant and progressive | intermittent, mild to moderate |
| | cough | absent or mild | persistent and severe |
| | sputum | absent or mild (clear, mucoid) | copious (mucopurulent, purulent) |
| | body weight | thin | obese |
| | central cyanosis | absent | present |
| | plethoric face | absent | present |
| | barrel chest | present | absent |
| | percussion note | hyperresonant | normal |
| | auscultation | decreased breath sounds | wheezes |
| CXR | bullae | present | absent |
| | peripheral markings | decreased | increased |
| | hemidiaphragms | flat | normal |
| | heart size | normal | large, boot shaped |
| arterial blood gases | hypoxia | absent or mild | moderate to severe |
| | hypercapnia | absent | moderate to severe |

**Clinical features which distinguish emphysema from chronic bronchitis**

**Fig. 31.3** Clinical features that distinguish emphysema from chronic bronchitis.

- Treatment of cor pulmonale: if appropriate.
- Home oxygen therapy: when indicated.

A trial of bronchodilator drugs is warranted in all patients with COPD. Although treatment follows a similar pattern to that seen in asthma (see Fig. 31.1), there are some differences. Inhaled antimuscarinic bronchodilators (e.g., ipratropium) are considered first choice in COPD, often combined with a short-acting $\beta_2$ agonist. Oral corticosteroids or high-dose inhaled steroids play an important role in a small minority of patients (perhaps 10–15%) who respond to a corticosteroid trial. This usually consists of 3 weeks of prednisone at 30–40mg/day with appropriate monitoring of the peak flow.

Infective exacerbations of COPD are treated with broad-spectrum antibiotics such as amoxicillin, trimethoprim, or tetracycline, aiming to cover the likely pathogens (pneumococci and *Haemophilus influenzae*). Type II respiratory failure often accompanies exacerbations of COPD; controlled oxygen therapy is discussed on p. 262.

Long-term administration of oxygen (at least 15 hours daily) may prolong survival in patients with severe COPD with cor pulmonale. Guidelines suggest that this treatment should be provided for patients who fulfil the following criteria:
- Ambulatory oxygen saturation monitoring <88% or partial pressure of oxygen ($pO_2$) <55mmHg.
- $FEV_1$ <1.5L and FVC (forced vital capacity) <2L.

Blood gas measurements should be stable on two occasions at least 3 weeks apart after the patient has received appropriate bronchodilator therapy. Increased respiratory depression is seldom a problem in patients with stable respiratory failure treated with low concentrations of oxygen, although it may occur during exacerbations.

Patients and relatives should be warned to call for medical help if drowsiness or confusion occur. Oxygen concentrators, rather than cylinders, are more economical for patients requiring oxygen for long periods and are now used routinely.

Less information is available on long-term oxygen in patients with a similar degree of hypoxemia and airflow obstruction but no hypercapnia. The current advice is that these patients should not be denied home oxygen, but the effects of long-term therapy have not yet been fully assessed.

## Tuberculosis

Tuberculosis (TB) is caused by bacteria belonging to the *Mycobacterium tuberculosis* complex. The disease usually affects the lungs, although in up to a third of cases other organs are involved. If properly treated, TB caused by drug-susceptible strains is curable in virtually all cases. If untreated, the disease may be fatal within 5 years in more than half of cases. Transmission usually takes place through the airborne spread of droplet nuclei produced by patients with infectious pulmonary TB.

Of the pathogenic species belonging to the *M. tuberculosis* complex, the most frequent and important agent of human disease is *M. tuberculosis* itself. Closely related organisms that also infect humans include *M. bovis* (the bovine tubercle bacillus, once an important cause of TB transmitted by unpasteurized milk and currently the cause of a small percentage of cases in developing countries).

*M. tuberculosis* is a rod-shaped, non-spore-forming, thin, aerobic bacterium measuring 0.5–3 μm.

Mycobacteria, including *M. tuberculosis*, do not stain readily and are often neutral on Gram stain. However, once stained, the bacilli cannot be decolorized by acid alcohol, a characteristic justifying their classification as acid-fast bacilli (AFB).

Tuberculosis is more common in Asians, patients with diabetes mellitus, the immunosuppressed, alcoholics, and vagrants.

## Clinical manifestations of tuberculosis

TB is usually classified as pulmonary or extrapulmonary. Before human immunodeficiency virus (HIV) infection, 80% of all cases of TB were limited to the lungs, but now two-thirds of HIV-infected patients with TB may have both pulmonary and extrapulmonary disease, or even extrapulmonary disease on its own.

### Pulmonary tuberculosis
Pulmonary TB can be classified as primary or postprimary (secondary).

### Primary pulmonary tuberculosis
Primary pulmonary TB results from an initial infection with tubercle bacilli. Where TB has a high prevalence, primary disease is often seen in children and is localized to the middle and lower lung zones. The lesion is usually peripheral and associated with hilar or paratracheal lymph node enlargement. In most cases, the lesion heals spontaneously and may later be seen as a small calcified nodule (Ghon's lesion).

Patients with impaired immunity who develop primary pulmonary TB may progress rapidly to clinical illness. This may result from spread of infection by the following:
- Pleural effusion: may lead to tuberculous empyema.
- Necrosis and acute cavitation of the primary lesion: known as progressive primary TB.
- Bloodstream dissemination: resulting in granulomatous lesions in various organs, or even miliary TB with tuberculous meningitis.

### Postprimary pulmonary tuberculosis
Postprimary disease is sometimes termed adult, reactivation, or secondary TB. It results from reactivation of latent infection and is usually localized to the apical and posterior segments of the upper lobes. The extent of lung changes can vary from small infiltrates to extensive cavitation. Widespread involvement of the lung with coalescing lesions produces tuberculous pneumonia.

The pathogenicity of TB varies, with a third of untreated patients dying from severe pulmonary TB within weeks or months, while the rest undergo spontaneous remission or proceed along a chronic course, often involving lung fibrosis.

### Symptoms and signs
Symptoms and signs of early TB are often nonspecific and include fever, night sweats, weight loss, anorexia, and lethargy. Most patients eventually develop cough with purulent sputum, and this may be associated with hemoptysis. Pleuritic chest pain can develop in

patients with subpleural lesions or from muscle strain due to persistent coughing. Clinical examination may be of limited use in pulmonary TB, but the following features may be present:
- Crackles: involved areas during inspiration.
- Wheeze: partial bronchial obstruction.
- Classic amphoric breath sounds: areas with large cavities.
- Pallor: anemia.
- Finger clubbing.

## Extrapulmonary tuberculosis
This most commonly involves lymph nodes, the pleura, genitourinary tract, bones and joints, meninges, and peritoneum.

# Diagnostic tests for tuberculosis
The key to the diagnosis of TB is a high index of suspicion. It should form part of the differential diagnosis in patients with febrile illnesses, cervical lymphadenopathy, or focal infiltrates on the chest x-ray.

The CXR may show the typical picture of upper lobe infiltrates, with or without cavitation. The diagnosis is commonly based on the finding of AFB by microscopy of a diagnostic specimen such as sputum or tissue (e.g., lymph node biopsy). Laboratory identification depends on either auramine–rhodamine staining and fluorescence microscopy or the more traditional light microscopy of specimens stained with Ziehl–Neelsen dye.

Patients with suspected pulmonary TB normally collect three sputum specimens for AFB smear and mycobacterial culture and sensitivity. Specimens are inoculated on to Lowenstein–Jensen medium. Most species of mycobacteria, including *M. tuberculosis*, are slow-growing so that 4–8 weeks may be required before growth is detected and antibiotic sensitivity can be assessed.

Other diagnostic tests for pulmonary TB include the following:
- Induced sputum by ultrasonic nebulization of hypertonic saline for patients unable to produce a sputum specimen spontaneously.
- Fiberoptic bronchoscopy with bronchial brushings or transbronchial biopsy of the lesion.
- Bronchoalveolar lavage of a lung segment containing an abnormality.

When extrapulmonary TB is suspected, specimens of involved sites may include the following:

- Cerebrospinal fluid: tuberculous meningitis.
- Pleural fluid and biopsy samples: pleural disease.
- Bone marrow and liver biopsy culture: good diagnostic yield in disseminated (miliary) TB.
- Early morning urine: renal TB.

In all cases specimens are sent for AFB microscopy and culture.

# Treatment
TB is treated in an initial phase using at least three drugs and a continuation phase using two drugs. Treatment requires specialized knowledge, particularly where the disease involves resistant organisms or nonrespiratory organs.

## Initial phase
Three drugs are used during the initial phase to reduce bacterial numbers rapidly and prevent the emergence of drug-resistant bacteria. The initial phase drugs are continued for 2 months. Where a positive culture for *M. tuberculosis* has been obtained but sensitivities are not available after 2 months, treatment with a third drug is continued until full susceptibility is confirmed.

## Continuation phase
After the initial phase, treatment is continued for a further 4 months with isoniazid and rifampicin; longer treatment may be necessary for meningitis or for resistant organisms.

Recommended drugs for a standard, unsupervised, 6-month regimen include:
- Isoniazid: for 6 months.
- Rifampicin: for 6 months.
- Pyrazinamide: for the first 2 months only.

## Immunocompromised patients
Immunocompromised patients may develop TB owing to reactivation of previously latent disease or to new infection. Multiresistant *M. tuberculosis* may be present, or the infection may be caused by other mycobacteria (e.g., *M. avium* complex), in which case specialist advice is needed. Culture should always be carried out and the type of organism and its sensitivity confirmed. Immunocompromised patients require three-drug therapy, often for a year.

## Monitoring treatment
Isoniazid, rifampicin, and pyrazinamide are associated with liver toxicity; therefore, hepatic

253

function should be checked before treatment with these drugs. Renal function should also be checked before treatment with antituberculous drugs and appropriate dosage adjustments made. Visual acuity should be tested before ethambutol is used because it can cause loss of visual acuity and visual field defects.

Major causes of treatment failure include incorrect prescribing by doctors and inadequate compliance by patients.

Drug-resistant TB should be treated by a specialist physician. Second-line drugs available for infections caused by resistant organisms or when first-line drugs cause unacceptable side effects include capreomycin, amikasin, cycloserine, newer macrolides (e.g., azithromycin and clarithromycin), and 4-quinolones (e.g., ciprofloxacin and ofloxacin). Duration of therapy is variable, with most chemotherapy continuing for 24 months after sputum culture becomes negative.

### Infection control for tuberculosis
By far the best way to prevent TB is the rapid diagnosis of infectious cases with appropriate treatment until cure. Additional strategies include BCG (bacillus Calmette-Guérin) vaccination and preventive chemotherapy.

### Vaccination
BCG was derived from an attenuated strain of *M. bovis* and was first administered to humans in 1921. Many BCG vaccines are now available worldwide, and all are derived from the original strain, but the vaccines vary in efficacy. The vaccine is safe and rarely causes serious complications.

BCG vaccination induces purified protein derivative (PPD) reactivity, but the magnitude of PPD skin test reactions after vaccination does not predict the degree of protection afforded. Currently vaccination is recommended only for PPD-negative infants and children who are at a high risk of intimate and prolonged exposure to patients with TB and who cannot take prophylactic isoniazid. In the U.K., BCG is offered to PPD-negative children at the age of 12 years, but it is not recommended in the U.S. This is because all patients who receive BCG vaccination will forever be PPD-positive. Therefore, screening TB tests are unable to be used in a population treated with the vaccine, possibly increasing the proportion of undiagnosed TB cases.

### Preventive chemotherapy
A major component of TB control involves contact tracing, skin testing, and the administration of isoniazid to contacts at high risk of active disease.

## Lung cancer

Lung cancer is the leading cause of cancer death in the U.S., with over 120,00 patients dying each year.

The term "lung cancer" is usually reserved for tumors arising from the respiratory epithelium (bronchi, bronchioles, and alveoli). Four major cell types account for 88% of all primary lung neoplasms:
- Squamous (epidermoid) carcinoma.
- Small cell (also called oat cell) carcinoma.
- Adenocarcinoma (including bronchioloalveolar).
- Large cell (also called large cell anaplastic) carcinoma.

The remainder includes undifferentiated carcinomas, carcinoids, bronchial gland tumors, and rarer tumor types (e.g., mesothelioma arising from the pleura). All cell types have different natural histories and responses to therapy; therefore, making a correct histologic diagnosis is the mandatory first step to correct assessment and treatment.

### Etiology
The majority of lung cancers are caused by carcinogens and tumor promoters inhaled via cigarette smoking. Overall, the relative risk of developing lung cancer is increased about 13-fold by active smoking and about 1.5-fold by long-term second-hand exposure to cigarette smoke. Probably there is a co-carcinogenic effect of smoking and industrial or environmental pollutants, e.g., radon gas from natural sources in the ground.

There is a dose–response relationship between the lung cancer death rate and the total amount of cigarettes smoked, such that the risk is increased 60–70-fold for a man smoking two packets a day for 20 years as compared with a non-smoker.

Conversely, the chance of developing lung cancer decreases with the cessation of smoking but may never return to the nonsmoker's level. The recent increase in lung cancer rate in women is also associated with a rise in cigarette smoking.

While human lung cancer is not thought of as a genetic disease, a variety of molecular genetic studies have shown that lung cancer cells have acquired a number of genetic lesions, including activation of dominant oncogenes and inactivation of tumour suppressor or recessive oncogenes. Of these the most important are as follows:

- Dominant oncogenes: point mutations in the coding regions of the *ras* family of oncogenes (adenocarcinoma of lung), amplification, rearrangement, and/or loss of transcriptional control of the *myc* family of oncogenes (non-small cell cancers and small cell lung cancer), and overexpression of the telomerase gene.
- Recessive oncogenes (tumor suppressor genes), cytogenetic and allele-typing analyses have shown deletions (allele loss) involving several chromosome regions.

The large number of lesions shows that lung cancer, like many other epithelial malignancies, is a multistep process that is likely to involve both carcinogens and tumor promoters.

Nicotine may play a central role in lung cancer pathogenesis as carcinogenic derivatives of nicotine are formed in cigarette smoke.

Other risk factors for developing lung cancer include asbestos, radon, arsenic, nickel, and ionizing radiation.

35% of solitary pulmonary nodules, 1–6cm in diameter, in adults aged 35 years and above, are malignant.

## Clinical findings in lung cancer

Although 5–15% of patients are detected while asymptomatic, usually on a routine chest radiograph, the vast majority of patients present with some signs or symptoms.

### Endobronchial growth of the primary tumor

This may result in cough, hemoptysis, wheeze and stridor, dyspnea, and postobstructive pneumonitis (fever and productive cough).

### Peripheral tumor growth

This could cause pain (pleural or chest wall involvement), cough, dyspnea, and symptoms of lung abscess due to tumor cavitation.

## Regional spread of tumor in the chest

Regional spread of tumor in the chest (by contiguous growth or metastasis to regional lymph nodes) may lead to tracheal obstruction, esophageal compression with dysphagia, recurrent laryngeal nerve paralysis with hoarseness, phrenic nerve paralysis with elevation of the hemidiaphragm and dyspnea, and sympathetic nerve paralysis with Horner's syndrome (ptosis, miosis, enophthalmos, and ipsilateral loss of sweating).

Pancoast's (or superior sulcus tumor) syndrome results from the local extension of a tumor growing in the apex of the lung with involvement of the 8th cervical and 1st and 2nd thoracic nerves. There is shoulder pain, which characteristically radiates in the ulnar distribution of the arm, often with destruction of the first and second ribs seen on CXR.

Other problems of regional spread include superior vena cava syndrome from vascular obstruction; pericardial and cardiac extension with resultant tamponade, arrhythmia, or cardiac failure; lymphatic obstruction with resultant pleural effusion; and lymphangitic spread through the lungs with hypoxemia and dyspnea.

### Transbronchial spread

Transbronchial spread (especially bronchioloalveolar carcinoma) produces growth along multiple alveolar surfaces with resultant impairment of oxygen transfer, dyspnea, hypoxia, and the production of copious sputum.

## Paraneoplastic syndromes

These syndromes describe symptoms and signs resulting from extrapulmonary organ dysfunction unrelated to space-occupying metastases. They occur in 15–20% of lung cancer patients and are commonly due to tumor secretory products. Important paraneoplastic syndromes associated with lung cancer are listed in Fig. 31.4. Occasionally resection of the primary tumor may result in resolution of the syndrome.

## Investigations

All patients with suspected lung cancer should have a complete blood count, liver function tests, and measurement of electrolytes, calcium, and creatinine, in addition to a CXR. However, the diagnosis of lung cancer depends on a histologic diagnosis either from cytology or tissue.

| Important paraneoplastic syndromes associated with lung cancer | | |
|---|---|---|
| **Organ/system** | **Syndrome** | **Lung cancer histology** |
| endocrine and metabolic | Cushing's | small cell |
| | SIADH | small cell |
| | hypercalcemia | squamous cell |
| | gynecomastia | large cell |
| connective tissue and bone | clubbing and HPOA | squamous cell, adenocarcinoma, and large cell |
| neuromuscular | peripheral neuropathy | small cell |
| | subacute cerebellar degeneration | small cell |
| | Eaton–Lambert (myasthenia) | small cell |
| | dermatomyositis | all |
| hematology | anemia | all |
| | DIC | all |
| | eosinophilia | all |
| | thrombocytosis | all |
| cardiovascular | thrombophlebitis | adenocarcinoma |
| | marantic (non-infective) endocarditis | adenocarcinoma |

**Fig. 31.4** Important paraneoplastic syndromes associated with lung cancer. (SIADH, syndrome of inappropriate antidiuretic hormone secretion; HPOA, hypertrophic pulmonary osteoarthropathy; DIC, disseminated intravascular coagulation.)

| The diagnostic yield of cytology and pleural biopsy in lung cancer | | |
|---|---|---|
| **Cytology/biopsy** | **Diagnostic yield** | **Comments** |
| sputum cytology | 40–60% | especially for central tumors |
| pleural fluid cytology | 40–50% | in patients with malignant pleural effusions |
| closed pleural biopsy (Abrams' needle) | 50–60% | with malignant effusion |
| pleural fluid cytology and closed pleural biopsy combined | 75–85% | with malignant effusion |

**Fig. 31.5** The diagnostic yield of cytology and pleural biopsy in lung cancer.

Techniques for obtaining a tissue diagnosis are varied and include the following:
- Fiberoptic bronchoscopy: central or endobronchial disease.
- Percutaneous needle aspiration: peripheral lesions.
- Mediastinoscopy.
- Lymph node biopsy.
- Biopsy of other metastatic site (e.g., the skin).
- Open lung biopsy via thoracotomy: when simpler investigations are negative.

The diagnostic yield of cytologic examination of different samples is shown in Fig. 31.5.

## Imaging for lung cancer

The CXR is abnormal in most patients. Common findings are hilar masses (squamous and small cell), peripheral masses (adenocarcinoma), atelectasis, infiltrates, cavitation (squamous cell), and pleural effusions. These changes are not specific for lung cancer and comparison between old and current CXRs is very important.

Computed tomography (CT) scanning, magnetic resonance imaging (MRI), and ultrasound examination are additional useful investigations in patients with invasion of the lung parenchyma, pleura, or mediastinal disease.

Additional imaging may be required to investigate symptoms or signs that suggest the possibility of distant metastatic spread. These include x-rays of suspected bone metastases (or isotope bone scan), and a CT head scan or MRI of the brain for patients with central nervous system abnormalities. PET scans can be used to look for distant metastases.

## Extent of disease and TNM staging

Small cell cancer is nearly always disseminated at presentation so the diagnosis of this histologic type excludes surgical resection, except in very rare circumstances where there is a single, small, peripheral lesion. In all other cell types surgery is possible, and the extent of disease is recorded by the TNM classification as shown in Fig. 31.6. The staging of disease using the TNM classification also helps to estimate the prognosis with treatment.

## Assessment of patient's functional status before surgery

The patient's general status and respiratory status needs to be assessed before surgery can be offered. This is usually assessed by the Karnofsky performance scale and by the following guidance regarding lung function testing (Fig. 31.7).

## Treatment

Major treatment decisions are made on the basis of whether a tumor is classified histologically as a small cell carcinoma or as one of the non-small-cell varieties (which include epidermoid, adenocarcinoma, large cell carcinoma, bronchioloalveolar carcinoma—a subtype of adenocarcinoma—and mixed versions of these). In general, small cell carcinomas have already spread at the time of presentation so that curative surgery cannot be performed, and they are managed primarily by chemotherapy with or without radiotherapy.

In contrast, non-small-cell cancers that are found to be localized at the time of presentation should be considered for curative treatment with either surgery or radiotherapy (Fig. 31.8). Also, the response of non-small-cell cancers to chemotherapy is usually not dramatic, making chemotherapy less important

| TNM classification for lung cancer | | |
|---|---|---|
| **T/N/M** | **Stage** | **Characteristics** |
| primary tumor (T) | T1 | <3 cm diameter surrounded by lung or pleura |
| | T2 | >3 cm diameter and/or collapse extending to hilum, invading pleura and more than 2 cm beyond the carina |
| | T3 | any size extending to chest wall but not involving mediastinal structures (e.g. heart and great vessels); tumor within 2 cm of carina |
| | T4 | any size invading mediastinum; malignant pleural effusion |
| lymph nodes (N) | N0 | no involvement |
| | N1 | ipsilateral hilar and peribronchial nodes |
| | N2 | ipsilateral mediastinal and subcarinal nodes |
| | N3 | contralateral mediastinal or hilar nodes; or any scalene or supraclavicular nodes |
| metastases (M) | M0 | none known |
| | M1 | distant metastases outside thorax |

**Fig. 31.6** TNM classification for lung cancer.

| Assessment of patient for lung cancer surgery | | |
|---|---|---|
| **Score** | **Karnofsky performance level*** | |
| 0–4 | not self-caring (0, dead; 2, very ill; 4; disabled) | |
| 5–7 | unable to work (5, often needs help; 7, self-caring) | |
| 8–10 | normal activity (8, some symptoms; 10, normal) | |
| **Surgery** | **Lung function criteria** | |
| pneumonectomy possible | preoperative $FEV_1$ | >2L or >60% predicted |
| | preoperative DLCO | >60% predicted |
| | predicted postoperative $FEV_1$ | >800mL or >40% predicted |
| | predicted postoperative DLCO | >40% |
| | maximal $VO_2$ during exercise | >15ml/kg/min |
| | patient age | 70 years or less |
| lobectomy possible | $FEV_1$ | >1.5L or 40% predicted |
| no lung resection possible | $FEV_1$ | <1.2L or inability to walk 100m on the level within 12min |
| | hypoxia | $pO_2 < 50mmHg$ when breathing air at rest or any rise in arterial $pCO_2$ |

**Fig. 31.7** Assessment of patient for lung cancer surgery. *Surgery is rarely curative in patients who are symptomatic from lung cancer.

| Treatment strategies for lung cancer | | |
|---|---|---|
| **Histology** | **Extent of disease** | **Treatment modality** |
| non-small cell lung cancer | stage 0–IIIa | surgery and/or postoperative radiotherapy (e.g. for node involvement) |
| | stage IIIb–IV | palliative radiotherapy for local complications or pain from bony metastases |
| small cell lung cancer | proven single peripheral lesion (rare) | curative surgery attempted |
| | limited stage | combination chemotherapy and radiotherapy |
| | disseminated at presentation (usual) | combination chemotherapy |

**Fig. 31.8** Treatment strategies for lung cancer.

in metastatic disease than it is in cases of small-cell lung cancer. Chemotherapy has been increasingly used as a neoadjuvant treatment, with chemotherapy and radiation given before surgical resection. The combination of carboplatin and paclitaxel is a preferred regimen.

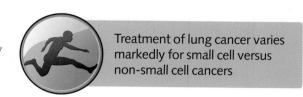

Treatment of lung cancer varies markedly for small cell versus non-small cell cancers

## Prognosis

Five-year survival rates in treated lung cancer patients are given in Fig. 31.9.

## Pneumonia

Pneumonia is an infection of the pulmonary parenchyma. Various bacterial species, mycoplasmas, chlamydiae, rickettsiae, viruses, fungi, and parasites can cause pneumonia. Thus it is not a single disease but a group of specific infections, each with a different epidemiology, pathogenesis, clinical presentation, and clinical course. Identification of the etiologic microorganism is of primary importance, since this is the key to appropriate antimicrobial therapy. However, because of the serious nature of the infection, antimicrobial therapy generally needs to be started immediately, often before laboratory confirmation of the causative agent.

## Etiology

Microbial pathogens enter the lung by one of several routes.

### Aspiration from the oropharyngeal flora

This is the most common mechanism for the production of pneumonia. Healthy individuals transiently carry common pulmonary pathogens in the nasopharynx such as *Streptococcus pneumoniae*, *S. pyogenes*, *Mycoplasma pneumoniae*, *Haemophilus influenzae*, and *Moraxella catarrhalis*.

### Airborne infection

Airborne infection is determined primarily by a particle diameter of less than 3–5 μm that contain one or perhaps two microorganisms. These droplets remain suspended in the atmosphere for long periods unless removed by ventilation or by filtration in the lungs of the individual breathing contaminated air. Inhaled particles of appropriate size may reach the alveoli and initiate infection.

Pneumonias typically acquired by droplet infection include TB, influenza, legionellosis, psittacosis, histoplasmosis, and Q fever.

### Blood-borne infection

Blood-borne infection, usually with *Staphylococcus aureus*, disseminates to the lungs in patients (e.g., intravenous drug abusers) who have either right- or left-sided bacterial endocarditis and in patients with infections in intravenous catheter.

## Epidemiology of pneumonia

The patient's living circumstances, occupation, travel history, pet or animal exposure history, and contacts with other ill individuals provide useful clues to the likely microbial cause for the pneumonia.

| Estimates of 5-year survival of treated patients with lung cancer | | |
|---|---|---|
| | Stage | 5-year survival |
| non-small cell lung cancer | 0 (T1 N0 M0); carcinoma *in situ* | 70–80% |
| | I (T1–2 N0 M0); no nodes or metastases | 50% |
| | II (T1–2 N1 M0); ipsilateral local nodes only | 30% |
| | IIIa (T1–3 N0–2 M0); more than T2 with ipsilateral mediastinal nodes | 10–15% |
| | IIIb (any T, any N, M0); invading vital mediastinal structure, or non-resectable nodes but no extrathoracic spread | <5% |
| | IV (any T, any N, M1); extrathoracic distant metastases | <2% |
| small cell lung cancer | patients rarely live for 5 years after diagnosis—median survival with combined chemotherapy, e.g. with cisplatin-containing regimens, is 40–70 weeks, compared with 6–20 weeks if untreated | |

**Fig. 31.9** Estimates of 5-year survival of treated patients with lung cancer.

In community-acquired pneumonia requiring hospital admission the most frequent pathogens are *S. pneumoniae*, *H. influenzae*, *Chlamydia pneumoniae*, and *Legionella pneumophila*. *M. pneumoniae*, which usually causes mild illness, is common among outpatients with community-acquired pneumonia.

In hospital-acquired pneumonia, enteric, aerobic, gram-negative bacilli and *Pseudomonas aeruginosa* are estimated to account for more than 50% of cases, while *S. aureus* is responsible for more than 10%.

Knowledge of the epidemiology of pneumonia is important because it guides antibiotic treatment used before the causative organism is identified.

## Clinical features of pneumonia
### Typical
The "typical" symptoms of pneumonia are sudden onset of fever, cough productive of purulent sputum and, in some cases, pleuritic chest pain. Signs of pulmonary consolidation (dullness, increased fremitus, bronchial breath sounds, and coarse crackles) may be found on physical examination and coincide with abnormalities on the CXR.

This type of pneumonia is usually caused by the most common bacterial pathogen in community-acquired pneumonia, *S. pneumoniae*, but can also be due to other bacterial pathogens, such as *H. influenzae*.

### Atypical
"Atypical" pneumonia usually causes a more gradual onset, a dry cough, and extrapulmonary symptoms (headache, muscle aching, fatigue, sore throat, nausea, vomiting, and diarrhea). Abnormalities on the CXR may be seen despite few signs of pulmonary involvement other than crackles on physical examination.

Atypical pneumonia is classically produced by *M. pneumoniae*, but it can also be caused by *L. pneumophila*, *Chlamydia*, oral anaerobes, and *Pneumocystis carinii*, as well as some less frequently encountered pathogens.

According to the American Thoracic Society (ATS), dividing patients into "typical" or "atypical" treatment groups probably is not beneficial because most patients exhibit both typical and atypical symptoms. It is more important to divide patients with pneumonia into four categories based on the likely pathogen involved and whether they are inpatients or outpatients (see below).

In hospital-acquired pneumonia the organism and its treatment are often different from that of the community acquired infection.

## Diagnosis of pneumonia
### Chest x-ray
A CXR can confirm the presence of the pulmonary infiltrate and assess the extent of infection. Other features which may be present include pleural involvement, pulmonary cavitation, or hilar lymphadenopathy. Cavitation suggests the following infective causes for the pneumonia—oral anerobic bacteria, enteric gram-negative bacilli, *S. aureus*, *Pseudomonas*, *Legionella*, TB, and fungi.

It should be noted that a normal CXR does not exclude pneumonia, especially early in the disease or in patients unable to mount an inflammatory response because of immunosuppression.

### Sputum microscopy and culture
Sputum microscopy and culture are important in acute bacterial pneumonia. Unfortunately, sputum is frequently contaminated by potentially pathogenic bacteria that colonize the upper respiratory tract without causing disease. Contamination, therefore, reduces the diagnostic specificity of lower respiratory tract specimens and so clinical judgment is required for interpreting the results.

Blood culture is especially important in diagnosing the likely pathogen and is frequently positive in patients with pneumonia.

### Fiberoptic bronchoscopy
Fiberoptic bronchoscopy is rarely performed for pneumonia but has become the standard invasive procedure used to obtain lower respiratory tract secretions from seriously ill or immunocompromised patients. Samples are collected with a protected double-sheathed brush, by bronchoalveolar lavage or by transbronchial biopsy at the site of the pulmonary consolidation.

## Treatment of pneumonia
Modifying factors have been shown to increase the risk of infection with certain organisms.

### Penicillin-resistant and drug-resistant pneumococci

- Age >65 years.
- Exposure to a child in a daycare center.
- Beta-lactam therapy within the past 3 months.
- Multiple chronic medical conditions.
- Immunosuppression (don't forget patients on steroid therapy).
- Alcoholism.

### Enteric gram-negative organisms

- Recent antibiotic therapy.
- Underlying cardiopulmonary disease.
- Multiple medical problems.
- Residence in a nursing home.

### Pseudomonas aeruginosa

- Any type of structural lung disease (e.g., bronchiectasis, interstitial lung disease).
- Corticosteroid therapy.
- Malnutrition.
- Broad-spectrum antibiotic therapy for >7 days in the past month.

### ATS guidelines for treatment of pneumonia

#### Group I

These are outpatients with no cardiopulmonary disease or modifying disease factors. They should be treated with azithromycin alone.

#### Group II

These are outpatients with cardiopulmonary disease and/or other modifying factors. Such patients should be treated with a beta-lactam plus a macrolide or doxycycline or with an antipneumococcal fluoroquinolone alone.

#### Group III

These are inpatients not in the ICU.

- Patients with cardiopulmonary disease and/or other modifying factors should be given an IV beta-lactam plus a macrolide or doxycycline or with an IV fluoroquinolone effective against pneumococci alone.
- Patients with no cardiopulmonary disease or modifying factors should be given IV azithromycin alone or monotherapy with a fluoroquinolone effective against pneumococci.

#### Group IV

These are ICU patients.

- Patients at no risk for *Pseudomonas* should be treated with an IV beta-lactam plus either an IV macrolide or an IV fluoroquinolone.
- Patients at risk for *Pseudomonas* should receive an IV antipseudomonal beta-lactam plus an IV antipseudomonal fluoroquinolone. Another therapy entails use of an antipseudomonal beta-lactam plus an IV aminoglycoside plus either an IV macrolide or a nonpseudomonal fluroquinolone.

## Respiratory failure

### Definition

Respiratory failure is defined as a dysfunction of gas exchange, resulting in abnormalities of oxygenation or carbon dioxide ($CO_2$) elimination severe enough to impair or threaten the function of vital organs.

Respiratory failure is said to be present in a patient breathing air at sea level when the $pO_2$ is less than 60mmHg as a result of lung disease. If hypoxia is combined with a normal or low $pCO_2$ (35–45 mmHg), this is type I respiratory failure, but if hypoxia is combined with a raised $pCO_2$, type II respiratory failure is present. Measurement of the ABGs is essential to the diagnosis of respiratory failure.

### Type I respiratory failure

This is essentially hypoxemia without $CO_2$ retention. Physiologic causes include the following:

- A low inspired oxygen concentration ($FIO_2$), e.g., at high altitude.
- Mismatch of alveolar ventilation (V) to alveolar perfusion (Q).
- A shunt where blood passes from the pulmonary artery to the left heart without passing through ventilated alveoli.

In medical practice the common causes of type I respiratory failure include the following:

- Pneumonia.
- Asthma.
- COPD (predominantly emphysema—"pink puffers").
- Pulmonary thromboembolism.
- Acute respiratory distress syndrome (ARDS) and noncardiogenic pulmonary edema.

- Cardiogenic shock.
- Tension pneumothorax.
- Pulmonary fibrosis.

### Treatment of type I respiratory failure

The main therapeutic objective in acute hypoxemic respiratory failure is to ensure adequate oxygenation of vital organs. Oxygen therapy is indicated when there is central cyanosis, tachycardia, systemic hypotension, and delirium. Consciousness can be lost suddenly without warning when the $pO_2$ falls below 30mmHg, even in previously healthy patients.

High concentrations of inspired oxygen ($FIO_2$ >50%) are safe in patients with type I respiratory failure, as there is no risk of $CO_2$ retention. However, pulmonary oxygen toxicity is a risk if the $FIO_2$ concentration remains over 60% for more than 48 hours continuously.

Other therapeutic objectives include the following:
- Specific therapy of the underlying cause (e.g., antimicrobial therapy for pneumonia, bronchodilators and steroids for asthma, or chest drain insertion for pneumothorax).
- General supportive care: adequate hydration, nutrition, and electrolyte balance, with measures to avoid stress gastritis, ulcers, deep venous thrombosis, and pulmonary embolism.

## Type II respiratory failure

In a healthy subject a rise in arterial $pCO_2$ causes an increase in ventilation by central stimulation of the respiratory centers in the medulla, resulting in an increase in breathing to lower the $pCO_2$. In type II respiratory failure this mechanism fails and signifies that, apart from lung disease, there is also an abnormality of the ventilatory control mechanisms.

Clinical features of type II respiratory failure include central cyanosis (indicating hypoxemia), but $CO_2$ retention can be assessed accurately only by the measurement of ABGs. There are, however, some clinical signs suggestive of $CO_2$ retention:
- Tachycardia.
- Distention of the forearm veins.
- A flapping tremor of the outstretched hands.
- Clouding of consciousness.
- Papilledema (rare).

These are unreliable signs because they can occur from other causes and their absence does not exclude significant $CO_2$ retention.

Common causes of type II respiratory failure include the following:
- COPD (predominantly chronic bronchitis—"blue bloater").
- Respiratory muscle failure (e.g., bilateral diaphragmatic palsy).
- Kyphoscoliosis and other structural thoracic disorders.
- Muscular dystrophy.
- Guillain-Barré syndrome (acute demyelinating polyneuropathy).
- Poliomyelitis.
- Myasthenia.
- Opiate overdose.
- Head injury.
- Sleep apnea.

### Treatment of type II respiratory failure

As in type I, the main therapeutic objective is to ensure adequate oxygenation of vital organs by administering oxygen therapy. However, in the most common clinical setting—an acute exacerbation of COPD—patients may have chronic $CO_2$ retention. They are therefore dependent on hypoxic drive for ventilation, so that with oxygen therapy there is a real risk of inducing hypoventilation, worsening of the respiratory dysfunction, and progressive respiratory acidosis. Oxygen therapy must be carefully controlled so that sufficient oxygen is supplied, usually 24% via face mask, to prevent death from hypoxemia but without precipitating severe respiratory acidosis. This needs repeated monitoring of ABGs.

Type II respiratory failure, as a consequence of causes other than COPD, is usually an indication for mechanical ventilation.

Other therapeutic objectives include the following:
- Specific therapy of the underlying cause (e.g., antimicrobial therapy for infective exacerbation of COPD or treatment of myasthenia).
- General supportive care is as for type I failure.
- Chemical (respiratory stimulants; e.g., doxapram), or mechanical ventilation should be considered if other measures fail.

### Prognosis in acute respiratory failure

The course of the disease and its prognosis depend to a great extent on the underlying pathology. In patients with COPD who do not require mechanical ventilation the immediate prognosis is good. Patients developing ARDS associated with septicemia have a very poor prognosis with mortality rates of about 90%. In general, patients requiring ventilation for respiratory failure have survival rates of about 60% to weaning off the ventilator, 40% to discharge from hospital, and about 30% 1-year survival.

Beware! Patients with type II respiratory failure can stop breathing if given high-dose oxygen.

## Miscellaneous respiratory conditions

### Cystic fibrosis

Cystic fibrosis (CF) is an autosomal recessive disorder that presents as a multisystem disease, and occurs in 1 in 3,000 live births in Caucasians. Signs and symptoms typically occur in childhood but up to 5% of patients are diagnosed as adults. Improvements in therapy now mean that about a third of patients reach adulthood and nearly 10% live beyond 30 years old.

The CF mutation causes an abnormal chloride receptor that affects exocrine secretion. CF is characterized by chronic airway infection that ultimately leads to bronchiectasis, exocrine pancreatic insufficiency, intestinal dysfunction, abnormal sweat gland function, and urogenital dysfunction.

#### Diagnosis

The diagnosis of CF rests on a combination of clinical criteria and analyses of sweat chloride values. Typically in adults, a chloride concentration of over 70mmol/L discriminates between CF patients and patients with other lung diseases. Molecular diagnoses can also be performed to confirm the diagnosis and to help with genetic counseling.

#### Treatment

The treatments for CF are to promote clearance of secretions (physiotherapy and bronchodilators), control infection in the lung (antibiotics), provide adequate nutrition (pancreatic enzyme and fat-soluble vitamin supplements), and prevent intestinal obstruction. Gene therapy with recombinant human DNAse may eventually become the treatment of choice.

### Allergic bronchopulmonary aspergillosis

Allergic bronchopulmonary aspergillosis (ABPA) may resemble hypersensitivity pneumonitis and presents with systemic symptoms and recurrent pulmonary infiltrates, but with eosinophilia. It is the association with asthma and the typical peripheral eosinophilia. Symptoms are typically episodes of obstruction associated with fever, malaise, and occasionally hemoptysis. The association with asthma and the typical peripheral eosinophilia (>1000/μL) distinguish it from hypersensitivity pneumonitis (or extrinsic allergic alveolitis).

ABPA is the most common example of the allergic bronchopulmonary mycoses and is sometimes confused with hypersensitivity pneumonitis because of the presence of precipitating antibodies to *Aspergillus fumigatus*. However, ABPA is an obstructive rather than a restrictive lung disease, and is associated with allergic (atopic) asthma. The bronchiectasis associated with ABPA is thought to result from a deposition of immune complexes in proximal airways. Diagnosis involves the spirometry, skin testing for *Aspergillus* sensitivity, blood eosinophilia, serum antibodies to *Aspergillus*, and central bronchiectasis on high-resolution CT scan. Adequate treatment usually requires the long-term use of systemic glucocorticoids.

### Bronchiectasis

Bronchiectasis is an abnormal and permanent dilatation of the bronchi. It can be focal, involving airways supplying a limited region of the lung, or diffuse, involving airways in a more widespread distribution. Whatever the distribution, the diagnosis is suggested by the clinical consequences of chronic or recurrent infection in the dilated airways and the associated copious purulent sputum that forms within these airways.

#### Etiology

During childhood, bronchiectasis was often a complication of measles or pertussis, but this is now rare as a result of effective immunization. Adenovirus and influenza are the main viral causes, and severe bacterial infections with necrotizing organisms (e.g., *Staph. aureus*, *Klebsiella*, TB, anaerobes) remain important causes of bronchiectasis.

## Clinical features

Patients typically present with persistent or recurrent cough and purulent sputum production. Hemoptysis occurs in more than half of cases and can cause massive bleeding. Physical examination of the chest overlying an affected area may reveal any combination of crackles and rhonchi, which reflect the damaged airways containing significant secretions. As with other chronic intrathoracic infections, clubbing may be present.

Patients with severe disease and chronic hypoxemia may develop cor pulmonale and right ventricular failure. Amyloidosis can result from chronic infection and inflammation, but it is now seldom seen in patients with bronchiectasis.

## Treatment

Treatment strategies are similar to those described for CF except that pancreatic insufficiency is not usually present. Appropriate treatment should be started when a treatable cause is found (e.g., antituberculous drugs for TB or steroids for ABPA).

## Interstitial lung diseases

Interstitial lung diseases (ILDs) represent a variety of conditions that involve the alveolar walls (septa), perialveolar tissue, and other adjacent structures. The ILDs are nonmalignant and are not caused by any defined infectious agents. Although an acute phase of illness may occur, the onset is often insidious, and the disease is usually chronic in duration.

## Etiology

One useful approach to classification is to separate ILDs into two groups, known and unknown causes. Each of these groups can be divided into subgroups, according to the presence or absence of histologic evidence of granulomas in interstitial or vascular areas.

Among the ILDs of known cause, the largest group comprises diseases due to exposure to occupational and environmental inhalant (e.g., inorganic dusts, organic dusts, and various irritative or noxious gases). These diseases can usually be recognized if the occupational history is pursued. The number of ILDs of unknown cause is very large, but the major ones within this group are idiopathic pulmonary fibrosis, sarcoidosis, and the ILD associated with collagen vascular disorders.

## Clinical features

In idiopathic pulmonary fibrosis, patients usually present with nonproductive cough, progressive dyspnea, fatigue, anorexia, weight loss, and arthralgias. The CXR often shows lower lung zone reticular or reticulonodular shadows, while pulmonary function tests show a restrictive pattern. This condition is also known as cryptogenic fibrosing alveolitis. Auscultation of the chest may be normal initially but, as the disease advances, dry crepitations or fine crepitations on inspiration, are usually heard at the lung bases. There may be tachypnea at rest, cyanosis, and clubbing. In later stages, cor pulmonale with right heart failure may develop.

## Diagnostic investigation

This is by histologic evaluation, microbial cultures, immunofluorescence, and electron microscopy studies. Samples are usually obtained by transbronchial biopsies, but if this does not yield sufficient tissue for diagnosis, a thoracoscopic-guided or even an open lung biopsy should be considered.

In addition to the CXR pattern noted above, a high-resolution CT scan may help distinguish the diagnosis as well. Pulmonary function testing should be performed in all patients and often shows a restrictive pattern. A tissue diagnosis is vital before embarking on immunosuppressive therapy (with prednisone and cyclophosphamide), as treatment has a high rate of possible complications.

## Pulmonary embolism

PE is responsible for 150,000–200,000 deaths each year in the U.S., with most patients dying shortly after the event. Three factors (Virchow's triad) predispose to venous thrombosis, namely local trauma to the vessel wall, hypercoagulability, and stasis (e.g., inherited disorder, drugs, malignancy). The origin of a PE is often from thrombi of the lower extremities. The clot can then dislodge, travel to the lungs, and lodge in a pulmonary vessel.

Many patients who suffer pulmonary thromboembolism have an underlying inherited predisposition that remains clinically silent until an acquired stressor occurs (e.g., surgery, especially total hip replacement), obesity, or pregnancy. The most frequent inherited predisposition to hypercoagulability is resistance to the endogenous anticoagulant protein, activated protein C. The phenotype of activated protein C resistance is associated with a single point mutation termed factor V Leiden.

Other inherited hypercoagulable states include deficiencies in protein C, protein S, antithrombin III, and disorders of plasminogen.

### Clinical features

Dyspnea is the most frequent symptom, and tachypnea is the most frequent sign in pulmonary embolism (PE). Dyspnea, syncope, hypotension, or cyanosis indicates a massive PE, while pleuritic pain, cough, or hemoptysis often suggests a small embolism located near the pleura. On examination, young or previously healthy individuals may simply appear anxious but otherwise seem well, even with a large PE.

Many drugs interact with warfarin to enhance or diminish its effect. Ask the patient to report any changes in treatment.

### Investigations

Investigations supporting the diagnosis of PE include the following:

- Electrocardiogram: tachycardia or the "typical" $S_1$ $Q_3$ $T_3$ pattern.
- D-dimer, ESR, LDH, AST.
- ABGs: hypoxemia.
- CXR: usually normal but may show atelectasis or a small wedge shadow.
- V/Q scan: unmatched V/Q defects.
- PE protocol CT scan.

If these investigations are negative but the clinical suspicion remains high, a search for corroborative evidence of thromboembolism is instigated by measuring D-dimer and looking for the presence of deep vein thrombosis with ultrasound or venography. Patients who have a negative D-dimer and low probability of having PE are effectively ruled out with this test.

Pulmonary angiography is performed to make a definitive diagnosis in certain circumstances (e.g., pregnancy or acutely ill patients who may require embolectomy).

### Treatment

The majority of patients are treated with intravenous heparin (low molecular weight or unfractionated) followed by oral warfarin for a period of 6 months. PE is a recurrent disease with an annual relapse rate of about 7%. When treatment is continued for only 6 weeks, the relapse rate is twice as high as with 6 months. Monitoring of maintenance warfarin treatment is performed 4–8 weekly in clinical practice, aiming to keep the international normalized ratio (INR) at about 3.0 (therapeutic range 2.0–3.5).

Patients who have recurrent thromboembolic events should be screened for the recognized hypercoagulable states mentioned above. They are also likely to need lifelong anticoagulation and should be considered for a caval filter if warfarin fails to prevent further emboli.

## Occupational lung disease

Many acute and chronic lung diseases are directly related to occupational exposure to inorganic and organic dusts. A number of different clinical syndromes may result and these are shown in Fig. 31.10.

## Sleep apnea

Sleep apnea is defined as an intermittent cessation of airflow at the nose and mouth during sleep. Periods of apnea of 10 seconds duration are considered important but in most patients the apneas last from 20 seconds to as long as 3 minutes.

Pulmonary embolism is life-threatening and common. If in doubt, heparinize and investigate fully.

### Sleep apnea syndrome

This refers to a clinical disorder that arises from recurrent apneas during sleep. The clinical importance of sleep apnea arises from the fact that it is a common cause of daytime sleepiness. In the U.S. it is thought that 3 million men and 1.5 million women meet at least one criterion for sleep apnea and that a 12-fold increase occurred during the 1990s. This syndrome is on the rise in the U.S. along with the epidemic of adult obesity.

Fig. 31.10 Common occupational lung diseases.

| Common occupational lung diseases | | |
| --- | --- | --- |
| **Disease** | **Etiology** | **Lung injury** |
| pneumoconiosis (chronic fibrotic lung disease) | coal dust silicosis asbestosis | diffuse nodular infiltrates on CXR |
| hypersensitivity pneumonitis | moudy hay (farmer's lung) avian proteins (bird fancier's lung) | restrictive pulmonary dysfunction |
| obstructive airways disorders | grain dust wood dust tobacco pollen synthetic dyes formaldehyde | occupational asthma |
| toxic lung injury | irritant gases | pulmonary edema bronchiolitis obliterans |
| lung cancer | asbestos | mesothelioma |
| | arsenic | all lung cancer types |
| | chromium | all lung cancer types |
| | hydrocarbons | all lung cancer types |
| pleural diseases | asbestos talc | may cause benign effusions and plaques may cause benign effusions and plaques |

## Classification

Sleep apneas are classified into three types:

- Central sleep apnea, in which the neural drive to all the respiratory muscles is transiently abolished.
- Obstructive sleep apnea, in which airflow ceases despite continuing respiratory drive because of occlusion of the oropharyngeal airway.
- Mixed apneas, which consist of a central apnea followed by an obstructive component.

## Treatment

Treatment of mild-to-moderate obstructive sleep apnea is by modest weight reduction, avoidance of alcohol, improvement of nasal patency, and avoidance of sleeping in the supine posture. Moderate-to-severe cases are treated by uvulopalatopharyngoplasty and nasal continuous positive airways pressure during sleep. It is important to tell patients with OSA that they have a 2- to 3-fold increase in automobile accidents, presumably because of daytime sleepiness.

## Acute respiratory distress syndrome

Acute respiratory distress syndrome (ARDS; or adult respiratory distress syndrome) is a condition featuring acute hypoxemic respiratory failure, due to pulmonary edema caused by increased permeability of the alveolar capillary barrier. Essential to the diagnosis are the following findings:

- A history of systemic or pulmonary insult (e.g., sepsis, shock, disseminated intravascular coagulation, high altitude, smoke inhalation).
- Respiratory distress: usually 12–48 hours after the initiating event.
- Bilateral pulmonary infiltrates: initially interstitial edema but rapidly becomes alveolar with air bronchograms in over 80% of cases.
- Severe hypoxemia refractory to oxygen treatment: due to shunting.
- Normal pulmonary capillary wedge pressure: this excludes cardiogenic pulmonary edema.

## Treatment

The treatment of ARDS includes the identification and treatment of any underlying cause (e.g., sepsis).

Supportive therapy almost always includes intubation and mechanical ventilation. The benefits of mechanical ventilation can be seen in the decreased work of breathing, recruitment of collapsed alveoli by using PEEP, and the reliable delivery of oxygen therapy. Positive end-expiratory pressure improves hypoxemia but does not affect the natural course of the disease.

Measures for avoiding a worsening of the pulmonary edema are aimed at reducing the intravascular volume (with diuretics) and keeping the hematocrit high (by transfusions of packed red blood cells).

New treatments for ARDS currently being assessed include the following:
- Lung surfactant.
- Monoclonal antibodies to tumor necrosis factor.
- Human recombinant interleukin-1 receptor antagonists.
- Inhaled nitric oxide.

### Prognosis
The prognosis is poor in ARDS with a mortality rate in excess of 50%, rising to 90% with associated sepsis. The major cause of death is nonpulmonary multiple organ failure. Patients who survive may be left with abnormal lung diffusing capacity.

## Pneumothorax
A pneumothorax is the presence of gas in the pleural space. The following distinctions are made between the different types of pneumothorax:
- Spontaneous pneumothorax: occurs without trauma to the thorax.
- Primary spontaneous pneumothorax: occurs in the absence of lung disease.
- Secondary spontaneous pneumothorax: occurs in the presence of pre-existing lung disease.
- Traumatic pneumothorax: penetrating or nonpenetrating chest injuries.

> Factors that predispose to pneumothorax include spontaneous factors (tall, thin, healthy men), trauma, airways obstruction, cystic fibrosis, pulmonary abscess and Marfan's syndrome.

- Tension pneumothorax: the pressure in the pleural space is positive throughout the respiratory cycle.

Primary spontaneous pneumothorax is usually due to the rupture of an apical pleural bleb that lays within or immediately under the visceral pleura. About 50% of patients with an initial primary spontaneous pneumothorax will have a recurrence.

### Clinical features
Clinical features of pneumothorax include the following:
- Chest pain on the affected side.
- Shortness of breath.
- Mild tachycardia.
- Decreased vocal fremitus, hyperresonance and diminished breath sounds may be detected if the pneumothorax is large.

A CXR will confirm the diagnosis by demonstrating a line of visceral pleura with absent lung markings beyond the line. The diagnosis may prove more difficult in secondary pneumothorax, especially if emphysematous bullae are present.

### Treatment
The treatment for primary spontaneous pneumothorax is a chest tube insertion with underwater seal drainage. Surgery by thoracoscopy or thoracotomy plus pleural abrasion is almost 100% successful in preventing further recurrences.

# 32. Gastrointestinal and Liver Disease

## Peptic ulcer disease

Peptic ulcer disease most commonly occurs in the duodenum, followed by the stomach, esophagus, and jejunum in Zollinger–Ellison syndrome, or after a gastroenterostomy, or in a Meckel's diverticulum with ectopic gastric mucosa. It occurs in up to 15–20% of the population at some time, and is more common in men. The incidence increases with age.

Although no cause is usually found, peptic ulceration is associated with gastric hypersecretion and impaired mucosal defences. *Helicobacter pylori* plays a central role. Exacerbating factors include stress (Curling's ulcer), smoking, alcohol, nonsteroidal anti-inflammatory drugs (NSAIDs), and steroids. Ulceration is also associated with Zollinger–Ellison syndrome, multiple endocrine neoplasia (MEN) type I, and hyperparathyroidism.

### Clinical features

The history is unreliable for separating duodenal ulcer (DU) from gastric ulcer (GU). Epigastric pain, often quite localized, is a frequent symptom. The pain may radiate to the back in posterior DU and is episodic, often waking the patient at night, whereas the pain with GU is worse during the day. The pain is relieved with antacids or milk. The pain of DU is often relieved by food, whereas with GU it is precipitated by food.

Other symptoms include nausea and heartburn secondary to acid reflux. Anorexia, vomiting, and weight loss should lead to the suspicion of gastric carcinoma. If there is persistent and severe pain, complications such as perforation or penetration into other organs should be considered.

Examination reveals epigastric tenderness. A mass suggests carcinoma, and a succussion splash suggests pyloric obstruction secondary to scarring.

### Investigation

Esophagogastroduodenoscopy (EGD) or upper GI endoscopy are the investigations of choice, although a trial of acid suppression may be given to younger patients as carcinoma is rarely present in those under 45 years old. Patients younger than 45 should have a serologic or breath test for *H. pylori*. All gastric ulcers should be biopsied to exclude malignancy, but DUs are nearly always benign; biopsies should be taken for *H. pylori*.

Most gastric carcinomas are on the greater curve and in the antrum. They may have a rolled edge and a translucent halo around them.

Acid secretion status may be assessed if Zollinger-Ellison syndrome is suspected, before and after stimulation with secretin.

### Management

The patient should be advised to modify exacerbating factors such as smoking, diet, and alcohol. NSAIDs should be stopped if not absolutely necessary.

Antacids relieve the pain of ulcers but do not necessarily promote healing and are best given when symptoms occur or are expected. Liquid preparations are more effective than tablets. They should preferably not be taken at the same time as other drugs as they may impair their absorption. They may also damage enteric coatings designed to prevent dissolution in the stomach. Prolonged high doses of calcium-containing antacids can cause hypercalcemia and alkalosis and can precipitate milk–alkali syndrome.

Aluminum hydroxide can lower serum phosphate levels and cause constipation, while magnesium carbonate can lead to diarrhea and belching. Some antacids contain a high sodium content and should not be used in patients on salt-restricted diets.

*H. pylori* should be eradicated because eradication promotes long-term healing of duodenal and gastric ulcers. This is best achieved by acid inhibition combined with antibiotic treatment. A proton pump inhibitor (see below) and clarithromycin, plus either amoxycillin or metronidazole, given twice daily for 2 weeks, produce *H. pylori* eradication in a large proportion of patients. Treatment failure may reflect poor compliance or antibiotic resistance, and antibiotic-induced colitis is a possible risk.

## H$_2$-receptor antagonists

These agents heal peptic ulcers by reducing gastric acid output as a result of H$_2$-receptor blockade. Examples include cimetidine, 400mg 2 times/day, or ranitidine, 150mg 2 times/day. (Note, however, that because of its involvement with hepatic 450 enzymes and predilection to raise serum creatinine secondary to blockage of creatinine secretion, cimetidine is rarely used.) Relapse rates are high on stopping treatment, and maintenance treatment may be required, especially in those with frequent severe recurrences and in the elderly. They are generally well tolerated, but cimetidine is occasionally associated with gynecomastia and acute psychosis. It also interacts with warfarin, phenytoin, and theophyllines.

## Proton pump inhibitors

These inhibit gastric acid by blocking the hydrogen/potassium adenosine triphosphate enzyme system (the "proton pump") of the gastric parietal cell. Examples include omeprazole, 20–40mg q.d., and lansoprazole, 30mg q.d. High doses may be used in Zollinger-Ellison syndrome. PPIs are becoming more and more popular as studies show that they are much more efficacious than H$_2$ blockers. Their popularity has also grown thanks to a generous advertising campaign by various pharmaceutical companies. Recently a PPI became available over the counter. Note, however, that the "new" version of this popular "colored" pill is nothing more than the enantiomer (chemical mirror image) and not a new medication.

Side effects include headaches, diarrhea, rashes, pruritus, and dizziness.

## Other drugs

*Misoprostol* is a synthetic prostaglandin analog and has antisecretory and protective properties, promoting peptic ulcer healing. It can prevent ulcers secondary to NSAIDs and is useful in patients in whom NSAIDs cannot be withdrawn. The usual dose is 800µg daily in divided doses. The main side effect is diarrhea.

*Sucralfate* may act by protecting the mucosa from acid–pepsin attack in peptic ulcers. It is a complex of aluminium hydroxide and sulphated sucrose but has minimal antacid properties.

*Tripotassium dicitratobismuthate* is a bismuth chelate effective in healing gastric and duodenal ulcers but not on its own in maintaining remission. It may be given in combination with two antibiotics to eradicate *H. pylori*, but other regimens are preferable.

## Surgery

Surgery is usually considered when medical treatment has failed or for complications that include persistent hemorrhage, perforation, or pyloric stenosis. Operations include partial gastrectomy or, now more commonly, highly selective vagotomy and pyloroplasty. Hemorrhage may be controlled endoscopically by injection or diathermy, laser photocoagulation, or heat probe. Perforations are usually oversewn with an omental plug.

Complications of surgery include:
- Recurrent ulceration.
- Abdominal fullness.
- Bilious vomiting.
- Diarrhea.
- Dumping syndrome. This is fainting and sweating after eating, possibly due to food of high osmotic potential being dumped into the jejunum and causing oligemia because of rapid fluid shifts. Late dumping is due to hypoglycemia and occurs 1–3 hours after taking food.

Metabolic complications include:
- Weight loss.
- Malabsorption.
- Bacterial overgrowth (blind loop syndrome).
- Anemia, usually due to iron deficiency following hypochlorhydria and stomach resection.

## Complications

The three main complications secondary to peptic ulceration are bleeding, perforation, and pyloric stenosis. Perforation is more common in DUs than GUs. Pyloric stenosis may also be prepyloric or in the duodenum. It occurs because of edema surrounding the ulcer or from scar formation on healing. The patient often has projectile vomiting with food ingested up to 24 hours previously. There may be visible peristalsis and a succussion splash. Vomiting may lead to dehydration and a metabolic alkalosis.

Fluid and electrolyte replacement is needed, as is gastric aspiration with a nasogastric tube. Surgery is indicated if the patient does not settle with conservative management.

## Gastrointestinal hemorrhage

The differential diagnosis, history, and examination of patients with gastrointestinal (GI) bleeding are given on p. 37. Emergency resuscitative measures may be needed before a full assessment is made. All patients with a significant bleed should be admitted to hospital. The vast majority will stop bleeding spontaneously within 48 hours.

Impending shock is indicated by:
- Pulse rate greater than 100 per minute.
- Hemoglobin less than 10g/dL.
- Systolic blood pressure below 100mmHg.

It requires intravenous fluids and transfusion.

### Management

Patients who have signs of shock suggested by tachycardia and low blood pressure or anemia should be given blood immediately to expand the circulating volume and restore cardiac output and blood pressure. Blood should be sent for grouping and type and screen, but if blood is not immediately available, colloid or crystalloids should be given. O Rhesus-negative blood may be given in severe bleeding. Fluids should be administered via a large-bore cannula through a peripheral vein or, ideally, through a central vein (jugular or subclavian) with central venous pressure (CVP) monitoring aiming to maintain the CVP at about 5–10 saline mmHg.

The rate of transfusion should be monitored closely by the general clinical status, as should the pulse and blood pressure, to ensure adequate replacement and to avoid overtransfusion and consequent heart failure.

Blood should also be taken for clotting studies, complete blood count (CBC), liver function tests (LFTs), and metabolic panel. The patient is given oxygen if bleeding is severe. The urea may rise due to

protein absorption from the gut, but the creatinine is usually normal unless there is coexistent renal failure.

Bleeds from GUs carry twice the mortality of bleeds from DUs. Adverse prognostic factors in patients with GI hemorrhage are listed in Fig. 32.1.

The hemoglobin concentration will remain normal for several hours after a significant hemorrhage.

If there are no signs of shock and the patient is not anemic, the patient may be managed conservatively with bed rest, nothing by mouth, and close monitoring of the pulse, blood pressure, and fluid balance. Blood should be typed and cross-matched, and normal saline should be given intravenously.

Once the patient is stable, endoscopy should be carried out within 24 hours. If varices are suspected, immediate endoscopy should be performed. The cause for the bleed will be apparent in over 80% of cases.

If there is active bleeding, a sclerosant can be injected, or bleeding vessels coagulated with a heat probe or with laser therapy. $H_2$-receptor antagonists or proton pump inhibitors are given to patients with ulcers for their long-term benefit, although there is little evidence of benefit in the acute situation. For persistent bleeding octreotide or somatostatin can be used for some benefit.

Surgery is indicated if it is not possible to control the bleeding with medical management, especially for persistent or recurrent bleeding, although this is

---

**Adverse prognostic factors in patients with gastrointestinal hemorrhage**

- age over 60 years
- recurrent hemorrhage
- initial presentation with shock
- more than 6 units of blood needed
- an active bleeding vessel seen on endoscopy
- bleeding from esophageal varices, which can lead to liver failure and hepatic coma

**Fig. 32.1** Adverse prognostic factors in patients with gastrointestinal hemorrhage.

now becoming less common. It is more often carried out in the elderly and for those with GUs compared to DUs.

## Management of bleeding esophageal varices

Resuscitative procedures and endoscopy should be carried out as above. Acute variceal sclerotherapy and banding are the treatments of choice. This arrests bleeding in 80% of cases and reduces early rebleeding. Holding measures before endoscopy is carried out include vasoconstrictor therapy, which aims to restrict portal inflow by splanchnic arterial constriction. Two drugs are used:

- Octreotide is a long-acting analog of the hypothalamic release-inhibiting hormone somatostatin and will produce splanchnic vasoconstriction without significant systemic vascular effects.
- Vasopressin (antidiuretic hormone) will cause generalized vasoconstriction. It can precipitate myocardial infarction in patients with ischemic heart disease; therefore, it must be given with NG to vasodilate cardiac vasculature.

Measures to prevent hepatic encephalopathy should be started, which include emptying the bowel with enemas or lactulose, and giving neomycin 1 g 6 hourly to reduce the number of bowel organisms. Vitamin K 10 mg IV is given, and platelets or fresh frozen plasma are given as needed.

If the bleeding continues, a Sengstaken–Blakemore tube can be passed through the esophagus, with balloons to compress the gastric and esophageal veins. Complications include aspiration pneumonia, esophageal rupture, and mucosal ulceration, and produce a 5% mortality rate.

To prevent recurrent variceal bleeding, measures include long-term injection sclerotherapy leading to obliteration of the varices by fibrous tissues. This reduces rebleeding but does not necessarily improve mortality. Complications include esophageal ulceration, mediastinitis, and strictures. Nonselective β-blockers (e.g., propanolol) decrease portal pressures and significantly reduce primary and secondary bleeding and mortality from large varices.

For patients with recurrent bleeding, a transjugular intrahepatic portosystemic shunt procedure (TIPS) can be performed to help alleviate the back pressure from the poral circulation. If bleeding can be stopped temporarily for 12 hours and

the patient has no pulmonary compromise, the 30-day survival rate is 90%.

Surgical procedures include esophageal transection with anastamosis, transthoracic transesophageal ligation of varices, and gastric transection with reanastamosis.

About half of those bleeding from varices for the first time will die. The risk of recurrence is about 80% in the next 2 years. Adverse prognostic factors are jaundice, ascites, hypoalbuminemia, and encephalopathy.

## Lower gastrointestinal bleeding

The differential diagnosis of lower GI bleeding is listed in Fig. 32.2.

Resuscitation should be carried out as for upper GI bleeds, and further investigations are carried out when the patient is stable. Examination should include a rectal examination to exclude carcinoma, sigmoidoscopy, and colonoscopy. Barium enema may add to information, and angiography can be carried out if vascular abnormalities are suspected.

Lower GI bleeding may be occult and chronic, presenting with iron-deficiency anemia and general lethargy and fatigue. If the history does not suggest a particular site in the GI tract responsible for the blood loss, a sensible working plan is upper GI endoscopy followed by colonoscopy. If no diagnosis is apparent, a small bowel follow-through (enteroclysis) is next performed, followed by angiography if needed. Isotope-labelled red blood cells may localize the site of bleeding.

---

**Differential diagnosis of lower gastrointestinal bleeding**

- anal fissure
- hemorrhoids
- inflammatory bowel disease
- infective colitis
- gastrointestinal carcinoma: sigmoid, cecum, rectum
- ischemic colitis
- diverticulitis
- intestinal polyps
- vascular abnormalities: angiodysplasia, arteriovenous malformations
- Meckel's diverticulum
- Peutz–Jeghers syndrome
- Osler–Weber–Rendu syndrome
- endometriosis

Fig. 32.2 Differential diagnosis of lower gastrointestinal bleeding.

## Inflammatory bowel disease

Inflammatory bowel disease usually implies both ulcerative colitis and Crohn's disease. It is likely that these conditions represent a spectrum of disease resulting from a combination of genetic and environmental factors, although they typically differ in their natural history and response to treatment.

### Ulcerative colitis

This is an idiopathic chronic relapsing inflammatory disease starting in the rectum and possibly spreading to involve all of the large intestine. It is more common in the Western world with a prevalence of about 150 in 100,000, and an incidence of about 10 in 100,000 annually, and is maximal at 15–40 years of age. There is no major sex difference.

### Etiology

The primary cause of ulcerative colitis is unknown, although 10–15% of patients have a first-degree relative with ulcerative colitis or Crohn's disease. It may result from a genetically determined, inappropriately severe, and/or prolonged inflammatory response to a dietary or microbial product. Abnormalities of colonic epithelial cell metabolism have also been reported in ulcerative colitis, and there are associations with certain drugs such as NSAIDs and antibiotics, and with stress, although the significance is uncertain.

There may be a history of atopy, autoimmune disease (e.g., chronic active hepatitis and systemic lupus erythematosus), and the presence of circulating immune complexes and antibodies to colonocytes and neutrophils (pANCA) in ulcerative colitis.

Ulcerative colitis occurs almost exclusively among nonsmokers, whereas about two-thirds of patients who have Crohn's disease smoke cigarettes.

### Clinical features

The disease may present with a single mild episode followed by remission for a prolonged period, or progressive symptoms over months with general ill health and chronic diarrhea, or as an acute severe episode. In general, the severity of diarrhea and systemic upset depends on the extent of the disease and depth of mucosal ulceration.

Active subtotal or total ulcerative colitis causes frequent bloody diarrhea, often with fever, malaise, anorexia, weight loss, abdominal pain, anemia, and tachycardia. With proctitis, characteristic symptoms are rectal bleeding and mucous discharge, but the stool is well formed and general health is maintained. The patient may present with a complication. Between relapses, the patient is usually symptomless.

### Complications
#### Local
Toxic megacolon, perforation, or rarely massive hemorrhage can occur. There is an increased risk of colonic carcinoma in patients with subtotal or total ulcerative colitis. The cumulative incidence is 10–15% at 20 years.

#### Extraintestinal
Extraintestinal complications of ulcerative colitis include the following:
- Skin: erythema nodosum, pyoderma gangrenosum, vasculitis.
- Eyes: uveitis, episcleritis, conjunctivitis.
- Joints: large joint arthropathy, sacroilitis, ankylosing spondylitis.
- Liver: pericholangitis, sclerosing cholangitis, cirrhosis, chronic active hepatitis, cholangiocarcinoma.
- Vasculature: arterial and venous thrombosis.

Extraintestinal manifestations of IBD are **A PIE SAC:** **a**phthous ulcers, **p**yoderma gangrenosum, **i**ritis, **e**rythema nodosum, **s**clerosing cholangitis, **a**rthritis, and **c**lubbing.

### Diagnosis
Sigmoidoscopy and rectal biopsy show inflamed mucosa. If the disease is active there may be pus and blood, visible ulceration, and bleeding on contact with the sigmoidoscope. Other types of colitis should be excluded, and stool microscopy and culture are needed to exclude infection.

Histology shows inflammatory cells infiltrating the lamina propria with crypt abscesses. There is little involvement of the muscularis mucosa, and there is a reduction of goblet cells.

Barium enema shows loss of the normal haustral pattern and the bowel looks like a smooth tube ("leadpipe"). Ulcers and pseudopolyps may be seen, edema of the colonic wall produces widening of the presacral space, and there may be narrowed areas secondary to strictures or carcinoma.

## Management
### General measures

A multidisciplinary approach is preferred with gastroenterologists, nursing staff, counselors, and stoma therapists, in collaboration with primary health-care teams. Support groups are available. Some patients may improve with avoidance of cow's milk, and some with proctitis benefit from fiber supplements. Specific nutritional, hematinic, and electrolyte deficiencies may require correction. NSAIDs and antibiotics should be avoided.

### Drugs

If the ulcerative colitis is not severe, the patient can usually be managed as an outpatient. Proctitis is treated with topical steroids and oral 5-aminosalicylic acid (5-ASA). Left-sided or extensive ulcerative colitis is treated with steroid enemas, oral 5-ASA, or oral steroid if the former treatment modalities fail. Patients with an extensive, severe attack should be admitted. Infection should be excluded, and intravenous fluids and electroytes given as needed. Transfusion may be required for extensive blood loss, and the patient should be given prophylactic subcutaneous heparin.

Antidiarrheal, antispasmodic, and anticholinergic drugs should be avoided as they can precipitate colonic dilatation. Patients are given intravenous hydrocortisone (400mg per day), followed by high-dose prednisone (30mgq 12 hours) and a corticosteroid enema. About 70% of patients improve substantially within 7 days. If there is an inadequate response, urgent colectomy is required, or cyclosporin may be tried as adjunctive treatment. Unfortunately, there is a high relapse rate on stopping the cyclosporin, and surgery is required. Newer treatment modalities added as adjunctive therapy for patients who have failed high-dose oral steroids include fish oil, antibiotics (ciprofloaxacin), and nicotine.

 Indications for surgery in IBD are **I CHOP:** **i**nfection, **c**arcinoma, **h**emorrhage, **o**bstruction, and **p**erforation.

To maintain patients in remission, oral 5-ASA is usually required unless relapse occurs less than once a year. For frequent relapses, oral azathioprine is of benefit.

*Corticosteroids*   Prednisone is used for acute flare-ups, and its side effects can be reduced by restricting its use to less than 3 months. It may be given intravenously, orally, or topically and as a suppository, liquid, foam, or enema.

*Aminosalicylates*   Examples include sulphasalazine 1–2g 3 or 4 times/day This consists of 5-ASA, linked by an azo bond to sulphapyridine. The 5-ASA, the active component, is released in the colon by bacterial action. About 20% of patients cannot tolerate sulphasalazine because of adverse effects, mostly related to the sulphapyridine. These include headache and fever, blood dyscrasias, bone marrow suppression, rashes, and oligospermia, making newer compounds preferable in young men.

Mesalazine contains 5-ASA alone and may have fewer side effects. Several other oral 5-ASA products are available with different mechanisms of drug delivery in the colon. Pentasa contains 5-ASA microgranules that delay release until they reach the small intestine and colon. Asacol is a 5-ASA product with a pH-dependent resin that dissolves only at a certain pH, more likely at the terminal ileum. Lastly, Colazal has an inert carrier to deliver the drug to the colon.

The aminosalicylates help maintain remission, reducing annual relapse rates from 70% to 30%. They are also available as enemas and suppositories.

*Immunosuppressive drugs*   Azathioprine may be used in patients who relapse repeatedly on steroid withdrawal after an acute episode or in whom aminosalicylates are ineffective for maintaining remission; it may take up to 4 months to effect a noticeable clinical benefit.

Serious adverse effects include bone marrow suppression and cholestatic jaundice, necessitating blood checks every other week for the first 3 months. Long-term safety data are still awaited.

Cyclosporin may be effective as an adjunct to steroids in refractory acute severe ulcerative colitis but has serious side effects, including hypertension, nephrotoxicity, epilepsy, and opportunistic infections. Close monitoring of the patient is needed.

Infliximab (anti-TNF alpha antibody) is the newest immunomodulator to show possible benefit in patients with ulcerative colitis. Currently studies are under way to determine whether it is efficacious to treat ulcerative colitis with this powerful immunomodulator.

*Antibiotics*    These may be used in severe attacks to prevent bacteremia and endotoxic shock. As noted above, some antibiotics are now being added to therapy regimens as adjuncts to immunosuppressive medications.

### Surgery

Surgery is curative for colonic disease though not for extraintestinal complications. Options include panproctocolectomy with ileoanal pouch, permanent ileostomy, or, rarely, subtotal colectomy with ileorectal anastamosis. It may be considered electively for chronic intractable ulcerative colitis, colonic carcinoma, persistent mucosal dysplasia, or growth retardation in children.

### Prognosis

About 70% of untreated patients relapse annually, and up to 30% eventually require surgery, although the overall mortality is close to that of the general population. The main risks to life are severe attacks of ulcerative colitis and colonic cancer. Patients with extensive ulcerative colitis of 10 years' duration or more are offered colonoscopy every 1 to 2 years to prevent colonic cancer, by taking multiple biopsies to look for mucosal dysplasia and to offer elective colectomy if appropriate or to detect cancer at a curable stage.

## Crohn's disease

Crohn's disease can affect any part of the GI tract from the mouth to the anus. It most frequently presents with ileocecal disease, followed by colonic, ileal alone, diffuse small intestinal, gastric, and esophageal involvement. The overall prevalence in the Western world is about 1 in 1000 and is more common in Caucasians than African-Americans.

### Clinical presentation

The patient has diarrhea and abdominal pain. There may be a fever, anemia, and weight loss. The patient may exhibit clubbing of the fingers, and there may be associated complications (e.g., joint, skin, or eye complications) as with ulcerative colitis.

The presentation depends on the site of disease and on the tendency to perforate or fistulate rather than to fibrose and stricture, which is probably determined by genetic factors. Terminal ileal disease presents with right iliac fossa pain, often with an associated mass. This may present acutely, mimicking appendicitis, or chronically, mimicking irritable bowel syndrome.

Colonic Crohn's disease is distinguishable from ulcerative colitis by the presence of skip lesions (multiple lesions with normal bowel in between), rectal sparing, perianal skin tags, or fistulas with or without granulomata on biopsy, although the distinction is unclear in up to a third of patients. Crohn's disease has transmural inflammation, which explains why the rates of fistulazation and stricture are more common than with ulcerative colitis.

## Complications
### Local

Perforation, stricture, fistula, abscess formation, or, rarely, massive hemorrhage can occur. There is an increased risk of colonic carcinoma in patients with Crohn's disease, although not nearly as high as in patients with ulcerative colitis. In addition, complications related to malabsorption are common. With increasing loss of the terminal ileum, bile salts are unable to be absorbed. The increase in steatorrhea can also cause malnutrition and hypocalcemia and eventually lead to osteoporosis. In addition, the loss of the terminal ileum prevents the absorption of vitamin $B_{12}$.

### Extraintestinal

Extraintestinal complications of Crohn's disease include the following:

- Skin: erythema nodosum, pyoderma gangrenosum, vasculitis.
- Eyes: uveitis, episcleritis, conjunctivitis.
- Joints: large joint arthropathy, sacroiliitis, ankylosing spondylitis.
- Liver: pericholangitis, sclerosing cholangitis, cirrhosis, chronic active hepatitis, cholangiocarcinoma.
- Vasculature: arterial and venous thrombosis.
- Renal stones and gallstones: in Crohn's disease.

275

## Investigations

Diagnosis is made by endoscopy with or without barium studies. Barium enema shows skip lesions, a coarse cobblestone appearance of the mucosa, and, later, fibrosis produces narrowing of the intestine ("string sign") with proximal dilatation.

Serum C-reactive protein is raised in about 95% of cases with active disease.

Magnetic resonance imaging (MRI) is useful for evaluation of fistulas and abscesses.

## Management

In most cases of active Crohn's disease, there are three therapeutic alternatives: surgery, corticosteroids, or diet. These options should be discussed with the patient. Steroids have no proven maintenance effect and inappropriate long-term use produces unacceptable adverse effects.

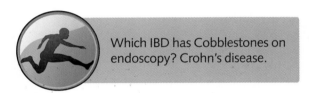

Which IBD has Cobblestones on endoscopy? Crohn's disease.

Therapy with 5-ASA maintenance probably reduces the risk of recurrence.

### Surgery

Postoperative fistulas used to be a common complication but are now rare, partly due to perioperative antibiotics, particularly metronidazole. Absolute indications for surgery include complete obstruction or peritonitis. After surgical resection, about half the patients remain symptom free for 5 years and half require further surgery within 10 years. Unlike patients with ulcerative colitis, whose disease is cured by the removal of the colon, surgery is only a temporizing measure in patients with Crohn's disease.

Perianal disease requires conservative management. Abscesses should be drained and fistulas treated with antibiotics, either metronidazole or ciprofloxacin. If there is coexistent active disease elsewhere, perianal disease may improve when the active disease is resected.

### Dietary therapy

Enteral feeding should be considered for patients with extensive small bowel disease, patients who have multiple or extensive small bowel resections, and patients who fail to respond to steroids. About two-thirds of patients achieve a satisfactory clinical and biochemical remission within about 3 weeks. The patient then gradually introduces components of the normal diet, although there is a 50% relapse rate 6 months after return to a normal diet.

Patients with stricturing disease should avoid fruit and vegetable fiber and may need vitamin C and folate supplements; also, vitamin $B_{12}$ supplements will be necessary after extensive small bowel surgery. Patients can experiment to find a diet that suits them best.

### Drugs

*5-ASA derivatives*   Treatment in mild cases is started with 5-ASA derivatives (e.g., mesalamine). If there is no response to these medications after 1 month of treatment, oral antibiotics (as noted below) can be added. Failure to improve with these two medications is an indication to start oral steroids. Immunosuppressive medications are added if improvement is not noted after 4 weeks of steroid therapy.

*Steroids*   Steroids may not modify the long-term course of the disease but are useful for acute episodes. High-dose prednisone is usually given, and tailed off over several weeks. Within 4 weeks about a third of patients are in remission and a further third are considerably improved. Formulations of steroids are now available that deliver the drug to the distal ileum.

*Azathioprine and other immunosuppressives* These may be used as an adjunct to steroids as with ulcerative colitis. They require close monitoring of the blood count. As well as maintaining remission, there is some evidence that they are helpful in healing fistulas.

*Metronidazole and other antibiotics*   A variety of bacteria and yeasts have been identified in Crohn's disease. Metronidazole is effective in colonic Crohn's disease, perianal disease, and in the prevention of recurrence following bowel resection. It should be given for 3 months. Longer maintenance doses carry a risk of peripheral neuropathy. Ciprofloxacin may also be of benefit.

*Antidiarrheals and cholestyramine*
Cholestyramine, an ion-exchange resin, is useful for chronic diarrhea after ileal resection due to

conjugated bile acids entering the colon. It should not be given at the same time as other medication because it impairs their absorption. Antidiarrhoeals such as loperamide are safe providing there is no evidence of obstruction.

*New immunomodulator treatments*   As with ulcerative colitis, studies are under way to determine the benefit of TNF-alpha antibodies and receptor fusion proteins that act to downregulate the immune system. Infliximab is a monoclonal antibody to TNF-alpha, and etanercept is a receptor fusion protein that binds to and inactivates TNF-alpha. In the upcoming months to years, further randomized, placebo-controlled trials will elucidate any possible benefit of these medications for patients with Crohn's disease.

### Prognosis
A minority of patients have extensive disease or frequent recurrences, and account for most of the 10% who ultimately die of the disease. Around 10–20% of patients remain asymptomatic for 20 years after the first or second episode of symptomatic disease. Most patients need surgery within the first few years and further resections at intervals of 10–15 years but have a good quality of life for most of this time.

## Gastrointestinal tumors

### Esophageal carcinoma
A total of 14,000 cases of esophageal carcinoma is diagnosed in the U.S. each year, and only 2% of patients generally survive beyond 5 years. Squamous carcinomas occur in the mid-esophagus. The incidence in the U.K. is 5–10 in 100,000 but higher in China and parts of Africa. It is more common in men, heavy drinkers, and smokers. Predisposing factors include Plummer–Vinson syndrome (see p. 141), achalasia, celiac disease, and tylosis (hyperkeratosis of the palms and soles).

Adenocarcinoma arises in columnar epithelium of the lower esophagus, resulting from long standing reflux. Columnar metaplasia, called Barrett's esophagus, increases the risk of adenocarcinoma by 40-fold. It is most common in older, white, obese male smokers. The incidence of adenocarcinoma of the esophagus has been increasing dramatically over the past 20 years.

### Clinical features
The incidence peaks in the seventh decade. Dysphagia is common, progressing from difficulty in swallowing solids to difficulty with liquids. Odynophagia (pain on swallowing) may ensue. The lesions may ulcerate and cause strictures. Direct invasion of surrounding structures and regional lymph node involvement are common. Weight loss, anorexia, lymphadenopathy, and aspiration pneumonia may be found.

### Investigations
Endoscopy with biopsy and barium swallow are the main diagnostic investigations. Computed tomography (CT) scanning or PET scans may show spread outside the esophagus.

### Management
Chemotherapy alone is not effective against esophageal carcinoma. Cisplatin combined with other agents has shown response rates in a minority of patients and often extend life by only several months.

Radiation therapy can be effective only for localized disease and is not recommended alone. The combination of cisplatin-based chemotherapy with radiation therapy has been shown to achieve long-term survival benefits. This treatment modality given before surgery has shown survival advantages, especially for localized disease. Only 30–40% of patients are candidates for surgery at the time of diagnosis. Strictures may be dilated if they cause dysphagia, and mesh stents can be placed. Laser photocoagulation via an endoscope is available in some centers. Treatment is mainly symptomatic and palliative.

### Gastric carcinoma
The incidence of gastric carcinoma is 15 in 100,000, and it is more common in men and the elderly. There is a link between gastric cancer and *H. pylori*, which may explain the higher prevalence in lower socioeconomic groups. Suggested dietary links include alcohol, spicy foods, and nitrates, which are converted to nitrosamines by bacteria. It occurs more often in Japan due to the higher fish intake, resulting in a high level of nitrosamines. It is more common in smokers, in patients with achlorhydria, and in patients with blood group A.

Other predisposing conditions include pernicious anemia, chronic gastritis with atrophy, areas of intestinal metaplasia, and partial gastrectomy.

Most cancers are adenocarcinomas and affect mainly the pylorus and antrum. They are polypoid or ulcerating lesions with rolled edges.

## Clinical features
In the early stages, the symptoms are similar to GU with epigastric pain, but the patient may present later with anorexia, nausea and vomiting, weight loss, and iron-deficiency anemia. Metastases occur to the liver, bones, brain, and lungs.

A palpable epigastric mass and upper abdominal tenderness may be present, and there may be a palpable lymph node in the left supraclavicular fossa (Virchow's node). Other signs include dermatomyositis and acanthosis nigricans.

## Investigation
Blood tests include a CBC to look for signs of chronic blood loss and LFTs for possible metastases. Diagnosis is made on gastroscopy with multiple biopsies. CT scans should be done to look for distant metastases. Paracentesis with cytologic studies should be performed if ascites is present.

## Treatment
The 5-year survival is about 10%, but the 5-year survival with gastrectomy (if found early) is up to 50%. Like esophageal carcinoma, treatment is difficult secondary to extensive disease at the time of diagnosis. Current therapy for early disease is usually chemotherapy with 5-FU, followed by a cycle of 5-FU plus radiation and then a final treatment with 5-FU. This regimen is followed by surgical resection. Patients may also require supportive care and palliative surgery.

# Colonic tumors
Colonic polyps are common and often found incidentally during investigation of coincidental GI symptoms such as pain, altered bowel habit, or bleeding hemorrhoids. They may be sessile or pedunculated, they vary from a few millimeters to up to 10cm in diameter, and they may be solitary or multiple.

Peutz-Jeghers syndrome consists of mucocutaneous pigmentation and polyps anywhere along the GI tract, most commonly in the small bowel. It has a Mendelian dominant inheritance.

Adenomatous polyps may bleed and lead to iron-deficiency anemia. Sessile villous adenomas of the rectum may present with profuse diarrhea and

hypokalemia. Once the polyp is removed endoscopically, continuous colonoscopic surveillance every 3–5 years is recommended due to the high probability of recurrence.

Familial adenomatous polyposis is Mendelian dominant. Patients have multiple polyps throughout the GI tract. In high-risk patients, colectomy with ileorectal anastamosis may be performed, with continued surveillance of the rectal stump.

The incidence of colonic adenocarcinoma is 52 per 100,000 in men and 36 per 100,000 in women. This averages out to approximately 150,000 new cases diagnosed in the U.S. per year. It is more common in the elderly and less common in Africa and Asia. It may be related to low fiber and high animal fat diets. Predisposing conditions include ulcerative colitis, HNPCC, and familial adenomatous polyposis (FAP). Genetic factors also play a role, with a 2- to 3-fold increased risk of developing colon cancer with one first-degree affected family member. Two-thirds of tumors occur with ulceration and spread by direct infiltration, invading the lymph nodes and blood vessels, leading to metastases.

## Clinical features
Left-sided tumors present with altered bowel habit and abdominal pain. They may be asymptomatic or present with an iron-deficiency anemia or with obstruction. Rectosigmoid tumors commonly bleed. Examination should always include a rectal examination.

## Investigation
CBC for anemia and metabolic panel for electrolyte abnormalities with diarrhea. Colonoscopy and barium enema will identify most tumors. Ultrasound is useful for staging and to detect liver metastases.

## Treatment
The primary treatment is surgical resection, although 10–15% of cases have metastasized at the time of diagnosis. The overall 5-year survival rate is about 30% but is over 90% with early resection. Adjuvant chemotherapy and radiotherapy increase survival in more advanced stages.

# Endocrine tumors of the gut
Although these are all very rare, they are sometimes discussed in examinations.

They arise from APUD (amine precursor: uptake and decarboxylation) cells, which secrete a number of hormones (e.g., gastrin, glucagon, and vasoactive intestinal peptide [VIP]). They may occur with other endocrine tumors as part of MEN syndromes.

### Zollinger-Ellison syndrome

This is usually due to a gastrin-secreting pancreatic adenoma, which stimulates excessive acid production and leads to multiple recurrent ulcers in the stomach and duodenum. About half are malignant and 10% are multiple.

Patients commonly get diarrhea due to the low pH in the upper intestine and steatorrhea due to the inactivation of lipase by the low pH. The diagnosis is made by a raised fasting serum gastrin level; the gastric acid output is also raised. Treatment is by removal of the primary tumor (provided there is no evidence of metastases) and omeprazole or octreotide.

### Insulinomas

These are tumors of the pancreatic islet β-cells; 5% are malignant and 5% are multiple. The patient presents with recurrent or fasting hypoglycemia, which may manifest in bizarre behavior, epilepsy, dementia, or confusion. The diagnosis is confirmed by the demonstration of hypoglycemia in association with inappropriate and excessive insulin secretion. Treatment is by surgical excision of the tumor. If surgery is not feasible, diazoxide or octreotide is useful.

### Vipomas

These tumors release VIP, which produces intestinal secretions, leading to watery diarrhea, hypokalemia, and sometimes achlorhydria. Diagnosis is by high serum levels of VIP. The tumor should be resected if possible. Octreotide is useful for controlling symptoms.

### Glucagonomas

These are tumors of the α-cells of the pancreas, which release glucagon. Symptoms include diabetes, diarrhea, a necrolytic migratory erythematous rash, weight loss, anemia, and glossitis.

### Carcinoid tumors

These tumors originate from the argentaffin cells of the intestine. They may appear in the appendix, terminal ileum, rectum, or other site in the GI tract. They have malignant potential; 80% of large tumors produce metastases. Presentations include appendicitis (10% of tumors arise in the appendix), GI obstruction and, in 5% of cases, carcinoid syndrome.

### Carcinoid syndrome

This occurs only when liver metastases are present. Clinical features include flushing (which may be prolonged and lead to telangiectases), abdominal pain, diarrhea, bronchospasm, and edema associated with pulmonary stenosis or tricuspid regurgitation. Symptoms are due to the release of pharmacologically active mediators (e.g., 5-hydroxytryptamine [5-HT], prostaglandins, and kinins).

Diagnosis is by measurement of 5-hydroxyindoleacetic acid (5-HIAA) in 24-hour urine collection, which is a metabolite (5-HT).

Abdominal CT scan or laparotomy may be needed to localize the tumor.

***Treatment*** Food and drink which precipitate flushing should be avoided (e.g., alcohol, coffee). Surgery is best for localized tumors and may be curative. Octreotide alleviates flushing and diarrhea. Other useful drugs include cyprohepatiine (an antihistamine with 5-HT and calcium channel-blocking properties), and methysergide (which also blocks 5-HT). Other procedures include enucleation of liver metastases, hepatic artery ligation, embolization, and 5-fluorouracil injection.

***Prognosis*** The median survival is 5–10 years after diagnosis.

## Malabsorption

Causes of malabsorption are given in Fig. 32.3.

### Clinical features

Symptoms include anorexia and weight loss, abdominal distention and borborygmi, pale, greasy stools with an offensive odor, tiredness, and paresthesias. There may be signs of wasting, abdominal distention, petechiae (vitamin K malabsorption), anemia, bone pain (hypocalcemia), edema and ascites (hypoproteinemia), clubbing, tetany, and peripheral neuropathy (vitamin B deficiency). There may also be signs of the underlying disease (e.g., jaundice or lymphadenopathy with lymphomas).

**Fig. 32.3** Causes of malabsorption.

| Causes of malabsorption | |
| --- | --- |
| **Cause** | **Examples** |
| mucosal disease | gluten-sensitive enteropathy<br>tropical sprue<br>intestinal lymphangiectasia<br>Whipple's disease |
| structural abnormalities | gastric surgery<br>intestinal resections<br>blind loops<br>diverticula, fistulae<br>small bowel malignancy<br>arterial insufficiency<br>systemic sclerosis |
| infections | acute enteritis<br>postinfective malabsorption<br>traveller's diarrhea<br>tuberculosis<br>parasites |
| impaired digestion | biliary and liver disease<br>pancreatic disease<br>Zollinger–Ellison syndrome |
| biochemical disorders | lactose intolerance<br>abetalipoproteinemia<br>hypogammaglobulinemia |
| iatrogenic | drugs<br>surgery<br>radiotherapy |
| disorders outside the gastrointestinal tract | endocrine disorders, e.g. thyroid disease, Addison's disease, hypoparathyroidism<br>collagen disorders<br>malignant disease<br>widespread skin diseases |

## Investigations

The following investigations are important in the patient with malabsorption:

- General blood tests: CBC may show a microcytic, macrocytic, or mixed picture. Albumin and calcium may be low. Electrolytes (e.g., sodium, potassium, and magnesium) may be low. LFTs are abnormal if liver pathology is responsible for the malabsorption, and prothrombin time may be increased.
- Specific blood tests: serum folate, vitamin $B_{12}$, and serum iron may help to confirm malabsorption.
- Fecal fat estimations: high fat content in stools.
- Endoscopy with biopsy and cytology can suggest the diagnosis in some cases.
- Glucose tolerance test: this is "flat."

- Radiology: plain x-ray may reveal fluid levels, pancreatic calcification or gallstones. Small bowel enemas are useful for Crohn's disease, lymphoma or diverticula. Jejunal biopsy is indicated in celiac disease. CT scan can show the pancreas and visualize the small bowel for signs of edema or fat staining.
- Pancreatic function tests: if pancreatic disease is suspected. Endoscopic retrograde cholangiopancreatography (ERCP) will give further information.
- Breath hydrogen tests: indicated in bacterial overgrowth.

## Specific diseases
### Celiac disease

Celiac disease is a gluten-sensitive enteropathy. In this disease there is an abnormal jejunal mucosa leading to malabsorption. The condition improves with a gluten-free diet but relapses when gluten is reintroduced.

Gluten is present in wheat, barley, rye, and oats.

Celiac disease is more common in Europeans, with an incidence of about 1 in 250 in the U.S. There is an increased incidence within families, and it is associated with HLA-B8 and DR3. It is also associated with a blistering subepidermal eruption of the skin (dermatitis herpetiformis). The etiology is thought to be due to $\alpha$-gliadin, a peptide present in gluten, which is injurious to the small bowel mucosa. Immunogenic mechanisms and possibly environmental factors (e.g., viral infections) may also play a role.

### Clinical features

The disease can present at any age. The peak incidence in adults is in the third and fourth decades, and it is more common in women. Symptoms may be nonspecific (e.g., lethargy and malaise). There is usually a history of diarrhea or steatorrhea, with abdominal discomfort, and there may be weight loss. Other features include mouth ulcers, anemia and, less commonly, tetany, osteomalacia, neuropathies, and myopathies.

There is an increased incidence of autoimmune disease (e.g., thyroid disease and insulin-dependent diabetes). Celiac disease may be complicated by GI lymphoma and gastric or esophageal carcinoma.

### Investigations

The following investigations are important in the patient with celiac disease:

- Jejunal biopsy: villous atrophy with chronic inflammatory cells in the lamina propria.
- CBC: may show anemia (folate, vitamin $B_{12}$, or iron deficiency).
- Antireticulin antibodies, antigliadin, anti-tissue transglutaminase, and antiendomysial antibodies: usually present.
- Serum albumin: hypoalbuminemia.
- Prothrombin time: may be prolonged due to vitamin K deficiency.

### Management

The condition improves on a gluten-free diet. Deficient vitamins are replaced. If symptoms persist, it may be that the patient is not complying with the diet.

## Bacterial overgrowth

Although bacterial overgrowth may occur spontaneously, especially in the elderly, it is normally associated with a structural abnormality of the small intestine (e.g., in diverticula or postoperative blind loops). Aspiration of jejunal contents reveals *Escherichia coli* or *Bacteroides* in concentrations greater than $10^6$/mL as part of a mixed flora. The bacteria can deconjugate bile salts, which can be detected in aspirates; this deficiency of conjugated bile salts leads to steatorrhea. The bacteria also metabolize vitamin $B_{12}$, leading to its deficiency.

### Management

Endoscopy or the [14C]-d-xylose breath test can be used to diagnose bacterial overgrowth. Hydrogen breath tests are usually not as good as the [14C]-d-xylose test. Underlying small bowel lesions should be corrected if possible. The condition may respond to intermittent courses of metronidazole (400mg 8 hourly), oxytetracycline (250mg 6 hourly), amoxicillin-clavulanate, cephalexin, or Bactrim.

## Tropical sprue

In this condition there is severe malabsorption, usually accompanied by diarrhea and malnutrition. It occurs in most of Asia and the Caribbean. The etiology is unknown, but it is thought to be infective. The onset can be insidious or acute with anorexia, weight loss, and abdominal distension, as well as diarrhea. There may be features of vitamin deficiency, especially vitamin $B_{12}$. Jejunal histology shows partial villous atrophy.

### Management

Severe cases may need intravenous fluids and electrolytes, and replacement of nutritional and vitamin deficiencies. Patients often improve when they leave an endemic area. Patients may be helped with tetracycline (250mg 6 hourly) and folic acid.

## Whipple's disease

This is a rare cause of malabsorption, usually affecting men over 50 years old. As well as steatorrhea, there is fever, weight loss, arthralgia, lymphadenopathy, and sometimes involvement of the heart, lung, and brain. Histologically, cells of the lamina propria are replaced by macrophages which contain periodic acid–Schiff (PAS) positive glycoprotein granules. The organism responsible is *Tropheryma whippelii*. Treatment is with antibiotics (e.g., tetracycline or chloramphenicol).

## Diseases of the gallbladder

### Gallstones

The incidence of gallstones rises with age and is more common in women on the oral contraceptive pill.

Bile contains cholesterol, bile pigments, and phospholipids, and it is the relative concentration of these that determines the kind of stone that is formed. Pigment stones are small and radiolucent, and they are occasionally associated with hemolytic anemia due to increased formation of bile pigment from hemoglobin.

Cholesterol stones are large, often solitary, and radiolucent. Mixed stones contain calcium salts, pigment, and cholesterol; 10% are radiopaque. (Compare with renal stones, of which about 90% are radiopaque).

Gallstones may be asymptomatic but may cause acute or chronic cholecystitis, biliary colic, or obstructive jaundice. Other presentations include cholangitis (infection of the bile ducts causing right upper quadrant pain, jaundice, and fever with rigors), pancreatitis, empyema, and gallstone ileus, in which the gallstone perforates the gallbladder, ulcerates into the duodenum, and passes on to obstruct the terminal ileum.

### Investigations

If pigment stones are suspected or found operatively, a hemolysis screen should be obtained. Plain abdominal x-ray and ultrasound should detect most stones. A cholecystogram or intravenous cholangiography may be performed in cases of uncertainty. Operative cholangiography will reveal stones in the bile ducts, which might otherwise be missed.

Gallstones are most common in people with the "six Fs":
- Fair.
- Fat.
- Fertile.
- Female.
- (Low) fiber diet.
- Forty.

### Management

If the patient is symptomatic, treatment is by cholecystectomy. Sphincterotomy via ERCP may release stones in the common bile duct. Other options include the medical dissolution of small, cholesterol-rich radiolucent stones (with ursodeoxycholic acid given for up to 2 years) or shockwave lithotripsy.

### Acute cholecystitis

This disease is most common in overweight, middle-aged women but may occur at any age. It usually follows the impaction of a stone in the cystic duct and leads to fever, rigors, epigastric or right upper quadrant pain, vomiting, local peritonism, or a gallbladder mass. If the stone moves to the common bile duct, jaundice may occur. Murphy's sign may be positive; this is pain on inspiration when two fingers are placed over the right upper quadrant, due to an inflamed gallbladder impinging on the examiner's fingers.

### Differential diagnosis

The differential diagnosis of acute cholecystitis includes the following:
- Appendicitis in a highly-situated appendix.
- Acute hepatitis.
- Right basal pneumonia.
- Perforated peptic ulcer.
- Pancreatitis.
- Myocardial infarction.

### Investigations

The white cell count is elevated. A chest x-ray (CXR), electrocardiogram (ECG), serum amylase and cardiac enzymes should be taken to help exclude differential diagnoses. Ultrasound will show a thickened gallbladder wall and stones.

### Management

Management is usually initially conservative, unless complications ensue (e.g., perforation of the gallbladder). The patient should be on bed rest, nil by mouth with intravenous fluids, and analgesia and antibiotics (e.g., cefuroxime or cefotaxime) should be given. Cholecystectomy is either performed after 48 hours or the inflammation is allowed to settle and the gallbladder is removed after 2–3 months.

### Chronic cholecystitis

Recurrent episodes of cholecystitis are usually associated with gallstones, leading to intermittent colic and chronic inflammation. Symptoms include abdominal discomfort, bloating, nausea, flatulence, and intolerance of fats.

The differential diagnosis includes myocardial ischemia, hiatus hernia and esophagitis, peptic ulcer disease, irritable bowel syndrome, chronic relapsing pancreatitis, and tumors of the GI tract. Treatment is by cholecystectomy.

## Diseases of the pancreas

### Carcinoma of the pancreas
Pancreatic carcinoma is one of the deadliest cancers and is the fourth leading cause of cancer deaths in the U.S. About 30,000 new cases are diagnosed each year; however, only 10–15% of cancers are respectable at the time of diagnosis. The incidence of pancreatic carcinoma is increasing. Risk factors include smoking and possibly diabetes. About three-quarters of tumors occur in the head; the rest occur in the body or tail. Secondary diabetes is uncommon. Pancreatitis may occur due to obstruction of the pancreatic duct. Jaundice, pruritus, dark urine, and clay-colored stools are also common in 50% of cases.

### Clinical features
Symptoms include dyspepsia or epigastric pain radiating to the back, anorexia and weight loss, fever, and obstructive jaundice with an enlarged gallbladder. There may be hepatomegaly from biliary obstruction or metastases. Thrombophlebitis migrans occurs in 10% of patients.

### Investigations
Ultrasound and CT scan may show the tumor, ERCP may confirm the diagnosis, and needle biopsy can be performed under CT control. As with other GI malignancies, GI ultrasound can also play a role in biopsy and local imaging. Tumor marker CA19–9 can be drawn prior to treatment to evaluate tumor response.

### Management
A minority of patients may be suitable for operative treatment although survival is not usually greater than 1 year, even after surgery. Patients with ampullary carcinoma often present early with jaundice, and surgical removal may therefore be more successful. Palliative treatment with endoscopy, surgery, chemotherapy, and radiation

should be offered to the patient who is not a surgical candidate.

Without treatment, survival is usually only a few weeks after diagnosis.

## Acute pancreatitis
### Etiology
Most cases are secondary to gallstones or alcohol. It may be also be idiopathic. Other causes include hypercalcemia, hyperlipidemia, post ERCP, and trauma.

### Clinical features
There may be a history of cholecystitis or other complications of gallstones. Alcohol intake should be ascertained. The patient complains of severe abdominal pain radiating to the back or shoulder, which may be relieved by sitting forward. There may be associated nausea and vomiting.

On examination there is abdominal tenderness with guarding and rebound tenderness. There may be a tachycardia, fever, jaundice, hypotension, and sweating. There may be bruising around the umbilicus (Cullen's sign) or in the flanks (Grey–Turner's sign).

### Differential diagnosis
This includes any cause of an acute abdomen (e.g., cholecystitis, mesenteric ischemia, and intestinal perforation). Myocardial infarction and dissecting aortic aneurysm should also be excluded.

### Investigations
The following investigations are important in the patient with acute pancreatitis:
- Serum amylase: markedly raised (over 1000 IU/mL). Amylase is also raised with cholecystitis and perforated peptic ulcer, but usually to a lesser extent. Serum lipase is also elevated and is more specific than amylase.
- Abdominal x-ray: gallstones, pancreatic calcification indicating previous inflammation, an absent psoas shadow due to retroperitoneal fluid, and a distended loop of jejunum ("sentinel loop").
- Serum calcium: may be low.
- White cell count: usually raised.
- ECG: to exclude myocardial infarction.
- Arterial blood gases: metabolic acidosis.
- CXR: widened mediastinum in aortic dissection; gas under the diaphragm in perforated peptic ulcer.
- Abdominal CT: assess severity.

The causes of pancreatitis can be recalled from the mnemonic **GET SMASH'D**: **g**allstones, **e**thanol, **t**rauma, **s**teroids, **m**umps, **a**utoimmune diseases, **s**corpion stings, **h**ypertriglyceridemia, and **d**rugs (e.g., azathioprine or diuretics).

## Management

Management is usually conservative. Intravenous fluids should be given to maintain the circulating volume, and a central venous catheter may be helpful for assessing the volume of fluid required. If the patient is in shock (systolic blood pressure <90 mmHg), plasma expanders will be required.

Pain relief is with intravenous or intramuscular opiates (e.g., pethidine, 50–150 mg 4 hourly, or pentazocine, 30–60 mg 4 hourly, meperidine, fentanyl, or morphine with an antiemetic such as prochlorperazine, 12.5 mg 8 hourly). A nasogastric tube should be inserted. Blood tests, especially metabolic panel, glucose, and calcium, should be monitored. TPN may be required.

Surgery should be considered for suspected hemorrhagic necrosis of the pancreas. Some give $H_2$-receptor antagonists, prophylactic antibiotics, or peritoneal lavage, although these measures are of unproven value.

## Prognosis

Ranson's criteria are used to predict the severity of acute pancreatitis (Fig. 32.4). Mortality is 5–10%, but recurrence is uncommon in patients who recover. Death may be from shock, renal failure, sepsis, or respiratory failure. Other complications include hypocalcemia due to the formation of calcium soaps, transient hyperglycemia, pancreatic abscess requiring drainage, and pseudocyst (i.e., fluid in the lesser sac presenting as a palpable mass), persistently raised serum amylase or liver function tests, and fever. Patients should be investigated to exclude gallstones, and alcohol should be avoided.

## Chronic pancreatitis

In chronic pancreatitis, recurrent acute attacks have altered the structure of the organ, leading to impaired exocrine or endocrine function. The main cause of chronic pancreatitis is chronic excessive alcohol intake. Other causes include gallstones, cystic fibrosis, and hemochromatosis. The patient is generally ill with weight loss and has recurrent abdominal pain radiating to the back. Steatorrhea is secondary to malabsorption from pancreatic insufficiency. Diabetes may occur due to involvement of pancreatic islet β-cells, and there may be intermittent or persistent obstructive jaundice.

## Investigations

These are similar to those for acute pancreatitis, although serum amylase is not helpful in the

| Ranson criteria to predict severity of acute pancreatitis | |
|---|---|
| **0 hours** | |
| Age | >55 |
| White blood cell count | >16,000/mm³ |
| Blood glucose | >200 mg/dL (11.1 mmol/L) |
| Lactate dehydrogenase | >350 U/L |
| Aspartate aminotransferase (AST) | >250 U/L |
| **48 hours** | |
| Hematocrit | Fall by ≥10 percent |
| Blood urea nitrogen | Increase by ≥5 mg/dL (1.8 mmol/L) despite fluids |
| Serum calcium | <8 mg/dL (2 mmol/L) |
| pO₂ | <60 mmHg |
| Base deficit | >4 MEq/L |
| Fluid sequestation | >6000 mL |

The presence of 1 to 3 criteria represents mild pancreatitis; the mortality rate rises significantly with four or more criteria.

Fig. 32.4 Ranson criteria to predict severity of acute pancreatitis. (Adapted from Ranson JHC, Rifkind KM, Roses DF, et al. Surg Gynecol Obstet 139:69, 1974.)

diagnosis because it is usually only slightly raised. This is due to the fact that in chronic pancreatitis the glands of the pancreas are "burned out" and so few are left to produce their product that, despite the ongoing inflammation, the blood levels of amylase and lipase may be low. In addition the following investigations should be performed:

- Plasma glucose: raised in diabetes.
- CT scan: may show dilated ducts.
- Abdominal films: calcified pancreatic ducts are often seen.
- MRI/ultrasound: may show dilated ducts, fluid collections, calcifications, or pseudocysts.
- ERCP: outlines the anatomy of the ducts and shows calculi.

Investigations of consequences or complications of pancreatitis should also be carried out (e.g., tests of malabsorption, jaundice, and pancreatic exocrine function).

## Management

Alcohol should be avoided, and the patient should be advised to follow a low-fat diet because of malabsorption. Fat-soluble vitamins, calcium, and pancreatic enzymes are given. Insulin is required if the patient develops diabetes, and the gallbladder should be removed if gallstones are present.

For recurrent attacks causing unremitting pain, pancreatectomy should be considered. Patients often have chronic persistent pain and can become addicted to opiates. NSAID therapy, in addition to amitriptyline or gabapentin, may allow patients to come off of narcotics. Invasive nerve ablation techniques and referral to a chronic pain clinic are also beneficial.

## Acute viral hepatitis

## Hepatitis A
### Epidemiology

Hepatitis A affects 1.4 million people worldwide annually. In the U.S., it is thought that 90,000 symptomatic cases occur each year, with 180,000 asymptomatic cases. Hepatitis A virus (HAV) is a member of the picornavirus family. The incubation period varies from 3–6 weeks. Transmission is by the fecal–oral route. Clinical disease with jaundice is uncommon in infants and young children, and the infection may go unnoticed. It may be acquired by eating partially cooked shellfish from estuaries contaminated by sewage.

### Serology

At the onset of symptoms, immunoglobulin (Ig)M anti-HAV antibody is present in serum. High titers persist for 3–12 months, so a positive test in a patient with acute hepatitis indicates recent acute infection. Previous infection, and therefore immunity, can be diagnosed by the presence of IgG anti-HAV without IgM anti-HAV.

### Outcome

Relapses and cholestatic jaundice may occur, but hepatitis A does not progress to chronic hepatitis. Patients with pre-existing liver disease, especially hepatitis C, have an increased risk of fulminant hepatic failure. Treatment is with supportive therapy and, rarely, hospitalization.

### Prevention and control

Prophylaxis can be obtained by immune serum immunoglobulin or active immunization. The latter induces higher levels of anti-HAV.

## Hepatitis B
### Epidemiology

The complete infectious virion (Dane particle) consists of the following:

- Hepatitis B surface antigen (HBsAg): the outer lipoprotein "surface" envelope.
- Hepatitis B core antigen (HBcAg): the internal core, which surrounds the viral genome of DNA.
- Hepatitis B e antigen (HBeAg): a subunit of HBcAg; it can be detected in serum and is a useful marker of circulating virions and infectivity.

Transmission is parenteral through cutaneous and mucosal routes, across breaks in the skin or mucous membranes, and the mean incubation period is 75 days. In developed countries hepatitis B occurs sporadically.

Risk factors are male homosexuality, low socioeconomic status, intravenous drug abuse, ethnic group, sexual promiscuity, residence in institutions, mental handicap, and employment in health professions. In endemic areas such as China and southern Africa, the disease is often acquired in childhood and can occur by inoculation of infectious blood during the birth process. Infection is characteristically anicteric, asymptomatic, and chronic.

## Serology

Following exposure to hepatitis B virus (HBV), HBsAg can be detected throughout the prodromal phase and is not usually cleared from the serum until convalescence. Other early markers include anti-HBc and HBeAg. A positive IgM anti-HBc test typically distinguishes acute from chronic hepatitis B. The presence of HBeAg implies high infectivity, but it is often no longer detectable by the time the patient consults the physician.

The loss of HBeAg is a good prognostic sign, indicating that the patient will clear HBsAg and will not develop chronic infection. The disappearance of HBeAg is usually followed by the appearance of serum anti-HBe. Anti-HBs is the last marker to appear in serum.

## Outcome

Acute infection may lead to fulminant hepatic failure. The disease may progress to chronic hepatitis, particularly in males and older people. It occurs in less than 5–10% of people with clinically apparent hepatitis B. Cirrhosis and hepatocellular carcinoma are complications of chronic hepatitis.

## Prevention and control

Patients who have chronic hepatitis B and evidence of active viral replication should be offered therapy with interferon alpha (IFN-$\alpha$). Combination therapy with lamivudine is often done as well. Infection can be prevented by active immunization.

# Hepatitis C
## Epidemiology

Hepatitis C (HCV) is an RNA virus and can be divided into many major types and subtypes. Transmission is most common after transfusion of whole blood products, and the mean incubation period is 9 weeks. Hepatitis C accounts for 20% of cases of acute hepatitis in the U.S. each year. There is a high prevalence in hemophiliacs, thalassemics, hemodialysis patients, transplant recipients, and intravenous drug abusers.

## Serology

Anti-HCV develops 1–3 months after the onset of clinical illness, and in some patients will not be detected for up to 1 year afterward. Identification of the viral RNA in serum is possible using the polymerase chain reaction. HCV antigens cannot be detected in serum.

## Outcome

The acute disease is often asymptomatic and leads to chronic infection in over 50% of patients. In about 20% of patients, cirrhosis may develop insidiously within 10 years, and patients may develop a clinical picture resembling autoimmune hepatitis. Systemic manifestations include cryoglobulinemia, porphyria cutanea tarda, and membranous glomerulonephritis. Hepatocellular carcinoma is recognized with chronic infection.

## Prevention and control

Patients who have had consistently elevated liver enzymes or who have shown significant fibrosis and cirrhosis on biopsy should be offered IFN therapy. Patients with a history of depression have an increased risk of suicide with IFN therapy, and caution should be used. Pegylated interferon therapy in combination with ribavirin for 48 weeks has been shown to reduce the presence of hepatitis C in up to 40% of patients and to extend survival. Blood bank screening for anti-HCV and genetically engineered factor VIII preparations for hemophiliacs limit the occurrence of hepatitis C.

# Hepatitis D
## Epidemiology

Hepatitis D (delta) virus (HDV) is an RNA virus. The virion particle is encapsulated by the coat protein of HBV (i.e., HBsAg). Thus infection by HDV occurs only in patients affected by hepatitis B. Transmission is similar to HBV, and the incubation period is 35 days. In developed countries, infection occurs mainly in drug addicts, hemophiliacs, and institutionalized persons.

## Serology

IgM anti-HD, IgG anti-HD, and HDAg can be detected.

## Outcome

The disease is not usually progressive, but outbreaks of fulminant hepatitis caused by HBV plus HDV are described. Chronic infection can occur.

## Prevention and control

The prevention of HBV infection will also prevent HDV infection as HDV cannot replicate in the absence of HBsAg.

## Hepatitis E
### Epidemiology

This RNA virus is transmitted via the fecal–oral route with a peak of epidemic infection 6–7 weeks after primary exposure and low secondary attack rate. It occurs predominantly in Africa, Asia, Central America, and the Middle East.

### Serology

Serologic tests are still in development.

### Outcome

This is usually self-limiting, and progression to chronic hepatitis does not occur. There is a high mortality rate (20%) in pregnant women.

### Prevention and control

This is dependent on high standards of public sanitation and sewage elimination.

## Clinical features of viral hepatitis

The clinical features of the various forms of acute viral hepatitis are similar. In the pre-icteric phase, the main symptoms include malaise, fatigue, listlessness, and lack of energy. Anorexia, nausea, and vomiting occur, which may be induced by fatty food. There is often a distaste for cigarettes. There may be right upper quadrant pain, change in bowel habit, myalgia, fever, and headaches.

In 10% of patients, acute hepatitis B may be accompanied by a serum sickness-like syndrome, which is characterized by low-grade fever, urticarial rash, and arthralgia.

The prodromal symptoms become less severe as jaundice appears. The urine darkens and the stools are pale. During the first week, the jaundice may deepen, and anorexia and fatigue may worsen in this period. There may be accompanying weight loss.

During recovery, symptoms gradually resolve although malaise and fatigue may persist and mild relapses can occur in 1–5% of patients. Exercise tolerance is generally depressed for some weeks; depression may be a prominent symptom.

Physical signs are usually minimal. Common findings are jaundice, hepatic tenderness, hepatomegaly, splenomegaly, and occasionally lymphadenopathy. Skin rashes may be noted.

Fulminant hepatitis leads to hepatic encephalopathy with severe jaundice, ascites, and edema, and is usually accompanied by hemorrhage caused by coagulopathies. The disturbance of consciousness reflects a combination of hepatic coma, hypoglycemia, and cerebral edema.

## Investigations

The following investigations are important in the patient with acute viral hepatitis:

- Liver enzymes, alanine aminotransferase (ALT), and aspartate aminotransferase: these are markedly elevated. Bilirubin concentration is also increased. During recovery, liver enzymes return to normal. A persistently raised ALT six months after the acute onset of hepatitis usually indicates progression of the disease.
- Prothrombin time: may be prolonged if fulminant hepatic failure occurs.
- Serum albumin concentrations: may fall slightly during the course of hepatitis, and serum globulin may rise.
- Hypoglycemia: may occur with fulminant hepatic failure.
- Serum $\alpha$-fetoprotein values: increased transiently in patients with acute viral hepatitis.
- CT scan and abdominal ultrasound can be used to help diagnose cirrhosis and hepatocellular carcinoma.

## Management

Most patients can be cared for at home, although hospital admissions may be required for diagnosis, social reasons, or if complications occur. Isolation precautions should be followed. All unnecessary drugs should be stopped. Acetaminophen is the preferred analgesic and is not hepatotoxic in low doses. Cholestyramine may alleviate itching.

For uncomplicated acute viral hepatitis, no specific treatment is required. Rest is recommended, and alcohol should be avoided.

## Chronic liver disease

### Chronic hepatitis

Clinically, chronic hepatitis is defined as any hepatitis lasting 6 months.

Chronic hepatitis may follow viral hepatitis, or develop with alcohol or drug use (e.g., isoniazid and methyldopa). Clinical features may include general malaise and lethargy, anorexia, hepatosplenomegaly, and signs of chronic liver disease. There may be remissions and exacerbations, and either complete recovery or progression to cirrhosis.

## Management of chronic liver disease

The principal problems in severe chronic liver disease are the degree of hepatocellular failure and the complications of portal hypertension.

### Management of variceal bleeds

This is described on p. 271.

## Ascites

Ascites is the presence of free fluid within the peritoneal cavity. Factors leading to the formation of ascites include salt and water retention as a result of cirrhosis, hypoalbuminemia resulting in decreased plasma colloid pressure, portal hypertension, and increased hepatic lymph production.

Clinically, there may be abdominal distention, shifting dullness, and a fluid thrill, if the ascites is tense. Associated features include hernias, separation of the abdominal musculature from the midline, abdominal wall venous distension, ankle edema, and distention of the neck veins. Abdominal ultrasound is the gold standard for the diagnosis of ascites and can also be helpful for paracentesis by marking an area unlikely to cause damage to structures upon insertion of the catheter. Abdominal ultrasound is also helpful in visualizing liver parenchyma and portal blood flow.

Investigations include diagnostic paracentesis. The ascites is clear and yellow unless it is infected, when it appears turbid. If the tap is non-traumatic, blood signifies intra-abdominal malignancy. The protein content is usually less than 1.5g/dL. Higher values indicate infection, hepatic venous obstruction, or malignancy. Fluid should be sent for cytology to look for malignant cells and for culture.

The patient should be on bed rest with restricted salt and fluids. The first choice of diuretic is spironolactone, 100–200mg per day. This can cause painful gynecomastia in men, and amiloride can be substituted. If there is a poor response to spironolactone, furosemide is added. Fluid balance, weight, and electrolytes should be monitored daily. Ascites can also be treated with therapeutic paracentesis and albumin infusion.

Overdiuresis may result in dehydration, uremia, and hyponatremia, and may precipitate hepatic encephalopathy, oliguria, and hepatorenal syndrome.

## Hepatic encephalopathy

Encephalopathy can either be reversible and episodic or lead to coma and death (Fig. 32.5). Liver failure results in diminished hepatic metabolism of substances derived from the gut, which can cause neurotoxicity. Clinical features include impaired conscious level, personality disturbances, inversion of the normal sleep pattern, slurred speech, constructional apraxia, flapping tremor (asterixis), hepatic fetor, brisk tendon reflexes, increased muscle tone and rigidity, and hyperventilation in deep coma.

### Management

Initial treatment aims to correct or remove the precipitating cause. These may include electrolyte abnormalities, sepsis, hypovolemia, hypoxia, bleeding, and constipation. Diuretics, sedatives, and opiates should be stopped, and intracranial pathology should be excluded, especially in alcoholic patients. CT scanning of the brain is useful to exclude subdural hematomas.

Measures should then be instituted to remove nitrogenous material and bacteria from the bowel. The patient is put on a low-protein, high-calorie diet. In alcoholics, intravenous thiamine is given to treat possible Wernicke's encephalopathy.

Once over the acute phase, routine measures include lactulose to ensure two soft bowel motions per day. Protein intake is restricted, and the patient is educated to avoid precipitating causes, including alcohol. In difficult cases of chronic encephalopathy,

| Grading of conscious level in hepatic encephalopathy | |
|---|---|
| Grade | Features |
| 1 | confusion, altered behavior, psychometric abnormalities |
| 2 | drowsy, altered behavior |
| 3 | stupor, obeys single commands, very confused |
| 4 | coma responding to painful stimuli |
| 5 | coma unresponsive to painful stimuli |

**Fig. 32.5** Grading of conscious level in hepatic encephalopathy.

a trial of bromocriptine is required. Recurrent acute-on-chronic encephalopathy is an indication for liver transplantation.

## Hemochromatosis

Hemochromatosis is due to excessive iron in the tissues and results from a genetic mutation that causes the body to absorb excessive dietary iron, which then becomes deposited in the tissues.

### Classification

Hemochromatosis may be classified as hereditary ("primary") or secondary.

Hereditary hemochromatosis is autosomal recessive. Secondary hemochromatosis may result from excessive iron administration (e.g., blood transfusion or iron tablets).

### Clinical features

Affected organs are the liver, endocrine system, heart, and joints. Most patients are asymptomatic or have nonspecific symptoms such as arthralgia and lethargy, until the effect of iron overload becomes apparent in the fifth or sixth decade. Joints are involved by chondrocalcinosis.

In the early stages, pain and swelling of the second and third metacarpophalangeal joints is characteristic. There is slate-gray skin, due to melanin, and iron deposition. Symptoms include asthenia, abdominal pain, impotence, arthralgia, and amenorrhea. Signs include hepatomegaly, splenomegaly, jaundice, and gynecomastia. The disease may lead on to cirrhosis.

The prevalence varies from 1 in 200 to 1 in 2000, and men are 5–10 times more affected than women, indicating that environmental and genetic factors modify disease expression. Women are usually affected at a later age, partly due to loss of iron during pregnancy or menstruation. Alcohol may exacerbate the problem by influencing iron metabolism and absorption.

### Pathology

Total body iron is increased in hemochromatosis from 4g up to as much as 60g. There is cellular damage and fibrosis, leading to a rusty colour of the liver, pancreas, spleen, and abdominal lymph nodes. The liver is usually enlarged and may be cirrhotic. Iron is found in all liver cell types and in cardiac myocytes, the adrenals, pituitary, pancreas, and testes. Chondrocalcinosis in the joints is associated with synovial hemosiderin and loss of intra-articular space.

### Investigations

- Serum iron is elevated and saturation of plasma transferrin is high. Serum iron is reduced in inflammatory conditions and is subject to diurnal variation.
- Serum ferritin is usually high.
- Definitive diagnosis of hemochromatosis depends on histology of liver biopsies.
- CT scanning and MRI can be used to detect increased tissue iron but are not routine.

### Course and prognosis

Complications include diabetes mellitus, cirrhosis, heart disease with arryhthmias, and liver cancer.

Life expectancy and hepatic and cardiac function in primary hemochromatosis are improved by iron depletion. The 5-year survival rate increases from 18% to 66%. Removal of iron does not prevent the development of cancer in patients with established cirrhosis.

Phlebotomy does not improve endocrine failure or joint disease.

### Treatment

Patients should have a phlebotomy regularly (e.g., 500mL weekly) until they develop a mild microcytic anemia. Care is needed in patients with severe hepatic disease since vigorous bleeding may be complicated by hypoproteinemia. Folate supplementation may be needed to optimize erythropoiesis. Seriously ill patients with overt cardiac hemochromatosis may require high-dose parenteral chelation therapy with desferrioxamine to reverse life-threatening disease.

Patients with established hemochromatosis should be investigated for cardiac involvement and pituitary as well as target organ endocrine failure, and replacement therapy should be instituted when necessary. Patients should be reviewed to monitor diabetic control, to care for joint disease, and to search for the development of complications (e.g., hepatocellular carcinoma).

Physical examination and screening tests to search for disordered iron metabolism should be carried out in family members to identify presymptomatic individuals so that iron can be removed before cirrhosis and other complications occur. Genetic studies may be of help.

# Primary biliary cirrhosis

Primary biliary cirrhosis (PBC) is a disease of unknown etiology, primarily affecting the middle-sized intrahepatic bile ducts as a nonsuppurative, destructive cholangitis, leading to bile duct damage, cholestasis, fibrosis, cirrhosis, and death from liver failure. It is more common in Europe than Africa and Asia with a prevalence of 3–35/ ·100,000 and an incidence of 6–15/million/ year.

## Clinical features

The disease is nine times more common in women. It usually presents in middle age with lethargy and pruritus. Pigmentation and xanthomata may be present, jaundice may develop, and portal hypertension may lead to ascites or esophageal varices. There may be stigmata of chronic liver disease. About 80% have hepatomegaly at presentation, and 50% have splenomegaly. The patient may be asymptomatic at presentation, or present with liver failure. The average life expectancy is 10 years from diagnosis.

PBC is associated with autoimmune conditions (e.g., Sjögren's syndrome, thyroid disease, Addison's disease, Raynaud's syndrome, systemic sclerosis, and celiac disease). It is also associated with malabsorption, extrahepatic malignancies, particularly of the breast, and hepatocellular carcinoma.

## Investigations

LFTs show an obstructive pattern with elevated serum alkaline phosphatase and gamma-glutamyl transpeptidase (GGT). As the disease progresses, serum bilirubin rises.

With regard to immunology, HLA-B8 and C4B2 are associated with a threefold increase in the risk of PBC. Serum immunoglobulins are raised, especially immunoglobulinM. Antimitochondrial antibody is positive in about 90%.

Ultrasound of the liver is important to exclude obstruction. It can also show evidence of portal hypertension and splenomegaly.

Histology of the liver will confirm the diagnosis. Initially there is asymmetrical destruction of middle-sized bile ducts and surrounding lymphocytic infiltrate. Granulomas may be present. Increasing fibrosis, and eventually cirrhosis, develops.

## Differential diagnosis

This includes autoimmune hepatitis, sarcoidosis, and drug reactions (e.g., phenothiazines).

## Treatment

Immunosuppressive agents may have a small effect. Bile salts (e.g., ursodeoxycholic acid) may help with cholestasis. Antifibrotic agents (e.g., colchicines) may be of help. Liver transplantation is indicated for intractable symptoms or end-stage disease.

Itching can be treated with cholestyramine. Alternatives include enzyme inducers (e.g., phenobarbitone) and opiate antagonists (e.g., naloxone or propofol). Patients with jaundice should receive supplementation with fat-soluble vitamins A, D, and K. Diarrhea is treated with a low-fat diet and pancreatic supplements.

# Hepatolenticular degeneration (Wilson's disease)

This is an autosomal recessive disorder of copper metabolism leading to deposition of copper in the following:

- Liver: cirrhosis with its ensuing complications.
- Basal ganglia: tremor and choreoathetosis.
- Cerebrum: dementia and seizures.
- Eyes: Kayser-Fleischer rings (a brown pigmentation of the periphery of the iris).
- Renal tubules: renal tubular acidosis.
- Bones: osteoporosis and osteoarthritis.
- Red blood cells: hemolytic anemia.

Clinical features are usually due to hepatic or CNS involvement.

## Investigations

There is a high concentration of copper in the blood, and low ceruloplasmin, the copper-binding protein. Cerebrospinal fluid studies also show increased copper concentrations, and levels can be monitored with treatment. Urinary copper excretion can also be monitored, and a penicillamine trial will increase copper excretion in patients with Wilson's disease. Liver biopsy, with cytology and hepatic copper quantification, can also help confirm the diagnosis of Wilson's disease.

## Management

The dietary intake of copper should be reduced, and penicillamine is given to aid the elimination of copper ions. Thirty percent of patients taking penicillamine have to stop because of side effects, which include skin changes, GI irritation, and aplastic anemia. Trientine is another copper chelator and has fewer side effects. Regular blood counts are mandatory due to potential agranulocytosis and thrombocytopenia with treatment. Other side effects include edema, proteinuria, hematuria, rashes, loss of taste, and muscle weakness. Relatives should be screened. The prognosis is generally good. For those with intractable liver disease, transplantation may be the only option. Of interest, psychiatric and neurologic complications gradually improve with transplantation.

## Alcoholic liver disease

Men who drink over 80g of alcohol per day (about 6–8 drinks) or women who drink over 40g per day have a significant risk of developing cirrhosis. However, cirrhosis is not inevitable. Only 10–20% of chronic alcoholics develop cirrhosis, even though they drink the same amount of alcohol over the same period as other alcoholics. Risk factors for developing cirrhosis include genetics, gender (women develop alcoholic hepatitis and cirrhosis at a younger age and after less intake than men), nutrition (alcohol is better tolerated under optimal dietary conditions), and a synergistic effect with hepatotropic viruses.

### Pathology

Initially there are fatty changes within the liver. With alcoholic hepatitis, there is liver cell necrosis and an inflammatory reaction. Cells contain alcoholic hyaline or Mallory's bodies. Later there is deposition of collagen around the central veins, which may spread to the portal tracts.

Cirrhosis may result, which is initially micronodular. Extensive fibrosis contributes to the development of portal hypertension. With continued cell necrosis and regeneration, the cirrhosis may progress to a macronodular pattern.

### Clinical features

The patient may initially be asymptomatic. With alcoholic hepatitis, there may be fatigue, anorexia, nausea, and weight loss. There may be signs of chronic liver disease (Chapter 10). Ascites may develop, and complicating hypoglycemia can precipitate coma.

Hepatic decompensation leads to encephalopathy and liver failure and can be precipitated by the factors listed in Fig. 32.6.

| Factors that can precipitate hepatic decompensation |
| --- |
| • constipation<br>• vomiting and diarrhea<br>• GI bleeding<br>• intercurrent infection<br>• alcohol<br>• morphine<br>• surgery<br>• electrolyte imbalance |

Fig. 32.6 Factors that can precipitate hepatic decompensation.

With advanced cirrhosis, there may be signs of malnutrition, ascites, encephalopathy, and a tendency to bleed. Signs include bilateral parotid enlargement, palmar erythema, Dupuytren's contractures, and multiple spider nevi. Men develop gynecomastia and testicular atrophy. Portal hypertension develops, leading to splenomegaly and distended abdominal wall veins.

There may be signs of alcohol damage in other organs (e.g., peripheral neuropathy, cardiomyopathy, proximal myopathy, or pancreatitis).

### Investigations

The mean corpuscular volume (MCV) and GGT are sensitive indices of alcohol ingestion. Important variables for predicting outcome include the prothrombin time, serum albumin, serum bilirubin, and hemoglobin.

Ultrasound will demonstrate fatty liver, and histology of liver biopsy will show the pathologic changes discussed above.

### Management

Patients should abstain from alcohol. General measures for the management of chronic liver disease should be initiated. Patients may need nutritional support, including vitamins B and C.

### Prognosis

Fatty liver alone carries a good prognosis if the patient abstains from alcohol. If the patient is encephalopathic and malnourished, the mortality is up to 50%. Ascites, peripheral edema, persistent jaundice, uremia, and the presence of collateral circulation are unfavorable prognostic signs.

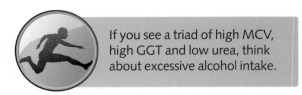

If you see a triad of high MCV, high GGT and low urea, think about excessive alcohol intake.

## Miscellaneous gastrointestinal disorders

### Gastroesophageal reflux disease

Reflux of gastric or duodenal contents into the esophagus causes heartburn and pain, often radiating to the back, which is worse on stooping or lying down, and with hot drinks. There may be bleeding from the esophagus resulting in anemia. There may be esophageal ulceration and stricture formation. Patients may have a "lump" in their throat or a brackish taste from hypersalivation. Dysphagia may result from chronic regurgitation. Eventually reflux can lead to esophagitis and bleeding from the esophagus, resulting in anemia. There may be esophageal ulceration and stricture formation. Chronic GERD may lead to intestinal columnar metaplasia of the distal esophagus called Barrett's esophagus, which predisposes the patient to adenocarcinoma. Barrett's esophagus is a premalignant chronic peptic metaplasia of the lower esophagus and may lead to dysphagia, vomiting, and hematemesis.

Predisposing factors include conditions that raise intra-abdominal pressure (e.g., tight clothes and obesity), a lax lower esophageal sphincter (e.g., with smoking and pregnancy), and drugs (e.g., tricyclic antidepressants and anticholinergic agents).

### Management

Patients should avoid tight clothes, stop smoking, avoid aggravating foods, and lose weight if overweight. Patients should be advised to prop themselves up in bed with pillows and put a block under the end of the bed to avoid slipping down. Drug treatment is initially with antacids or alginates, which coat the esophagus. Metoclopramide will increase the tone of the lower esophageal sphincter and relieves nausea. $H_2$-receptor antagonists are prescribed for severe symptoms. Proton pump inhibitors are the treatment of choice for erosive esophagitis. Anemia should be investigated and

managed appropriately. For patients who fail medical management, Nissen 360-degree fundoplication usually provides relief of symptoms.

## Irritable bowel syndrome

Irritable bowel syndrome is the most common diagnosis made in GI clinics, although there is no accepted definition. It occurs mainly in young women. There is intermittent colicky abdominal pain, which is relieved by bowel action, diarrhea or frequent passage of small amounts of stool, and bloating. The diarrhea may alternate with periods of constipation. Some people have a sense of incomplete evacuation or "rectal dissatisfaction." Symptoms may be precipitated by certain foods, drugs (e.g., antibiotics), or stress.

### Investigation

The diagnosis is one of exclusion. It is important not to miss more serious disease (e.g., inflammatory bowel disease or malignancy). It is prudent to check the CBC and erythrocyte sedimentation rate, fecal occult blood, and perform a sigmoidoscopy. Older patients, or patients in whom colonic carcinoma is suspected, warrant a barium enema.

### Treatment

Symptoms may improve with a high-fiber diet, with bran or with other agents which increase stool bulk. Specific aggravating foods should be avoided. In some patients there may be important psychologic aggravating factors which respond to reassurance. Antimotility drugs such as loperamide may relieve diarrhea, and antispasmodic drugs (e.g., mebeverine, 135 mg t.i.d.) may relieve pain. Opioids with a central action such as codeine are best avoided because of the risk of dependence. A new medication, tegaserod, was recently approved by the FDA to treat IBS. This medication is a derivative of serotonin that acts as a partial agonist at the 5-HT4 receptor. The most common side effects include diarrhea, abdominal pain, and headache.

## Pseudomembranous colitis

Pseudomembranous colitis is caused by colonization of the colon with *Clostridium difficile*, which produces toxins. It usually follows antibiotic therapy and should be suspected in patients in hospital who develop diarrhea after a period of antibiotics. It is usually of acute onset but may run a chronic course. The most frequently implicated antibiotic is clindamycin but few antibiotics are free of this side effect. Clinical features include diarrhea, fever and abdominal cramps.

## Diagnosis

Diagnosis is by identification of the toxin in stool specimens. Sigmoidoscopy reveals an erythematous, ulcerated mucosa, which is covered by a membrane. Sigmoidoscopy, however, is not essential for the diagnosis.

## Management

Suspected antibiotics should be stopped and patients should be isolated. Oral vancomycin or metronidazole is used as specific treatment.

## Diverticular disease

A diverticulum is an outpouching of the wall of the gut. Diverticula can occur anywhere in the gut but are most common in the colon, especially the sigmoid colon. Diverticulosis implies the presence of diverticula, and diverticulitis implies that there is inflammation within a diverticulum. They are due to high intracolonic pressure with weakness of the colonic wall. The weaknesses often occur at a site of blood vessel entry into the mucosa. The mucosa, therefore, herniates through the muscle layers of the gut. The incidence increases with age and affects up to a third of the population although most people are asymptomatic. It is more common in women then men.

## Clinical features

There may be colicky left-sided abdominal pain and tenderness, nausea, and flatulence. The pain may be relieved with defecation, and there may be a change in bowel habit with constipation or diarrhea. With diverticulitis, pain is more severe, and the patient is febrile. Diverticula may perforate and lead to localized or generalized peritonitis or fistula formation. Fistulas may communicate between the colon and bladder (vesicocolic fistula), leading to pneumaturia and recurrent urinary tract infection. They may also form between the colon and vagina or small bowel. Rectal bleeding may occur and is usually sudden and painless. Subacute obstruction may occur due to stricture formation. For recurrent diverticular bleeds, resection of the offending segment of colon is often necessary.

## Management

In acute diverticulitis, treatment is with bed rest, analgesia, and antibiotics. The patient may have to be kept NPD and given intravenous fluids. Abscesses may need to be drained, and peritonitis following perforation or obstruction may necessitate resection and colostomy. Patients with profuse rectal bleeding may require transfusion and colonic resection. Treatment of fistulas is surgical.

For diverticulosis, a high-fiber diet is recommended, and bran supplements and bulk-forming agents can be prescribed. Antispasmodics may provide symptomatic relief when colic is a problem. Drugs which slow intestinal motility (e.g., codeine and loperamide) could exacerbate symptoms and are contraindicated.

## Glomerulonephritis

Glomerular disease is often found to be confusing because there is a poor correlation between the clinical findings and the histology. Systemic disorders that can involve the glomerulus are listed in Fig. 33.1.

### Clinical features

Clinical features of glomerular disease include the following:

- Proteinuria (see also Chapter 13): up to 150mg of proteinuria daily is normal, but this may increase in pregnancy, febrile states, and following exercise. It may be preglomerular, as in the overproduction of small-sized proteins which pass freely across the glomerular basement membrane (e.g., Bence Jones protein in myeloma). It may be postglomerular with tubular damage. Gross proteinuria, which leads to hypoalbuminemia and edema, is called *nephrotic syndrome*.
- Hematuria.
- Raised blood urea or creatinine.
- *Nephritic syndrome*: this is a combination of proteinuria, hematuria and impaired renal function, often in association with oliguria and hypertension.

Most patients present with nephrotic syndrome, asymptomatic proteinuria, or hematuria. Presentation with oliguria or a nephritic syndrome is less common.

The causes of secondary nephrotic syndrome (i.e., not of direct renal origin) are summarized by the mnemonic **DAVID**: **d**iabetes mellitus, **a**myloidosis, **v**asculitis, **i**nfections, and **d**rugs.

### History

The history should include asking about hematuria and proteinuria (e.g., is there frothy urine?). There may also be a history of previous nephritis. Ask about associated systemic diseases (e.g., arthritis, diabetes, hypertension, or evidence of malignancy). A full drug history should be taken, including exposure to toxins.

Hearing impairment is present in Alport's syndrome (a hereditary nephritis with progressive glomerulonephritis, ocular abnormalities, and neural hearing loss), and there may be a family history of renal disease. Ask about recent upper respiratory tract infections and valvular heart disease.

### Consequences of glomerular dysfunction

The consequences of glomerular dysfunction include the following:

- Iron deficiency secondary to hematuria in a patient with limited iron reserves.
- Protein loss. The absolute level of plasma albumin necessary to induce edema varies from patient to patient.
- Hypovolemia resulting in postural hypotension or prerenal failure.
- Altered drug metabolism, usually secondary to hypoalbuminemia, leading to reduced binding and increased circulating levels of free drug.
- Hyperlipoproteinemia and hypercholesterolemia.
- Hypercoagulability due to urinary loss of anticoagulation proteins (e.g., protein S, protein C).
- Cardiovascular disease, including increased risk of venous and arterial thrombosis.
- Changes in serum immunoglobulins: IgG often falls and IgM is often raised in many patients with severe proteinuria. In IgA nephropathy up to 50% of patients have abnormally high serum IgA levels.
- Hormonal changes, including low circulating levels of 25-hydroxycalciferol and 1,25-

| Sytemic disorders that can involve the glomerulus |
|---|
| • diabetes |
| • amyloidosis |
| • systemic lupus erythematosus |
| • rheumatoid arthritis |
| • ankylosing spondylitis |
| • neoplasia |
| • myeloma |
| • vasculitic syndromes |
| • liver disease |
| • sarcoidosis |
| • partial lipodystrophy |

**Fig. 33.1** Systemic disorders that can involve the glomerulus.

dihydroxycholecalciferol. This results in decreased bone mobilization and gut absorption of calcium, and hence hypocalcemia.
- Increased risk of infection due to urinary losses of some immunoglobulins, as noted above.
- Pancreatitis precipitated by high serum triglyceride levels.

## Investigations

The following investigations are important in the patient with glomerular disease:
- Electrolyes, blood urea nitrogen (BUN), serum creatinine.
- Plasma albumin and creatinine, creatinine clearance, and 24-hour urinary protein excretion serve as a baseline and can be used to monitor progress and response to treatment.
- Urine microscopy for red blood cell casts indicating glomerular disease.
- Blood glucose: to exclude diabetes mellitus (DM).
- Anti-DNA and antinuclear antibodies in systemic lupus erythematosus (SLE).
- Antiglomerular basement membrane (anti-GBM) antibodies for the diagnosis of anti-GBM disease.
- Hepatitis B surface antigen to exclude hepatitis B.
- Tests for rheumatoid arthritis (e.g., Rose-Waaler and Latex tests).
- Serum immunoelectrophoresis to exclude myeloma.
- Antineutrophil cytoplasmic antibodies are often present in microscopic polyarteritis and Wegener's granulomatosis.
- Cryoglobulins.
- Serologic tests for syphilis.

- Serum complement levels: C3 may be low in postinfectious glomerulonephropathy, mesangiocapillary glomerulonephropathy, and SLE; C4 may be depleted in SLE and mesangiocapillary glomerulonephropathy.
- Chest x-ray: this may show pulmonary edema, malignancy, pulmonary hemorrhage, and cavitation in Wegener's granulomatosis.

## Histologic classification, treatment, and prognosis

The terms "focal" and "diffuse" refer to the kidney as a whole, i.e., some or all of the glomeruli are involved. "Segmental" and "global" refer to individual glomeruli, i.e., part or all of each glomerulus is involved. Because of clinical overlap, the diagnosis is confirmed only after renal biopsy. Biopsies should not be taken if there is only one functioning kidney, bilateral small kidneys, or a bleeding disorder.

### General principles of management

In glomerulonephritis with a specific etiology, specific action can be taken (e.g., withdrawal of an offending drug or treatment of a malignancy or infection). Adequate protein and calorie intake is most important. Potent acting loop diuretics may be needed to produce natiuresis and reduce edema. It may be necessary to give an infusion of salt-poor albumin to maintain plasma volume at the same time. (Note: The latter treatment is controversial.)

Patients tend to have hyperlipidemia and are at high cardiovascular risk. If there is any evidence of coronary artery disease, treatment with a statin should be started. Hypertension should be controlled, and nephrotoxic agents should be stopped. If renal function does not improve, treatment of chronic renal failure should be considered.

### Minimal change nephropathy

This is most common in boys under 5 years of age and accounts for 90% of children in the U.S. who present with nephrotic syndrome. Renal biopsy is therefore not always indicated and is usually reserved for patients who do not respond to steroid therapy. Light microscopy is normal, but electron microscopy reveals retraction and fusion of the epithelial foot processes at the glomerular basement membrane. There are no deposits of immunoglobulin or complement on immunofluorescence. There is usually severe and selective proteinuria, which remits with corticosteroid therapy. In patients with frequently relapsing disease, a course of cyclophosphamide for a maximum of 8 weeks can be considered.

Patients often relapse after infections, especially upper respiratory infections. While most of these exacerbations can be treated on an outpatient basis, severe edema can lead to intravascular hypovolemia and prerenal renal failure. In such cases inpatient treatment with albumn infusion (to draw fluid back into the vasculature) is most appropriate.

## Focal segmental glomerulosclerosis

This is the most common cause of nephrotic syndrome in adults. Histology shows a proliferation of sclerotic lesions, but electron microscopy and immunofluorescence findings are variable. Nephrotic syndrome is the usual presentation, and progressive renal impairment occurs in 80–90% of patients. It is associated with SLE, polyarteritis nodosa (PAN), subacute bacterial endocarditis, Henoch–Schönlein purpura, sickle cell anemia, type 1 diabetes, HIV infection, and Wegener's granulomatosis.

Adults are treated initially with high-dose prednisone, then continued on cyclosporine. Patients who have become steroid-dependent may benefit from tacrolimus. In patients not responsive to steroids, the 5-year renal survival rate is about 50%.

## Diffuse mesangial proliferation

This is associated with IgA deposition (Berger's disease), seen on immunofluorescence, and cellular proliferation within the glomerular mesangium. It usually presents with intermittent hematuria in the second and third decades of life. There may be an associated upper respiratory tract or gut infection.

It is also associated with SLE, cirrhosis, hepatitis B infection and Henoch–Schönlein purpura. About one-third of patients will eventually require dialysis or transplantation.

## Membranous nephropathy

This is most common in adults with a peak age at onset of 40–50 years. It may be idiopathic with strong human lymphocyte antigen associations, or it may occur in association with drugs such as gold and penicillamine, neoplasms, or infections such as hepatitis B. Patients usually present with proteinuria or nephrotic syndrome.

Histologically there is thickening of the glomerular wall, with subepithelial deposits of antigen-antibody complexes visible on electron microscopy. Immunofluorescence shows deposition of IgG and C3. About one-third of patients improve spontaneously, a third have persistent proteinuria, and a third progress to renal failure. Women and children have a better prognosis than men. When renal function is declining quickly, corticosteroids and azathioprine may be effective.

## Mesangiocapillary glomerulonephritis

This presents with hematuria, proteinuria, nephrotic syndrome, or renal impairment. There appears to be a layer of tissue beneath the glomerular basement membrane, giving it a double contour on light microscopy. In type I, there may be subendothelial extension of mesangial matrix and cells containing immune deposits and C3, and in type II or dense deposit disease there may be electron dense material incorporated into the membrane.

Overall, type I lesions have a 50% 5-year survival rate, and type II is generally regarded as having a worse outcome.

## Diffuse proliferative glomerulonephritis

This often occurs in association with acute infections, classically with streptococcus. It often heals completely after an acute nephritic illness. Light microscopy shows hypercellular glomerular tufts with proliferation of mesangial cells which have a neutrophilic and mononuclear cell infiltrate. Complexes containing IgG can be seen on immunofluorescence along the glomerular basement membrane and in the mesangium.

## Crescentic glomerulonephritis

This is usually rapidly progressive, and presents with hematuria, oliguria, and hypertension. It results from the proliferation of epithelial cells. It may occur in SLE, anti-GBM disease, and vasculitides but often occurs in the absence of underlying disease. The prognosis is usually poor, but it is potentially curable if treatment is instituted at a sufficiently early stage. Treatments consists of pulse methylpednisolone and should be started as early as possible in the course of the disease. Some evidence also supports the use of cyclophosphamide for 6 months.

## Antiglomerular basement membrane disease

There is the even and linear deposition of IgG along the glomerular basement membrane, with a variable inflammatory response. At its most destructive, this produces a neutrophilic cell infiltrate, heavy fibrin deposition, and extensive epithelial crescent formation.

Goodpasture's syndrome is anti-GBM disease associated with pulmonary hemorrhage. Note, however, that patients with SLE, Henoch–Schönlein purpura, Wegener's granulomatosis, and microscopic polyarteritis can also have pulmonary hemorrhage. Goodpasture's syndrome is strongly associated with cigarette smoking.

Treatment with plasma exchange and immunosuppressive drugs remove and suppress the antibody, together with the reversal of its renal and pulmonary effects.

### Wegener's granulomatosis and microscopic polyarteritis

The incidence of these uncommon conditions appears to be increasing. They are strongly associated with circulating antibody directed at cytoplasmic components of normal neutrophils. Early recognition is important as treatment may prevent progression. Combination of prednisone and immunosuppressive therapy produces a survival rate of 80% at 5 years.

## Acute renal failure

Acute renal failure (ARF) is a rapid decline in glomerular filtration rate (GFR) sufficient to cause uremia. Oliguria (below 15mL per hour) is often a feature, although nonoliguric renal failure can also occur, particularly in patients with severe burns, nephrotoxic damage, or oliguric renal failure that has been converted to nonoliguric renal failure by aggressive management with fluids, diuretics, and other agents.

Remember that a doubling of the creatinine is the result of loss of 50% of renal function. Therefore, if a patient who has a baseline creatinine of 0.4mg/dL comes to the hospital with a creatinine of 1.0mg/dL (still within normal limits), the patient is in renal failure. This situation arises in the elderly, who, because of loss of muscle mass have very low creatinine at baseline. Always check old lab values to determine baseline when they are available.

### Etiology

It is useful to classify ARF into prerenal, renal, and postrenal causes (Fig. 33.2). However, the etiology is often multifactorial. For example, in postsurgical

ARF, fluid depletion, systemic infection, and nephrotoxic drugs may all play a role. ARF may also complicate chronic renal failure.

### Clinical features

The clinical features depend on whether there is pre-existing chronic renal impairment and whether the cause is pre-, renal-, or post-renal failure. A full history should be taken, focusing on previous renal disease, a history of hypertension or analgesic abuse, symptoms of prostatism, recent diarrhea, vomiting or blood loss, and recent operations.

Symptoms of renal failure include:
- Thirst.
- Polyuria.
- Nocturia.
- Anorexia.
- Nausea and vomiting.
- Fatigue.
- Itching.
- Confusion.
- Oliguria.
- Dehydration.
- Signs of volume overload (e.g., pulmonary edema and ankle or sacral edema) with nephrotic syndrome.
- Signs of volume depletion (e.g., postural hypotension, a rapid small volume pulse, reduced tissue turgor).

The examination should focus on both the cause and consequences of the renal failure. The patient may have a yellow-brown pallor of uremia, and brown lines at the ends of the finger nails. If acidotic, there is deep sighing (Kussmaul's) respiration. There may be palpable kidneys with polycystic kidney disease or hydronephrosis. There will be a palpable bladder with outflow obstruction.

Pericarditis occurs in advanced uremia, and twitching, hiccoughs, and uremic frost also occur late. Check the blood pressure (are there other signs of malignant hypertension, and/or is there a postural drop suggesting volume depletion?) and look for bruising.

Perform a rectal examination for prostatic hypertrophy or carcinoma, and a vaginal examination for pelvic masses.

### Investigations

Urea, creatinine, and electrolytes should be assessed, in addition to strict recording of fluid intake and

| Causes of acute renal failure | |
|---|---|
| prerenal failure (ischemic) | extracellular volume loss: GI loss (e.g. severe diarrhea or vomiting), urinary loss (polyuria with salt-losing kidneys), burns<br>intravascular volume loss or redistribution: sepsis, hemorrhage (e.g. postpartum or at operation), hypoalbuminemia<br>decreased cardiac output: heart failure (e.g. postmyocardial infarction), cardiac tamponade, cardiac surgery<br>miscellaneous: hypercalcemia, hepatorenal syndrome, rhabdomyolysis |
| renal failure | postischemic acute tubular necrosis: shock, trauma, sepsis, hypoxia<br>nephrotoxic acute tubular necrosis: antibiotics, analgesics, contrast media, heavy metals, solvents, proteins<br>glomerulonephritis: acute diffuse proliferative nephritis<br>acute pyelonephritis<br>acute interstitial nephritis: antibiotics, analgesics, leptospirosis, *Legionella*, viral infections<br>vasculitis: polyarteritis<br>intratubular obstruction: myeloma (Bence–Jones protein), urate<br>coagulopathies: acute cortical necrosis, hemolytic uremic syndrome, thrombotic thrombocytopenic purpura, postpartum renal failure<br>miscellaneous: malignant hypertension |
| postrenal failure | renal tract obstruction: stones, tumor (prostatic or pelvic), prostatic hypertrophy, surgical mishap (e.g. accidental ligation of ureters), periureteric fibrosis, bladder dysfunction<br>major vessel occlusion: renal artery thrombosis, renal vein thrombosis |

**Fig. 33.2** Causes of acute renal failure. (GI, gastrointestinal.)

output. This will confirm renal impairment and serve as a useful baseline for monitoring the patient's progress. If the patient is acidotic, serum bicarbonate will be low. It is crucial to check the potassium as hyperkalemia can be life-threatening, and immediate measures to lower the potassium need to be taken.

Urine should be sent for microscopy, culture, and sensitivity. In patients with acute tubular necrosis there will be casts, whereas these are absent in prerenal failure.

Patients with established acute tubular necrosis cannot concentrate the urine or conserve sodium. Consequently urinary sodium is usually over 20mEq/L; the urine is dilute (osmolality below 310mEq/L) with a urine/plasma osmolality ratio below 1.1:1; and urinary urea is below 150mEq/L with a urine/plasma urea ratio below 3:1.

Conversely, in prerenal failure, urinary sodium is below 20mEq/L; the urine is concentrated (osmolality over 450mEq/L) with a urine/plasma osmolality ratio over 1.5:1; and urinary urea is over 330mEq/L with a urine/plasma urea ratio over 8:1.

In prerenal failure the serum BUN to creatinine ratio is also increased. During times of intravascular hypovolemia, the kidney preferentially retains urea to increase the osmotic load to which the loop of Henle is exposed. By increasing the urea concentration, more water is pulled out of the loop of Henle as it dips toward the renal medulla. This allows the body to conserve more water and alleviates the hypovolemia. Prerenal states can lead to a BUN/creatinine ratio >30:1.

In addition, the following investigations are important in the patient with ARF:
- Complete blood count: a normochromic normocytic anemia suggests pre-existing chronic renal impairment.
- Coagulation panel for coagulopathies.
- Urine for Bence–Jones protein; serum immunoglobulins and electrophoresis.
- Blood cultures to look for infection.
- Electrocardiogram (ECG) for the precipitating cause (e.g., myocardial infarction) or complications such as pericarditis or hyperkalemia.
- Abdominal x-ray: look for renal size; normal kidneys are $13 \pm 2$ cm; small kidneys suggest pre-existing renal disease; the kidneys may be large in polycystic disease; stones in the renal tract may be visible.

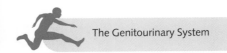

- Abdominal ultrasound will demonstrate kidney size, as well as stones and dilatation of the pelvicalyceal system in outflow obstruction.
- Isotope renography will demonstrate kidney function.
- CT scan, especially noncontrast, can be very helpful in evaluating kidney stones, renal cell carcinoma, cysts, and even renal vein thrombosis.
- Renal biopsy should be performed in patients to confirm the diagnosis of glomerulonephritis or vasculitis. The biopsy can help direct treatment.

## Management

Immediate thoughts should be to correct hypovolemia, exclude obstruction, and assess the presence of previous intrinsic renal disease. Fluids should be replaced and electrolytes should be corrected quickly. Monitoring with a central venous pressure line is essential for proper assessment of fluid balance. Appropriate antibiotics should be given for septicemia or other infections. Bilateral nephrostomy tubes will relieve obstruction. Surgery can then be performed later.

If there is established acute tubular acidosis, intravenous fluids may still be needed. Vasoactive agents (e.g., dopamine and dobutamine) may be necessary to achieve a blood pressure which is appropriate for the patient's age and history. Correction of hypoxia and acidosis may also improve cardiac and renal function.

If oliguria persists after adequate circulation is established, or if the patient has established renal failure and is volume overloaded, intravenous furosemide should be given, either as slow boluses or as an intravenous infusion. Strict fluid balance should be kept with daily weights and regular assessment of fluid, electrolyte, and nutritional requirements. In general, patients should be given 500ml of fluid per 24 hours as well as the volume of urine output from the previous 24 hours. In patients with fluid retention a weight loss of 0–1kg per day should be aimed for.

Note, however, that fluid overload may occur in patients without any change in weight, as negative nutritional balance may cause a loss of 1–2kg per day. Careful examination is necessary to detect fluid accumulation, which should be counteracted by further sodium and water restriction. Patients should be on a low-protein, high-carbohydrate diet. In many cases, the patient's appetite is poor and calorie supplements may be required.

### Treatment of hyperkalemia

Because this may be life-threatening, reduction of potassium should be the top priority if it is above 7 mEq/L, particularly if ECG changes are present. These ECG changes can be reversed temporarily by boluses of 10ml of 10% calcium gluconate solution. The patient should also be on a cardiac monitor.

Potassium should be redistributed intracellularly by the correction of acidosis with sodium bicarbonate 100–150mmol/L and the administration of glucose 50–100mg. Insulin may be necessary to control hyperglycemia. It is usually necessary to give these drugs in small volumes in order to avoid fluid overload. Polystyrene sulphonate resin (Kayexalate), 20g 6 hourly orally, or as an enema (30g), will maintain a low potassium.

Do not give calcium chloride IV through the same canula as sodium bicarbonate—it forms chalk!

### Indications for dialysis in renal failure

Indications for dialysis in renal failure are as follows:
- Persistent hyperkalemia (e.g., serum potassium above 6.5mEq/L).
- Severe acidosis (e.g., bicarbonate below 15mEq/L).
- Symptomatic uremia (e.g., confusion and hiccoughs).
- Pericarditis.
- Pulmonary edema or progressive fluid retention.

### Prognosis

The prognosis of patients with ARF depends on the cause. Patients with nonoliguric ARF have a lower mortality rate. A particularly high mortality rate is found in older patients and those who have severe burns, severe pancreatitis, hepatorenal syndrome, intra-abdominal sepsis, pre-existing cardiovascular disease, or serious complications, such as pulmonary infection. Patients who recover generally return to health and independent living, and this justifies an aggressive approach to treatment.

## Chronic renal failure

Chronic renal disease can be shown by any significant rise in creatinine that is sustained for 3 months. A GFR <15mL/min is generally termed end-stage renal disease (ESRD) or renal failure. Features that suggest chronic rather than acute renal failure include a long history of urinary symptoms and chronic ill health, anemia, osteodystrophy, and small kidneys.

### Causes

Finding the cause of renal failure is important because some are reversible and treatment can delay or prevent progression to ESRD. In addition, the prognosis can be better determined, risks of rejection with renal transplantation can be assessed, and diagnosis of familial disease may benefit other members of the family by early diagnosis, treatment, and genetic counseling.

Common causes include the following:

- Glomerulonephritis: the most common single cause of ESRD, accounting for more than a third of cases.
- Infection: mainly due to obstruction or vesicoureteric reflux.
- Obstruction: most cases are due to prostatic hypertrophy and stones.
- Renovascular causes: renovascular atheroma and consequent ischemia are becoming increasingly recognized, reflecting the ageing population. Risk factors include age, a history of cardiac, cerebral or peripheral vascular disease, smoking, hypertension, and diabetes.
- Drugs: analgesic nephropathy should be considered in patients with chronic painful conditions but may also be taken for "social" reasons. Nonsteroidal anti-inflammatory drugs (NSAIDs) can cause ESRD.
- Interstitial nephritis: this may be idiopathic but also secondary to NSAIDs and chronic diuretic therapy with furosemide.
- DM: both insulin-dependent and non-insulin-dependent diabetes can lead to ESRD.
- Hypertension: the incidence of ESRD seems to be decreasing due to better identification and treatment of hypertension. It is more common in the black population.
- Inherited disease: the two most common conditions are polycystic kidney disease and Alport's disease.
- Idiopathic causes.
- Less common causes are amyloidosis, myeloma, SLE, PAN, gout, hypercalcemia, and retroperitoneal fibrosis.

### Clinical features

These are outlined in the features of ARF.

Specific questions in the history should include symptoms of prostatism, previous urinary tract infections, a drug history (especially of analgesics), and family history (polycystic kidneys?).

There may be signs of anemia and brown lines on the finger nails. The skin is classically "lemon yellow," and there may be bruising. There may be a pericardial rub or signs of neuropathy, and hyperventilation secondary to acidosis may be present. The blood pressure may be elevated. Examine for signs of obstruction (e.g., a palpable bladder), and perform a rectal examination for prostatic hypertrophy or pelvic masses. The kidneys are large in polycystic disease.

### Investigations

The following are important investigations in the patient with chronic renal failure:

- Urine: microscopy for casts and culture to exclude infection. Urinary electrolytes and osmolality should be determined. 24-hour urinary protein and creatinine clearance should be measured.
- Urea and electrolytes will help determine the degree of renal dysfunction and acidosis. Serum calcium may be low secondary to hyperphosphatemia or acquired vitamin D resistance. The acidosis protects the patient from tetany by increasing the ionized portion of the reduced calcium. Serum phosphate is high and plasma uric acid is often raised although clinical gout is uncommon.
- A fasting blood glucose should be done to exclude diabetes. Other investigations include those to elucidate an underlying cause for the renal failure such as a myeloma screen.
- Plain abdominal film will define kidney size, and ultrasound will exclude obstruction. X-rays of the chest and hands may show evidence of secondary hyperparathyroidism.
- Renal biopsy should be considered once prerenal and postrenal disease have been excluded, especially if renal size is normal, suggesting more acute disease.

More than 50% of glomeruli may be lost before the U&Es become abnormal.

## Management

The aims of treatment are to prevent further deterioration in renal function and to prevent or treat the complications of renal failure. Renal function should be monitored with reciprocal plots of serum creatinine (Fig. 33.3). Whenever an abrupt decline or acceleration in the slope is noted, its cause must be determined and rectified.

Possible causes include uncontrolled hypertension, infection, hypovolemia or fluid overload, urinary tract obstruction, drugs, and pregnancy. Always question whether the drugs that the patient is on are necessary, in particular NSAIDs, and angiotensin-converting enzyme (ACE) inhibitors in patients with renovascular disease. Other drugs to avoid include tetracycline, polymyxin, nitrofurantoin, aminoglycosides, and potassium-sparing diuretics (e.g., amiloride and spironolactone).

### Prevention of decline in renal function

Hypertension should be tightly controlled (to about 130/85 mmHg).

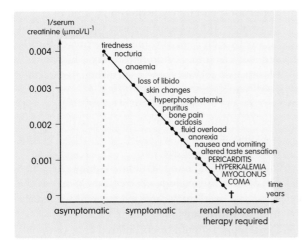

**Fig. 33.3** Inverse creatinine plot with typical progressive onset of the nonspecific symptoms and signs of chronic renal failure.

Restriction of dietary phosphate intake may delay the decline in renal function, although it is difficult to achieve as it is often accompanied by a concomitant decrease in calcium intake, which can accelerate the development of renal osteodystrophy.

A low-protein diet may also reduce the decline in renal function and can reduce the symptoms of uremia. Protein intake is reduced from a normal 85 g per day to 40 g per day. If protein intake is lowered further, essential amino acids should be added and the overall calorie intake should be high enough to suppress the breakdown of body protein using carbohydrate supplements if necessary. Total serum protein, albumin, transferrin, vitamin $B_{12}$, and red blood cell folate levels should be measured at regular intervals.

Potassium restriction may be necessary to prevent hyperkalemia, along with sodium restriction to prevent fluid retention.

ACE inhibitors slow down the decline in renal function associated with diabetic nephropathy.

### Prevention of complications
#### Hypertension

Regular measurements of blood pressure are necessary as the onset of hypertension is insidious. Control of hypertension can slow the deterioration of renal function and prevent cardiovascular complications. High doses of furosemide are often required and, in resistant cases, minoxidil is a potent antihypertensive agent. All classes of antihypertensives may be used but ACE inhibitors are contraindicated in renal artery stenosis.

#### Renal osteodystrophy

Renal osteodystrophy is due to a combination of disturbed vitamin D metabolism and secondary hyperparathyroidism. Serum alkaline phosphatase is raised. Management is by the normalization of serum phosphate by diet and oral phosphate-binding agents such as calcium carbonate. Serum calcium should be maintained in the normal range with synthetic vitamin D analogues. Frequent monitoring of serum calcium is required for the early detection of hypercalcemia, which will further decrease renal function.

#### Systemic acidosis

Systemic acidosis accompanies declining renal function and may contribute to increased potassium levels. Sodium bicarbonate supplements will help to maintain serum bicarbonate levels within the normal range.

### Anemia

In renal failure there is a normochromic normocytic anemia. Evidence of blood loss should be sought if there is an inappropriately low hemoglobin. Vitamin $B_{12}$ and folate deficiency should be corrected with diet and supplements if needed. Recombinant human erythropoietin will increase the hemoglobin and improve symptoms attributable to anemia, but it can cause hypertension and convulsions.

### Nausea and vomiting

This often responds to protein restriction or antiemetics (e.g., metaclopramide). Dialysis should be considered if these measures are unsuccessful.

### Pruritus

This can lead to excoriation of the skin, bleeding, and secondary infection. The correction of serum calcium and phosphate may help, and antipruritic agents such as chlorpheniramine may also be of value.

### Peripheral neuropathy

Dialysis should produce an improvement.

### Hyperuricemia

Treatment with allopurinol may be required.

### End-stage renal disease

ESRD is identified on biochemical and clinical grounds as that point when, despite conservative measures, the patient will die without the institution of renal replacement by dialysis or transplantation. Specific indications for dialysis in ESRD include symptomatic uremia, hyperkalemia, metabolic acidosis, peripheral neuropathy, pericarditis, central nervous system disorders, and poor control of ESRD by conservative treatment. Problems with dialysis include infection, hypotension, hemorrhage, and the maintenance of fluid and electrolyte balance.

Renal transplantation is becoming increasingly common. Patients are on immunosuppressive drugs (e.g., cyclosporin, prednisolone, and azathioprine), which have their own problems such as susceptibility to opportunistic infections, skin malignancies, and cyclosporin-induced nephrotoxicity.

Other complications of transplantation include rejection, obstruction at the ureteric anastamosis, and persisting hypertension.

## Urinary tract infection

Urinary tract infections (UTIs) are one of the most common infections encountered in general practice. Women are more prone to UTIs than men, except during the first few months of life and in old age. Approximately 25–35% of all women have symptoms of UTI at some stage in their lives.

UTI is a general term referring to the presence of micro-organisms in the urine. Significant bacteriuria is defined as urine that yields more than 100,000 organisms per mL on culture. The causes of UTI are given in Fig. 33.4.

### Lower urinary tract infections

Lower UTIs may take the following forms:
- Cystitis: a symptomatic infection of the bladder in the presence of significant bacteriuria.
- Asymptomatic bacteriuria: the patient has no symptoms, but urine culture yields a growth of over 100,000 per mL.
- Acute urethral syndromes: symptomatically similar to cystitis but the urine culture may be sterile.

### Upper urinary tract infections

Upper UTIs may take the following forms:
- Acute pyelonephritis: an inflammatory process within the renal parenchyma, most commonly caused by bacterial infection.
- Chronic pyelonephritis: this is usually the result of long-standing bacterial infection, which usually occurs in childhood. Urinary tract obstruction and vesicoureteric reflux are associated with eventual parenchymal scarring, which is characteristic of chronic pyelonephritic kidneys.

---

**Precipitating causes of urinary tract infection**

- stones
- obstruction
- polycystic kidneys
- papillary necrosis
- diabetes mellitus
- analgesic nephropathy
- sickle cell disease
- sexual intercourse
- pregnancy
- bladder catheterization

**Fig. 33.4** Precipitating causes of urinary tract infection.

The causes of sterile pyuria (a common exam question) are:
- Tuberculosis of the urinary tract.
- Analgesic nephropathy.
- Neoplasms.
- Catheterization.
- Fevers in children.
- Intra-abdominal inflammation (e.g., appendicitis).
- Surgery involving the urinary tract.

Infection usually occurs by ascent of the invading organism from the urethra into the bladder. Colonization of the ureters may then occur, and from there to the kidneys. This is facilitated by vesicoureteric reflux. The hematogenous route of infection is less common but may occur secondarily to bacteremia, septicemia, or endocarditis.

The most common pathogen is *Escherichia coli*. Other organisms include *Proteus*, *Klebsiella*, staphylococci, and streptococci. *Pseudomonas* may be present after catheterization. In patients with long-term catheters mixed infections can be a significant problem.

### Clinical features

Symptoms of lower UTI are suprapubic pain, frequency, nocturia, dysuria, and strangury. Upper UTIs such as acute pyelonephritis or renal abscesses present with fever, rigors, loin pain, vomiting, and weight loss.

### Investigations

Obvious predisposing factors such as pregnancy or diabetes should be considered. Indications for further investigations include relapsing infections, childhood onset, male sex, urological symptoms, persistent hematuria, unusual organisms (such as *Pseudomonas*), and frequent recurrence of infections.

Initial investigations should involve an ultrasound scan, which will determine renal size, cysts, obstruction, and residual urine; abdominal x-rays involving the kidneys, ureters, and bladder will detect radiopaque stones.

An intravenous urogram (IVU) often complements the above investigations, and gives a better demonstration of parenchymal scars and calyceal clubbing. A micturating cystogram is used to detect vesicoureteric reflux, and bladder and urethral abnormalities, especially in children. Scarring may also be demonstrated on isotope and computed tomography (CT) scanning.

### Management

Treatment is usually started after urine has been sent for culture and antibiotic sensitivities, but before results are available. Antibiotics may then be changed if necessary according to the results. High fluid intake should be encouraged. More than 80% of lower UTIs respond to a 48-hour course of an antibiotic such as trimethoprim or amoxycillin. If the urinary tract is structurally abnormal, a 5–10 day course of therapy is indicated. Follow-up microscopy and culture should be carried out to ensure eradication of organisms and pyuria (especially in pregnant women, who should be treated with amoxicillin). Patients with a sulfa allergy can be treated with flouroquinolone.

Patients with acute pyelonephritis usually require admission to hospital for intravenous fluids and antibiotics. Acetaminophen will reduce the temperature, but stronger analgesia may be required.

Patients with frequent reinfection require a high fluid intake, and frequent and complete voiding should be encouraged. Long-term, low-dose prophylaxis using antibiotics such as trimethoprim, 100mg, or nitrofurantoin, 50mg per day, may be of benefit, but the need for continued treatment should be reassessed after 6 months.

If infection is related to sexual intercourse, the patient should void after intercourse and may benefit from a single dose of an antibiotic.

## Fluid and electrolyte balance

In a 70-kg man, the total fluid volume is 42L (i.e., 60% of the body weight). The intracellular fluid volume is 28L or two-thirds of the total body fluid, and the extracellular fluid volume is 14L or one-third of the total body fluid. The intravascular component is 3 liters (plasma contributing to 5L of blood).

The average total fluid intake in 24 hours is 2500mL (1500mL drunk, 800mL in food, and 200ml via the metabolism of food). The output matches this via urine, insensible loss, and stool.

Sodium ingestion is about 80mEq in 24 hours and potassium is also 80mEq in 24 hours.

**Fig. 33.5** Causes of hyponatremia. (ADH, antidiuretic hormone; CNS, central nervous system; GFR, glomerular filtration rate; GI, gastrointestinal; i.v., intravenous.)

| Causes of hyponatremia | |
|---|---|
| **Cause** | **Examples** |
| sodium and water retention | secondary hyperaldosteronism, e.g., cardiac failure hypoproteinemia, e.g., nephrotic syndrome reduced GFR, e.g., renal failure |
| sodium and water depletion | losses from GI tract, renal and skin (see above) |
| normal total body sodium (excessive ADH effect) | CNS disease, e.g., encephalitis drugs, e.g., chlorpropamide, carbemazepine glucocorticoid deficiency inappropriate ADH secretion |
| artifact | blood taken from arm with i.v. fluids marked hyperlipidemia or hypoproteinemia |

## Salt and water balance

Water depletion results from reduced intake or increased losses. Examples of the former include an inability to get water (e.g., unconsciousness or extreme weakness), inability to swallow (e.g., causes of dysphagia), and nausea. Increased losses usually occur via the skin (e.g., fever, thyrotoxicosis), lungs (e.g., hyperventilation), and urine (e.g., diabetes insipidus).

Water and sodium depletion tend to occur together. Causes of mixed depletion of water and sodium include loss from the following:

- Gastrointestinal tract (e.g., vomiting, watery diarrhea, fistulous drainage, and paralytic ileus).
- Urinary tract (e.g., overuse of diuretics, osmotic diuresis [in DM], chronic renal failure, and renal tubular damage such as the relief of obstruction), and Addison's disease.
- Skin (e.g., excessive sweating, exfoliative dermatitis, and burns).
- Others (e.g., ascites and inferior vena caval thrombosis).

Clinically, hyponatremia (Fig. 33.5) leads to confusion and fits. Hypernatremia (Fig. 33.6) leads to thirst, confusion, and coma.

Water deficiency may show as hypotension. The pulse will be thready and fast, the skin is dry and turgor is reduced, and there is peripheral vasoconstriction. The urea, hemoglobin, packed cell volume, and plasma protein tend to rise. Water excess (Chapter 12) leads to hypertension, cardiac failure, edema, headache, anorexia, nausea, muscle weakness, and later confusion, fits, and coma. Investigations show hemodilution (reduced packed cell volume).

| Causes of hypernatremia | |
|---|---|
| low total body sodium | extrarenal, e.g., sweating, diarrhea renal—osmotic diuresis |
| normal total body sodium | high temperatures diabetes insipidus |
| high total body sodium | steroid excess, e.g., Cushing's. Conn's iatrogenic, e.g., hypertonic sodium infusions self-induced, e.g., ingestion of sodium chloride tablets |

**Fig. 33.6** Causes of hypernatremia.

## Management of hyponatremia

Treat the underlying cause. If the patient is not dehydrated fluid intake should be restricted to 500–1000mL in 24 hours; diuretics should also be considered. If the patient is dehydrated, an infusion of 0.9% saline can be given.

Too rapid an increase in sodium may lead to central pontine myelinolysis, or severe shrinking of the brain cells, which can lead to death.

## Management of hypernatremia

Treat the underlying cause. Water is given orally or as intravenous 5% dextrose guided by the urine output and plasma sodium. In severe hypernatremia, 0.9% saline should be used initially to avoid too rapid a drop in sodium concentration (to avoid cerebral edema).

## Hypokalemia

The causes of hypokalemia are given in Fig. 33.7. The clinical features of hypokalemia are muscle

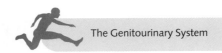
| Causes of hypokalemia | |
|---|---|
| Cause | Examples |
| losses | gastrointestinal: chronic laxative abuse, diarrhea and vomiting, villous papilloma of the colon<br>renal: diuretics (e.g. thiazides and furosemide), hyperaldosteronism, glucocorticoid excess (including treatment with steroids, and ACTH-secreting tumors), renal tubular acidosis, Bartter's syndrome<br>inadequate replacement: postoperative, diuretic phase of acute renal failure |
| redistribution of potassium | alkalosis<br>insulin overdose<br>familial periodic paralysis |
| secretion of atrial natriuretic peptide | paroxysmal SVT |

**Fig. 33.7** Causes of hypokalemia (ACTH, adrenocorticotrophic hormone; SVT, supraventricular tachycardia.)

| Causes of hyperkalemia | |
|---|---|
| Cause | Examples |
| excessive oral intake | potassium supplements |
| diminished renal excretion | renal failure<br>potassium sparing diuretic in combination with renal failure, e.g. amiloride, spironolactone |
| redistribution of potassium | hemolysis, e.g. incompatible blood transfusion, DIC<br>acidosis<br>tissue necrosis, e.g. burns |
| artifact | delay in separation of plasma or serum, improper storage conditions |

**Fig. 33.8** Causes of hyperkalemia (DIC, disseminated intravascular coagulation).

weakness, apathy, anorexia, confusion, ileus, increased cardiac excitability, digitalis toxicity, thirst, polyuria, renal lesions (e.g., Fanconi's syndrome), interstitial inflammation, and fibrosis in severe prolonged depletion. The ECG changes are described in Chapter 29.

### Management
The underlying cause should be identified and treated. If hypokalemia is mild, oral potassium supplements are given. These are rarely required for patients on thiazides. If the patient is severely hypokalemic, the cautious infusion of intravenous potassium should be considered (but not more than 20mEq per hour).

## Hyperkalemia
The causes of hyperkalemia are given in Fig. 33.8. The management of hyperkalemia is described on p. 300.

Hyperkalemia causes large T waves on the ECG, hypokalemia causes small ones—large pot, lots of tea; small pot, no tea.

## Hypercalcemia
The causes of hypercalcemia are given in Fig. 29.21.

## Hypocalcemia

The causes of hypocalcemia are given in Fig. 33.9.

### Management

Treat the underlying cause. If mild, give oral calcium supplements. If severe, give 10mL 10% intravenous calcium gluconate over 3 minutes and repeat as necessary.

## Miscellaneous genitourinary conditions

### Adult polycystic kidney disease

This is an autosomal dominantly inherited disease, the gene lying on chromosome 16. Patients are usually between the ages of 30 and 50. Cysts develop in the kidney and lead to progressive renal failure. About 30% of patients also have cysts in the liver.

### Clinical features

Hematuria or abdominal pain are presenting features in about a third of patients. The patient may have signs or symptoms of chronic renal failure. There is an association with subarachnoid hemorrhage. Examination reveals large irregular palpable kidneys, and the patient is often hypertensive. There may be bruits from intracranial vascular anomalies.

### Investigations

Ultrasound shows multiple cysts. IVU shows large kidneys and "spider calyces."

### Management

Blood pressure should be controlled and infections treated. Renal failure is progressive and may necessitate dialysis or renal transplantation. Screening first degree relatives and genetic counseling is recommended.

## Hepatorenal syndrome

This mainly occurs in patients with obstructive jaundice. Renal failure may be precipitated by surgery to relieve the jaundice, overvigorous diuretic therapy, diarrhea, or paracentesis for ascites, although there may be no precipitating factor found. Histology of the kidney is usually normal early on but may advance to produce an acute tubular necrosis.

The mechanism of the renal failure is not fully understood but may be due to or peripheral vasodilatation mediated through nitric oxide, leading to hypotension. This then activates the renin–angiotensin system and other humoral mechanisms to cause constriction of renal vessels.

Opiates should be avoided preoperatively, and euvolemia should be ensured with intravenous fluids. Urine output and serum electrolytes should be monitored. If renal failure occurs, the prognosis is usually poor.

The differential diagnosis includes leptospirosis, which may cause hepatic and renal failure. The organism can be grown from urine and blood and is penicillin-sensitive.

| Causes of hypocalcemia | |
| --- | --- |
| Cause | Examples |
| hypoproteinemia | nephrotic syndrome |
| renal disease | chronic renal failure |
| inadequate intake of calcium or vitamin D | malabsorption |
| hypoparathyroidism | — |
| target organ resistance | pseudohypoparathyroidism |
| neonatal hypocalcemia | — |
| others | acute pancreatitis, cystinosis, cytotoxic drugs |

**Fig. 33.9** Causes of hypocalcemia.

## Hemolytic uremic syndrome (HUS)/thrombotic thrombocytopenic purpura (TTP)

HUS is a disorder usually affecting infants under 3 years old. The etiology is unknown, but the syndrome often follows an infective illness such as gastroenteritis or upper respiratory tract infection. The infection may trigger endothelial damage and cause clotting disturbances characteristic of the condition. There is intravascular hemolysis with red blood cell fragmentation. Fibrin deposition is seen in renal arterioles. Thrombocytopenia also occurs and the condition is similar to thrombotic thrombocytopenic purpura in adults. See Chapter 37 for more details.

It is now understood that both HUS and TTP can consist of the symptomatic pentad of thrombocytopenia, fever, mental status change, hemolysis, and renal failure. This pentad no longer defines the difference between the two states.

Treatment is with heparin, prostacyclin, fresh frozen plasma, plasma exchange, and dialysis for renal failure. Most children recover spontaneously.

## Urinary tract malignancies
### Renal cell carcinoma

Renal cell carcinoma is the most common renal tumor in adults and is twice as common in men. The peak age of onset is between 50 and 60 years of age. It may be solitary, multiple, or occasionally bilateral. Clinically, patients present with hematuria, loin pain, and an abdominal mass. Other features may include fever, polycythemia, anemia, hypercalcemia, and left-sided varicocele associated with left renal vein obstruction. A tendency to grow into the inferior vena cava (IVC) is a typical characteristic. About a quarter of patients present with metastases.

Investigations include urinalysis for red cells, chest x-ray for metastases, ultrasound, IVU, and CT or magnetic resonance imaging of the abdomen. Angiography will reveal the circulation of the tumor.

Treatment is by nephrectomy. Metastases may regress after the primary tumor is removed. Radiotherapy has no proven value. Progesterone may be of help in controlling metastatic disease. The overall 5-year survival rate is about 40% but is better if the tumor is confined to the renal parenchyma and worse if there are metastases or lymph node involvement.

### Nephroblastoma

This is seen in infants. It presents as an abdominal mass or occasionally with hematuria. Treatment is with nephrectomy, radiotherapy, and chemotherapy and is often curative.

### Transitional cell carcinoma

This occurs mainly in people over 40 and most commonly affects the bladder. It is four times more common in men than women. Predisposing factors include cigarette smoking, exposure to industrial carcinogens, exposure to drugs (e.g. phenacetin and cyclophosphamide), and chronic inflammation (e.g., schistosomiasis).

Patients usually present with painless hematuria, although pain may occur. There may be symptoms similar to UTI. Investigations include urine cytology, IVU, cystoscopy, abdominal CT scanning, and retrograde urography.

Treatment options include local resection with follow-up cystoscopy, cystectomy, radiotherapy, and local or systemic chemotherapy.

### Prostatic carcinoma

Prostatic carcinoma is the third most common malignancy in men. The incidence increases with age, and the disease may be very indolent. Patients are often asymptomatic but may present with symptoms of prostatism (e.g., hesitancy, frequency, and postmicturition dribbling) or with symptoms arising from metastatic spread, especially to bone. There is a hard, irregular prostate on rectal examination.

Investigation includes prostate-specific antigen (PSA), transrectal ultrasound, and prostatic biopsy, which shows an adenocarcinoma. Evidence of metastases should also be sought.

Treatment for local disease may be by transurethral resection of the prostate, radical prostatectomy, or radiotherapy. Metastases can be treated with orchidectomy, luteinizing hormone-releasing hormone analogues, and antiandrogens (e.g., cyproterone acetate).

## Cerebrovascular disease

### Stroke

A stroke is a focal neurologic deficit due to a vascular lesion that lasts for more than 24 hours. About 80% are due to infarction secondary to thrombosis or embolism, and 20% are due to intracerebral hemorrhage. The overall incidence is about 150 in 100,000 but rises with age so that the incidence at 75 years is 1000 in 100,000. It is the third leading cause of death in the U.S.

Risk factors for stroke are summarized in Fig. 34.1. The main cause of thrombotic strokes are thromboembolism from arteries and emboli from the heart. Uncommon causes of thrombosis are vasculitis, polycythemia rubra vera, and meningovascular syphilis. Thrombus *in situ* may also occur following hypotension. Cerebral hemorrhage is usually due to rupture of microaneurysms in perforating arteries or intracerebral vessels.

Less common causes of hemorrhagic stroke include hemorrhage, tumor, abscess, or secondary to blood dyscrasias.

The sudden onset of any symptom usually suggests either a vascular or neurologic etiology.

### Clinical features

Signs and symptoms usually appear rapidly, whereas a gradual progression over days suggests a tumor. Clinical features relate to the distribution of the affected artery, although in practice this may not be clear-cut due to collateral circulation and the development of cerebral edema. The most common presentation is hemiplegia due to infarction of the internal capsule.

### Types of infarction

***Cerebral hemisphere infarcts***   Cerebral hemisphere infarcts may be classified by vascular territory:

- Anterior cerebral artery infarcts: proximal to the medial striate branch, they cause contralateral hemiplegia; distal to the medial striate branch, they cause contralateral paralysis with sparing of the arm and face.
- Middle cerebral artery infarcts: causes contralateral hemiplegia, often sparing the leg, and hemianopia. Aphasia is present if the dominant hemisphere is affected.
- Posterior cerebral artery infarcts: causes contralateral hemianopia.
- Motor signs are upper motor neuron.

***Lacunar strokes***   Lacunar strokes are due to small areas of infarction usually occurring around the basal ganglia, thalamus, and pons. Clinical features include pure motor or sensory signs, a mixed motor and sensory picture, ataxia, and dysarthria. They may also be asymptomatic and found at post-mortem examination.

***Brainstem infarcts***   Clinical features include hemi- or quadriplegia, sensory loss, diplopia, facial weakness and numbness, nystagmus, dysphasia, and coma due to damage to the reticular formation.

The locked-in syndrome results from upper brainstem infarction. The patient is conscious but unable to respond.

The most common brainstem vascular syndrome is lateral medullary syndrome (Wallenberg's syndrome), which is due to thromboembolism of the posterior inferior cerebellar artery. The patient presents with sudden vertigo and vomiting. Ipsilateral signs include 9th and 10th nerve lesions, Horner's syndrome, spinothalamic sensory loss in the face, diplopia, and cerebellar signs in the limbs. Contralateral signs include spinothalamic sensory loss in the body.

| Risk factors for stroke | |
|---|---|
| major risk factors | hypertension<br>atrial fibrillation<br>previous transient ischemic attacks<br>diabetes mellitus<br>ischemic heart disease<br>peripheral vascular disease<br>oral contraceptive pill |
| other risk factors | smoking<br>obesity<br>excessive alcohol intake<br>polycythemia<br>arteritis<br>bleeding disorders<br>hyperlipidemia*<br>low cholesterol[†] |

**Fig. 34.1** Risk factors for stroke. *Hyperlipidemia is associated with cerebral infarction. [†]Low cholesterol may be associated with cerebral hemorrhage.

## Investigations

The following investigations should be performed in patients who have suffered a stroke:

- Complete blood count (CBC): polycythemia or thrombocytopenia.
- Coagulation studies: bleeding disorders.
- Erythrocyte sedimentation rate (ESR): giant cell arteritis.
- Blood glucose: hyper- or hypoglycemia may lead to impaired consciousness.
- Chest x-ray (CXR): primary tumor; left atrium enlarged with mitral stenosis.
- Syphilis serology.
- Noncontrast computed tomography (CT) scan: this will distinguish between hemorrhagic and ischemic infarction if done within 2 weeks and should be done acutely to rule out hemorrhage whenever thrombolytics are considered; also aids diagnosis of other conditions in cases of uncertainty, such as tumor or subdural hematoma; should always be performed in cerebellar stroke as hematoma requires urgent evacuation.
- MRI: can show ischemia within 15–30 minutes. Different types of MRI can be performed, including MR angiography (MRA), depending on the information needed.
- Carotid duplex scan: stenoses.

## Management
### Prevention

Risk factors such as hypertension, smoking, diabetes mellitus (DM), high cholesterol, and atrial fibrillation should be identified and managed appropriately. Following stroke, the blood pressure may be high for some days, and a decision about the use of antihypertensive drugs is not usually made for about 2 weeks.

Cholesterol should be lowered to reduce coronary risk because myocardial infarction is the major cause of death during the period following the acute stage of stroke or transient ischemic attacks (TIAs). Anticoagulation should be considered for patients with atrial fibrillation and thromboembolic stroke.

If there is a severe internal carotid artery stenosis (of more than 70%) and the patient has had TIAs within the past 6 months, endarterectomy should be considered.

### Treatment

If the patient is unconscious or severely impaired, a decision about the most appropriate degree of intervention needs to be made in liaison with relatives and the patient, if possible. Factors to consider include prognosis, quality of life, and the patient's wishes. Raised intracranial pressure should be suspected if the blood pressure rises, the pulse falls, and there is papilledema.

An urgent CT scan should be considered. If urgent noncontrast CT scan shows no hemorrhage, the patient should be treated with alteplase (recombinant tissue-type plasminogen activator [rt-PA] up to 3 hours after the stroke. After 3 hours, the risk of giving the agent outweighs the benefits. The quicker the patient can be given the thrombolytic, the better the outcome in terms of long-term morbidity and mortality. Patients treated within the first 90 minutes had the best outcomes.

All blood pressure medications should be held in order to ensure proper brain perfusion. Increases in the ICP sometimes force the systemic blood pressure higher than normal. In the presence of an acute bleed, the ICP should be measured. For ischemic stroke, blood pressure should not be treated unless it is severe (>220 systolic or >120 diastolic). This is often true for up to 2 weeks following acute presentation as well.

Stroke patients should be on a low threshold for intubation. With altered mental status, aspiration is a risk. In addition, hyperventilation can help decrease ICP. Often the stroke will affect the respiratory drive itself, and mechanical ventilation is necessary in acute stabilization.

Hydration should be maintained, and this should be done parenterally if there is no gag reflex.

The patient should be turned regularly to prevent pressure sores. If incontinent, urinary catheterization should be considered. Physical therapy will prevent contractures and hasten mobility.

Speech therapy and occupational therapy are important later on.

Aspirin, 81–325 mg daily, or clopidogrel, 75 mg daily, for people with thrombotic stroke, reduces the rate of further strokes and vascular deaths. Complications (e.g., pneumonia, depression, and constipation) should be managed appropriately.

Patients may also be started on another antiplatelet medication such as clopidogrel or dipyridamole, with or without continuing daily aspirin. For patients who fail aspirin therapy by having another TIA or stroke while on the medication, a second antiplatelet medication should be started. Patients with atrial fibrillation who are not on anticoagulation should have heparin therapy started after any neurologic event.

## Prognosis

Features associated with a poor prognosis include impaired consciousness, severe hemiplegia, incontinence, a defect in conjugate gaze, and increasing age. About 20–25% of patients with thromboembolic infarction and 75% of patients with intracerebral hemorrhage die at 1 month. Recurrent strokes are common. About a third of survivors make a complete recovery and a third are left with severe disability.

## Transient ischemic attacks

These are focal neurologic deficits due to vascular events that resolve within 24 hours with a complete clinical recovery. They are usually due to emboli from the carotid or vertebrobasilar arteries, but emboli may also arise from the heart or other vessels. The annual incidence is about 50 per 100,000.

Other possible causes are arteritis (e.g., giant cell arteritis, polyarteritis nodosa [PAN], systemic lupus erythematosus [SLE], syphilis, arterial trauma) and hematologic causes (e.g., polycythemia rubra vera and sickle cell disease).

## Clinical features

There is a sudden focal neurologic deficit, which gradually resolves over minutes or hours, leading to complete recovery within 24 hours. In the internal carotid artery territory, platelet emboli obstruct blood flow, leading to loss of function in part of the brain. The platelet aggregates then break up, restoring blood flow and hence function. This may lead to dysphasia and dysarthria, contralateral hemiparesis, hemisensory loss, homonymous hemianopia, and ipsilateral amaurosis fugax. The latter is due to emboli passing through the retinal arteries, leading to a sensation of a curtain passing across the vision.

TIAs in the vertebrobasilar system may again result from emboli or from a pinching of the vertebral arteries by osteophytes arising from the cervical vertebrae. Symptoms include diplopia, vertigo, nausea and vomiting, ataxia, hemiparesis or hemisensory loss, tetraparesis, deafness, cortical blindness, occasionally loss of consciousness, and transient global amnesia.

Sources of emboli should be sought. Risk factors are the same as for stroke and should be identified and managed appropriately.

## Differential diagnosis

This includes all conditions that may cause transient neurologic symptoms. Epilepsy is usually distinguished by features such as jerking, and migraine is usually associated with headache, which is rare in TIAs. Hypoglycemia, multiple sclerosis (MS), and intracranial lesions should be excluded.

## Investigations

These should identify risk factors, find the cause of the TIA, and exclude other causes of symptoms, as for stroke. Carotid Doppler studies or angiography may identify stenoses (Fig. 34.2).

## Treatment

Risk factors should be controlled, particularly hypertension. Cholesterol should be lowered to reduce coronary risk. Aspirin 75–300 mg daily reduces the risk of subsequent nonfatal stroke, myocardial infarction, and vascular deaths. More recent evidence suggests that dipyridamole MR, 200 mg daily, has a protective effect for subsequent neurologic events, which are additional to the protective effect of aspirin.

**Fig. 34.2** (A) Carotid angiogram showing a severe atheromatous plaque leading to stenosis of the internal carotid artery. (B) The same vessel is shown after angioplasty and stent insertion.

Anticoagulation should be considered if TIAs continue despite antiplatelet treatment, or if there is a known cardiac source of embolism. Carotid endarterectomy is indicated for recurrent TIAs in the appropriate distribution if the responsible carotid stenosis is over 70% of the luminal diameter.

## Prognosis
Patients with TIAs in the carotid distribution fare worse than those with TIAs in the vertebrobasilar territory. The risks of stroke and myocardial infarction are significantly increased, at about 5% per year each.

# Extracerebral hemorrhage
## Subarachnoid hemorrhage
Subarachnoid hemorrhage (SAH) is due to bleeding into the subarachnoid space. The annual incidence is 15 in 100,000. Most cases are due to rupture of a congenital berry aneurysm in the circle of Willis and its adjacent branches (Fig. 20.2); 15% are multiple.

Berry aneurysms are associated with coarctation of the aorta, polycystic kidneys, and Ehlers-Danlos syndrome. About 5–10% of SAHs are due to arteriovenous malformations, but in 15% of patients no cause is found.

Risk factors include cigarette smoking, alcohol, hypertension, and anticoagulation. Bleeds may occasionally be due to ruptures, mycotic aneurysm from endocarditis, and bleeding diatheses.

### Clinical features
The classic history is of a feeling like a sudden blow to the back of the neck. This is usually followed by faintness, nausea, vomiting, and sometimes loss of consciousness. The increase in ICP can even lead to seizures, hyponatremia, and ECG changes.

Examination reveals photophobia, neck stiffness, and a positive Kernig's sign. If bleeding continues, the level of consciousness deteriorates. There may be signs of raised intracranial pressure or pressure effects on surrounding structures (e.g., cranial nerve palsies). There may be a bruit over the skull due to an arteriovenous malformation.

### Investigations
Noncontrast CT scan usually shows blood in the subarachnoid space, and it can also identify arteriovenous malformations. A lumbar puncture shows raised pressure, uniform blood staining in consecutive samples, and xanthochromia (yellow color), which persists for several days. MRA, contrast CT, or angiography will show the aneurysm and should be carried out if surgery is considered.

### Management
The supportive care mentioned above for stroke should be offered to patients with SAH as well. ICP is often elevated in patients with SAH. Often a ventriculotomy needs to be placed to allow direct measurement of ICP so that blood pressure can be controlled appropriately. If the patient is conscious, perfusion is adequate and the blood pressure can be lowered. IV labetalol is often the drug of choice because it can be more precisely titrated than oral agents.

Immediate treatment is bed rest, analgesia, and supportive measures. About a third of patients rebleed, most commonly about two weeks after the initial event. Angiography should therefore be performed before then if the aneurysm is to be clipped.

Blood pressure should be monitored and lowered if severely raised. The lowering of blood pressure should be done with caution. Patients with SAH may have an increased ICP, which will lower perfusion pressure within the brain. While a high blood pressure increases the risk for a rebleed, lowering the blood pressure too much can lead to infarction. When in doubt, an ICP monitor can be placed to determine the exact ICP and perfusion pressure.

Nimodipine, 60mg 4 hourly, is used to prevent vascular spasm following SAH and reduces mortality. It is related to nifedipine, but the smooth muscle relaxant effect preferentially acts on cerebral arteries. It should be started within 4 days and continued for 21 days.

Seizure medications obviously should be given to convulsing patients. For patients without seizures but increased ICP, medication prophylaxis is often given and continued for 6 months.

### Prognosis
Nearly half of patients with SAH are dead or moribund before reaching hospital. A further 30% will rebleed in the next few days.

Patients who have severe neurologic deficits have a poor prognosis. Of patients who survive 1 year, about a third will have made a full recovery.

## Subdural hematoma
These are due to bleeding from bridging veins between the cortex and venous sinuses. An initial small hemorrhage gradually enlarges by absorbing

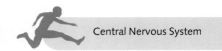
fluid osmotically from the cerebrospinal fluid (CSF). It is more common in the elderly, epileptics, and alcoholics. Although it is often secondary to trauma, the initial event may not be recalled.

Symptoms develop insidiously. They include headache, confusion, a fluctuating level of consciousness, and sometimes a personality change. There may be focal neurologic signs (which may develop many days after the initial insult), signs of raised intracranial pressure, or secondary epilepsy.

CT scan should show the hematoma, which may be bilateral. Treatment is by removal of the hematoma, which often leads to a full recovery if performed early.

Hematomas may resolve spontaneously, and in the very elderly they can be monitored with serial CT scans.

## Extradural hematoma

This results from tearing of the middle meningeal artery or its branches following head injury. The classic picture is of a sudden brief loss of consciousness followed by a lucid interval. The patient's consciousness level then deteriorates, and the ipsilateral pupil dilates, followed by bilateral fixed dilated pupils and death. Treatment is by evacuation of the clot through Burr holes or craniotomy.

## Management of conditions causing headache

The differential diagnosis of headache is given in Chapter 15. Headache is a common symptom, which may either be of trivial significance or the expression of serious disease. The clinical approach to headache depends on a detailed analysis of symptoms and a thorough general and neurologic examination.

## Acute headache

The most common cause of acute severe headache is acute meningeal irritation as a result of SAH or meningitis. Headache also occurs with encephalitis, hydrocephalus, and head injury. CT scanning is usually the first investigation used to exclude a mass lesion, hematoma, or hydrocephalus. Lumbar puncture may be necessary to examine the CSF for SAH and meningitis. Occasionally acute migraine can produce a meningitic picture.

## Recurrent and chronic headache
### Tension headache

Tension headaches are extremely common and classically present as intermittent attacks of diffuse tightness, pressure or heaviness over the vertex, or in the neck or occiput. It may occasionally be unilateral. The headache may be relieved by analgesics but is not accompanied by vomiting or visual disturbance. When the headaches are constant and occur daily, analgesics are ineffective, and excessive medication may itself induce headache. Tension headaches are most common in middle-aged women.

Acetaminophen, aspirin, and NSAIDs can be used as abortive therapy by patients with tension headaches. Biofeedback, tricyclic antidepressants, and Botox injections are used as prophylactic measures.

Inquiries should be made for the common and often concealed fear of a brain tumor or stroke.

### Migraine

Migraine affects about 10% of the population and is slightly commoner in women than men (ratio of 1.5:1). Migraine runs in families, and attacks tend to occur without aura. About 75% of people have their first attack before the age of 20 years.

#### Clinical features

The frequency of headaches varies from one to two each week to a few attacks scattered over a lifetime. The prodrome may consist of yawning, euphoria, or depression and sometimes a craving for, or a distaste of, food in the 24 hours before the headache.

This is followed by an aura 30–60 minutes before the headache. It is usually visual, consisting of teichopsiae (flashes of light), scotomata, and fortification spectra (zigzag castellations). There may be micropsia and metamorphosia. Circumoral tingling and paresthesias in the hands may also occur. In hemiplegic migraine, a hemiparesis, sometimes with dysphasia, occurs.

The headache is commonly unilateral. It usually starts in the day and is classically throbbing or pulsating. Associated features include nausea and vomiting, diarrhea, chills, faintness, and fluid retention. There may be photophobia and sonophobia. The headache is usually worse with movement and lasts for 24–48 hours.

Occasionally, especially in older people, the aura may occur without the headache—"migraine sine cephalgia."

## Pathology
The mechanism of migraine attacks is not well understood, but a reduction in cerebral blood flow leads to the aura. This is followed by an increased blood flow associated with vasodilatation leading to headache. The process involves neurohumoral triggers, including 5-hydroxytryptamine (5-HT) and norepinephrine.

The cerebral mechanism is responsive to mood, emotions, tiredness, relaxation, hormonal changes, and peripheral stimuli (e.g., bright lights and noise). There is often a seasonal and/or diurnal pattern.

## Management
Precipitating factors should be identified and avoided, such as certain foods, including cocoa, cheese, citrus fruits, and alcohol. Acute attacks should be treated with simple analgesia (e.g., aspirin, acetaminophen, or codeine), combined with an antiemetic (e.g., domperidone or metoclopramide and serotonin agonists [triptans]). The triptans are used almost exclusively with analgesics. Ergot-based drugs are rarely used because of questions about their efficacy.

Ergotamine is used in patients who do not respond to analgesics. It relieves migraine headache by constricting cranial arteries, but the aura is not affected and vomiting can be made worse. Common side effects include nausea, vomiting, abdominal pain, and muscular cramps. It should not be used for hemiplegic migraine in patients with peripheral vascular disease, or in coronary heart disease. The frequency of administration should be limited to no more than twice a month to avoid habituation.

Sumatriptan and other 5-HT antagonists are of value for treatment of acute attacks. They should not be given to patients with ischemic heart disease or previous myocardial infarction, coronary vasospasm, or uncontrolled hypertension.

## Prophylaxis
Prophylactic drugs are indicated in patients who have two or more attacks each month and include β-blockers, and tricyclic antidepressants. The need for continuing therapy should be reviewed every 6 months.

Beta blockers, such as propanolol, are effective, but their use is limited by contraindications and interaction with ergotamine.

Calcium channel blockers (CCBs) can be used to prevent not only the migraine pain but also the aura. While studies using CCBs do show some benefit, tolerance can develop to the medication.

Tricyclic antidepressants, such as amitriptyline, can be effective in low doses, even in patients who are not depressed.

Other newer options include antiseizure medications such as valproate or gabapentin.

## Cluster headache
Cluster headaches are 10 times more common in men than women. Attacks usually start in adulthood. Headaches are of agonizing severity around one eye and often occur at night. Attacks last for 30–120 minutes and usually occur every day for 4 weeks to 3 months. There is then usually a total remission until the next cluster ensues a year or two later.

The pain may radiate to the face, jaw, neck, and shoulder, and the eyes may water and become red. The nostrils may also run or feel blocked. Meiosis occurs in 20% of attacks, and in about 5% a permanent partial Horner's syndrome occurs. Attacks can be precipitated by vasodilators (e.g., alcohol, nitrites, and CCBs).

Treatment is with ergotamine given in anticipation of the attacks, or pizotifen, lithium, steroids, or verapamil can be used for prophylaxis. Oxygen affords prompt relief in some patients. Sumatriptan will stop attacks in 5–10 minutes in 70% of patients.

## Brain tumors and other space-occupying lesions
These present with headaches in about 50% of patients but are uncommon causes of headache overall. The following symptoms may be present:
- Raised intracranial pressure: headache, vomiting, and papilledema.
- Generalized or focal epilepsy.
- Progressive focal signs: hemiparesis, hemianopia, and dysphasia.

- Mental changes: depression, apathy, dementia, and hallucinosis.

Headaches often occur in the mornings and are worse with coughing, exertion, or a change in posture. Focal signs are suggestive of tumors. Investigations should include CT scanning to show primary or secondary tumor.

## Temporal (giant cell) arteritis

This disease usually occurs in patients over 60 years old. The classic features include engorged, reddened, tender, nonpulsatile temporal arteries (Fig. 34.3), but this is not invariably present. The headache is severe and often worse at night and may be accompanied by sweats, fever, malaise, and pain in

**Fig. 34.3** Temporal arteritis with typical thickening of the right temporal artery. This patient presented with temporal pain and sudden visual impairment in the right eye but responded to prompt treatment with systemic steroid. (Courtesy of Dr. C.D. Forbes and Dr. W.F. Jackson, Color Atlas and Text of Clinical Medicine, Mosby, 1993.)

the jaw during eating ("masseter claudication"). It may be associated with polymyalgia rheumatica. Involvement of the vertebral arteries may lead to TIAs or stroke, and disease of the ophthalmic arteries may lead to retinal ischemia or infarction, which is irreversible.

### Investigation

The ESR is markedly raised at around 100mm per hour. A biopsy of the temporal artery should be taken within 24 hours of starting steroid therapy. "Skip lesions" may lead to false negatives, and so a long biopsy specimen should be obtained. Inflammatory cells infiltrate the tunica, and the internal elastic lamina is commonly destroyed or disrupted. Intraluminal thrombosis may also be found.

### Treatment

Treatment is with high doses of prednisone (60mg daily). This relieves the headache within 24 hours and averts the risk of blindness, which occurs in up to 50% of patients if untreated. The prednisone is gradually reduced to a maintenance level, and the dose is monitored by symptoms and serial ESRs. Treatment may have to be continued for many years.

## Glaucoma

Localized pain in the eye and forehead may be a recurrent source of headache, and glaucoma should be considered in hypermetropic, middle-aged, or elderly patients. In acute attacks, there may be vomiting, blurred vision, cloudiness of the cornea, and discoloration of the iris with a dilated pupil and circumorbital injection. Tonometry will confirm the elevated intraocular pressure.

Standard treatments include miotics, acetazolamide, and iridectomy, which should be supervised by an ophthalmologist.

## Paget's disease of the skull

This is a common condition presenting with diffuse headaches, somnolence, deafness, and enlargement of the skull. Headaches result from local bony changes with vascular hyperemia. Hydrocephalus may later be an additional factor of importance.

## Trigeminal neuralgia

This condition of unknown cause is seen most commonly in the elderly and is more common in women. In young patients, MS should be suspected. It is unilateral in 96% of patients and consists of paroxysms of stabbing pain in the distribution of the trigeminal nerve. The face may screw up with pain; hence the alternative name of tic douloureux.

The pain may be brought on by touching a specific trigger zone such as the side of the nose and is thus provoked by factors such as eating, shaving, or talking. If left untreated, the condition usually progresses with shorter periods of remission.

Treatment is with carbamazepine, phenytoin, or occasionally clonazepam or baclofen. Surgical procedures, such as sectioning of the sensory root or thermocoagulation of the ganglion, are reserved for failure of medical therapy.

Other neuralgias include glossopharyngeal neuralgia and auriculotemporal neuralgia, which are precipitated by swallowing. Postherpetic neuralgia occurs in patients with previous herpes zoster.

## Atypical facial pain

This refers to episodes of prolonged facial pain for which no cause can be found. It is more common in women and is often bilateral. It is associated with depression and may respond to tricyclic antidepressants.

## Benign intracranial hypertension

This is also known as pseudotumor cerebri. The etiology is often unknown, but it may be related to steroids in some patients. A few cases are secondary to thrombosis of the dural venous sinuses. The condition occurs mainly in overweight young women, and there may be a history of menstrual irregularities or recent pregnancy. Symptoms include headache and vomiting. There is marked papilledema which, if longstanding, can lead to optic atrophy and infarction of the optic nerve, causing blindness.

CT scan shows no mass lesion, and the ventricles are of normal or small size. Thiazides or furosemide may reduce the intracranial pressure, and repeated lumbar puncture may induce a remission. In resistant cases, or if visual acuity deteriorates, a ventriculoperitoneal CSF shunt may be necessary.

## Parkinsonism

Parkinsonism comprises the syndrome of tremor, rigidity, and bradykinesia. Parkinson's disease is only one type of parkinsonism.

First described by James Parkinson in 1817, it is now known to be due to a relative deficiency of the neurotransmitter dopamine, resulting in a neurohumoral imbalance. Pathologically, there is progressive degeneration of the basal ganglia, predominantly affecting the substantia nigra, and the appearance of eosinophilic inclusion bodies (Lewy bodies). The cause of the degeneration is unknown.

People with Parkinson's disease are less likely to be smokers. The incidence increases with age and affects 1 in 200 people over 70 years old. It affects men and women equally, and there does not appear to be a genetic predisposition.

## Clinical features

Early on the patient may complain of fatigue, muscular discomfort, or restlessness. Fine movements may be difficult.

### Tremor

Initially this is intermittent and may only appear when the patient is tired. It commonly affects one hand, spreading to the leg on the same side and later to the other limbs. The frequency of the tremor is 3–6 beats per second, and it is most marked at rest (whereas a cerebellar tremor is more marked on intention). There is a "pill-rolling" movement of the thumb over the fingers.

### Rigidity

There is resistance to passive movement, which may be smooth throughout its range ("lead pipe" rigidity). When combined with tremor, resistance to passive movement is jerky and termed "cogwheel" rigidity.

### Bradykinesia

Bradykinesia means difficulty in initiating movements and varying posture. It may be difficult to rise from a chair. Writing becomes small (micrographia), spidery, and cramped. The face is expressionless and mask-like (Fig. 34.4), and the voice is monotonous and unmodulated. There is a shuffling, festinating gait, and the patient stoops (Fig. 34.5). The arms do not swing, and the frequency of spontaneous blinking reduces.

To examine for bradykinesia, ask the patient to unbutton and button his or her shirt.

**Fig. 34.4** Parkinson's disease is characteristically associated with a mask-like face which is devoid of emotion. The patient often drools and has monotonous speech. (Courtesy of Dr. C.D. Forbes and Dr. W.F. Jackson, Color Atlas and Text of Clinical Medicine, Mosby, 1993.)

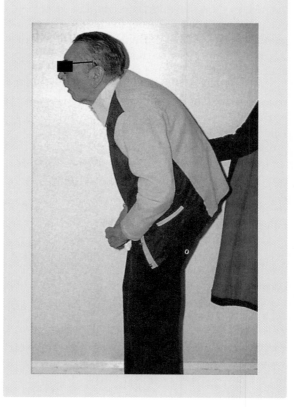

**Fig. 34.5** Typical posture in Parkinson's disease. (Courtesy of Dr. Kamal, St. George's Hospital, Lincoln.)

## Other features

Due to a disorder of the normal pattern of swallowing, saliva gathers and drips from the half-open mouth. Constipation and urinary difficulties are common. Rigidity may be accompanied by pain in the muscles. Late in the disease, dementia may occur. Depression is common.

## Other causes of parkinsonism

Other causes of parkinsonism include the following:
- Drugs (e.g., neuroleptics).
- Atherosclerosis: look for symptoms and signs of atherosclerosis in other regions (e.g., TIAs or intermittent claudication).
- Postencephalitis: following outbreaks of encephalitis lethargica (as in 1917–25).
- Progressive supranuclear palsy: a symptom complex comprising a parkinsonism-like illness, dementia, and a failure of upward gaze.

- Shy-Drager syndrome: parkinsonism, orthostatic hypotension, and atonic bladder.
- Poisoning with heavy metals or carbon monoxide.
- Wilson's disease (hepatolenticular degeneration).
- "Punch drunk" syndrome: brain damage in boxers.

## Management

The disease is treated symptomatically. Physical therapy can improve the gait and help build confidence. Physical aids such as high chairs and rails may help with daily activities.

## Drugs

The aim of drug therapy is to correct the neurohumoral imbalance. This may greatly improve the quality of life but does not prevent progression of the disease. Ten to twenty percent of patients are unresponsive to treatment.

Drugs may cause confusion in the elderly, and it is important to start treatment with low doses and use small increments.

## Dopaminergic drugs

### Levodopa

Levodopa (L-dopa) is used with a dopa decarboxylase inhibitor and is the treatment of choice for idiopathic Parkinson's disease. It is less helpful for elderly patients or those with longstanding disease who may not tolerate the high doses required to overcome their deficit. It is also less valuable in patients with postencephalitic disease, who are particularly susceptible to side effects.

Parkinsonism caused by generalized degenerative brain disease does not normally respond to levodopa. It should not be used for neuroleptic-induced parkinsonism.

Levodopa is the amino acid precursor of dopamine and acts mainly by replenishing depleted striatal dopamine. It helps bradykinesia and rigidity more than tremor. It is generally administered with an extracerebral dopa decarboxylase inhibitor (e.g., benserazide or carbidopa). These prevent the peripheral breakdown of levodopa to dopamine, but unlike levodopa do not cross the blood-brain barrier. Effective brain concentrations of dopamine can thus be achieved with lower doses of levodopa.

Sinemet is the combination of L-dopa and carbidopa. Medications should be ingested 1 hour before a meal, since these drugs should not have to compete with other amino acids for absorption.

The reduced peripheral formation of dopamine decreases peripheral side effects (e.g., nausea, vomiting, and cardiovascular effects). There is less delay in the onset of therapeutic effect and a smoother clinical response. There is, however, an increased incidence of abnormal involuntary movements.

Side effects of levodopa include nausea and vomiting, which may be limited by domperidone. Late side effects include the sudden unpredictable swings of the "on-off" syndrome, dyskinesia, and "end-of-dose" deterioration. In the last, the duration of benefit after each dose becomes progressively shorter. This may be improved with modified-release preparations.

### Selegiline

This is a monoamine oxidase B inhibitor used in severe parkinsonism in conjunction with levodopa to reduce end-of-dose deterioration. Early treatment with selegiline may delay the need for levodopa therapy but does not delay disease progression.

### Bromocriptine

This is one of the ergot derivatives, which act by direct stimulation of surviving dopamine receptors. It should be reserved for patients in whom levodopa alone is no longer adequate or who, despite careful titration, cannot tolerate it. It is important to note that, if the patient has never had a response to L-dopa, it is unlikely that bromocriptine will be beneficial. Some studies have shown that bromocriptine and ropinirole provide more lasting benefits compared with L-dopa therapy. Occasionally bromocriptine may cause neuropsychiatric side effects and retroperitoneal fibrosis.

### Ropinirole

Ropinirole is a dopamine $D_2$ receptor agonist that improves the symptoms and signs in Parkinson's disease. Its side effects are similar to those of dopamine.

### Amantadine

This improves mild bradykinetic disabilities as well as tremor and rigidity. Few patients derive much benefit, and tolerance develops to its effects.

### Apomorphine

Apomorphine is a potent stimulator of dopamine receptors, which is sometimes helpful in stabilizing patients experiencing unpredictable "off" periods with levodopa treatment.

## Antimuscarinic drugs

Examples of antimuscarinic drugs used in the treatment of Parkinson's disease include trihexyphenidyl and benztropine. They are less effective than levodopa in idiopathic Parkinson's disease, although they may be used to supplement its action.

Antimuscarinic drugs may be used first in patients with mild disease, especially when tremor is the predominant symptom. They are also of value in postencephalitic parkinsonism. They correct the relative central cholinergic excess thought to occur in parkinsonism as a result of dopamine deficiency. They also reduce the symptoms of drug-induced parkinsonism seen with antipsychotic drugs.

Side effects include blurred vision, dry mouth, tachycardia, urinary retention, and constipation.

319

## Multiple sclerosis

Multiple sclerosis (MS), also called disseminated sclerosis, is an inflammatory, demyelinating disorder. It is the most common cause of neurologic disability in young adults in the U.S. The prevalence of MS varies worldwide and is much higher in temperate zones. The overall prevalence in the U.S. is 60 in 100,000.

There is a female preponderance with a male: female ratio of 1:1.5. The mean age of onset is 30 years, but there is a bimodal distribution with a major peak at 21–25 years and a lesser peak at 41–45 years.

### Etiology

The cause of MS is unknown. Evidence suggests that in a genetically susceptible individual an environmental agent is responsible. The causative agent is likely to be a virus, and it is possible that a range of viruses may be involved. First-degree relatives have an increased chance of developing MS.

### Pathology

The hallmark of MS is the presence of multiple lesions disseminated in site and time. These are characterized by demyelination with relative preservation of the axons, gliosis, and varying degrees of inflammation. Sites of predilection include the optic nerve, spinal cord, periventricular areas, and the brainstem. Each small lesion is orientated around a venule, which, in the acute stages, shows perivascular cuffing with lymphocytes and plasma cells.

Axonal loss is seen in established lesions and may result in an expansion of the extracellular space. Chronic lesions show marked astrocytic gliosis. There are also a number of immunologic abnormalities.

### Clinical features

The diagnosis depends on the demonstration of physical signs that can only be explained by lesions in at least two sites in the central nervous system (CNS). There is a wide spectrum of disease activity, and the course of the disease is extremely variable. The onset is monosymptomatic in 85% of patients, while in the remainder there is clear evidence of involvement at a number of sites. Common presentations include optic neuritis, symptoms referable to the brainstem and cerebellum (including diplopia and ataxia), sensory disturbance of the limbs, and leg weakness.

Cerebellar lesions lead to **VANISH'D**: **v**ertigo, **a**taxia, **n**ystagmus, **i**ntention tremor, **s**lurred speech, **h**ypotonic reflexes, and **d**ysdiadochokinesia.

### Optic neuritis

The patient develops increasingly blurred vision in one eye, which may progress to complete uniocular blindness during a period of a few hours or 2–3 days. Central vision is usually more severely affected. The affected eye may be painful, and color vision is almost always affected. The optic nerve head appears normal unless the plaque is very anterior, when the disc may be swollen. Vision usually improves after 3–4 weeks and often returns to normal within 2 months. Transient blurring of vision lasting minutes, associated with exercise or raised body temperature (Uthoff's phenomenon), may occur. After an isolated episode of optic neuritis, patients are at an increased risk of MS. In addition, the risk in one study increased with each decade following the episode of MS.

### Diplopia

This is a common symptom, caused by a brainstem plaque involving fibers of the 3rd, 4th, or 6th cranial nerves, or by a lesion in the medial longitudinal bundle, causing an internuclear ophthalmoplegia.

### Motor weakness

Motor weakness is more common in the arms than in the legs, reflecting involvement of the thoracic spinal cord.

### Sensory symptoms

These include paresthesia and dysesthesia, proprioceptive disorders resulting in sensory ataxia and incoordination, and diminished vibration sense. Flexion of the neck may lead to an electric shock sensation in the back and limbs (Lhermitte's sign) and is associated with a lesion in the cervical cord.

## Cerebellar signs

Cerebellar signs include nystagmus, dyssynergia (fragmentation of voluntary movements resulting in intention tremor), dysdiadochokinesia, incoordination of the heel-shin test, titubation (continuous rhythmical tremor of the head and trunk), and dysarthria.

## Other manifestations

Other manifestations include the following:

- Cognitive impairment: especially of memory, sustained concentration, and abstract conceptual reasoning.
- Psychiatric abnormalities: most commonly depression; about 10% of patients suffer psychotic symptoms; euphoria may be present in severely disabled patients.
- Pain: this occurs in up to 50% of patients; trigeminal neuralgia is 300 times more common in patients with MS than in the general population.
- Paroxysmal symptoms: these include tonic seizures, and rapid flickering contraction in the facial muscles (myokymia).
- Bladder disturbance: this occurs in 50–75% of patients and is the presenting symptom in 10%; frequency, urgency, and incontinence are the most common symptoms; sexual dysfunction is common.
- Uncommon manifestations: "useless hand" syndrome (an upper limb ataxia), lower motor neuron signs, swallowing and respiratory problems, and extrapyramidal movement disorders.

# Diagnosis and differential diagnosis

The diagnosis of MS is based on clinical findings and the exclusion of conditions producing a similar clinical picture.

Initially, individual plaques may cause diagnostic difficulty and must be distinguished from compressive, inflammatory, and mass or vascular lesions. Inflammatory conditions include isolated angiitis of the CNS, SLE, primary Sjögren's syndrome, Behçet's disease, and PAN.

The differential diagnosis also includes infectious diseases (e.g., Lyme disease and brucellosis), multiple emboli, and granulomatous disorders (e.g., sarcoidosis and Wegener's granulomatosis).

## Investigations

The following investigations are important in the patient with MS:

- Examination of CSF shows a pleocytosis, raised protein, and immunoglobulin (Ig)G. Oligoclonal IgG is seen in 90% of patients with clinically definite MS, but is not specific for MS as it is also seen in a wide range of inflammatory and infectious disorders.
- Delay in the visually evoked response follows optic neuropathy, which may be subclinical. It is useful in providing evidence of a second lesion in patients whose neurologic deficits are only attributable to a single lesion.
- Magnetic resonance imaging (MRI) is very useful and can show plaques in the vast majority of patients with clinically definite disease.

## Prognosis

The progression of MS is very variable. There are four distinctive clinical presentations:

- Relapsing-remitting: intermittent relapses followed by remissions. With each ensuing attack, the remissions are less complete, so that within 10–20 years the patient is physically disabled.
- Progressive-relapsing: rapid deterioration with numerous relapses and only partial remissions in the first year or two of illness.
- Secondary progressive: infrequent attacks with long periods of remission.
- Primary progressive: continuous deterioration without remission.

Once the particular pattern has been established, the disease tends to develop along its declared path. After 5 years, 70% of patients are still employed. After 20 years, only 35% are employed, and 20% are dead from complications.

## Management

No cure for MS has been found. Adrenocorticotrophic hormone or corticosteroids have an established role in acute relapses but do not alter the course of the disease. Intravenous pulses of steroids may be effective in acute disease, but there is no justification for subjecting patients to the hazards of long-term corticosteroid therapy.

Beta-interferon may be used for patients with relapsing–remitting MS who are able to walk unaided. It is indicated for reducing the frequency and degree of severity of clinical relapses. There is no evidence of an effect on the progression of the disease, the duration of exacerbations, or on disability. Not all patients respond, and an

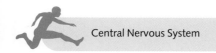 

accelerated deterioration has been observed in some. It should not be used in those with a history of severe depressive illness, inadequately controlled epilepsy, or decompensated hepatic impairment. Side effects include irritation at the injection site, and influenza-like symptoms, although these decrease with time.

Interferon beta-1b is available in subcutaneous and intramuscular forms. Subcutaneous Betaseron was the first interferon beta-1b used to treat MS. Every other day therapy resulted in reduction of acute episodes and decreased rate of progression at 2 years. Patients, however, often formed antibodies against the drug that limited its efficacy. Later it was found that weekly intramuscular Avonex resulted in more improvements in disease progression compared to subcutaneous therapy. Rebif is another approved subcutaneous interferon beta-1b treatment approved in the U.S. It has the benefit of producing less of an antibody response than Betaseron. Multiple side effects of interferon beta-1b include flu-like symptoms, local site reactions, thyroid dysfunction, liver dysfunction, anemia, and leucopenia.

The use of steroids for specific MS therapy has revolved around high-dose IV corticosteroids for acute attacks. Some benefit seems to result from oral methylprednisolone, with a 10-day taper following IV therapy.

A synthetic polymer, glatiramer acetate, given as a daily subcutaneous injection, is also currently used in the U.S. to treat relapsing-remitting MS. Side effects include local injection site reaction and transient post-injection chest pain or flushing.

In patients with progressive disease, different modalities are used. More potent immunomodulators such as cyclosporine, methotrexate, azathioprine, cyclophosphamide, and IVIG are used in conjunction with steroids and interferon. However, these potent immunosuppressants, while they may halt progression of the disease during use, are too powerful to be administered for extended periods.

Symptomatic treatment is of great importance. Physical therapy and occupational therapy maintain maximum function. Spasticity may respond to baclofen, dantrolene, or vigabatrin. The intention tremor resulting from the involvement of the cerebellum may respond to isoniazid and pyridoxine, or to β-blockers. Trigeminal neuralgia and paroxysmal symptoms may respond to carbamazepine, and chronic dysesthetic pain may respond to tricyclic antidepressants.

The management of patients with bladder disturbance has been revolutionized by the introduction of clean intermittent self-catheterization. Anticholinergic agents, particularly oxybutynin, may alleviate urinary frequency. In men with erectile dysfunction, intracorporeal papaverine may be helpful.

## Meningitis

Meningitis is inflammation of the membranous coverings of the brain and spinal cord. It may be caused by the following:
- Infection: bacteria, viruses, and fungi.
- Malignant cells.
- Blood following SAH.
- Air, drugs, or contrast media during encephalography.

The term "meningitis" is usually reserved for infection of the meninges by organisms.

### Pathophysiology
In acute bacterial meningitis, a dense exudate forms over the base of the brain and extends towards the convexity along the sulci. It may affect emerging cranial nerves giving rise to ocular palsies. Sulcal pockets of the exudate may become encysted or it may occlude the foramina of Magendie and Luschka with consequent hydrocephalus.

In tuberculous meningitis, the meninges over the base of the brain are most severely affected. A tough gelatinous exudate often involves the cranial nerves and the blood vessels. The subsequent arteritis may lead to occlusion of the vessel and infarction of the tissues which it supplies. In the case of miliary dissemination, choroidal tubercles can often be found in the optic fundus.

Viral meningitis consists mainly of a lymphocytic inflammatory reaction in the CSF without the formation of pus or adhesions.

### Predisposing factors
Outbreaks of meningitis tend to occur with overcrowding, poverty, and malnutrition. Infection may spread in institutions such as prisons or college dorms. Secondary meningitis can occur after head injury, sinusitis, mastoiditis, or extension of infection from the ears and nasopharynx.

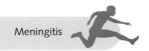

Immunocompromised patients, such as those with acquired immunodeficiency syndrome (AIDS), carcinoma, or those on cytotoxic drugs, and following splenectomy, are at increased risk. People with congenital meningeal defects or CSF shunts are also prone to infection.

## Clinical features

The features of meningitis are headache, neck stiffness, and clouding of consciousness. Bacterial meningitis is spread by droplet infection, and the organism lodges and multiplies in the nasopharynx. It enters the bloodstream, giving rise to a generalized septicemia, pyrexia, malaise, and rigors. Signs of cerebral irritability include photophobia, increased tendon reflexes, vomiting, and convulsions. In patients with *Neisseria meningitidis*, petechia, palpable purpura, and other skin manifestations may appear.

Kernig's sign (Fig. 34.6) may be positive, i.e., pain on passively extending the knee with the hips fully flexed. A petechial rash may occur, especially with meningococcal meningitis.

In tuberculous meningitis, symptoms may initially be nonspecific with malaise, anorexia, headache, and a variable mild fever. These symptoms may persist for days but gradually an unremitting deterioration occurs. There may be personality changes and intermittent dulling of consciousness before signs of meningism are obvious. The appearance of focal neurologic signs suggests a complication (e.g., venous sinus thrombosis, cerebral edema, or hydrocephalus).

## Differential diagnosis

Any cause of headache (Chapter 15) or infection should be considered. Of particular note are severe migraine, acute encephalitis, and SAH.

## Investigations

Blood should be taken for CBC, metabolic panel, glucose, and culture. Cultures should also be taken from the urine and nose. A head CT scan should be obtained with a history of head injury.

Lumbar puncture is the key investigation and should be performed as soon as possible. If the patient is profoundly ill, intravenous antibiotics should be given first.

A CT scan should be carried out if raised intracranial pressure is suspected or if there are focal neurologic signs, to rule out a space-occupying lesion. If normal, a lumbar puncture should be performed.

CSF changes in meningitis are summarized in Fig. 34.7.

## Treatment

High doses of appropriate antibiotics should be given immediately after a lumbar puncture is performed, or before it if the patient is very ill. The treatment of viral meningitis is supportive. Causative organisms include echovirus, mumps, coxsackievirus, herpes simplex and zoster, measles and influenza. Other causes of aseptic meningitis include SLE, syphilis, Lyme disease, leptospirosis, *Listeria*, *Brucella*, and partially treated bacterial meningitis.

Gram-staining of CSF may demonstrate organisms. *Pneumococcus* is a gram-positive

**Fig. 34.6** (A) Eliciting Kernig's sign. (B) Testing for neck stiffness.

| Changes in the cerebrospinal fluid in meningitis | | | | |
|---|---|---|---|---|
| | **Normal** | **Viral** | **Bacterial** | **Tuberculous** |
| appearance | clear | clear/turbid | turbid | turbid/fibrinous |
| predominant cell | <5 mononuclear cells/mL | 10–100 mononuclear cells/mL | 200–3000 polymorphs/mL | 10–300 mononuclear cells/mL 0–300 polymorphs/mL |
| protein | 0.2–0.4g/L | 0.4–0.8g/L | 0.5–5g/L | 0.5–5g/L |
| glucose | >2/3 plasma level | >2/3 plasma level | <2/3 plasma level | <2/3 plasma level |

**Fig. 34.7** Changes in the cerebrospinal fluid in meningitis.

| Treatment of meningitis | |
|---|---|
| **Organism** | **Treatment** |
| *Neisseria meningitidis* | benzylpenicillin or cefotaxime |
| *Streptococcus pneumoniae* | cefotaxime<br>benzylpenicillin if organism is penicillin sensitive<br>add vancomycin if organism is highly resistant to penicillin or cephalosporins |
| *Haemophilus influenzae* | ceftriaxone |
| *Listeria* | amoxycillin and gentamicin |
| *Escherichia coli* | third-generation cephalosporin |
| *Staphylococcus aureus* | benzylpenicillin and nafcillin or vancomycin |
| *Mycobacterium tuberculosis* | isoniazid, rifampicin, pyrazinamide, and ethambutol<br>pyridoxine prevents the neurotoxic effects of isoniazid |
| *Cryptococcus neoformans* | amphotericin B and flucytosine |

**Fig. 34.8** Treatment of meningitis.

intracellular diplococcus, and meningococcus (*Neisseria meningitidis*) is a gram-negative coccus. Ziehl-Neelsen staining may show acid-fast bacilli suggesting tuberculosis.

If bacterial meningitis is suspected, high doses of intravenous antibiotics should be started. If the organism is not known, adults should be given intravenous benzylpenicillin, 2.4g 4 hourly, and IV chloramphenicol, 50–100mg/kg 6 hourly, in liaison with the infectious disease specialist. Also consider a third-generation cephalosporin, such as cefotaxime, 2gIV q 6–8 hours. If the organism is known, specific antibiotics can be given (Fig. 34.8).

## Causative organisms

This is likely to vary with the patient's age:
- In neonates: *E. coli* and β-hemolytic streptococci are common.
- In children: *Haemophilus influenzae* and meningococcus predominate.
- Young adults: prone to meningococcus.
- Older adults: prone to pneumococcus (*Streptococcus pneumoniae*).
- Immunocompromised patients and the elderly: prone to pneumococcus, *Listeria*, gram-negative organisms, and cryptococcus.

Pain is treated with opiates and an appropriate antiemetic. Intravenous fluids are given if the patient is in shock, aiming to increase blood pressure and urine output.

Contacts of patients with meningitis due to *N. meningitidis* or *H. influenzae* should be given rifampicin for 2 days.

Prognosis of meningitis depends on how soon antibiotics were started. A delay of 4 hours in the ED led to an increased mortality rate of 15% in one study. Mortality can be as high as 20%, with significant morbidity for survivors.

Cases of meningitis must be reported to the Department of Public Health.

## Epilepsy

Epilepsy refers to a group of conditions in which paroxysms of abnormal electrical activity of cerebral neurones results in seizures. As many as 1 in 20 of the general population have a fit at some time in their lives, and between 0.5% and 1.0% of the U.S. population has epilepsy.

### Classification

Seizure disorders can be divided into two main groups: idiopathic generalized epilepsies and localization-related epilepsies.

### Idiopathic generalized epilepsies

These are mostly genetic in origin and are often associated with a characteristic spike and wave on electroencephalogram (EEG).

#### Tonic–clonic (grand mal) seizures

Before the seizure the patient may be irritable and experience minor disturbances such as myoclonic jerks. There may be a strange feeling (aura) before the seizure, which has a sudden onset. The tonic phase involves powerful muscular contractions. The patient is struck unconscious and falls rigidly to the ground. Teeth are clenched; cyanosis may occur. After about a minute, the clonic phase starts, consisting of violent convulsive movements. There may be tongue biting and urinary or fecal incontinence. The patient then becomes drowsy or will sleep for several hours. The reflexes are depressed, with a positive Babinski sign. The patient may be confused on waking (postictal confusion).

#### Absence attacks (petit mal)

These start in childhood and are accompanied by a characteristic EEG pattern of three spike-and-wave discharges per second. It is due to a congenital neuronal instability. There are brief interruptions of consciousness, sometimes accompanied by rhythmical blinking of the eyelids. To an observer, the child may appear to be dazed or daydreaming. Recovery is immediate, and there are no sequelae. Children can have hundreds of these episodes per

day. In evaluating a child with suspected petit mal seizures, ask about such indicators as school performance; these seizures can be detrimental to school work.

#### Myoclonic epilepsy

This is a form of idiopathic epilepsy developing in early childhood. Various types of generalized seizures occur, including sudden jerking movements of the limbs (myoclonus).

### Localization-related epilepsy

These have a focus of activity (e.g., a tumor or scar tissue caused by trauma or stroke), from which epileptic activity begins and then spreads. They may lead to generalized tonic-clonic seizures. The nature of the attack varies according to the primary site of the lesion. Examples include focal motor attacks, focal sensory attacks, and temporal lobe epilepsy.

#### Focal motor attacks

These arise in the precentral motor cortex and consist of clonic movements in localized groups of muscles such as the hand or face. They may continue for hours, in which case it is called epilepsia partialis continuans. The discharge may spread along the precentral gyrus causing a march of clonic movements throughout the body (Jacksonian seizure). After the seizure there may be a short-lived weakness of the affected parts of the body (Todd's paresis).

#### Focal sensory attacks

These start in the postcentral sensory cortex, and either localized or spreading paresthesias occur.

#### Temporal lobe epilepsy

This may consist of hallucinations of any of the five senses and of memory. Gustatory and olfactory hallucinations are usually unpleasant. *Jamais vu* is a sudden feeling of unfamiliarity while the patient is in his or her own environment and *déjà vu* is a vivid sense of familiarity with the current situation.

In automatism, the patient remains conscious but "dreamy" and may continue with normal activities. The patient cannot remember these events after the attack.

### Etiology

Although most seizures are idiopathic, a cause for the epilepsy and precipitating factors should be looked into. These include the following:
- Metabolic causes: hypoxia, hyper- or

hypoglycemia, hypocalcemia, uremia, alcoholism, hypo- and hypernatremia, liver failure, pyridoxine deficiency.
- Drugs and toxins: alcohol, lead, and drugs (e.g., phenothiazines, monoamine oxidase inhibitors, tricyclic antidepressants, amphetamines, lidocaine, nalidixic acid [a quinolone antibiotic]).
- Trauma and surgery (e.g., perinatal trauma or head injury).
- Space-occupying lesions.
- Cerebral infarction.
- Other organic brain diseases: SLE, PAN, sarcoidosis, vascular malformations.
- Infections: encephalitis, syphilis, and human immunodeficiency virus.
- Degenerative brain disorders: Alzheimer's disease, Creutzfeld–Jacob disease.

## Precipitants of epilepsy
Seizures may be precipitated by flashing lights. Other possible precipitants include fever, irregular meals, menstruation, hyperventilation leading to alkalosis, lack of sleep, emotional disturbances, and pregnancy.

## Differential diagnosis
In taking a history it is important to keep in mind a differential diagnosis of conditions causing transient loss of consciousness. These include the following:
- Syncope: this is due to cerebral ischemia. The onset is gradual, and the patient slips to the floor. Recovery occurs after 1–2 minutes and is gradual. The patient is back to normal within a few minutes.
- Drop attacks: these involve a sudden weakness of the legs, making the patient fall. They are most commonly due to vertebrobasilar artery insufficiency.
- Hypoglycemia: the onset is prolonged, and the patient is confused, sweating, and light-headed. A time relationship to meals may be established.
- Narcolepsy: irresistible diurnal attacks of sleepiness. The patient may experience visual or auditory hallucinations when falling asleep (hypnogogic hallucinations). The patient wakes within a few minutes, feeling well.
- Cataplexy: a sudden loss of muscle tone so that the patient crumples to the ground.
- Micturition, defecation, and cough syncope: fainting after the respective acts.

- Carotid sinus syncope: this is due to supersensitivity of the carotid sinus to external pressure.
- Postural hypotension: either autonomic or secondary to drugs.
- TIAs, especially in the posterior cerebral circulation.
- Cardiac arrhythmias: due to impaired cardiac output; the loss of consciousness is sudden and the patient goes pale; there may be flushing on regaining consciousness.
- Psychogenic (hysterical seizures): there is usually some apparent gain for the patient, although he or she is seldom aware of the motivation. The seizures usually only occur in front of an audience. There is often active opposition on attempting to examine the patient. There may be strange cries and flailing limbs in an attempt to mimic true epilepsy.

## Investigations
After a careful history and examination to consider differential diagnoses, blood tests include CBC, metabolic panel, serum calcium, liver function tests, and glucose. A CXR and ECG should be performed.

The diagnosis should not be based solely on the EEG because 10–15% of the general population may have an "abnormal" EEG, and approximately 15% of people with epilepsy never have specific epileptiform discharges.

CT scanning as the sole basis of diagnosis is also unreliable. The frequency of abnormalities found in CT scans in people with epilepsy varies greatly. A CT scan is indicated in a patient with late-onset epilepsy who has focal seizures, because it may detect a tumor.

## Treatment
The aims of drug treatment are to prevent seizures while keeping the patient free of side effects. Antiepileptic drugs should be prescribed singly, using the lowest dose to obtain complete seizure control with minimum side effects. A single drug will suffice in approximately 80% of patients; the remainder need a second drug to achieve acceptable control. Localization-related epilepsy is more likely to be refractory.

Carbamazepine, phenytoin, and barbiturates all induce hepatic enzymes and therefore speed up the metabolism of estrogens and progestogens, making the oral contraceptive pill unreliable. Valproate does not affect oral contraceptive efficacy.

Treatment should be based on the type of seizure. For instance, certain medications are more effective in treating partial seizures than others (see below).

Patients who have had an isolated seizure related to a metabolic or infectious cause can usually be spared treatment with anticonvulsant medications.

Risk factors for recurrent seizures include:
- A mass lesion shown on CT or MRI (e.g., stroke, neoplasm).
- A focal neurologic deficit.
- Past brain injury or cognitive impairment.
- Abnormal EEG.

Epileptics should be encouraged not to drink alcohol, since more than 3 drinks can increase the risk of seizure. By law in many states, physicians are required to report seizures, and driving limitations may be imposed. Epilepsy can have profound social consequences, including discrimination and exclusion from certain jobs (e.g., the armed forces). Personal implications include feelings of insecurity.

Patients who have had a seizure-free period of 2 years should be given a trial period off the medication. About 60% will have to return to taking medication. Patients who have refractory disease, especially those with a specific brain lesion, should be considered for surgery. Although studies are lacking, reported cases in the hands of a specialty center are generally encouraging.

### First-line drugs
#### Idiopathic generalized epilepsy
Phenytoin is often recommended as the treatment of choice because carbamazepine is ineffective for the treatment of absence or myoclonic seizures. Phenytoin, valproate, and carabmazepine are equally as effective for idiopathic generalized tonic–clonic seizures. Common unwanted effects of valproate include weight gain, hair thinning, and tremor. Hepatotoxicity, thrombocytopenia, and pancreatitis may occur. Note that loading a patient with phenytoin after a seizure (usually 20mg/kg) can lead to hypotension. Use of fosphenytoin can prevent this side effect. Ethosuximide and valproate are useful alternatives in children with absence seizures only.

### Localization-related epilepsies
Carbamazepine, sodium valproate, phenytoin, and phenobarbitol are equally effective. However, they differ in their side-effect profiles and ease of use, and because of this carbamazepine and valproate have become the drugs of first choice. Carbamazepine may cause CNS side effects (e.g., dizziness, nausea, headaches, and drowsiness), which may be avoided by slowly increasing the dose. It induces hepatic microsomal enzymes and so increases the metabolism of phenobarbitol, valproate, lamotrigine, corticosteroids, oral contraceptives, theophylline, and warfarin. It also inhibits the metabolism of phenytoin. Idiosyncratic reactions include the Stevens-Johnson syndrome, exfoliative dermatitis, and hepatitis.

### Second-line drugs
Phenytoin is useful but often difficult to use because of its unpredictable pharmacokinetics, and so the best dose is difficult to determine. Phenobarbitol affects cognition and behavior and is no longer considered a first-line drug. Primidone is partly metabolized in the liver to phenobarbitone and is no longer recommended.

### Add-on drugs
Vigabatrin, lamotrigine, and gabapentin are used as add-on therapies for partial or secondarily generalized seizures. They are equally effective. Vigabatrin may cause drowsiness, fatigue, irritability, weight gain, and psychosis. Lamotrigine can precipitate carbamazepine toxicity, so if unwanted effects such as diplopia occur, the dose of carbamazepine should be reduced. It causes a mild maculopapular rash in 5% of patients, the incidence of which can be reduced by starting at a low dose. Gabapentin is renally excreted so the dose should be reduced in patients with renal impairment. The most common side effects are somnolence, dizziness, and ataxia.

The benzodiazepines, such as clonazepam, may also be used. Clobazem can be used as an add-on for people with refractory epilepsy. Taken continuously it can cause dependence. Clonazepam is useful in children with myoclonic or tonic–clonic seizures. Sedation and tachyphylaxis are common, and withdrawal seizures may occur. It should be used only rarely.

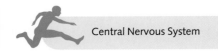

## Treatment of status epilepticus

Status, as it is known, is defined as continuous seizure activity for over 5 minutes (some still define status as seizure activity lasting over 30 minutes). It can lead to rhabdomyolysis, lactic acidosis, aspiration pneumonitis, and respiratory failure. Neuronal death can occur after 30 to 60 minutes of continuous seizure activity. Treatment should start with 0.2 mg/kg of diazepam, followed by 20 mg/dk of phenytoin.

## Intracranial tumors

Cerebral tumors represent about 10% of all malignancies. They may be primary or secondary mainly from the bronchus, breasts, kidneys, colon, ovary, prostate, or thyroid. The main sites of origin of brain tumors are shown in Fig. 34.9. Other tumors are rare.

## Clinical features

Symptoms arise from the direct effects of the mass on surrounding structures, the effects of raised ICP, or by provoking seizures. Similar symptoms may be produced by any mass lesion (e.g., hematomas, aneurysms, abscesses, tuberculomas, granulomas, and cysts).

Direct effects depend on the site of the tumor:
- Frontal lobe: personality changes, apathy, and impairment of intellectual function. There may be anosmia, contralateral hemiparesis, or dysphasia (Broca's area).

- Parietal lobe: contralateral homonymous field defects and hemisensory loss. There may be apraxia, spatial disorientation, and dysphasia if the temporoparietal region is affected. Signs include "parietal drift" or falling of the outstretched contralateral arm, asteriognosis (inability to recognize an object placed in the hand), and sensory inattention.
- Temporal lobe: symptoms and signs are those of temporal lobe epilepsy (see p. 325).
- Occipital lobe: contralateral hemianopia.
- Cerebellopontine angle: progressive ipsilateral perceptive deafness, numbness of the ipsilateral side of the face, facial weakness, vertigo, and ipsilateral cerebellar signs (see p. 321).

## Raised intracranial pressure

Symptoms include a throbbing headache (which is worse in the morning and with stooping, coughing, and sneezing), nausea and vomiting, and papilledema. A shift of intracranial contents produces symptoms similar to direct mass effects. There may be impairment of consciousness, progressing to coma, respiratory depression, and "false localizing signs," e.g., a 6th nerve lesion, as it is compressed on the petrous temporal bone.

## Investigations

The main investigations are a skull x-ray, EEG, CT brain scan, and MRI. If metastases are suspected, investigations for the primary neoplasm should be carried out. Lumbar puncture is contraindicated because of the risk of herniation of the cerebellar tonsils through the foramen magnum ("coning"). Biopsy should be considered, especially if an abscess is suspected.

## Management

This is by surgical excision if possible. Radiotherapy is usually recommended for gliomas and for radiosensitive metastases. Dexamethasone will reduce cerebral edema. Epilepsy is treated with anticonvulsants.

## Prognosis

The overall 1-year survival rate for patients with primary intracerebral tumors is less than 50%. There may be complete recovery from meningiomas if they are removed completely.

| The origins of brain tumors | |
|---|---|
| **Site** | **Example of tumor derived** |
| glia | gliomas (50%) ollgodendrogliomas, ependymomas |
| meninges | meningiomas (25%) |
| blood vessels | angiomas angloblastomas |
| the Schwann cells of the cranial nerves | acoustic neuromas |
| pituitary gland | craniopharyngioma |

**Fig. 34.9** The origins of brain tumors.

## Miscellaneous neurologic disorders

### Motor neuron disease

This is a disease of unknown cause involving progressive degeneration of the anterior horn cells, lower cranial nuclei (hence the external ocular movements are normal), and neurons of the motor cortex and pyramidal tracts. Both upper and lower motor neurons can be affected, but there are no sensory abnormalities.

It is slightly more common in men with a peak incidence between the ages of 50 and 70 years. The prevalence in the U.S. is about 6 in 100,000. Clinically there are three classical patterns of disease:

- Amyotrophic lateral sclerosis (50%): combined lower motor neuron wasting and upper motor neuron spasticity and hyperreflexia. Weakness starts in the legs and spreads to the arms.
- Progressive muscular atrophy (25%): anterior horn cell involvement leading to lower motor neuron weakness, wasting, and fasciculation of distal muscles, which spreads proximally.

- Progressive bulbar palsy (25%): lower motor neuron weakness and wasting of the tongue and pharynx, leading to dysarthria and dysphagia.

Combinations of the above may occur.

### Management

Management is symptomatic. The aim is to help the patient with activities of daily living and to reduce symptoms. Opiates should be considered for joint pains and distress. Death usually occurs between 2 and 5 years after diagnosis.

### Peripheral neuropathy

The causes of peripheral neuropathy are summarized in Fig. 34.10. The four most common causes are DM, malignancy, vitamin $B_{12}$ deficiency, and drugs. Treatment is aimed at the underlying cause.

### Guillain-Barré syndrome

This condition (also called acute postinfective polyneuropathy) affects motor nerves more than sensory nerves, and follows days or weeks after an infectious illness such as cytomegalovirus and Epstein-Barr virus. There is inflammation, edema,

| Causes of peripheral neuropathy | |
|---|---|
| **Cause** | **Example** |
| idiopathic | |
| drugs and chemicals | isoniazid, amiodarone<br>lead, mercury |
| metabolic | diabetes mellitus<br>amyloidosis<br>uremia<br>acute intermittent porphyria |
| deficiency states | deficiencies of vitamin $B_{12}$, $B_1$ (beriberi) and niacin (pellagra)<br>alcoholism |
| infections | leprosy<br>diphtheria<br>tetanus<br>botulism |
| miscellaneous | Guillain-Barré syndrome<br>collagen diseases, e.g. PAN, RA<br>malignancy<br>sarcoidosis<br>myxedema |
| congenital | rare hereditary ataxias and neuropathies |

**Fig. 34.10** Causes of peripheral neuropathy (PAN, polyarteritis nodosa; RA, rheumatoid arthritis).

and demyelination of peripheral nerves and roots. Clinically, there is paresthesia and numbness followed by a flaccid paralysis, which is progressive and ascending but may come on rapidly and affect all four limbs simultaneously. The trunk, respiratory, and cranial nerves may be affected. Complications include respiratory failure, pulmonary embolism, and cardiac dysrhythmias.

## Investigations

The CSF shows a very high protein concentration (up to 10g/L) with a normal cell count. The vital capacity should be measured 4–6 hourly to anticipate respiratory depression. EMG studies typically show slow conduction velocities, prolonged latencies distally, and partial motor conduction block.

## Management

Treatment is supportive. Attention should be paid to fluid balance and nutrition, and prevention of pressure sores, deep vein thrombosis, and pneumonia (physiotherapy). Ventilation may be necessary if respiratory failure occurs. Around 90–95% of patients recover within 3–6 months. Treatment modalities include supportive care for possible respiratory failure, IVIG, and plasma exchange.

# Muscle disorders

For more on muscle disorders, see polymyositis on p. 371.

## Myasthenia gravis

This is an autoimmune disease with a reduction in the number of functioning postsynaptic acetylcholine receptors, leading to muscle weakness. About 90% of patients have detectable antiacetylcholine receptor antibodies. It is associated with thymic tumors, hyperthyroidism, rheumatoid arthritis, and SLE.

### Clinical features

The condition affects young adults and women twice as commonly as men. There is painless muscle weakness, which worsens on repetitive contraction. It is usually most marked in the face and eyes, producing ptosis, diplopia, and a "myasthenic snarl" on smiling. The voice may weaken on continued speaking, and dysphagia may occur. Proximal muscles and upper limbs are more often affected than distal muscles and lower limbs. Reflexes tend to be brisk.

Since respiratory muscles can be affected, it is important to determine the pulmonary reserve for patients with MG because they may quickly need emergent intubation. An easy way to test respiratory capacity is to have the patient maximally inhale, then count out loud while exhaling. If the patient cannot count to 20 while exhaling one breath, this may be a sign of impending respiratory failure.

### Investigations

Edrophonium (Tensilon), 10mg, is given intravenously (with cardiac monitoring and resuscitation facilities). This improves muscle power for 3–4 minutes. It is an anticholinesterase, which enhances neuromuscular transmission in myasthenia gravis. It prolongs the action of acetylcholine by inhibiting the action of the enzyme acetylcholinesterase. There is raised antiacetylcholine receptor antibody.

### Management

Symptomatic control is with a longer-acting anticholinesterase (e.g., pyridostigmine or neostigmine). The dose is slowly titrated against muscle power. Side effects include nausea, vomiting, increased salivation, diarrhea, and abdominal cramps. In overdosage there may be excessive bronchial secretions and sweating, involuntary defecation and micturition, bradycardia, agitation, and weakness, eventually leading to fasciculation and paralysis. Thymectomy increases the percentage of patients in remission.

Immunosuppression with prednisone on alternate days may achieve remission. If there is no remission and weakness is severe, azathioprine may be helpful. In intractable cases, plasmaphoresis gives about 4 weeks of benefit. The condition is usually relapsing or slowly progressive, and respiratory muscle involvement can lead to death. The 5-year survival rate with a thymoma is about 30%.

## Myotonic dystrophy (myotonia dystrophica)

This is an autosomal dominant condition characterized by myotonia, i.e., the inability of the muscles to relax normally after contraction. The peak onset is between the ages of 20 and 30 years. There is muscle wasting and weakness of the facial muscles with frontal balding, ptosis, a wry smile or "sneer" and a "hound dog" appearance.

There is also weakness of the shoulder girdle and quadriceps, cataracts, testicular or ovarian atrophy, cardiomyopathy with conduction disturbances, and mental impairment. Reflexes are lost. The myotonia increases with fatigue, cold, and stress. It may improve with procainamide or phenytoin, and there may be associated DM.

## Muscular dystrophies

These are a group of genetically determined diseases characterized by progressive degeneration and weakness of certain muscle groups.

### Duchenne muscular dystrophy (pseudohypertrophic)

This is the most common type and is x-linked recessive. The incidence is 25 in 100,000 male births. The condition presents at around 5 years of age with clumsiness in walking and difficulty in climbing stairs Examination reveals a lordotic posture and "waddling" gait due to proximal muscle weakness. The calves are hypertrophied. Investigations show a markedly raised creatine kinase concentration. Electromyography and muscle biopsy show characteristic changes. Death usually occurs before the age of 20 years from intercurrent illnesses (e.g., chest infection). There is no specific treatment.

### Facioscapulohumeral dystrophy (Landouzy-Dejerine syndrome)

This is autosomal dominant. The onset is around puberty with wasting and weakness of the upper limb girdle and face. Life expectancy is normal.

### Limb girdle dystrophy (Erb's syndrome)

This is autosomal recessive and presents at around 20–40 years. The shoulders and muscles of the pelvic girdles are affected, and the condition is progressive with death in middle age.

## Disorders of the spinal cord

### Syringomyelia

This is due to a longitudinal cyst in the cervical cord. As it enlarges it may extend into the dorsal horns and white matter. Clinical features are insidious and include the following:

- Weakness and wasting of the small muscles of the hand.
- Dissociated sensory loss in the hand: loss of pain and temperature sensation only. This may involve the trunk and arm.
- Trophic changes (e.g., ulceration and scarring) and swollen fingers due to subcutaneous hypertrophy.
- Loss of tendon reflexes.
- Pain in the arm.
- Spastic paraplegia: upper motor neuron signs.
- Charcot's joints in the upper limbs: destruction of the joints by too great a range of movement when normal sensation is lost.

Treatment is by surgical decompression or aspiration.

### Syringobulbia

This is usually due to the extension of the cyst into the midbrain. It may involve the trigeminal nerve root, the motor nuclei of the lower cranial nerves, and the cervical sympathetic tract. Symptoms include the following:

- Facial pain or sensory loss: 5th cranial nerve.
- Vertigo and nystagmus: 8th cranial nerve.
- Facial, palatal, or laryngeal palsy: 7th, 9th, 10th, and 11th cranial nerves.
- Wasting of the tongue: 12th cranial nerve.
- Horner's syndrome: sympathetic tract.

| Causes of spinal cord compression | |
|---|---|
| **Cause** | **Example** |
| vertebral (extradural) | collapsed vertebrae, e.g. metastatic cancer (bronchus, breast, thyroid, kidney, prostate), osteoporosis, myeloma<br>spondylosis with disc prolapse<br>Pott's disease (tuberculosis)<br>Paget's disease<br>abscess<br>reticuloses |
| intradural, extramedullary | meningioma<br>neurofibroma |
| intramedullary | glioma |

**Fig. 34.11** Causes of spinal cord compression.

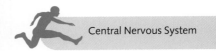

## Subacute combined degeneration of the cord

This is due to vitamin $B_{12}$ deficiency and refers to demyelination of the posterior and lateral columns. The onset is usually insidious and associated with a sensory peripheral neuropathy. Clinical features include the following:

- Loss of vibration and proprioception senses, and positive rombergism: posterior columns.
- Weakness, hypertonia, and extensor plantars: upper motor neuron.
- Absent knee jerks and reduced touch sensation: peripheral neuropathy.

Treatment is with vitamin $B_{12}$ injections intramuscularly.

## Spinal cord compression

Spinal cord compression is a medical emergency. Symptoms include root pain often precipitated by movement or straining, spastic paraparesis with upper motor neuron signs and weakness, sensory loss, with sphincter disturbances at a later stage. Investigation is by x-ray of the spine, and CT or MRI to show the spinal cord. Investigations should also include those of the underlying cause.

Treatment is by decompression, which should be performed as soon as possible to prevent irreversible damage. Radiotherapy may be useful in malignant disease.

Causes of spinal cord compression are summarized in Fig. 34.11.

# 35. Metabolic and Endocrine Disorders

## Diabetes

Diabetes mellitus (DM) is a persistent state of hyperglycemia due to diminished availability or effectiveness of insulin. The diagnosis is made on finding two random plasma glucose concentrations greater than or equal to 200mg/dl (11.1mmol/L) or two fasting plasma glucose levels greater than or equal to 126mg/dl (7.8mmol/L).

A new classification is called impaired fasting glucose (IFG). If the fasting glucose is at least 110mgdl (6mmol/L) but below 126mg/dl (7.8mmol/L), the patient may have IFG. IFG is an indication for an oral glucose tolerance test, although this is rarely carried out in practice. The patient is given 75mg of glucose. If the glucose after 120 minutes is above 126mg/dl (7.8mmol/L) but below 200mg/dl (11.1mmol/L), then the patient has IFG.

The cause of diabetes is not known but it is partly genetic and partly environmental—30% of identical twins and 10% of siblings develop diabetes. There is an association with human leukocyte antigen (HLA)-D3 and HLA-DR4. Environmental triggers may include viral infections. Diabetes affects about 2% of the population.

### Classification

Type I, or insulin-dependent diabetes mellitus (IDDM), typically starts in young people who are usually thin and have an abrupt onset of signs and symptoms associated with low circulating insulin. IDDM is due to autoantibodies to pancreatic β cells causing a low concentration of circulating insulin.

Patients with type II, or non-insulin-dependent diabetes mellitus (NIDDM), are usually older and overweight, and the onset is more insidious. NIDDM is due to reduced insulin production and reduced sensitivity of peripheral tissues to circulating insulin. Patients may require insulin if hyperglycemia persists, despite maximal doses of oral hypoglycemic agents, and in times of stress such as severe infections or after myocardial infarction.

Secondary DM may be caused by the following:
- Drugs (e.g., thiazide diuretics and steroids).
- Gestational DM: patients develop impaired glucose tolerance or frank diabetes during pregnancy.
- Pancreatic disease (e.g., pancreatectomy, carcinoma of the pancreas, pancreatitis, cystic fibrosis, hemachromatosis).
- Endocrine causes: Cushing's syndrome, acromegaly, pheochromocytoma.

### Clinical presentation

Diabetes may be asymptomatic and found on routine screening, but about half of all diabetics are undiagnosed. Patients may present with nonspecific symptoms such as weight loss and lethargy, and they are more prone to infection (e.g., carbuncles and thrush). Polyuria and polydipsia are characteristic. The patient may present for the first time with diabetic ketoacidosis, i.e., smelling of ketones, hyperventilating, dehydrated, and even drowsy, confused, or comatose (Fig. 35.1).

### Complications

The chronic complications of DM are summarized in Fig. 35.2.

### Vascular system

Disease in both the large and small vessels is more common in people with diabetes and occurs in all vascular beds, leading to an increased incidence of myocardial infarction, stroke, renal failure, retinopathy, and peripheral vascular disease. It is therefore important to control other cardiovascular risk factors such as hypertension, smoking, and hyperlipidemia. Myocardial infarction is twice as common in diabetics as in the general population.

In small vessel disease, pedal ischemia and gangrene can occur despite the presence of palpable pedal pulses.

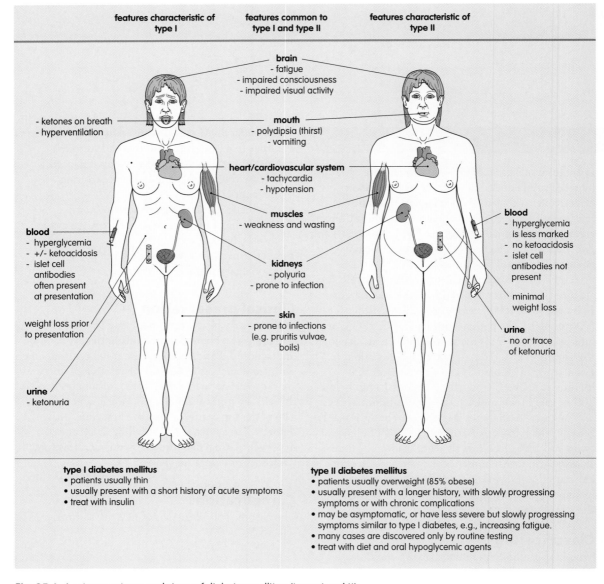

**type I diabetes mellitus**
- patients usually thin
- usually present with a short history of acute symptoms
- treat with insulin

**type II diabetes mellitus**
- patients usually overweight (85% obese)
- usually present with a longer history, with slowly progressing symptoms or with chronic complications
- may be asymptomatic, or have less severe but slowly progressing symptoms similar to type I diabetes, e.g., increasing fatigue.
- many cases are discovered only by routine testing
- treat with diet and oral hypoglycemic agents

**Fig. 35.1** Acute symptoms and signs of diabetes mellitus (types I and II).

## Eyes

Blindness occurs in up to 20% of patients with IDDM. Good diabetic control reduces the incidence of eye complications. Large fluctuations in blood glucose concentration (and hence the glucose concentration of the vitreous humor) cause osmotic shifts across the lens resulting in transiently blurred vision. This is common when the diabetes is first treated. Cataracts occur at a younger age in diabetics.

In a patient with gangrene and a palpable dorsalis pedis pulse, think of microvascular disease.

**Fig. 35.2** Chronic complications of diabetes mellitus.

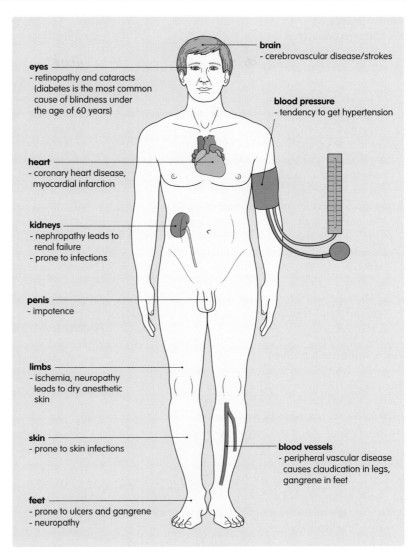

**brain**
- cerebrovascular disease/strokes

**eyes**
- retinopathy and cataracts (diabetes is the most common cause of blindness under the age of 60 years)

**blood pressure**
- tendency to get hypertension

**heart**
- coronary heart disease, myocardial infarction

**kidneys**
- nephropathy leads to renal failure
- prone to infections

**penis**
- impotence

**limbs**
- ischemia, neuropathy leads to dry anesthetic skin

**skin**
- prone to skin infections

**blood vessels**
- peripheral vascular disease causes claudication in legs, gangrene in feet

**feet**
- prone to ulcers and gangrene
- neuropathy

## Background retinopathy

This is characterized by hemorrhages ("blots"), hard exudates, and microaneurysms ("dots"), which are bulges in the capillary walls. Vision is rarely affected unless macular edema develops, in which case referral to an ophthalmologist should be made.

## Preproliferative retinopathy

The above changes are usually more marked. In addition, there are soft "cotton-wool" exudates, which are small deep retinal infarcts.

## Proliferative retinopathy

There is new vessel formation, mainly near the optic disc in response to relative hypoxia in the vitreous. Other features such as cluster hemorrhages and soft exudates are present. Urgent referral to an ophthalmologist for laser therapy should be made because the new vessels are fragile and may bleed into the vitreous leading to sudden blindness. Fibrosis then ensues and can lead to retinal detachment and thrombotic glaucoma.

## Maculopathy

Although sometimes difficult to see on fundoscopy, this should be suspected if there is a decrease in visual acuity. Patients should visit an ophthalmologist.

## Neuropathies

### Somatic neuropathies

Somatic neuropathies may take the following forms:

- Peripheral neuropathies: this commonly affects the lower limbs, with numbness and paresthesias of the feet, spreading up the leg. Symptoms are predominantly sensory with early loss of vibration sense and absent ankle jerks. In advanced cases, the loss of pain sensation may lead to the development of punched-out chronic ulcers at pressure points, in areas of thick callus. Foot pulses may be easily palpable; the foot may become infected and eventually gangrenous.
- Mononeuritis: this is due to occlusion of an artery supplying the nerve. Commonly involved nerves include the 3rd cranial nerve, ulnar nerve, and lateral popliteal nerve. More than one nerve can be involved; hence mononeuritis multiplex.
- Diabetic amyotrophy: this is painful asymmetrical weakness and wasting of the quadriceps muscles. It may recover.

### Autonomic neuropathies

This may lead to symptoms of postural hypotension (i.e., dizziness on standing), impotence, nocturnal diarrhea, and urinary retention. There may be lack of awareness of symptoms of hypoglycemia, which is also more frequent in patients on β-blockers.

## Kidneys

About a quarter of diabetics diagnosed before the age of 30 years develop renal failure. Renal failure is hastened by concomitant poor blood pressure control. Predisposing factors include the following:

- Atherosclerosis and hypertension: leading to renal ischemia.
- Infection: glycosuria predisposes to infection, which is more common throughout the urinary tract.
- Renal papillary necrosis: caused by infarction of the papillae, resulting in hematuria and renal impairment. The papillae may slough and cause obstruction.

Most of the renal problems are secondary to glomerular lesions; there is thickening of the basement membrane. This may be diffuse and present in the majority of diabetics, or nodular as in the Kimmelstiel–Wilson lesion, which is pathognomonic of DM and consists of homogenous, acellular, eosinophilic nodules.

## Skin

Complications occurring in the skin include the following:

- Lipoatrophy: this is fat necrosis at insulin injection sites. The patient should be advised to vary the injection sites because the absorption of insulin at sites of atrophy is unpredictable. Transfer to human insulin may help.
- Necrobiosis lipoidica diabeticorum: these are yellowish areas on the skin with telangiectasia. Biopsy shows atrophy of subcutaneous collagen. They are pathognomonic of diabetes.
- Infections, such as boils, are more common.
- Granuloma annulare.

## Infections

Common infections are of the urinary tract and skin, and candidiasis. Tuberculosis (TB) is also more common in diabetics.

# Management of diabetes

The aim of treatment is to achieve the best possible control of plasma glucose without making the patient obsessional and to avoid disabling hypoglycemia. The patient is best managed as part of a multidisciplinary team with doctors, nurses, ophthalmologists, dieticians, and podiatrist. A good rapport should be established and the patient should be educated about good diabetic control, how to abort hypoglycemic attacks, and the symptoms to watch out for with hyperglycemia.

New patients may be deliberately made hypoglycemic so that they know what symptoms to expect and how to abort the attack.

## Diet

Calorie intake should be adjusted to achieve or maintain an ideal body weight. The diet should be low in fat (to help delay the progression of atherosclerosis), low in refined sugars but high in complex carbohydrates like starch, and high in fiber, which, among other benefits, helps to lower postprandial hypoglycemia.

## Oral hypoglycemic agents

These drugs should be used in addition to, not instead of, diet. The two main classes are sulfonylureas and biguanides, although other classes have recently been introduced, including— Thiazolidinediones and eg (Rosiglitazone, Pioglitazoe)—Meglitinides.

## Sulfonylureas

These act mainly by augmenting insulin secretion and therefore some residual pancreatic β-cell activity is required. There are several sulfonylureas, but all are probably equally as effective. Chlorpropamide, however, has more side effects and a very prolonged duration of action, leading to possible hypoglycemia in some patients. It may also cause facial flushing after alcohol. Elderly patients are particularly prone to the dangers of hypoglycemia when long-acting sulfonylureas are used, and so chlorpropamide and glibenclamide should be avoided and replaced by shorter-acting drugs.

The sulfonylureas tend to encourage weight gain. Caution is needed in the elderly and those with hepatic and renal insufficiency because of the hazard of hypoglycemia. Side effects are generally mild and infrequent and include gastrointestinal (GI) disturbances and headache. Some patients acquire sensitivity reactions, which include transient rashes, rarely progressing to erythema multiforme and exfoliative dermatitis.

Second-generation sulfonylureas have become much more commonly used than the first-generation medications noted above. Glipizide, glyburide, and glimepride are usually taken once daily in either their standard or long-acting formula.

## Biguanides

Metformin is the only available biguanide. It exerts its effect mainly by decreasing gluconeogenesis and by increasing peripheral utilization of glucose. Some residual islet cell function is required. It is usually reserved for people with NIDDM who are overweight and in whom diet and sulfonylureas fail to control diabetes adequately, but it may be used as a first-line agent in overweight patients; hypoglycemia is not usually a problem. GI side effects are common, and lactic acidosis may also occur, although usually only in patients with renal impairment, in whom it should not be used.

## Other agents

Acarbose, an inhibitor of intestinal α-glucosidases, delays the digestion of starch and sucrose and hence the increase in blood glucose levels which follow a carbohydrate-containing meal.

Guar gum can reduce postprandial plasma glucose concentrations in diabetes, probably by retarding carbohydrate absorption. It is also used to relieve symptoms of the dumping syndrome.

## Insulin

Approximately 25% of diabetics require treatment with insulin (a polypeptide hormone). It is inactivated by GI enzymes and must therefore be given by injection, usually subcutaneously. Mixtures of available insulin preparations may be required to maintain good control, and these will vary for individual patients. Requirements may be affected by variations in lifestyle, infections, and concomitant drugs.

Patients should aim for blood glucose concentrations between 100–120mg/dl (4–10mmol/L) for most of the time, while accepting that on occasions they will be above or below these values. They should be advised to look for "peaks" and "troughs" of blood glucose and to adjust their insulin dosage only once or twice weekly. Overall it is ideal to aim for a glycosylated hemoglobin ($HbA_{1c}$) level of below 7% (normal range is 4–6%).

The insulin preparations may be short-acting (lispro insulin), regular, or long-acting. Most patients are best started on insulins of regular action twice daily; a short-acting insulin can later be added to cover any hyperglycemia which may follow breakfast or evening meals (Fig. 35.3).

## Continuing assessment

The aims of continued assessment of diabetics are education, assessment of glycemic control, and assessment of complications.

Many patients now monitor their own blood glucose concentrations using blood glucose strips, preferably with an electronic meter. These records should be examined, together with any hypoglycemic symptoms, and $HbA_{1c}$. Visual acuity should be checked, together with an examination of the optic fundi (after dilatation of the pupils) for retinopathy. The feet should be examined for neuropathy, ischemic changes, and infection. Nephropathy should be looked for by monitoring the urea and electrolytes (U&Es) and by testing for albuminuria.

## Diabetes and surgery

Diabetic patients should be first on the operating list, and fasted on the morning of surgery. Oral agents should be stopped 24 hours before surgery, and restarted postoperatively unless the patient is ill or the blood glucose is very high, necessitating a period on insulin.

| Insulin pharmacokinetics | | | |
|---|---|---|---|
| Insulin type | Onset | Peak | Duration |
| Lispro or Aspart | 5–15 min | 45–75 min | 2–4 h |
| Regular | ~30 min | 2–4 h | 5–8 h |
| NPH or Lente | ~2 h | 6–10 h | 18–28 h |
| Ultralente | ~4 h | 10–20 h | 12–20 h |
| Insuline glargine | ~2 h | No discernible peak | 20–24+ h |

**Fig. 35.3** The approximate times to onset of action, peak activity, and duration of action of the major types of insulin.

For patients already on insulin, the usual insulin should be given the night before the operation. An intravenous infusion of 500 mL of 5% glucose with 10 mmol KCl should be started early on the day of the operation and run at a constant rate to the patient's fluid requirements. A 1 unit/mL solution of soluble insulin in 0.9% saline should also be infused intravenously using a syringe pump. The rate varies according to the patient's blood glucose concentration, which should be measured every 2 hours until stable and every 6 hours thereafter. When the patient starts to eat and drink, he or she may be restarted on the normal insulin regimen.

# Diabetic coma
## Hypoglycemia
Symptoms of hypoglycemia include sweating, hunger, and tremor. Very low glucose concentrations may cause drowsiness, fits, transient neurologic symptoms, and loss of consciousness.

## Etiology
The etiology of hypoglycemia includes the following:
- Drugs: excessive insulin or sulfonylureas (especially chlorpropamide). Large doses may be taken deliberately, particularly by medical and paramedical staff. Alcohol binges, especially with decreased food intake, may also lead to hypoglycemia.
- Endocrine causes: pituitary insufficiency, Addison's disease, and insulinomas.
- Post-gastrectomy and functional hypoglycemia.
- Liver failure.
- Inherited enzyme defects.
- Neoplasms (e.g., retroperitoneal fibrosarcomas).
- Immune hypoglycemia (e.g., anti-insulin receptor antibodies in Hodgkin's disease).
- Malaria.

## Investigations
Blood glucose and simple tests to exclude possible causes (e.g., liver function tests [LFTs]) and thick and thin blood films for malaria.

Insulinoma can be confirmed by infusing intravenous insulin and measuring C peptide. Normally insulin suppresses C peptide but this suppression does not occur in patients with insulinomas.

## Management
If the patient is conscious, three or four lumps of sugar should be given with a little water, and this should be repeated as necessary. If the patient is unconscious, 50 mL of 50% glucose should be given intravenously. Glucagon intramuscularly can be given as an alternative—this is a polypeptide hormone produced by the α-cells of the pancreatic islets of Langerhans. It increases plasma glucose by mobilizing glycogen stored in the liver.

For patients who have taken a long-acting preparation, a continuous intravenous glucose infusion for 24 hours may be required. If an underlying cause is found it should be treated on its own merits.

## Diabetic ketoacidosis
Diabetic ketoacidosis usually presents as a gradual deterioration over hours or days, often precipitated by an infection such as pneumonia or urinary tract infections. The patient may be an undiagnosed diabetic. The patient is dehydrated and may be confused, vomiting, and hypotensive. The breath has a characteristic smell of ketones (like nail-polish remover).

## Management
Dehydration, hypoglycemia, electrolyte imbalances, and infections should be treated. Blood should be

taken for glucose, metabolic panel, complete blood count (CBC), blood cultures, and arterial blood gases (ABGs), and the urine should be tested for ketones and sent for microscopy and culture. A chest x-ray (CXR) should be requested.

A nasogastric tube may be passed to prevent gastric dilatation and aspiration, and 0.9% saline IV should be started immediately. Large volumes of fluid may be required as patients are usually 6–9 L fluid depleted, and the infusion should be started at 1 L per half hour in young people. The potassium may be low, and intravenous insulin will exacerbate this by shifting potassium into cells—intravenous fluids should therefore be supplemented with potassium.

Electrolytes should be checked hourly, aiming for a plasma potassium concentration between 4 and 5 mmol/L. Soluble insulin mixed with normal saline should be given intravenously by syringe pump. The rate is usually 4–12 units per hour according to the blood glucose level. When the blood glucose level has normalized and the patient is rehydrated and eating, the patient may be returned to subcutaneous insulin.

Urine output, blood glucose, blood pressure, pulse, and U&Es are monitored hourly. Patients are at risk of deep vein thrombosis (DVT), so prophylactic subcutaneous heparin, such as heparin, 5000 units 2 times/day, or enoxaparin, 20 units daily, may be given. Some centers give bicarbonate if the acidosis is very severe. However, the acidosis will resolve with the above treatment, and its administration is potentially dangerous because it may exacerbate hypokalemia. A source of infection should always be sought, with a low threshold for treatment.

## Hyperglycemic hyperosmolar nonketotic coma

The onset of this is gradual over days. The patient is often elderly and may not be a known diabetic. Polyuria leads to dehydration. The blood glucose is very high and plasma osmolality is increased. There is no acidosis or ketonuria as there is no change to ketone metabolism. Patients require small doses of intravenous insulin and hypotonic saline, although long-term insulin may not be required. Central venous pressure monitoring may be required. Patients are at a high risk of DVT and are given prophylactic subcutaneous heparin. The mortality rate is up to 50%.

## Lipid disorders

Hypercholesterolemia is widely prevalent in Western societies. In the U.S., it was found that, of patients who have coronary artery disease (CAD) before the age of 55, 80–88% had elevated blood lipid levels as opposed to 40–48% of the age-matched controls without CAD. There is a positive association between serum cholesterol and coronary heart disease, although cholesterol concentration alone is of limited predictive value. Of more importance is the patient's overall coronary risk, of which cholesterol is one risk factor. Hence, some patients will have "normal" cholesterol concentrations, but may be at high coronary risk by virtue of additional risk factors such as diabetes or left ventricular hypertrophy. Conversely, some patients, notably young women, will be at low coronary risk even with "high" cholesterol concentrations.

There is now good evidence that lowering serum cholesterol in high-risk patients leads to a reduction in coronary events, and these people should therefore be targeted for treatment. Drug treatment of people at low risk is undesirable as the adverse effects of treatment may outweigh any potential benefits.

Lipids are insoluble in water, and so cholesterol and triglyceride are transported in the bloodstream bound to proteins as lipoproteins. There are five principal types of protein in the blood, and they can be separated in the laboratory by their density and electrophoretic mobility.

*Chylomicrons* are very large particles, mainly containing triglyceride. They provide the main mechanism for transporting the digestion products of dietary fat to the liver and peripheral tissues. The endothelial enzyme lipoprotein lipase removes triglyceride from the particle. The remaining chylomicron remnant is taken up by the liver.

*Very low density lipoproteins* (VLDL) are synthesized and secreted by the liver and contain most of the endogenously synthesized triglyceride. As they pass round the circulation, triglyceride is progressively removed by lipoprotein lipase, leaving a particle called an *intermediate density lipoprotein* (IDL).

IDLs can bind to the hepatocyte and be catabolized, or have further triglyceride removed, producing *low density lipoprotein* (LDL) particles.

LDLs are the main carrier of cholesterol and deliver it to both the liver and to peripheral cells. The circulating LDL concentration is regulated by hepatic LDL receptors, and by the rate limiting enzyme in the cholesterol synthetic pathway, 3-hydroxy-3-methylglutaryl coenzyme A (HMG-CoA) reductase. Some cholesterol synthesized by the liver is converted into bile salts and excreted in the bile, where they are reabsorbed through the terminal ileum and recirculated.

*High density lipoproteins* (HDLs) are produced in both the liver and intestine. They take up cholesterol from cell membranes in peripheral tissues to the liver by "reverse cholesterol transport." HDL cholesterol therefore has a cardioprotective effect and concentrations are inversely proportional to coronary risk.

## Classification of hyperlipidemia

The most common form of hyperlipidemia is polygenic with high serum cholesterol concentrations and normal triglyceride concentrations. Other forms are much less common.

Familial combined hyperlipidemia has a prevalence of 1 in 200 and is associated with high cholesterol and triglyceride concentrations.

Familial hypercholesterolemia has an autosomal dominant inheritance and is due to LDL receptor deficiency, resulting in an increase in LDL particles in the circulation. The prevalence is about 1 in 500. Homozygotes can have serum cholesterol levels of up to 1000mg/dL or more and may develop coronary artery disease in their teenage years.

Familial hypertriglyceridemia is also an autosomal condition and can cause pancreatitis. Patients may have eruptive xanthomata. Triglyceride may also be raised in diabetes, alcoholism, and obesity.

Other classes of dyslipidemia are rare.

### Secondary hyperlipidemia

Causes include DM, excess alcohol, hypothyroidism, cholestasis, chronic renal impairment, nephrotic syndrome, and synthetic estrogens.

## Management

Causes of secondary hyperlipidemia should be treated. Where there is no secondary cause, dietary measures should be tried first. However, the average fall in total cholesterol concentration with a general lipid lowering diet is only 2%. Drug treatment is aimed at high-risk patients. For every 1% reduction in total cholesterol concentration (by diet or drug treatment), coronary heart disease risk is reduced by 1–2%.

## Drugs
### Statins

The statins—atorvastatin, cerivastatin, fluvastatin, lovastatin pravastatin, and simvastatin—competitively inhibit HMG-CoA reductase, an enzyme involved in cholesterol synthesis, especially in the liver. There is evidence that statins produce important reductions in coronary events in high-risk patients, and their use is outlined below. They should be used with caution in those with a history of liver disease. Side effects include reversible myositis.

Treatment should be stopped if there are symptoms of myopathy and creatinine phosphokinase is markedly elevated. Patients should therefore be advised to report unexplained muscle pain, tenderness, and weakness. Other side effects include headache, altered LFTs and GI effects (e.g., abdominal pain, nausea, and vomiting).

### Fibrates

Examples include clofibrate, fenofibrate, and gemfibrozil. Their main action is to decrease serum triglyceride but they also tend to reduce LDL cholesterol and raise HDL cholesterol. They can all cause a myositis-like syndrome, especially in patients with impaired renal function.

### Anion-exchange resins

These include cholestyramine and colestipol, and act by binding bile acids, preventing their reabsorption; this promotes hepatic conversion of cholesterol into bile acids. They reduce LDL cholesterol but can aggravate hypertriglyceridemia. Anion-exchange resins interfere with the absorption of fat-soluble vitamins. Supplements of vitamins A, D, and K, and of folic acid may be required when treatment is prolonged.

Side effects are mainly GI effects and include change in bowel habit, nausea, vomiting, and abdominal pain. Other drugs should be taken at least 1 hour before, or 4–6 hours after cholestyramine or colestipol to reduce possible interference with absorption.

### Nicotinic acid group
The value of nicotinic acid is limited by its side effects, especially vasodilatation. In high doses it lowers both cholesterol and triglyceride concentrations by inhibiting synthesis. It also increases HDL cholesterol.

### Fish oils
These may be useful in hypertriglyceridemia. They can, however, aggravate hypercholesterolemia.

### The use of statins
Before considering treatment with statins, other methods to reduce the risk of coronary heart disease (CHD) should be instigated. This includes stopping smoking, dietary advice to control weight and lower lipids, advice on regular physical activity, control of hypertension, and other pharmacologic measures, such as aspirin therapy, where appropriate. The current recommendation for lipid-lowering with statins in the U.S. is to prioritize patients according to risk.

### Secondary prevention
The first priority is patients who have had a myocardial infarction with serum cholesterol ≥200mg/dL (4.8mmol/L) or LDL ≥70mg/dL (3.2mmol/L). The second priority is patients with angina or other clinically overt atherosclerotic disease who have total cholesterol 200mmol/L. This includes patients with peripheral vascular disease or symptomatic carotid disease or who have had a bypass or angioplasty.

### Primary prevention
The third priority is treatment of people without clinically apparent vascular disease but who nevertheless have a high risk of developing overt CHD, equivalent to those requiring secondary prevention (that is a risk of major CHD events of 3% per year or more) and with LDL above 190mg/dL or 160mg/dL for those with two or more risk factors, based on the average of at least two measurements taken several weeks apart.

People may have this level of risk because of a combination of other CHD risk factors, particularly diabetes or hypertension. Formal estimation of CHD risk is essential when identifying subjects for primary prevention of CHD. This group for primary prevention encompasses a further 3.4% of the population aged 35–69 years. At present there is little evidence of benefit or harm from starting statin treatment in people over the age of 70 years. Treatment of people free of vascular disease with a risk of developing overt CHD of less than 3% a year and a total cholesterol of 200ng/dL would entail treating a high proportion of adults. At present cost-effectiveness is low.

Treatment should be started at a low dose and increased as necessary to reduce LDL to less than 100mg/dL in high-risk patients and to less than 125mg/dL for those without CHD risk factors.

## Metabolic bone disease

Vitamin D metabolism is shown in Fig. 35.4.

## Osteoporosis
Bone normally consists of 60% mineral and 40% matrix or organic matter. In osteoporosis there is a loss of bone matrix and reduction in bone mass, although the deposition of calcium salts, or mineralization, occurs normally. There is therefore a reduction in the amount of bone mineral per unit volume of anatomical bone. This prevalence increases with age and overall affects about 5% of the population.

### Etiology
There are a number of risk factors associated with osteoporosis. They can be divided into physiologic and pathologic factors, as follows.

#### Physiologic factors
- Age.
- Early menopause.
- Immobility.
- Smokers.
- Thin people.
- Excess alcohol intake.

#### Pathologic factors
- Steroids.
- Cushing's disease.

**Fig. 35.4** Metabolism of vitamin D.

- Multiple myeloma.
- Thyrotoxicosis.
- Hypogonadism.
- Primary biliary cirrhosis.
- Rheumatoid arthritis.

Osteoporosis is sometimes subclassified into two types. Individuals with type I (postmenopausal osteoporosis) are middle-aged. Trabecular bone is more commonly affected leading to crush fractures of the vertebrae. It is principally due to estrogen deficiency.

In type II (senile osteoporosis), individuals are usually over 70 years old. Cortical bone is most commonly affected, resulting in fractures of the long bones (e.g., of the femoral neck). The mechanism is thought to be due to secondary hyperparathyroidism due to reduction in calcium and vitamin D intake and synthesis.

### Clinical features

Osteoporosis is not painful in itself; the pain results from fractures. Vertebral crush fractures may lead to back pain, loss of height, and kyphosis.

## Investigations

The following investigations should be considered in osteoporosis:

- Serum calcium, phosphate, and alkaline phosphatase: normal.
- Bone x-rays: show skeletal rarefaction.
- Bone densitometry (e.g., DEXA scan).
- Exclusion of other disease associated with osteoporosis.

## Management

As there is no effective cure, prevention is the key to management. High-risk individuals should be identified. Hormone replacement therapy (HRT) is beneficial in high-risk postmenopausal women. A combined preparation should be given to women, as unopposed estrogens increase the risk of endometrial carcinoma, while androgens should be given to hypogonadal men. Exercise should be encouraged and increasing dietary calcium intake may be beneficial. Bisphosphonates are of benefit in preventing fractures in susceptible individuals. Calcitonin and fluoride may be useful, although they are not of proven benefit.

## Paget's disease

In Paget's disease there is uncontrolled bone turnover with local excessive osteoclastic resorption. This is followed by disordered osteoblastic activity, leading to new bone formation, which is structurally abnormal and weak (Fig. 35.5). The etiology is unknown although viruses have been implicated. The incidence increases with age—it is uncommon in the under 40s but by the age of 90 years about 10% of the population in temperate climates is affected. It is also commoner in Anglo-Saxons and there appears to be a familial incidence.

## Clinical features

The axial skeleton and femur are most commonly affected. The condition is most commonly asymptomatic but can cause bone pain and tenderness, and there may be deformities of affected bones, such as an enlarged skull and bowed (saber) tibia.

Complications include:
- Progressive occlusion of the foramina of the skull (e.g., deafness due to nerve compression, basilar invagination, and cervical cord stenosis with paraparesis).
- Optic atrophy.
- Fractures of long bones.
- Hypercalcemia: if the patient is immobile.
- High-output cardiac failure from shunting.
- Osteogenic sarcoma.
- Osteoarthritis of related joints.

## Investigations

Serum alkaline phosphatase is markedly raised but serum calcium and phosphate are normal; 24-hour urinary hydroxyproline output is raised and reflects the increased bone turnover. There may be mild hypercalcemia in immobile patients.

X-rays of affected bones show a mosaic of osteolytic and sclerotic lesions, thickening of trabeculae, and thick cortices with an enlarged irregular outline.

## Treatment

Asymptomatic patients do not require specific treatment. Analgesia is given for pain, but specific treatment is given for bone pain, bone deformities, hypercalcemia, or for complications. Drug treatment is with bisphosphonates or calcitonin.

### Bisphosphonates

Bisphosphonates are adsorbed on to hydroxyapatite crystals, so slowing both their rate of growth and dissolution, and reducing the increased rate of bone turnover associated with the disease. Disodium etidronate is most commonly used. A single daily dose of 5 mg/kg is given for up to 6 months. This may be repeated after an interval of 3 months if there is

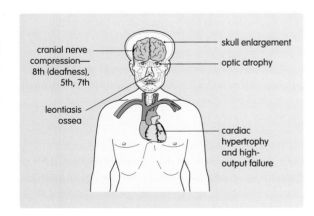

**Fig. 35.5** Complications of Paget's disease of the bone.

cranial nerve compression— 8th (deafness), 5th, 7th

leontiasis ossea

skull enlargement

optic atrophy

cardiac hypertrophy and high-output failure

evidence of reactivation. Side effects include focal osteomalacia and fractures.

## Calcitonin

Calcitonin is involved with parathyroid hormone (PTH) in the regulation of bone turnover and hence in the maintenance of calcium balance and homoeostasis. The prolonged use of porcine calcitonin can lead to the production of neutralizing antibodies.

Salcatonin (synthetic salmon calcitonin) is less immunogenic and thus more suitable for long-term therapy. The dose for Paget's disease ranges from 50 units three times weekly up to 100 units daily, in single or divided doses. Treatment is for 3–6 months. Side effects include nausea, faintness, and flushing.

# Osteomalacia

Osteomalacia results from inadequate mineralization of bone and occurs after fusion of the epiphyses. Rickets is the result if this occurs during the period of bone growth.

## Etiology

The etiology of osteomalacia includes the following:
- Lack of dietary vitamin D.
- Ineffective conversion of 7-dehydrocholesterol (provitamin $D_3$) to previtamin $D_3$ by ultraviolet light in the dermis. This is due to lack of sunlight.
- Intestinal malabsorption (e.g., gluten-sensitive enteropathy and postgastrectomy states).
- Vitamin D resistance: in chronic renal disease most commonly due to ineffective conversion of 25-hydroxyvitamin $D_3$ to 1,25-dihydroxyvitamin $D_3$, inherited deficiency of renal 1$\alpha$-hydroxylase, or end-organ receptor abnormality (rare).
- Drug-induced: chronic anticonvulsant therapy may induce liver enzymes, leading to the breakdown of 25-hydroxyvitamin $D_3$.
- Excessive renal phosphate loss due to Fanconi's syndrome or a specific defect in renal phosphate handling.

## Clinical features

In patients with osteomalacia, there may be bone pain and tenderness. Fractures, especially of the femoral neck, may occur. There is a proximal myopathy, resulting in a waddling gait and difficulty in rising from a chair.

In rickets, there are deformities of the legs (bow-legs and knock-knees), the chest (ricketic rosary), and the skull. There may also be features of hypocalcemia (e.g., tetany).

## Investigations
### Biochemistry
- Serum calcium and phosphate: tend to be decreased.
- Serum alkaline phosphatase activity: increased.
- Urinary calcium excretion: low.
- Plasma 25-hydroxyvitamin $D_3$: low except in resistant cases.
- 1,25-dihydroxyvitamin $D_3$: low in renal failure.
- Parathyroid hormone is high because of secondary hyperparathyroidism due to hypocalcemia.

### X-rays
X-rays of bone in rickets show cupped, ragged metaphyseal surfaces. In osteomalacia, there is loss of cortical bone and pseudofractures (Looser's zones), which are small translucent bands perpendicular to the bone and extending inwards from the cortex. They are best seen on the lateral border of the scapula, the femoral neck, and in the pubic rami.

### Bone scan
A bone scan shows a generalized diffuse increase in uptake of isotope.

## Treatment
Dietary vitamin D deficiency can be prevented by taking an oral supplement of 10µg of ergocalciferol daily. Vitamin D deficiency caused by intestinal malabsorption or chronic liver disease usually requires vitamin D in pharmacologic doses, such as calciferol tablets up to 1mg (i.e., 10,000 units) daily. The hypocalcemia of hypoparathyroidism often requires doses of up to 2.5mg (100,000 units) daily in order to achieve normocalcemia.

The newer hydroxylated vitamin D derivatives—alfacalcidol and calcitriol—have a shorter duration of action and therefore have the advantage that problems associated with hypercalcemia due to excessive dosage are shorter lived and easier to treat.

In patients with chronic renal impairment alfacalcidol or calcitriol should be prescribed. All patients receiving pharmacologic doses of vitamin D should have their serum calcium levels checked at intervals, and whenever nausea and vomiting are present.

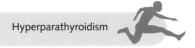

Breast milk from women taking pharmacologic doses of vitamin D may cause hypercalcemia if given to an infant.

## Renal osteodystrophy

The term "renal osteodystrophy" is used to cover the various forms of bone disease that develop in chronic renal failure. These include the following:

- Delayed epiphyseal closure in children and young adults.
- Rickets or osteomalacia.
- Osteitis fibrosa cystica (brown tumors) due to secondary or tertiary hyperparathyroidism.
- Generalized or localized osteosclerosis.

There is usually a metabolic acidosis. Serum calcium is low but serum ionic calcium is normal unless steps are taken to treat the acidosis actively. This can precipitate a severe attack of tetany. Serum phosphate and chloride are raised, which leads to ectopic calcification.

### Management

Hydroxylation of 25-hydroxyvitamin $D_3$ is impaired and so treatment is with the hydroxylated derivatives of vitamin D. Phosphate binders (e.g., aluminium hydroxide) will lower serum phosphate and reduce the risk of metastatic calcification. Dialysis will help to return serum calcium and phosphate levels to normal.

Renal transplantation should restore calcium metabolism to normal, although this may take some months as the parathyroid glands may not always switch off immediately after a long period of secondary hyperparathyroidism. Occasionally, subtotal parathyroidectomy is required.

## Hyperparathyroidism

Hyperparathyroidism results from excess circulating parathyroid hormone (PTH), which increases serum calcium by increasing calcium absorption from the gut, increasing mobilization of calcium from bone, and reducing renal calcium clearance.

Primary hyperparathyroidism is usually due to a single benign adenoma but may less commonly be due to multiple adenomas, carcinoma, or hyperplasia. It may be associated with other endocrine abnormalities as part of the multiple endocrine neoplasia (MEN) syndromes. Ectopic

PTH production may be produced by carcinoma from the lung and kidney.

Secondary hyperparathyroidism is due to raised PTH levels secondary to hypocalcemia; the hypocalcemia persists. Causes include chronic renal failure and deficiency of vitamin D (e.g., due to inadequate intake or malabsorption).

Tertiary hyperparathyroidism is the continued secretion of excess PTH after prolonged secondary hyperparathyroidism. The parathyroids act autonomously and cause hypercalcemia, despite the absence of the original cause of the secondary hyperparathyroidism.

## Clinical features

Symptoms may be due to bone disease and can result in fractures. There may be renal stones and nephrocalcinosis due to hypercalciuria, resulting in renal failure. Abdominal pain may be non-specific or due to constipation, peptic ulcer, or pancreatitis. Other features include anorexia, nausea and vomiting, thirst, polyuria, muscle fatigue, and psychiatric disorders, including depression and confusion.

## Investigations

In primary hyperparathyroidism serum calcium is raised. Fasting blood samples should be taken without venous compression. Serum phosphate is low, and alkaline phosphatase is high, reflecting increased bone turnover. There is a mild renal tubular acidosis with a high serum chloride level, and serum PTH is raised. In secondary hyperparathyroidism of renal failure, serum calcium is low but phosphate is high.

 For the clinical features of hypercalcemia remember **bones** (bone pain), **stones** (renal stones), **groans** (peptic ulcer), and **moans** (psychiatric disease).

X-rays show subperiosteal resorption, being most marked in the hands, and evidence of osteitis fibrosa cystica. A CXR should be done to look for bilateral hilar lymphadenopathy of sarcoidosis, or carcinoma producing PTH. A skull x-ray shows a "pepperpot" appearance.

## Treatment

Parathyroidectomy is indicated for persistent hypercalcemia above 11 mg/dL or for symptomatic hypercalcemia. The parathyroid glands may be localized by computed tomography (CT) scan or isotope scans. All four glands should be biopsied; single adenomas can be removed.

If the glands are hyperplastic, three-and-a-half glands are removed, leaving the last half *in situ*. Serum calcium and magnesium should be checked frequently postoperatively as removal of the glands may lead to rapid hypocalcemia and hypomagnesemia.

## Hypoparathyroidism

Hypoparathyroidism is usually secondary to thyroid surgery. Primary (idiopathic) hypoparathyroidism is an autoimmune disorder associated with vitiligo, Addison's disease, pernicious anemia, and other autoimmune diseases. The DiGeorge syndrome is a familial condition with parathyroid agenesis. It is associated with intellectual impairment, cataracts, and calcified basal ganglia.

Pseudohypoparathyroidism is a syndrome of end-organ resistance to PTH. It is associated with intellectual impairment, short stature, a round face, and short metacarpals and metatarsals. Pseudopseudohypoparathyroidism describes the appearance present in pseudohypoparathyroidism but without the calcium abnormalities.

## Clinical features

Circumoral paresthesias, cramps, anxiety, and tetany are followed by convulsions, laryngeal stridor, dystonia, and psychosis. Trousseau's sign may be present—carpopedal spasm when the brachial artery is occluded with a blood pressure cuff. Chvostek's sign may also be present—twitching of the facial muscles when the facial nerve is tapped.

## Investigations

Serum calcium is low, phosphate is high, and alkaline phosphatase is normal. Additional tests include serum urea and creatinine, serum PTH level, parathyroid antibodies, and vitamin D metabolite levels.

X-rays of the hands show short fourth metacarpals in pseudohypoparathyroidism.

## Treatment

Emergency treatment is with 10mL 10% intravenous calcium gluconate, repeated as necessary. Intravenous magnesium chloride may also be required if there is hypomagnesemia.

Long-term treatment is with alfacalcidol or calcitriol. Serum calcium should be monitored to prevent hypercalcemia.

## Crystal arthropathy

### Gout

Gout is a result of the deposition of sodium urate crystals in joints and soft tissues due to an abnormality of uric acid metabolism. It affects about 4 in 1000 people in the U.S. It is commoner in men, drinkers, and in higher socioeconomic classes, and about a third have a positive family history. The underlying biochemical abnormality is an overproduction or underexcretion of uric acid, resulting in hyperuricemia. The main causes are given in Fig. 35.6.

### Clinical features
#### Acute gout
This typically starts in the first metatarsophalangeal joint with an acute onset of a red, hot, swollen, extremely painful big toe (Fig. 35.7). It may be precipitated by alcohol, diet, starvation, diuretics, or after surgery. Other commonly affected joints include the ankle, wrist, knees, and bursae. The

---

**Causes of gout**

- idiopathic
- drugs: diuretics, low-dose aspirin
- chronic renal impairment
- hypertension
- primary hyperparathyroidism
- hypothyroidism
- alcohol
- glucose-6-phosphate deficiency

rapid cell turnover:
- myeloproliferative disorders, e.g. polycythemia rubra vera
- lymphoproliferative disorders, e.g. leukemia
- severe psoriasis

**Fig. 35.6** Causes of gout.

**Fig. 35.7** Acute gout of the first metatarsophalangeal joint.

patient may have high blood pressure, renal impairment, or peripheral vascular disease. The renal disease may be secondary to uric acid stones.

### Chronic tophaceous gout
This leads to joint erosion and disruption leading to chronic disability. There are tophi in the ear lobes or around joints (particularly hands and elbows), which are soft tissue deposits of urate.

### Investigations
The following investigations are important in patients with gout:
- Synovial fluid examined under polarized light microscopy shows needle-shaped, negatively birefringent crystals.
- X-rays may be normal in acute gout but show punched-out erosions and joint disruption in chronic gout.
- Serum uric acid may be high, but there are a large number of false-positive and false-negative results. It is more useful for monitoring treatment.

### Management
#### Acute attacks
These are normally treated with high doses of non-steroidal anti-inflammatory drugs (NSAIDs) such as naproxen, 500 mg 2 times/day, or ibuprofen, 400 mg t.i.d. They should be used with care in patients with peptic ulcer disease, heart failure, hypertension, and renal impairment.

Colchicine is probably as effective as NSAIDs, but excessive doses cause diarrhea. Other common side effects include nausea and vomiting, and abdominal pain. They do not cause fluid retention and may be given to patients with hypertension, heart failure and renal impairment, and patients on anticoagulants.

#### Prophylactic treatment
The patient should be advised about weight reduction, reducing alcohol consumption, avoiding precipitating foods such as red meat, and avoiding precipitating drugs if possible.

Drug treatment should be continued indefinitely once the decision to prevent further attacks had been made. The initiation of treatment may precipitate an acute attack, therefore colchicine or NSAIDs should be used prophylactically for at least 1 month after the hyperuricemia has been corrected.

Allopurinol inhibits xanthine oxidase, which catalyzes the conversion of hypoxanthine to xanthine, and of xanthine to uric acid. It is especially useful in patients with renal impairment or urate stones where uricosuric agents cannot be used. It is usually given once daily (initially 100 mg after food) and gradually increased to a maintenance dose of about 300 mg daily. Lower doses are given in patients with renal impairment. It may cause skin rashes.

Uricosuric drugs include probenecid and sulphinpyrazone. They may be used instead of allopurinol or with it in cases that are resistant to treatment. Aspirin antagonizes the effect of uricosuric drugs. It is important to ensure a good urine output as they may lead to crystallization of urate in the urine.

## Hypercalcemia

The causes of hypercalcemia have already been given in Fig. 29.21. The two most common pathologic causes are primary hyperparathyroidism and malignant disease. However, the commonest cause of borderline hypercalcemia is probably faulty technique, i.e., excessive venous stasis when collecting blood samples. An abnormally high result should therefore be repeated.

The physiologically relevant measurement is of ionized calcium. This can be determined by correcting serum total calcium levels for serum protein or albumin concentrations. The higher the protein concentration, the more calcium is protein bound, and the lower the proportion of ionized calcium.

## Clinical features

These are discussed under hyperparathyroidism.

## Management

Severe hypercalcemia is a medical emergency and in extreme cases can lead to drowsiness, altered consciousness, and coma; adequate rehydration with intravenous saline is essential. Furosemide should also be given if necessary. Drugs that promote hypercalcemia should be discontinued and dietary calcium should be restricted. Intravenous bisphosphonates are given for hypercalcemia of malignancy (e.g., intravenous etidronate 7.5 mg per kg per day for 3 days).

High-dose prednisolone is effective for hypercalcemia secondary to myeloma, sarcoidosis, and excess vitamin D but otherwise is of little value. It may take some days to achieve the desired effect. Intravenous calcitonin has an acute but short-lived effect. It is rarely effective where intravenous bisphosphonates have failed to reduce serum calcium adequately. Sodium cellulose phosphate, which binds calcium in the gut, has been used but is rarely helpful, and any associated increase in serum phosphate may be harmful.

After treatment of severe hypercalcemia the underlying cause must be established and treated appropriately.

## Pituitary disorders

## Nonfunctioning pituitary tumors and hypopituitarism

The incidence of pituitary tumors varies from 0.2–3 in 100,000 population, and the prevalence is about 9 in 100,000. Prolactin (PRL)- and adrenocorticotrophic (ACTH)-secreting tumors occur most commonly in 25–35 year olds, growth hormone (GH)-secreting tumors in 35–50 year olds, and nonfunctioning tumors usually present after the age of 60 years.

The signs and symptoms of functioning tumors are related to hormonal hypersecretion. They may cause acromegaly via GH, amenorrhea–galactorrhea syndrome via PRL, or Cushing's disease via ACTH. Nonfunctioning tumors can extend beyond the sella turcica and produce symptoms related to the mass of the tumor. These may be related to pressure on the anterior pituitary, resulting in hypopituitarism, or symptoms related to extrasellar tumor growth, resulting in headaches, bitemporal hemianopia due to pressure on the optic chiasma, other visual field defects and cranial nerve disturbances, personality changes, focal neurologic symptoms and signs, and epilepsy.

Investigations include skull x-ray, magnetic resonance imaging (MRI), or CT scanning of the brain, and endocrinologic assessment, as outlined in Chapter 29.

Management may be surgical or medical. Transsphenoidal surgery improves visual field defects in up to 70% of patients. However, the recurrence rate of non-functioning tumors is about 20% after 5 years. Drug therapy includes dopamine receptor agonists (e.g., bromocriptine), which inhibits PRL release and induces shrinkage of PRL-secreting adenomas. Somatostatin analogs inhibit GH release and induce a lesser degree of tumor shrinkage in most GH-secreting adenomas.

## Hypopituitarism

This may result from hypothalamic or pituitary disease. The most common cause includes the mass effect of pituitary adenomas, with additional loss of pituitary function after surgery and pituitary irradiation. Other causes include hypothalamic tumors and cysts, peripituitary tumors (e.g., gliomas and meningiomas, craniopharyngiomas), infiltrative diseases (e.g., sarcoidosis), and vascular and metastatic lesions in and around the pituitary fossa.

### Clinical features

These can be worked out from knowledge of the effects of the various pituitary hormones:

- GH: fatigue, loss of energy, increased abdominal adiposity, and reduced muscle strength and exercise capacity.
- Luteinizing hormone (LH) and follicle-stimulating hormone (FSH): in women there is oligomenorrhea, infertility, dyspareunia, breast atrophy, loss of pubic and axillary hair, and hot flushes; in men, there is loss of libido, impotence, infertility, flushes, regression of secondary sexual characteristics, soft testicles, and fine wrinkles on the face.

- Thyroid-stimulating hormone (TSH): fatigue, muscle weakness, sensitivity to cold, constipation, apathy, weight gain, and dry skin.
- ACTH: fatigue, anorexia, weight loss, pallor, weakness, nausea and vomiting, hypoglycemia, apathy, and loss of pubic and axillary hair.
- Vasopressin: polyuria and polydipsia with nocturia.

Tests of pituitary function are given in Chapter 29.

## Management

Hormone replacement involves the use of multiple hormones. Careful instruction and patient compliance are mandatory for long-term recovery.

# Acromegaly

Acromegaly is an insidious disease resulting from excessive circulating levels of GH in adults. The incidence is about 5 per million per year, and the prevalence is 50 per million.

Acromegalic gigantism results from acromegaly in young individuals before epiphyseal fusion and is very uncommon.

## Etiology

The most common cause is a benign pituitary tumor secreting GH. Pituitary carcinoma is an uncommon cause. Carcinoid tumors which secrete hypothalamic GH-releasing hormone are another uncommon cause.

## Clinical features

The clinical features of acromegaly are summarized in Fig. 35.8.

### Facial appearance

Features are coarse, with enlargement of the supraorbital ridges, a broad nose, and thickening of the soft tissues. The lips are thick, with prognathism, and increased dental separation, and macroglossia. There is excessive sweating, and in women there may be hirsutism.

### Hands

The hands enlarge and become spade-like. Carpal tunnel syndrome may occur as a result of compression of the median nerve.

### Arthritis

This occurs prematurely, especially in the spine and weight-bearing joints.

### Cardiovascular problems

These are often the cause of mortality. Coronary artery disease, hypertension, and diabetes are more common than in the normal population. Cardiomyopathy may occur.

### Effects of the pituitary tumor

Headaches, visual field defects, and cranial nerve palsies may occur. Hyperprolactinemia is common, and hypopituitarism can also occur.

## Diagnosis

GH levels are elevated although they may rise with stress. Therefore, GH is measured during a glucose tolerance test. In healthy individuals, GH is undetectable during the test.

Other investigations include the following:

- Assessment of visual fields: bitemporal hemianopia.
- Skull x-ray and CT or MRI of the brain.
- Hand x-ray: tufting of the terminal phalanges and increased joint spaces due to hypertrophy of the cartilage. The heel pad is usually thickened.
- Glucose or glucose tolerance test.
- CXR and electrocardiogram (ECG): left ventricular hypertrophy secondary to hypertension.

 The diagnosis of acromegaly may become more obvious by comparing old photographs of the patient with present appearance.

## Management

The aim of treatment is to relieve symptoms, reverse somatic changes, and reverse metabolic abnormalities. Treatment is by surgery, radiotherapy, or drugs.

### Surgery

The transsphenoidal route is usually used. Up to 90% of microadenomas are cured. The success rate is lower for larger tumors. Complications include hypopituitarism, meningitis, intraoperative bleeding, and death.

### Radiotherapy

This is often used if attempts at surgery do not reduce GH levels sufficiently. Hypopituitarism may

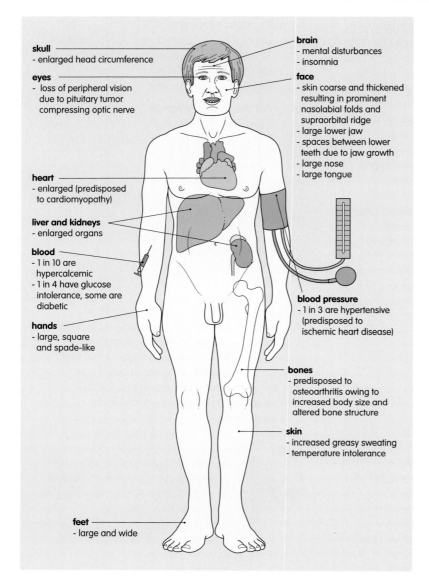

**Fig. 35.8** Signs and symptoms of acromegaly (caused by excessive growth hormone secretion in adults).

**skull**
- enlarged head circumference

**eyes**
- loss of peripheral vision due to pituitary tumor compressing optic nerve

**brain**
- mental disturbances
- insomnia

**face**
- skin coarse and thickened resulting in prominent nasolabial folds and supraorbital ridge
- large lower jaw
- spaces between lower teeth due to jaw growth
- large nose
- large tongue

**heart**
- enlarged (predisposed to cardiomyopathy)

**liver and kidneys**
- enlarged organs

**blood**
- 1 in 10 are hypercalcemic
- 1 in 4 have glucose intolerance, some are diabetic

**hands**
- large, square and spade-like

**blood pressure**
- 1 in 3 are hypertensive (predisposed to ischemic heart disease)

**bones**
- predisposed to osteoarthritis owing to increased body size and altered bone structure

**skin**
- increased greasy sweating
- temperature intolerance

**feet**
- large and wide

occur, and regular tests of pituitary function should be performed.

### Medical therapies

The most effective treatment is with octreotide, a somatostatin analog. Somatostatin inhibits GH secretion. Side effects include colicky abdominal pain and diarrhea, but this usually settles with continued treatment. Gallstones occur in about a third of patients. Bromocriptine also reduces GH and PRL levels.

### Prognosis

Untreated, mortality is more than twice that in healthy individuals. Death is secondary to cardiovascular and cerebrovascular disease.

## Prolactin disorders

Prolactin (PRL) is the hormone most commonly secreted by pituitary tumors. Secretion of PRL is under tonic inhibitory control by hypothalamic dopamine, such that interruption produces hyperprolactinemia. Thyrotrophin-releasing hormone and vasoactive intestinal polypeptide exert less important stimulatory effects on pituitary prolactin release. Elevation of serum prolactin occurs physiologically during pregnancy and lactation. Pathologically, hyperprolactinemia is more common in women than men. Most are due to microprolactinomas.

## Clinical features

In women, the most common symptoms are oligomenorrhea, galactorrhea, infertility, and occasionally hirsutism. In men, symptoms include reduced libido, impotence, infertility, and galactorrhea. Symptoms caused by large tumor size are more common in men and include headache, visual field defects, and cranial nerve palsies. Varying degrees of hypopituitarism may be present.

## Etiology

The causes of hyperprolactinemia are summarized in Fig. 35.9.

## Investigations

Elevated prolactin levels should be confirmed on repeat testing. Other blood tests include thyroid function tests (TFTs) and a pregnancy test in women. A careful drug history should always be taken.

Radiologic assessment of the pituitary tumor should be carried out with skull x-rays and MRI or CT scans of the brain. Full assessment of pituitary function should be undertaken if a macroadenoma is suspected, and visual fields should be assessed.

## Management

The dopamine agonist bromocriptine is most commonly used, which produces a fall in serum PRL in more than 90% of patients and reduces tumor size in patients with macroadenomas.

Cabergoline is a more recent longer-acting dopamine receptor agonist.

For patients intolerant of drugs, surgery and radiotherapy can be tried.

Tumors may enlarge rapidly in pregnancy. However, bromocriptine does not appear to have any adverse effects in mother or child when used before or during pregnancy.

## Diabetes insipidus

This rare disease is due to deficiency of vasopressin—central diabetes insipidus. The differential diagnosis includes nephrogenic diabetes insipidus (i.e., a lack of renal response to adequate circulating vasopressin) and primary polydipsia or excessive drinking. Clinically the patient presents with polyuria,

| Causes of hyperprolactinemia | |
|---|---|
| **Cause** | **Examples** |
| physiologic | pregnancy, lactation, stress |
| drugs | antiemetics, e.g. metoclopramide, prochlorperazine phenothiazines tricyclic antidepressants |
| primary hypothyroidism | — |
| pituitary tumors | prolactinoma growth-hormone secreting tumors non-functioning tumors |
| polycystic ovary syndrome | — |
| uncommon | sarcoidosis |
| hypothalamic lesions | Langerhans' cell histiocytosis hypothalamic tumors |
| chest wall stimulation | repeated self-examination of breasts post herpes zoster |
| liver or renal failure | — |

**Fig. 35.9** Causes of hyperprolactinemia.

nocturia, and polydipsia. Investigation is outlined in Chapter 12.

## Causes of diabetes insipidus
### Central diabetes insipidus
Familial central diabetes insipidus is inherited as autosomal dominant or as part of the **DIDMOAD** syndrome (**d**iabetes **i**nsipidus, **d**iabetes **m**ellitus, **o**ptic **a**trophy, and **d**eafness).

Causes of acquired central diabetes insipidus are given in Fig. 35.10.

### Nephrogenic diabetes insipidus
Familial nephrogenic diabetes insipidus is X-linked recessive and autosomal recessive.

Causes of acquired nephrogenic diabetes insipidus are given in Fig. 35.11.

## Treatment
For cental diabetes insipidus, desmopressin is the treatment of choice because it has minimal pressor activity but prolonged antidiuretic potency compared to native vasopressin. It may be administered orally, intranasally, or parenterally.

Metabolic and electrolyte disturbances should be corrected if they are responsible for nephrogenic diabetes insipidus. In familial forms, thiazide

diuretics or indomethacin can reduce urine output by up to 50%.

For patients with primary polydipsia, water restriction and treatment of any associated psychiatric disorder are required.

## Thyroid disorders

For a diagram of the hypothalamus–pituitary–thyroid axis refer to Fig. 29.18.

## Hypothyroidism
Hypothyroidism results from deficiency of thyroxine ($T_4$) or tri-iodothyronine ($T_3$). The prevalence is 15 in 1000 females and 1 in 1000 males.

### Etiology
Primary thyroid failure may take the following forms:

- Autoimmune (Hashimoto's thyroiditis): this is 15 times more common in women than men and tends to affect the middle-aged and elderly. Patients may present with a firm, nontender goiter, hypothyroidism, or both. It is associated with vitiligo, pernicious anemia, IDDM, Addison's disease, and premature ovarian failure.
- Idiopathic atrophic hypothyroidism: incidence increases with age and is 10 times more common in women than men. The etiology is probably autoimmune.
- Previous treatment for hypothyroidism: operative or radioiodine.
- Congenital hypothyroidism: the prevalence in the U.S. is 1 in 4000 infants. It is diagnosed in the first week of life by routine screening, measuring TSH or $T_4$. It is usually due to thyroid agenesis or dyshormonogenesis, which are both due to autosomal recessively inherited enzyme defects. The most common is Pendred's syndrome, characterized by congenital hypothyroidism, goiter, and nerve deafness in homozygotes.
- Iodine-deficient hypothyroidism: this is a major cause of hypothyroidism and goiter worldwide, although most iodine-deficient people are euthyroid, even though they have a goiter.
- Iatrogenic hypothyroidism: long-term iodine therapy, for example in expectorants, may result in hypothyroidism. Other drugs include amiodarone and lithium carbonate.

| Causes of acquired central diabetes insipidus | |
|---|---|
| **Causes** | **Examples** |
| trauma | head injury and neurosurgery |
| tumors | craniopharyngioma or secondary tumors |
| granulomas | tuberculosis, sarcoid, histiocytosis |
| infections | encephalitis or meningitis |

**Fig. 35.10** Causes of acquired central diabetes insipidus.

| Causes of acquired nephrogenic diabetes insipidus |
|---|
| • metabolic: hypokalemia, hypercalcemia |
| • chronic renal failure |
| • lithium toxicity |
| • postobstructive uropathy |
| • diabetes mellitus |

**Fig. 35.11** Causes of acquired nephrogenic diabetes insipidus.

Secondary thyroid failure is caused by diseases of the hypothalamus or pituitary. These are very rare.

## Clinical presentation

The onset is insidious and the symptoms often nonspecific and vague. Common presenting symptoms include tiredness, lethargy, weight gain, cold intolerance, hoarseness, and dryness of the skin. However, virtually any organ system can be affected (Fig. 35.12).

## Investigations

The following investigations are important in patients with hypothyroidism:

- Free or total $T_4$ are reduced, and serum TSH is high.
- $T_4$ may be normal with a high serum TSH. This indicates subclinical hypothyroidism.
- If secondary hypothyroidism is suspected, the free and total $T_4$ are reduced and the TSH is also low. This picture is also obtained in sick people without thyroid disease, and patients on steroids and anticonvulsants.
- Antibodies to thyroglobulin or thyroid peroxidase (microsomal antibodies): typically strongly positive in Hashimoto's thyroiditis.
- Cholesterol: raised.
- CBC: anemia and raised mean corpuscular volume.
- ECG: sinus bradycardia, low voltage complexes.

## Treatment

Thyroxine sodium is the treatment of choice for maintenance therapy. Usual maintenance doses are between 100–200 µg daily. The initial dose is usually 50 µg, increased as necessary over a few weeks, and even lower doses (25 µg) are started in elderly patients or patients with cardiac disease to avoid worsening angina or precipitating a myocardial infarction. Treatment is monitored by serum TSH and serum $T_4$ and is nearly always lifelong, except in cases of subacute or silent thyroiditis.

## Myxedema coma

This is uncommon. It is typically seen in the elderly and precipitated by infection, treatment with sedatives, or inadequate heating in cold weather. Most patients have hypothermia and are hypotensive with heart failure, hyponatremia, hypoxia, and hypercapnia.

Treatment is with $T_3$ intravenously because of its rapid action. Supportive measures are also needed including intravenous fluids, antibiotics, ventilation, and slow rewarming. $T_4$ can be substituted after 2–3 days if there is a clinical improvement.

## Thyrotoxicosis

Thyrotoxicosis results from an excess of circulating free $T_4$ and free $T_3$. It affects about 10 in 1000 women and 1 in 1000 men. Hyperthyroidism indicates thyroid gland overactivity, resulting in thyrotoxicosis.

| Effects of hypothyroidism by body system | |
| --- | --- |
| **Body system** | **Effects** |
| cardiovascular | bradycardia, hyperlipidemia, angina, heart failure, pericardial and pleural effusions |
| neuromuscular | aches and pains, carpal tunnel syndrome, deafness, cerebellar ataxia, depression and psychoses, delayed relaxation of reflexes |
| hematologic | iron-deficiency anemia, macrocytic anemia, pernicious anemia, normochromic normocytic anemia |
| dermatologic | dry skin, myxedema (which is local infiltration of the skin with mucopolysaccharides), erythema ab igne, vitiligo, alopecia |
| gastrointestinal | constipation, ileus, ascites |
| reproductive | infertility, menorrhagia, galactorrhea |
| developmental | growth retardation, mental retardation, delayed puberty |

**Fig. 35.12** Effects of hypothyroidism by body system.

## Etiology

### Primary hyperthyroidism

*Graves' disease*   This accounts for 70–80% of all cases of hyperthyroidism. It is caused by the production of autoantibodies that stimulate the TSH receptor. There is a painless diffuse goiter in more than 90% of patients. In addition to the general features of thyrotoxicosis, pathognomonic features include ophthalmopathy, pretibial myxedema, and thyroid acropathy.

The ophthalmopathy includes grittiness and increased tear production, periorbital edema, conjunctival edema (chemosis), proptosis, diplopia, impaired visual acuity, and corneal ulceration. It is clinically obvious in 60% of patients with Graves' disease but subclinical ophthalmopathy can be detected in more than 90% by CT scan or MRI, revealing fusiform enlargement of the extraocular muscles caused by lymphocytic infiltration, edema, and later fibrosis.

Pretibial myxedema occurs in 1–5% of patients with Graves' disease and comprises of painless thickening of the skin in nodules or plaques, generally over the shin.

Thyroid acropathy occurs in less than 1% of patients and resembles finger clubbing.

*Other causes of primary hyperthyroidism*   Toxic multinodular goiter and toxic adenoma account for most of the remaining causes. Less common causes include metastatic thyroid cancer, genetic causes such as the McCune–Albright syndrome and TSH receptor mutations, and ectopic thyroid tissue (e.g., struma ovarii).

### Secondary hyperthyroidism

This is very uncommon. Causes include pituitary adenoma-secreting TSH, and trophoblastic tumors secreting human chorionic gonadotrophin

### Thyrotoxicosis without hyperthyroidism

This may occur with destructive thyroiditis, such as in postpartum thyroiditis, subacute (de Quervain's) thyroiditis, and amiodarone-induced thyroiditis, and with excessive thyroxine administration, or self-administered thyroxine, particularly in doctors and nurses.

## Clinical presentation

The symptoms and signs of thyrotoxicosis are shown in Fig. 35.13. General symptoms include:
- Weight loss.
- Increased appetite.
- Heat intolerance and sweating.
- Fatigue and weakness.
- Hyperactivity, irritability.
- Tremor.

Less common symptoms include:
- Depression.
- Oligomenorrhea.
- Pruritus.
- Diarrhea.
- Polyuria.

Signs include:
- A goiter, possibly with a murmur over it.
- Tremor.
- Tachycardia and atrial fibrillation.
- Warm moist skin.
- Lid retraction and lid lag.
- Muscle weakness.
- Proximal myopathy.
- Cardiac failure.

## Investigations

In thyrotoxicosis TSH is suppressed. It can also be suppressed in euthyroid patients with Graves' ophthalmopathy, large goiters, recent treatment for thyrotoxicosis, or severe nonthyroid illness.

$T_4$ is raised although excess estrogens, protein-losing states, drugs, and hereditary abnormalities can alter the binding of $T_4$ to thyroxine-binding globulin, making total $T_4$ levels inaccurate in these situations. Free $T_4$ assays are therefore preferable.

If the TSH is suppressed and free $T_4$ is normal, $T_3$ should be measured to diagnose $T_3$ toxicosis.

In Graves' disease, 80% of people have serum autoantibodies against thyroglobulin and thyroid peroxidase/microsomal antigen. However, these also occur in autoimmune thyroiditis, and in 15% of healthy women and 5% of healthy men.

## Treatment

Treatment options include drugs, radioiodine, and surgery. Most patients under 50 years old receive a course of antithyroid drug as initial treatment. Patients with large goiters usually relapse after antithyroid drugs. Relapse after a period of drug therapy should be treated with [131]I or subtotal thyroidectomy; [131]I is generally given to older patients in whom recurrent thyrotoxicosis may be dangerous. Subtotal thyroidectomy is often recommended in young patients with large goiters to remove the neck swelling. All options should be

**Fig. 35.13** Symptoms and signs of thyrotoxicosis (caused by hyperthyroidism). The features shown in italics are exclusive to thyrotoxicosis caused by Graves' disease.

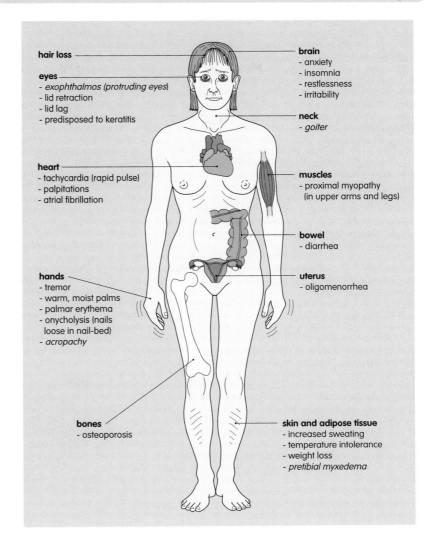

**hair loss**

**eyes**
- *exophthalmos (protruding eyes)*
- lid retraction
- lid lag
- predisposed to keratitis

**heart**
- tachycardia (rapid pulse)
- palpitations
- atrial fibrillation

**hands**
- tremor
- warm, moist palms
- palmar erythema
- onycholysis (nails loose in nail-bed)
- *acropachy*

**bones**
- osteoporosis

**brain**
- anxiety
- insomnia
- restlessness
- irritability

**neck**
- *goiter*

**muscles**
- proximal myopathy (in upper arms and legs)

**bowel**
- diarrhea

**uterus**
- oligomenorrhea

**skin and adipose tissue**
- increased sweating
- temperature intolerance
- weight loss
- *pretibial myxedema*

discussed with the patient and a joint decision should be arrived at.

### Antithyroid drugs

In the U.S. methimazole is the most commonly used drug. Propylthiouracil (PTU) may be used in patients who suffer sensitivity reactions to methimazole. Both drugs act primarily by interfering with the synthesis of thyroid hormones.

Methimazole is given in a daily dose of 30–40mg and maintained at this dose until the patient becomes euthyroid, usually after 4–8 weeks. The dose may then be progressively changed to a maintenance dose of 5–15mg daily, adjusted according to response. Rashes are common and PTU may then be substituted. Pruritus and rashes can also be treated with antihistamines without discontinuing therapy, although patients should be advised to report any sore throat immediately because of the rare complication of agranulocytosis.

PTU is given in a dose of 450mg every 8 hours and maintained at this dose until the patient becomes euthyroid. The dose is then lowered to a maintenance dose of 50–150mg daily.

A combination of methimazole, 20–60mg daily, with thyroxine, 50–150μg daily, may be used in a blocking replacement regimen. Treatment is usually for 18 months—this regimen is not suitable during pregnancy.

Iodine may be given 10–14 days before surgery in addition to carbimazole to assist control and to reduce vascularity of the thyroid.

Propanolol is useful for the rapid relief of thyrotoxic symptoms because antithyroid drugs may take several weeks to produce an improvement in symptoms. They are also useful for the control of supraventricular arrhythmias secondary to thyrotoxicosis.

### Radioiodine

Radioactive sodium iodide ($Na^{131}I$) is concentrated by the thyroid and causes cell damage and cell death. Hypothyroidism may therefore develop at any stage after treatment, and so the patient should be under regular follow-up. It is used increasingly for the treatment of thyrotoxicosis at all ages, particularly where medical therapy or compliance is a problem, in patients with cardiac disease, and in patients who relapse after thyroidectomy. Contraindications include pregnancy and breastfeeding. Pregnancy is safe 4 months or more after treatment.

### Subtotal thyroidectomy

The aim of surgery is to remove sufficient thyroid tissue to cure hyperthyroidism. One year later about 80% of patients are euthyroid, 15% hypothyroid, and 5% have relapsed. Complications include hypoparathyroidism, recurrent laryngeal nerve damage, and bleeding into the neck causing laryngeal edema.

### Thyrotoxic crisis (thyroid "storm")

This is an uncommon, life-threatening exacerbation of thyrotoxicosis with a mortality of 50%. Precipitating factors include thyroid surgery, radioiodine, withdrawal of antithyroid drugs, iodinated contrast agents, and acute illnesses (e.g., stroke, infection, trauma, and diabetic ketoacidosis). It requires emergency treatment with oxygen, intravenous fluids due to profuse sweating, propanolol (5mg IV) for control of tachycardia, hydrocortisone (100mg 6 hourly IV), which inhibits $T_4$ conversion to $T_3$ in the tissues, as well as oral iodine solution, which may need to be administered by nasogastric tube. PTU is also given at doses of 300–400mg every 8 hours to block any further synthesis of thyroid hormones.

### Subacute (de Quervain's) thyroiditis

Various viruses (e.g., enterovirus or coxsackievirus) can cause subacute thyroiditis. Patients present with a small, tender goiter and initially thyrotoxicosis caused by release of stored thyroid hormones. There may be a history of preceding "flu-like" illness. Some weeks later there is a period of hypothyroidism followed by the recovery of normal thyroid function 3–6 months after onset.

The erythrocyte sedimentation rate is raised and there is low radioisotope uptake by the thyroid. Treatment is with NSAIDs for mild symptoms, and with high-dose prednisone for moderate or severe thyroiditis. The dose is gradually tailed off in subsequent weeks.

## Goiter and thyroid cancer

"Goiter" means an enlarged thyroid gland. Diffuse goiters can be due to simple, nontoxic goiters, Graves' disease, Hashimoto's thyroiditis, subacute thyroiditis, or thyroid lymphoma. Goiters with a single nodule may be due to adenoma or carcinoma, and multiple nodules secondary to multinodular goiter or Hashimoto's thyroiditis. Goiters are four times more common in women than men and are present in about 7% of the population. Etiologic factors include underlying autoimmune disease and iodine deficiency.

The most common thyroid carcinoma is P-apillary (P-opular). It also has P-sammoma bodies on histology. It causes P-alpable lymph nodes (lymphatic spread).

## Clinical features

Most patients are asymptomatic. The history should include the following:

- Duration of goiter: long-standing goiters suggest benign disease.
- Goitrogenic drugs (e.g., lithium).
- Prior exposure to radiation: risk factor for benign and malignant thyroid nodules.
- Age: increased risk of cancer in the over 65s.
- Sex: thyroid cancer is more common in men than women.
- Family history: if positive for goiter, this suggests autoimmune thyroiditis. A positive family history for thyroid cancer suggests familial thyroid cancer or MEN.
- Tenderness: subacute thyroiditis.
- Local symptoms: dysphagia, dyspnea, and hoarseness; all are uncommon.

## Investigations

The following investigations are important in patients with goiter and thyroid cancer:

- TFTs: hyper- or hypothyroidism.
- Calcitonin secretion: increased in medullary thyroid cancer, and should be measured in patients with a positive family history.
- Thyroid size: assessed using plain x-rays, which may show tracheal deviation, or CT scan.
- Respiratory function tests: upper airways obstruction.
- Radionuclide imaging: can distinguish "hot nodules" (high uptake of radioisotope) from "cold nodules" (due to lack of concentration of radioisotope). Unfortunately, there are no specific features that indicate the benign or malignant nature of a thyroid nodule. Malignant nodules are more likely to be cold than hot, although most cold nodules are benign. Even so, the presence of a hot nodule does not exclude malignancy.
- Ultrasound scan: differentiation of solid from cystic lesions of the thyroid; it cannot distinguish benign from malignant nodules, although a solid nodule is more likely to contain malignant cells.
- Fine-needle aspiration cytology: can be done in outpatients and is well tolerated; cytology is not completely reliable as false-positive and false-negative results occur.

## Thyroid malignancy

### Papillary thyroid carcinoma

This accounts for 70–80% of thyroid malignancies and is more common in women; the peak age of onset is 20–30 years. It may be locally invasive or multifocal, treatment is by surgical excision, and the 10-year survival rate is 95%.

### Follicular thyroid carcinoma

This occurs in older people. Distant metastases develop in 20% of patients. Treatment is by thyroidectomy and radioiodine ablation of the thyroid remnant. The 10-year survival rate is 20%.

### Anaplastic carcinoma

Anaplastic carcinoma is uncommon. The peak incidence is at 60–70 years. The mean survival is only 6 months from diagnosis.

### Medullary thyroid carcinoma

This is rare. It secretes calcitonin and other hormones. It may be associated with pheochromocytoma. The prognosis is poor. Family members should be screened.

### Lymphoma

Lymphoma may be primary or as part of a systemic disease. There is an increased risk in patients with autoimmune thyroiditis. Radiotherapy is the treatment of choice.

## Disorders of the adrenal glands

Histologically, the adrenal glands are divided into the medulla, which secretes epinephrine and norepinephrine, and the cortex, which is divided into three zones:

- The inner zone or zona reticularis produces sex hormones.
- The middle zone or zona fasciculata produces cortisol. Production is stimulated by ACTH produced by the pituitary gland. In turn, cortisol influences, by negative feedback, both corticotropin-releasing hormone production in the hypothalamus and pituitary release of ACTH.
- The outer zona glomerulosa produces aldosterone which is regulated through the renin–angiotensin system.

### Cushing's syndrome

Cushing's syndrome is the result of chronic exposure to excess glucocorticoid. This is most commonly iatrogenic secondary to glucocorticoid administration given to treat inflammatory diseases. Other causes include the following:

- As a result of ACTH hypersecretion by a pituitary corticotrophic adenoma (60–70%).
- Primary adrenocortical tumors (30%).
- Ectopic ACTH syndrome caused by a variety of ACTH-secreting nonpituitary tumors (5–10%), such as small cell lung carcinoma.

The annual incidence of spontaneous Cushing's syndrome is about 1 in 100,000, and it is 3–5 times more common in women than men.

### Clinical features

The clinical features of Cushing's syndrome include the following:

- Centripetal fat deposition producing the typical moon facies and buffalo hump (dorsocervical fat pad).

- Skin thinning, and purple striae over the abdomen and flanks. Bruising is common and wounds heal slowly.
- Lower limb edema.
- Proximal muscle wasting.
- Osteoporosis, particularly of the vertebral bodies, leading to compression fractures.
- Impaired defense against infections.
- Hypertension.
- Mild hirsutism in women.
- Amenorrhea and infertility in women and impotence in men.
- Electrolyte disturbances with hypernatremia and hypokalemia.
- Impaired glucose tolerance or frank diabetes.

## Investigations

Investigations for Cushing's syndrome are discussed in Chapter 29. They include 24-hour urinary free cortisol measurement, dexamethasone suppression tests, assessment of corticotrophic function, and imaging techniques.

## Management

### Cushing's disease

Transsphenoidal surgery is the first line of treatment and is curative in about 80% of patients. Drugs are used if surgery fails. Metyrapone inhibits steroidogenesis and is the drug of choice. Op'DDD has a specific adrenolytic action and is used for patients intolerant to metyrapone.

Rarely, bilateral adrenalectomy is necessary, although this has a risk of leading to Nelson's syndrome, resulting in hyperpigmentation from excess β-lipotrophin activity (melanocyte-stimulating hormone and ACTH) which is not suppressed by a high blood cortisol.

### Adrenocortical tumors

Surgical removal of an adrenocortical tumor is curative. Bilateral adrenalectomy necessitates replacement therapy with cortisol, 20–40mg daily, and fludrocortisone, 0.1mg daily.

### Ectopic ACTH syndrome

Surgical resection of the tumor cures the hypercortisolism, although this is often not possible.

## Addison's disease

Addison's disease is primary adrenocortical failure. The prevalence is about 100 per million per year, and the incidence is about 5 per 1 million per year.

## Causes

Causes of Addison's disease include the following:

- Autoimmune adrenal destruction: this accounts for up to 90% of cases. Women are affected 2–3 times more often than men. Patients may have other autoimmune endocrine deficiencies.
- Infections: especially tuberculosis; cytomegalovirus and fungal infections associated with AIDS are now becoming common.
- Adrenal hemorrhage/infarction: this may be associated with sepsis, particularly meningococcal septicemia—the Waterhouse-Friderichsen syndrome. The presentation is usually acute.
- Metastatic carcinoma: especially from the breast.
- Inherited disorders: there are several familial disorders of adrenal function, all of which are rare.

## Clinical features

Symptoms and signs of Addison's disease are predominantly caused by cortisol deficiency, although deficiencies of aldosterone and adrenal androgen will also be present to varying extents (Fig. 35.14). The main symptoms are insidious and nonspecific: fatigue, weight loss, orthostatic dizziness, and anorexia. Patients may present with GI symptoms (e.g., abdominal pain, nausea, vomiting, and diarrhea). Hyperpigmentation of the skin and mucous membranes may occur as a result of high ACTH concentrations.

## Investigations

The following are important investigations in patient with Addison's disease:

- Serum cortisol concentration: low.
- Adrenal autoantibodies are detected in about 50% of patients.
- Serum ACTH levels: raised in Addison's disease and low in secondary failure.
- Serum electrolytes: usually normal but in an impending crisis there may be hyponatremia, hyperkalemia, and raised blood urea.
- Short and long synacthen tests: described in Chapter 29.
- TFTs: may show low thyroxine and raised TSH.
- Screening for other autoimmune diseases.

## Management

In emergencies, intravenous saline and glucose are required. Intravenous hydrocortisone, 100mg 6 hourly, is given. Underlying infection must be treated.

**Fig. 35.14** Symptoms and signs of adrenal insufficiency. (ACTH, adrenocorticotrophic hormone.)

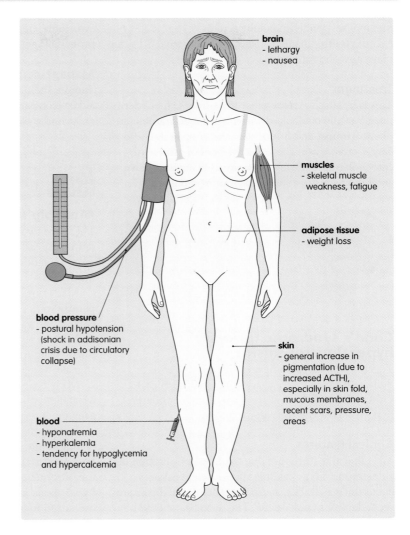

**brain**
- lethargy
- nausea

**muscles**
- skeletal muscle weakness, fatigue

**adipose tissue**
- weight loss

**blood pressure**
- postural hypotension (shock in addisonian crisis due to circulatory collapse)

**blood**
- hyponatremia
- hyperkalemia
- tendency for hypoglycemia and hypercalcemia

**skin**
- general increase in pigmentation (due to increased ACTH), especially in skin fold, mucous membranes, recent scars, pressure, areas

Maintenance therapy is with hydrocortisone, usually 20mg in the mornings and 10mg in the evenings. The dose of hydrocortisone should be increased during intercurrent illnesses and during surgery. Enzyme-inducing drugs (e.g., phenytoin and rifampicin) may also increase patient requirements for hydrocortisone. Fludrocortisone is used to replace aldosterone because aldosterone taken orally undergoes first pass metabolism through the liver. The dose is adjusted to maintain blood pressure and potassium levels. The usual dose is about 0.1mg daily.

## Pheochromocytoma

This is a rare tumor arising from the chromaffin tissues of the sympathetic nervous system, producing catecholamines. It may be associated with medullary carcinoma of the thyroid, parathyroid adenoma, and neurofibromatosis.

### Clinical features

Symptoms and signs are due to the release of epinephrine and norepinephrine and include episodic hypertension, cardiomyopathy, weight loss, and hyperglycemia. During a period of crisis there may be pallor, palpitations, panic, sweating, nausea, tremor, pain (headache or chest pain), and rarely paroxysmal thyroid swelling. The blood pressure may rise to very high levels and may precipitate a cerebrovascular accident or myocardial infarction.

### Investigations

Urine is collected for 24 hours for measurement of epinephrine and norepinephrine, or of their

359

metabolites vanillylmandelic acid or hydroxymethylmandelic acid. An abdominal CT scan may show the tumor.

### Treatment

This is by surgical removal of the tumor. The patient must be fully α-blocked with phenoxybenzamine or phentolamine, and β-blocked with propanolol before surgery to prevent the consequences of release of catecholamines during operation. Changes in pulse and blood pressure should be monitored closely.

In pheochromocytoma 90% are benign, 90% are in the adrenal medulla, and 90% of these are unilateral.

### Conn's syndrome (primary hyperaldosteronism)

This is a very rare condition, which is due to a unilateral adrenocortical adenoma in 75% of cases. Other causes include adrenal carcinoma or bilateral hyperplasia of the zona glomerulosa.

### Clinical features

The clinical features are due to excess production of aldosterone. Hypokalemia and muscle weakness occur during attacks, and polyuria and polydipsia are secondary to hypokalemia. The diagnosis should be suspected in a patient with hypertension and hypokalemia when not on a diuretic. Sodium tends to be mildly raised, but there is usually no edema.

### Investigation

Serum potassium is low and should be measured whilst the patient is not on drugs. Urinary potassium is increased for serum blood level. There is usually a metabolic alkalosis. Serum sodium is raised.

Serum renin is low and 24-hour urinary aldosterone and serum aldosterone are raised.

Secondary hyperaldosteronism is a result of high circulating renin. Causes include nephrotic syndrome, heart failure, hepatic failure, and bronchial carcinoma.

### Management

Tumors should be resected. Spironolactone is an aldosterone antagonist, which can be given in primary or secondary aldosteronism.

## Miscellaneous endocrine conditions

### Multiple endocrine neoplasia

There are two main syndromes, both autosomal dominant and both rare. Tumors originate from two or more endocrine glands which produce peptide hormones.

MEN type I refers to benign adenomas of parathyroid, pancreatic islets, pituitary, adrenal cortex, and the thyroid.

MEN type IIa refers to the association of pheochromocytoma, medullary carcinoma of the thyroid, and parathyroid adenoma or hyperplasia.

MEN type IIb is the same as IIa but with a Marfanoid phenotype and intestinal and visceral ganglioneuromas.

Family members should be screened. In type I, fasting serum calcium should be measured. In type II, pentagastrin and calcium infusion tests with measurement of serum calcitonin will pick up C-cell hyperplasia. Urinary metanephrines should be measured for pheochromocytoma.

Multiple endocrine neoplasia is a common exam question. MEN I is three Ps (pituitary, parathyroid, and pancreas), MEN II is two Cs (catecholamines, i.e., pheochromocytoma, and carcinoma of the medullary of the thyroid) and parathyroid (for MEN IIa) or mucocutaneous neuromas (for MEN IIb).

# 36. Musculoskeletal and Skin Disorders

## Arthritis

### Rheumatoid arthritis

Rheumatoid arthritis (RA) is a systemic disease producing a symmetrical inflammatory polyarthropathy with extra-articular involvement of many organs. It affects 2–3% of the population and is three times more common in women than men. The peak age of onset is between 30 and 40 years, although it can start at almost any age. There is often a family history and there is an association with HLA-DR4. The etiology is unknown but it is thought to be autoimmune.

### Clinical features

RA usually presents with an insidious onset of swollen, painful, and stiff hands and feet, progressing to involve the larger joints. Less common presentations include a relapsing and remitting monoarthritis of different large joints, a persistent monoarthritis, systemic features (myalgias, low-grade fever, weight loss, depression) before joint problems are apparent, and an acute onset of widespread arthritis, especially in the elderly.

General features of the disease include general malaise and fatigue; signs affecting the joints are described in Chapter 16. The metacarpophalangeal (MCP) joints, proximal interphalangeal (PIP) joints, and wrists are most commonly affected (Fig. 36.1). Initially there is joint swelling, which may progress to subluxation of joints and deformities. There is wasting of small muscles resulting from disuse atrophy, vasculitis and peripheral neuropathy. There may be tenosynovitis and bursitis; rheumatoid nodules are present in about 20% of patients. The feet are similarly affected.

Atlantoaxial subluxation may give rise to neurological signs, spinal cord compression and death. Other organs affected are summarized in Fig. 36.2.

Four of the seven following factors, if positive, predict RA:

1. Morning stiffness.
2. Symmetrical involvement.
3. MCP joint involvement.
4. Swelling of 3 or more joints for 6 weeks.
5. Rheumatoid nodules: found in the subcutaneous tissue.
6. Radiographic evidence of pannus formation and joint erosion.
7. Rheumatoid factor (70–80% of patients).

### Investigations

These are discussed in Chapter 16. They should include:

- Complete blood count (CBC): anemia is common.
- Erythrocyte sedimentation rate (ESR) and C-reactive protein (CRP).
- Rheumatoid factor and other autoantibodies.
- Joint x-rays. MRI may show decalcification and erosion.
- Aspiration of synovial fluid, if appropriate.

### Management

The aims of treatment are to control symptoms, to maintain a normal life and to modify the underlying disease process and inflammation. Functional status should be assessed. Proven disease should be treated aggressively since much of the joint damage of RA occurs early in the disease. Patients should be educated about their chronic illness, its progression, and techniques for pain control. Physical therapy will help to keep joints mobile, strengthen muscles, and prevent deformities. Surgery may be required to correct deformities (e.g., repair of tendons, joint prostheses, and arthrodeses). Resting the joints will relieve pain, and splints can help prevent deformities.

### Drug treatment

Initial measures should include analgesia with acetaminophen alone or with a low dose of an opioid analgesic. The pain and stiffness due to inflammation responds to nonsteroidal anti-inflammatory drugs

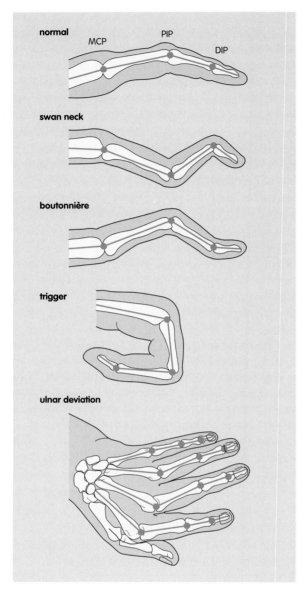

normal

MCP    PIP

DIP

swan neck

boutonnière

trigger

ulnar deviation

**Fig. 36.1** Finger and hand abnormalities in rheumatoid arthritis (DIP, distal interphalangeal joint; MCP, metacarpophalangeal joint; PIP, proximal interphalangeal joint).

(NSAIDs) (see below). Drugs are available that may affect the disease process itself and favorably influence the outcome. These include penicillamine, gold salts, antimalarials, immunosuppressants, and sulphasalazine. They are sometimes referred to as disease-modifying antirheumatic drugs or DMARDs.

Corticosteroids may also be able to reduce the rate of joint destruction.

*Nonsteroidal anti-inflammatory drugs*   About 60% of patients will respond to any NSAID, and those who do not may well respond to another. An analgesic effect should be obtained within a week, whereas an anti-inflammatory effect may not be achieved for up to 3 weeks. If appropriate responses are not obtained within these times, another NSAID should be tried.

The main differences among the NSAIDs are in the incidences and types of side effect; efficacy should always be weighed against possible side effects. They should be used with caution in the elderly, during pregnancy and breastfeeding, and in coagulation defects.

NSAIDs may cause deterioration of renal function and may worsen cardiac failure via fluid retention. They should not be used in patients with active peptic ulceration. Common side effects include gastrointestinal (GI) discomfort, nausea, diarrhea, and peptic ulceration.

*Corticosteroids*   Treatment with corticosteroids should be reserved for specific indications (e.g., when the patient is febrile and toxic-looking, when other anti-inflammatory drugs are unsuccessful). Prednisone, 7.5–20mg/day, may substantially reduce the rate of joint destruction in moderate to severe RA of less than 2 years' duration. This dose should only be maintained for 2–4 years. Steroids should be tapered as fast as possible given their inherent ability to cause osteoporosis. Oral corticosteroids may be most beneficial as a bridge between unsuccessful NSAID therapy and the use of DMARDs listed below. Corticosteroids may also be given intra-articularly to relieve pain, increase mobility, and reduce deformity in one or a few joints.

*Disease-modifying antirheumatic drugs*
DMARDs do not produce an immediate therapeutic effect but require 4–6 months for a full response. If there is no objective benefit within 6 months they should be stopped. The drugs may also improve extra-articular manifestations of RA (e.g., vasculitis). Some may retard erosive damage as judged radiologically. The drugs are normally used in RA when treatment with NSAIDs alone provides inadequate control.

*Gold salts*   These are given intramuscularly or orally. They should be discontinued in the presence

**Fig. 36.2** Organ systems affected by rheumatoid arthritis (CRP, C-reactive protein; ESR, erythrocyte sedimentation rate; RA, rheumatoid arthritis).

| Organ systems affected by rheumatoid arthritis | |
| --- | --- |
| **Organ system** | **Effects** |
| eyes | Sjögren's syndrome occurs in 15% of patients<br>scleritis causes a painful red eye, and may lead to uveitis and glaucoma<br>scleromalacia perforans is an uncommon complication where a rheumatoid nodule in the sclera perforates |
| nervous system | carpal tunnel syndrome (most common)<br>peripheral neuropathy causing glove and stocking sensory loss and occasionally motor weakness<br>mononeuritis multiplex due to vasculitis of vessels supplying nerves<br>atlantoaxial subluxation resulting in spinal cord compression |
| lymphoreticular system | generalized lymphadenopathy and splenomegaly may be present<br>Felty's syndrome |
| blood | normochromic normocytic anemia or iron-deficiency anemia (see Chapter 25)<br>ESR and CRP are raised<br>thrombocytosis may be found |
| respiratory system | pleural effusions (more common in men)<br>rheumatoid nodules<br>diffuse fibrosing alveolitis<br>Caplan's syndrome (the presence of large rheumatoid nodules and fibrosis in patients with RA exposed to various industrial dusts) |
| cardiac | pericarditis and pericardial effusions may occur |
| skin | vasculitis may produce nail-fold infarcts, ulcers, and digital gangrene peripheral edema may be present and is due to increased vascular permeability |
| kidneys | secondary amyloidosis may affect the kidneys leading to proteinuria, nephrotic syndrome, and renal failure |

of blood disorders (e.g., anemia) or proteinuria. Blood and urine tests should therefore be carried out regularly during treatment. Rashes with pruritus may occur after some months of intramuscular treatment and may necessitate discontinuation of treatment. The most common side effect of oral therapy is diarrhea, which may respond to bulking agents or a temporary reduction in dosage.

***Penicillamine*** Penicillamine has a similar action to gold salts. Blood counts and urine tests should be checked frequently.

Adverse effects include:
- Thrombocytopenia.
- Neutropenia.
- Aplastic anemia.
- Proteinuria associated with immune complex nephritis.

- Nausea.
- Anorexia.
- Fever.
- Skin reactions.
- Taste loss.

***Antimalarials*** Chloroquine and hydroxychloroquine have a similar action to gold salts and penicillamine and are better tolerated. Retinopathy is a rare side effect.

***Sulphasalazine*** This has a beneficial effect in suppressing the anti-inflammatory activity of RA. Side effects include rashes, GI intolerance, and occasionally bone marrow suppression.

***Immunosuppressants*** These are useful in patients who do not respond to the drugs above. Agents include azathioprine, methotrexate, cyclosporin, and cyclophosphamide. While methotrexate is the mainstay treatment in this category, some new immunomodulators are being used in RA. Etanercept, infliximab, and adalimumab (which play a role in the physiology of TNF-alpha, a pro-inflammatory cytokine) are now being used for patients with contraindications to methotrexate or as an add-on drug for patients already taking methotrexate. Clinical trials have shown significant improvement with etanercept. These studies have shown that the onset of symptom relief is rapid in patients who failed to respond to DMARDs. However, the positive effects were lost upon discontinuation of the drug. Infliximab and adalimumab have also shown efficacy in treating methotrexate-resistant RA. Risks with TNF-alpha antagonists are a local injection site reaction and serious infections due to immunosuppression. These infections are typically due to TB, *Mycobacterium avium*, and fungal disease.

***Interleukin-1 receptor antagonist (IL-1ra)*** In vivo, this is a naturally occurring inhibitor of IL-1. It normally inhibits the formation of prostaglandins, decreases metalloprotease activity, and may inhibit the migration of monocytes. Recombinant human IL-1ra (anakinra [Kineret]) has been clinically studied in double-blind trials and has shown significant improvement in RA symptoms and radiologic disease progression. Risks associated with the drug are similar to those associated with TNF-alpha antagonists: injection site reaction and increased risk of infection.

## Osteoarthritis

Osteoarthritis (OA) is the most common joint condition and affects about half of the population by the age of 60 years; it is more common in women. OA is a degenerative disorder affecting mainly the weight-bearing joints (e.g., the hips and knees). It is a disease of cartilage, which becomes eroded and progressively thinned as the disease proceeds. Risk factors include age, family history, obesity, and systemic features (e.g., sex and growth hormones). It may also be secondary to other joint conditions and trauma.

### Clinical features

Clinical signs and symptoms are described in Chapter 16. Joints commonly affected by OA are summarized in Fig. 36.3. There is pain in affected

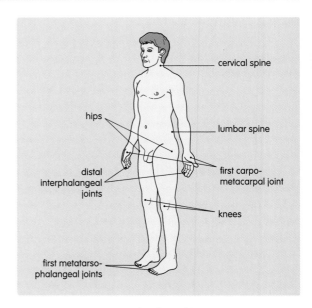

**Fig. 36.3** Joints commonly affected by osteoarthritis.

joints, which is worse with movement and toward the end of the day, superimposed on a background of pain at rest. The joints are stiff, immobile, and deformed with bone tenderness and enlargement. Pain and stiffness are often noted after a period of rest.

On examination, there may be swelling due to bony protuberances or joint effusions, crepitus on movement, signs of inflammation, limited joint movement, and deformities. The pattern of joint involvement tends to be asymmetrical. In the hands, the most commonly affected joints are the distal interphalangeal (DIP) joints (Heberden's nodes), proximal interphalangeal (PIP) joints (Bouchard's nodes), and first carpometacarpal joints giving an appearance of "square hands" (Fig. 36.4). Unlike RA, there is no systemic illness or extra-articular manifestations of the disease.

### Investigations

There are no biochemical abnormalities, but ESR, RF, and possible microscopic evaluation of synovial fluid should be undertaken to rule out other causes of joint pain. Diagnosis is based on clinical findings and radiological changes of loss of joint space, subchondral sclerosis and cysts, and marginal osteophytes.

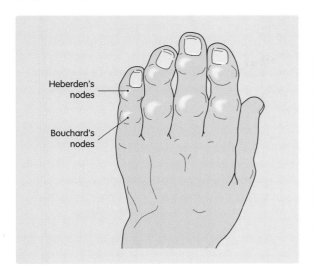

**Fig. 36.4** Osteoarthritis in a hand, showing Heberden's nodes at the distal interphalangeal joints and Bouchard's nodes at the proximal interphalangeal joints.

## Management

Treatment options include combinations of drugs, physical treatments (e.g., weight reduction and heat application), exercises, hydrotherapy, aids (e.g., walking sticks and special shoes), and surgery (e.g., arthrodesis, arthroplasty, joint replacement). Initially, simple analgesics (e.g., acetaminophen) should be prescribed for the pain. NSAIDs are given if simple analgesia is not effective. Intra-articular corticosteroids can be used for inflammatory exacerbations.

## Spondyloarthropathies

This term describes a group of related diseases with some common features. There is an association with HLA-B27 with familial clustering of cases. These include:

- Ankylosing spondylitis.
- Reiter's syndrome and reactive arthritis.
- Enteropathic arthropathies.
- Psoriatic arthritis.
- Juvenile chronic arthritis.
- Undifferentiated spondyloarthropathy.

## Ankylosing spondylitis

This most commonly affects young men, with a prevalence of about 1 in 2000 to 1.4%, depending on racial group. AS is much less common in African-Amerians than in Caucasians. HLA-B27 is present in over 90% of patients.

**Fig. 36.5** Advancing ankylosing spondylitis. Eventually the trunk may become fixed in a fully flexed position, so that the patient cannot see directly ahead—the classic "question mark" posture.

### Clinical features

The onset is insidious with sacroiliitis causing pain in the buttocks radiating down the back of the legs. There is progressive spinal fusion with loss of movement, low back pain, and morning stiffness that improves with exercise.. Eventually the patient has a fixed kyphotic spine, hyperextended neck and spinocranial ankylosis, and a reduction in chest expansion leading to a "question mark" posture (Fig. 36.5). Peripheral joints may be affected and tend to affect larger joints in an asymmetrical distribution. Other features include:

- General malaise.
- Uveitis: in about one-third of cases.
- Ulcerative colitis: more common than uveitis.
- Aortic regurgitation: due to aortitis.
- Respiratory failure: secondary to kyphoscoliosis and fibrosing alveolitis.

### Investigations

The following investigations should be performed in the patient with ankylosing spondylitis:

- ESR and C-reactive protein (CRP): often raised.
- HLA-B27: provides useful supporting evidence, but it is also present in the normal population.
- X-rays: sacroiliitis indicated by irregular margins and sclerosis of adjacent bone; "bamboo" spine with squaring of the vertebrae and calcification and ossification of intervertebral ligaments.

### Management

Treatment includes analgesia with NSAIDs. Patients should be encouraged to exercise to prevent deformity and to maintain movement and relieve symptoms. Sulphasalazine or methotrexate can improve symptom due to peripheral arthritis. Anti-TNF-alpha therapy (etanercept, infliximab, and adalimumabab) is also used for patients who still have unacceptable active disease after NSAID treatment. Radiotherapy may be tried in a minority of patients with intractable symptoms, although the majority of patients will be able to maintain a normal lifestyle. The disease may be progressive, it may remit, or there may be recurrent episodes. In extreme cases, ventilation may be impaired due to immobility of the spine and rib cage.

### Reiter's syndrome

Reiter's syndrome consists of the triad of seronegative arthritis, nonspecific urethritis (NSU), and conjunctivitis. It is 20 times more common in men than women and usually affects young adults. It follows NSU with a history of unprotected sexual intercourse about 1 month prior to presentation. Less commonly, it may follow GI infection with *Shigella*, *Salmonella*, *Yersinia*, or *Campylobacter*.

### Clinical features

The arthritis is often of acute onset, polyarticular, and asymmetrical, particularly affecting the lower limbs. It may be associated with non-articular

inflammatory lesions including plantar fasciitis and Achilles tendinitis. Other clinical features include:

- Urethritis: associated with penile discharge and dysuria; there may be circinate balanitis (an erythematous circular lesion on the penis with a pale center).
- Conjunctivitis: usually mild and bilateral; iritis and anterior uveitis may also occur.
- Mouth ulcers.
- Keratoderma blennorrhagica: a pustular hyperkeratotic lesion on the soles of the feet.
- Nail dystrophy and subungual keratosis.
- General malaise.
- Low-grade fever. Cardiovascular, respiratory, and neurological complications are rare.

### Investigations

The diagnosis is clinical and autoantibodies are negative. HLA-B27 is positive in 60% of patients.

### Management

Treatment is symptomatic with analgesia (e.g., NSAIDs) and rest of affected joints. Effusions can be aspirated. As in other joint diseases, infliximab (a TNF-alpha antagonist) is effective in treating Reiter's symptoms. Maintenance therapy has also been proven to be safe. In chronic cases, sulphasalazine or methotrexate can be tried. In most cases, the acute arthritis settles within 1–2 months; about 50% of patients develop recurrent symptoms.

### Reactive arthritis

This term describes arthritis following enteric or venereal infection, as in Reiter's syndrome, but the other features of Reiter's syndrome are absent.

### Psoriatic arthritis

This is a seronegative arthritis occurring in 10% of patients with psoriasis. The most common pattern is involvement of the small joints of the hand, particularly the DIP joints, in an asymmetrical pattern (Fig. 36.6). Other variants are described in Chapter 16. There is nail pitting and onycholysis.

Treatment is with analgesia and anti-inflammatory drugs. Immunosuppressive drugs such as cyclosporine and methotrexate may be effective and are used in severe cases. Like other spondyloarthropathies, psoriatic arthritis may respond to treatment with TNF-alpha antagonists (infliximab and etanercept).

**Fig. 36.6** Psoriatic arthritis involving the distal interphalangeal joints. There is "pitting" of the nails, and there may be anycholysis.

**Fig. 36.7** Systemic lupus erythematosus showing the classic "bat" or "butterfly wing" rash.

## Enteropathic arthropathies

This occurs in patients with inflammatory bowel disease and usually affects the knees and ankles as a monoarthritis or asymmetrical oligoarthritis. The aetiology is unknown but immune complexes in the joint may play a part. Management should be aimed at the underlying bowel disease, which will improve the arthritis. NSAIDs and joint aspiration will provide symptomatic relief.

## Systemic lupus erythematosus

Systemic lupus erythematosus (SLE) is a multisystem, autoimmune connective tissue disorder. The prevalence in the U.S. is 40–50 cases per 100,000. It is nine times more common in women and also more common in African-Americans. The peak age of onset is between 20 and 40 years. The etiology is unknown but is probably multifactorial. Predisposing factors include a genetic predisposition and environmental triggers (e.g., drugs such as hydralazine, ultraviolet light, viral infections, and immunologic mechanisms).

## Clinical features

SLE is characterized by vasculitis—the clinical features of the disease are mainly due to the effects of the vasculitis in different body systems. The most common early features are fever, arthralgia, malaise, tiredness, and weight loss. The following systems may be involved.

## Musculoskeletal system

This is involved in over 90% of cases. There is arthralgia, the symptoms of which are clinically similar to RA, although examination is often normal. There may be myalgia and myositis, and, rarely, there is a deforming arthropathy due to capsular laxity (Jaccoud's arthropathy). Aseptic necrosis affecting the hip or knee may also rarely occur. Osteoporosis is a common feature.

## Cutaneous system

This is involved in about 80% of cases. Classically there is a "butterfly" rash over the bridge of the nose and spreading over both cheeks (Fig. 36.7). Other features include photosensitivity, alopecia, livedo reticularis, Raynaud's phenomenon, nail-fold infarcts, purpura, urticaria, and oral ulceration.

Discoid lupus is a benign variant of SLE, with skin involvement only. There are discoid erythematous plaques on the face that progress to scarring and pigmentation. Patients with widespread skin disease may develop SLE.

## Central nervous system

The central nervous system (CNS) is involved in 60% of cases. Psychiatric disturbances include depression, delirium, and occasionally psychosis. Other features include:

- Epilepsy.
- Cerebrovascular accidents: often associated with antiphospholipid antibody syndrome.
- Cranial nerve lesions.
- Cerebellar ataxia.
- Aseptic meningitis.
- Peripheral neuropathies.

The effects are due to arteritis and ischemia or immune complex deposition.

## Respiratory system

The respiratory system is involved in about 50% of cases. Pulmonary manifestations include:

- Pleurisy with pleural effusions.
- Pneumonia and atelectasis.
- Interstitial lung disease: restrictive defects with diffuse reticular-nodular shadowing in the chest x-ray.

## Renal system

The renal system is involved in about 50% of cases. This is associated with a poor prognosis. Proteinuria is common. There may be minimal change, and membranous or proliferative glomerulonephritis. Clinically, the patient may present with nephrotic or nephritic syndrome, hypertension, or chronic renal failure.

## Cardiovascular system

The cardiovascular system is involved in 40% of cases. There may be:

- Increased coronary artery disease.
- Pericarditis with pericardial effusion.
- Myocarditis with consequent heart failure.
- Aortic valve lesions.
- Nonbacterial endocarditis of the mitral valve (Libman-Sacks endocarditis).

## Blood and lymphatic systems

The ESR is markedly raised. There may be:

- Normochromic normocytic anemia.
- Hemolytic anemia.
- Leukopenia.
- Thrombocytopenia.
- Generalized lymphadenopathy.
- Hepatosplenomegaly.

## Drug-induced lupus

Drug-induced lupus may occur with hydralazine in slow acetylators, and with procainamide, isoniazid, chlorpromazine, and anticonvulsants. It remits when the drug is stopped. Renal and CNS involvement is rare.

## Investigations

The following investigations are important in patients with SLE:

- ESR: raised.
- CRP: usually normal.
- There may be anemia, leukopenia, or thrombocytopenia.
- Antinuclear antibody: positive in almost all cases; anti-double-stranded DNA is present in about 75% of cases and is specific for SLE.
- Serum complement levels: reduced; immunoglobulins raised.
- Radiology: CXR is useful for suspected pleural involvement, effusion. Renal ultrasound can be used to look for size and obstructive pathology. MRI is used to evaluate neurologic deficits, and echocardiography can be used if Libmann-Sacks endocarditis is suspected.
- Renal biopsy: if there is involvement of the kidneys, renal biopsy shows characteristic histologic changes.

## Management

Patients with mild disease can be managed with aspirin or NSAIDs for joint pain. Anemia can be corrected with transfusion, and sun block will protect from photosensitivity. For acute exacerbations, steroids are given in high doses and gradually tailed off, depending on symptoms, signs, and changes in ESR.

Immunosuppressive drugs are used for patients with more serious disease (e.g., if there is renal or CNS involvement), as they have a steroid-sparing effect. Drugs used include azathioprine, chlorambucil, and cyclophosphamide. Lupus nephritis is treated with pulse cyclophosphamide.

In some patients in whom NSAIDs are ineffective in controlling joint pain or in whom skin manifestations predominate, the antimalarial drug chloroquine may be useful. Chloroquine can cause irreversible retinal degeneration so vision should be formally assessed at regular intervals.

Some women are prone to recurrent abortions, which are associated with lupus anticoagulant.

Specialist care should therefore be available in pregnancy.

## Polymyalgia rheumatica

Polymyalgia rheumatica (PMR) is a clinical syndrome characterized by proximal muscle pain and stiffness. The incidence increases with age and the prevalence is as much as 2% in patients aged over 60 years. It is 2–3 times more common in women than men, more common in Northern Europe than Southern Europe, and is rare in non-Caucasians. PMR and giant cell arteritis (see p. 316) are closely linked, but either can occur in isolation.

### Clinical features
Discriminating characteristics for PMR include:
- Bilateral shoulder pain with or without stiffness.
- Bilateral upper arm tenderness.
- Illness of less than 2 weeks' duration.
- Morning stiffness that lasts for more than 1 hour.
- Depression with or without weight loss.
- Age greater than 65 years.
- An initial ESR of at least 40mm/hour.

The distribution tends to be symmetrical, and systemic features such as sweating and malaise are common. True weakness does not occur, although power and range of movement may be limited by pain.

### Differential diagnosis
The differential diagnosis of PMR includes:
- Late-onset RA.
- OA.
- Soft tissue rheumatic conditions: rotator cuff disease, nonspecific back pain, trochanteric bursitis.
- Multiple myeloma (due to elevated ESR): however, stiffness is not usually a major feature.
- Hypothyroidism: due to myalgia and malaise.
- Parkinson's disease: may occasionally cause confusion due to loss of mobility.
- Connective tissue diseases, polymyositis, and proximal myopathy.
- Occult malignancy if systemic features are marked.
- Infection.

### Investigations
The following investigations are important in patients with PMR:
- ESR: usually over 40mm per hour; very high values can occur.
- Acute-phase proteins: increased (e.g., CRP).
- Alkaline phosphatase: raised in about 30% of patients.
- Platelets: tend to be increased.
- Mild normochromic normocytic anemia: common.
- Temporal artery biopsy: rarely helpful.
- Tests to exclude conditions capable of mimicking PMR: rheumatoid factor, myeloma screen, thyroid function tests, creatine kinase if muscle weakness is suspected, autoantibodies if there are features suggesting connective tissue disease.

### Management
Eighty percent of symptoms improve within a few days with corticosteroids. The ESR falls to normal within 2–3 weeks, and the CRP becomes normal within 1 week. An initial daily dose of 7.5–20mg of prednisone is usually adequate to control symptoms. The dose should be continued for 1 month and slowly reduced over the following month to about 10mg daily. It is advisable to reduce the dose by no more than 1mg per month.

There is no indication for prophylactic high-dose steroids to prevent blindness as with giant cell arteritis. Patients, however, should be warned to look out for additional symptoms such as headache or blurred vision. Steroids should be reduced slowly over the subsequent months.

Approximately 50% of patients manage to discontinue steroids within 2 years. Management should be based mainly on the clinical picture, although a rise in ESR in someone who is otherwise well should prompt more frequent monitoring. Relapses are most common in the first year, but the incidence falls steadily thereafter. They are often associated with a reduction in steroid dose. Adding a NSAID to cover aching and stiffness may be of help.

In patients who are becoming cushingoid, a steroid-sparing immunosuppressant (e.g., azathioprine) should be considered under expert supervision. In a few patients it is impossible to withdraw steroids altogether; it is acceptable to maintain them indefinitely on prednisone, 2–3mg/day.

## Prognosis

The prognosis is good provided the steroid dosage is not excessive. Most patients can be reassured that treatment can usually be discontinued after 2–4 years with a low rate of recurrence thereafter.

## Other connective tissue disorders

## Systemic sclerosis

Systemic sclerosis is a multisystem disease that mainly occurs in middle-aged women. It presents with Raynaud's phenomenon in more than three-quarters of cases. The etiology is unknown. Familial cases occur with HLA-B8 and HLA-DR3 at increased frequency. There are abnormalities of both humoral and cellular immunity. Early in the disease the skin is edematous, and the blood vessels show arteritis and thickening. There is an increase in collagen and progressive fibrosis of viscera.

### Clinical features

There is general malaise, lassitude, fever, and weight loss. The following systems may be involved.

### Cutaneous system

Systemic sclerosis is also termed scleroderma, reflecting the thickening and hardening of the skin associated with increased collagen content. Patients classically have a beaked nose, telangiectasia, and tight skin around the mouth, causing difficulty in opening the mouth wide (Fig. 36.8). The skin becomes smooth and waxy, and atrophic with pigmentation or depigmentation. There is sclerodactyly and the fingers are "sausage shaped." Raynaud's phenomenon is common. There may also be subcutaneous calcification.

Morphea is a benign condition affecting only the skin, especially on the the trunk and limbs. Plaques evolve to produce waxy, thickened skin and induration. These may enlarge, or new lesions may appear over time. Resolution is associated with hyperpigmentation. Only rarely does morphea proceed to systemic sclerosis.

### Gastrointestinal system

Esophageal involvement is very common. There is delayed peristalsis, dilatation, or stricture formation, leading to dysphagia or heartburn in about half of affected patients. Dilatation and atony of the small bowel may lead to bacterial overgrowth and hence malabsorption and steatorrhea.

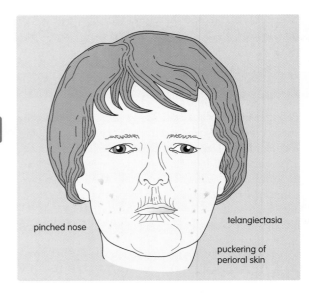

**Fig. 36.8** Systemic sclerosis, showing pinched nose, multiple telangiectasia, and tightening of the skin around the mouth. The skin may also be waxy and shiny.

### Respiratory system

There is interstitial fibrosis, which either affects the lower lobes of the lungs or is diffuse. This may cause a restrictive defect and may progress to respiratory failure. There may be aspiration pneumonia and pulmonary hypertension.

### Musculoskeletal system

There may be polyarthralgia and flexion deformities due to fibrosis of tendons. Myopathy and polymyositis can occur.

### Cardiovascular system

Myocardial fibrosis can cause arrhythmias and conduction defects. Pericardial effusions can occur and cardiomyopathy can lead to heart failure. Cardiac involvement often carries a poor prognosis.

### Renal system

Renal involvement due to an obliterative endarteritis of renal vessels can lead to progressive renal failure and hypertension, which may be fatal.

### Eyes

Sjögren's syndrome may occur.

## CREST syndrome

CREST syndrome is a form of systemic sclerosis, including **c**alcinosis of subcutaneous tissues, **R**aynaud's phenomenon, **e**sophageal dysmotility, **s**clerodactyly, and **t**elangiectasia. The prognosis is generally better than systemic sclerosis *per se*. It is associated with anticentromere antibodies.

## Investigations

The following investigations are important in patients with systemic sclerosis:

- Antinuclear antibodies: present in 80% of patients; rheumatoid factor is positive in 30%. Antitopoisomerase-1 antibodies (Scl-70) are highly specific but not sensitive for scleroderma.
- ESR: often raised.
- CBC: may show a normochromic normocytic anemia or a hemolytic anemia.
- Hand x-rays: may show calcinosis.
- Barium swallow or esophageal manometry: motility problems.

## Management

Treatment is symptomatic. Electrically heated gloves may help with Raynaud's phenomenon. Antacids, $H_2$ receptor antagonists, or proton pump inhibitors will help relieve heartburn. Physical therapy may help when joints are affected, and NSAIDs can be given for joint pain.

## Prognosis

The course of the disease is variable but is usually slowly progressive. Death usually occurs from lung or cardiac complications. The overall mean 5-year survival rate is about 70%.

## Polymyositis and dermatomyositis

Polymyositis is a disorder of muscle and is of unknown etiology. Immunologic and viral factors have been suggested. Pathologically there is necrosis of muscle fibers with regeneration and inflammation. When accompanied by a rash, it is known as dermatomyositis. It can occur at any age, with a peak incidence at around 50 years old, with women twice as likely to be affected as men. About 20% of cases are associated with an underlying malignancy of bronchus, breast, stomach, or ovary. The incidence of malignancy increases with age and is more common in men.

## Clinical features

The clinical feature of polymyositis and dermatomyositis include the following:

- Muscle weakness and proximal muscle wasting (but no morning stiffness as in polymyalgia rheumatica).

- Onset: acute or chronic with progressive weakness.
- Muscle pain and tenderness: about 50% of patients.
- Fibrosis: flexion deformities of the limbs.
- Arthralgia and arthritis: about 50% of patients.
- Skin involvement: purple "heliotrope" color around the eyes and sometimes the rest of the face; violaceous, edematous lesions over the knuckles; telangiectasia, nail-fold infarcts.
- Muscle involvement: can affect the esophagus leading to dysphagia.
- Raynaud's phenomenon.
- Lung fibrosis.
- Cardiomyopathy.
- Sjögren's syndrome.

The risk of underlying malignancy with dermatomyositis or polymyositis is 30% at age 30, 40% at age 40, etc.

## Investigation

- Muscle enzymes: creatine phosphokinase and aldolase are raised and can be used to follow the course of the disease.
- Characteristic electromyographic changes.
- Muscle biopsy: necrosis of muscle fibers with swelling and disruption of muscle cells; fibrosis, thickening of blood vessels, and inflammatory changes.
- ESR: usually raised and there may be a normochromic normocytic anemia; antinuclear antibodies; Pos-1 antibodies may be positive.
- Investigations for underlying malignancy.

## Management

High-dose steroids should be prescribed in the acute phase. These can be gradually tapered. Immunosuppressive drugs (e.g., methotrexate or azathioprine) may be required if there is a poor response to steroids. Physical therapy may help to restore muscle power.

## Prognosis

Adults fare better than children unless there is an underlying malignancy. The disease may be progressive or may wax and wane. Death usually occurs from respiratory or cardiac failure.

## Sjögren's syndrome

This is the association of a connective tissue disease with keratoconjunctivitis sicca (dry eyes) or xerostomia (dry mouth). There is an association with HLA-B8 and HLA-DR3. Involvement of other secretory glands may cause dyspareunia, dry skin, dysphagia, otitis media, and pulmonary infection. Other features include:

- Arthralgia and polyarthritis.
- Raynaud's phenomenon.
- Esophageal motility abnormalities and dysphagia.
- Renal tubular defects.
- Pulmonary fibrosis.
- Polyneuropathy.
- Hepatosplenomegaly.
- Vasculitis.

There is an increased incidence of lymphoma. Sjögren's syndrome is associated with other organ-specific, autoimmune diseases (e.g., thyroid disease, myasthenia gravis, primary biliary cirrhosis and chronic active hepatitis).

Pathologically there is a lymphocytic and plasma cell infiltrate of the secretory glands.

### Investigations

The following investigations are important in patients with Sjögren's syndrome:

- Anti-Ro and anti-La antibody titers: high levels.
- Immunoglobulins: raised.
- Rheumatoid factor: always present.
- Schirmer's test: this is a method of quantifying conjunctival dryness. A strip of filter paper is put under the lower eyelid, and the distance along the paper that tears are absorbed is measured. This should be more than 10mm in 5 minutes.

## Mixed connective tissue disease

This is a term used when the symptoms and signs do not fit neatly into one of the well-defined syndromes. It affects women more than men and presents in young adults. There are high titers of antibody to an extractable nuclear antigen such as ribonucleoprotein (RNP). The condition may respond to steroids. Immunologic tests for this disorder and others are summarized in Fig. 36.9.

## Polyarteritis nodosa

Polyarteritis nodosa (PAN) is one of the "vasculitides." It is a necrotizing vasculitis which causes aneurysms of medium-sized arteries. It is four times more common in men than women, and the peak incidence is between the ages of 20 and 50 years. The association with hepatitis B surface antigen suggests that the vasculitis is secondary to deposition of immune complexes.

### Clinical features

Polyarteritis nodosa, like most other rheumatic diseases, presents with systemic symptoms. Clinical features include the following:

- General: fever, malaise, weight loss, myalgia.
- Renal: the main cause of death. Patients may present with hypertension, proteinuria, an acute nephritic syndrome, nephrotic syndrome, or renal failure.
- Cardiac: this is the second most common cause of death. Coronary arteritis may lead to angina and myocardial infarction. There may be pericarditis.
- Pulmonary: pulmonary infiltrates and late-onset asthma. The Churg–Strauss syndrome is associated with allergic angiitis and granuloma formation, accompanied by an intense eosinophilic infiltration that affects the pulmonary arteries and causes asthma and pneumonia.
- GI tract: abdominal pain from visceral infarction; malabsorption from chronic ischemia.
- CNS: mononeuritis multiplex, sensorimotor polyneuropathy, fits, subarachnoid hemorrhage, psychoses.
- Skin: tender nodules, nail-fold infarcts, urticaria, purpura, livedo reticularis.
- Joints: arthralgia or a nondeforming polyarthritis.

### Investigations

Investigations include:

- ESR and CRP: usually raised; normochromic normocytic anemia, leucocytosis, and eosinophilia in 30% of cases.
- Biopsy: affected organs may be biopsied, demonstrating fibrinoid necrosis and cellular infiltration in the arteries.
- Angiography: may demonstrate microaneurysms in affected viscera.

### Management

Treatment is symptomatic, and with steroids and immunosuppressive agents. The course of the disease may be rapidly or slowly progressive. Renal failure is the main cause of death. The overall 5-year survival rate is 40%.

**Fig. 36.9** Immunologic tests. (ANA, antinuclear antibody; GAD, glutamate decarboxylase; MCTD, mixed connective tissue disease; SLE, systemic lupus erythematosus).

| Immunological tests | |
|---|---|
| **Test** | **Associated disorder** |
| antinuclear factor (ANA) | SLE: fits, confusion, neuropathy, aseptic meningitis<br>Sjögren's syndrome: gritty eyes, neuropathies, MCTD |
| anti double-stranded DNA antibodies | SLE |
| rheumatoid factor | rheumatoid arthritis: cervical spine subluxation, neuropathies, vasculitis, SLE, MCTD |
| anti-Ro (SSA), anti-La (SSB) antibodies | Sjögren's syndrome |
| antiphospholipid antibodies (e.g. anticardiolipin) | antiphospholipid syndrome |
| anti-ribonucleoprotein antibodies | MCTD; myositis, trigeminal nerve palsies |
| Jo-1 antibodies | polymyositis |
| antineutrophil cytoplasmic antibodies (ANCA) | pANCA (peripheral): polyarteritis nodosa<br>cANCA (classical): Wegener's granulomatosis |
| antiacetylcholine receptor antibodies | myasthenia gravis |
| anti-GM1 antibodies | multifocal motor neuropathy, Guillain-Barré syndrome |
| anti-GAD antibodies | stiff-man syndrome |
| anticentromeric antibodies | scleroderma |
| anti-topoisomerase-1 (Sci-70) | scleroderma |

## Primary skin diseases

### Psoriasis

Psoriasis is a papulosquamous, proliferative, inflammatory skin disease that affects 2% of the population. It may present at any age with a peak incidence in the late-20s with polygenic inheritance. Triggers include stress, trauma, infection, and drugs (e.g., lithium, chloroquine and β-blockers).

The main lesion in plaque psoriasis is a salmon-pink plaque topped by a silvery scale, most frequently found over the extensor surfaces of the limbs (e.g., elbows and knees). Involvement of the scalp with a thickened hyperkeratotic scale is also common. Plaques may be round or "guttate" (like rain drops), geographical or circinate (ring-like). Removal of the scales leaves pinpoint bleeding sites (Auspitz's sign).

In flexural psoriasis, lesions have a pinkish glazed appearance, are clearly demarcated, and are nonscaly.

The most common sites of involvement are the groin, perianal and genital regions, and inflamammary folds. Other sites include elbows and scalp.

In guttate psoriasis, small lesions can appear anywhere on the body without pattern.

Pustular psoriasis affects the palms or soles with well-demarcated scaling and erythema. The pustules are white, yellow, green, or brown when dried.

Arthropathy occurs in about 10% of patients. Other extradermal manifestations include nail pitting, corneal nodules, edema, and liver damage.

### Management

Psoriasis that involves <5% of the body area can be treated by a primary care physician; extensive cases should ideally be treated by a dermatologist. Treatment should be based on body surface area and severity of disease. Often localized therapy can be used.

For mild conditions, treatment other than reassurance and an emollient may be unnecessary. In more troublesome cases, local application of salicylic acid, coal tar, calcipotriol or dithranol may have a beneficial effect.

### Salicylic acid
This enhances the rate of loss of surface scale. Side effects include irritation or toxicity when large areas are treated.

### Anthralin/coal tar
Coal tar has anti-inflammatory and antiscaling properties, but its use is limited by its unpleasant appearance and odor, and it may not be used on the face. However, when the lesions are extensive, coal tar baths are useful.

### Dithranol
This is very effective in psoriasis. It can cause severe skin irritation and should therefore be started at low concentrations and gradually built up.

### Ultraviolet B radiation therapy
This is helpful in mild-to-moderate, guttate, or chronic plaque psoriasis.

### Topical corticosteroids
These remain the major form of treatment for psoriasis. Corticosteroids are anti-inflammatory, antiproliferative, and immunosuppressive. They have a natural ability to thin skin, which is normally as a side effect. Note that on the face and intertriginous areas of the body less concentrated preparations are necessary.

### Calcipotriol
Calcipotriol is a vitamin D derivative that can be applied topically for mild-to-moderate psoriasis. It does not have an unpleasant odor.

### Photochemotherapy using psoralens with long-wave ultraviolet irradiation
Photochemotherapy using psoralens with long-wave ultraviolet (UV) irradiation (or PUVA) is effective in some patients. Special lamps are required. Short-term side effects include burning; long-term effects may include cataract formation, accelerated ageing of the skin (solar elastosis), and the development of skin cancer.

### Acitretin
This is a retinoid (vitamin A derivative) given orally for severe resistant or complicated psoriasis. Side effects include dry and chapped lips, mild transient increase in the rate of hair fall, pruritus, paronychia, and nose bleeds. It is teratogenic.

### Cytotoxic drugs
Cytotoxic drugs (e.g., methotrexate and cyclosporin) can be used for severe resistant psoriasis. Promising results in patients with moderate-to-severe psoriasis have also been found with the use of TNF-alpha inhibitors. Infliximab and etanercept have shown promise in randomized trials. Another immunomodulator with promise is alefacept, a recombinant protein that binds to the CD2 on memory effector T lymphocytes. This inhibits the actions of T cells within the psoriatic plaque.

## Eczema (dermatitis)
The terms eczema and dermatitis are often used interchangeably. The disorder affects 10% of the population. Clinically, lesions are often vesicular, rupturing to leave a raw, weeping surface. They may be diffuse, irritating, and sometimes painful. There may be itching and secondary infection. Lesions can be chronic and may involve scaling with lichenification.

### Atopic eczema
This often starts in infancy, with the vast majority of patients growing out of it by the age of 12 years. Breastfeeding may help prevent atopic eczema. Clinical symptoms include itching and inflammation. Investigations include prick tests to common allergens and raised serum IgE.

### Irritant contact dermatitis
The hands are often affected by erythema, vesiculation, and fissuring. Irritants include detergents, bleaches, soaps, etc. It may be a problem in certain occupations (e.g., hairdressers and engineers).

### Allergic contact dermatitis
This requires previous sensitization. Patch testing produces a marked, prolonged response even to dilute quantities of the allergen. The pattern of eczema depends on the site of contact. There is often a sharp cut-off where contact ends, although spread to other sites may occur (autosensitization). Thin, moist skin is the most vulnerable. Common allergens include:
- Dyes.
- Nickel: buttons and zips.
- Chromates: cement and leather.
- Lanolin: cosmetics.
- Rubber.

- Resins: glues.
- Plants.
- Topical antibiotics.
- Antiseptics.

## Seborrheic dermatitis
This is a scaly, crusty, red, itchy eruption appearing on oily areas of the skin (e.g., the face, flexures, and scalp [dandruff]).

## Management
Where possible, the cause should be established and removed. A patient with suspected contact dermatitis should be patch-tested to establish the diagnosis. Atopic eczema usually requires the regular application of an emollient with short courses of a mild-to-moderate topical corticosteroid, the least potent that is effective. In more severe eczema, more potent steroids may be needed and, if itching is a major problem, consideration should be given to the administration of antihistamines and possibly antibiotics to prevent secondary bacterial infection.

For dry, fissured, scaly lesions, treatment is with emollients and emulsifying ointment as soap substitutes. For weeping eczema, treatment is with topical corticosteroids, wet dressings of potassium permanganate, and topical antibacterials. Coal tar is used occasionally in chronic atopic eczema. Cyclosporin may be used for severe resistant atopic dermatitis.

## Acne vulgaris
This is a papulopustular inflammatory condition, usually affecting the face and trunk, which affects about 90% of adolescents. Overproduction of sebum leads to blockage of the sebaceous duct, producing the primary lesion (the comedo or "blackhead"). Open comedo is blackhead and closed; comedo is white head. Colonization by *Propionibacterium acnes* is probably an important factor. Healing may leave residual scarring.

Lichen planus is summed up by four Ps: peripheral, pruritis, polygonal, and purple.

## Management
A sympathetic approach is needed. Dispel myths that the patient is dirty or that acne is caused by eating chocolate or greasy food. Advise patients to wash the face with soap and water frequently to degrease the skin. Both comedones and inflamed lesions respond well to benzoyl peroxide or azelaic acid.

Topical antibiotics are used for mild-to-moderate acne and include erythromycin, tetracycline, and clindamycin. Prolonged periods of oral antibiotics (e.g., for 6 months) are also effective. Topical retinoids are used as well in increasing concentrations. The ideal therapy is often a combination of different topical treatments with or without oral antibiotics. In addition, oral isotretinoin (accutane) is a retinoid used for severe acne unresponsive to systemic antibiotics. It acts primarily by reducing sebum secretion. The drug is teratogenic.

## Lichen planus
Lesions occur in patients between 30 and 60 years old. Lichen planus is more common in females. Lesions are purple, polygonal, and planar or flat-topped papules. The cause is unknown but may be related to disturbances of immune function. Lichen planus-like reactions occur with certain drugs, such as sulphonamides, sulfonylureas, methyldopa, thiazides, β-blockers, and drugs that alter immune function (e.g., antimalarials, gold salts, penicillamine).

The distribution of lesions is mainly peripheral and symmetrical. Scarring occurs with chronic disease. Linear lesions may follow trauma or scratching (Koebner's phenomenon). Lesions may occur on the buccal mucosa or in the nails. The presence of Wickham's striae help to distinguish the disease. These are fine white lacy lines coursing over the papule. Postinflammatory hyperpigmentation is also a useful diagnostic sign.

The lesions usually last for 12–18 months if untreated. Systemic steroids may be required to suppress intractable itching. Less acute disease can be managed with topical corticosteroids with an antihistamine at night to control the itching.

## Pityriasis rosea
This is a self-limiting, nonrecurrent, scaling, maculopapular eruption, occurring mainly in children and young adults. The cause is probably viral, and some drugs may produce similar features (e.g., gold salts or penicillamine). It is preceded by a red oval lesion 2–6cm in diameter—this is the herald patch. The rash that follows may cover the entire trunk,

upper thighs, and arms. The reddish-brown discrete macules tend to follow the lines of the ribs in a linear fashion ("Christmas tree" distribution). The eruption is only mildly pruritic and usually clears within 6–8 weeks without treatment.

## Rosacea

This is a chronic inflammatory eruption over the flush areas of the face (cheeks, nose, and chin) with erythema, papules, pustules, and telangiectasia. It mainly affects fair-skinned, middle-aged women and can be triggered by hot drinks, stress, sunlight, spicy foods, alcohol, and topical steroids.

Rhinophyma (an enlarged nose) is common and more often seen in men.

Management is by avoiding precipitating factors and taking oxytetracycline for at least 3 months. Metronidazole may be of help if tetracycline is not effective. Isotretinoin can be tried in resistant cases.

## Skin manifestations of systemic disease

### Erythema nodosum

These are painful, nodular lesions, usually on the anterior shins which go through similar color changes to a bruise. New crops of lesions emerge while earlier lesions are fading. It is five times more common in women, with a peak incidence between 20 and 50 years.

### Causes of erythema nodosum

- Sarcoidosis.
- Drugs (e.g., sulfonamides, oral contraceptive pill, dapsone).
- Bacterial infections (e.g., streptococcus, tuberculosis).
- Crohn's disease and ulcerative colitis.
- Behçet's disease.
- Leptospirosis.
- Fungal infections (e.g., *Histoplasma*).
- Viral infections.
- Malignancies.

### Erythema multiforme

These are "target" lesions, or circular lesions in a symmetrical distribution with central blistering. They usually occur on the limbs. The lesions may be preceded by a prodrome of fever, sore throat, headache, arthralgia, and gastroenteritis.

In Stevens-Johnson syndrome there is systemic illness, and lesions are present in the mouth, eye, and genital regions. Stevens-Johnson syndrome can progress to toxic epidermal necrolysis (TEN).

### Causes of erythema multiforme

- Drugs (e.g., barbiturates, sulfonamides, penicillin, salicylates).
- Systemic infections, especially viral (e.g., herpes simplex).
- Vitamin deficiency, especially niacin, and vitamins A and C.
- Collagen disorders.

### Erythema marginatum

This is associated with rheumatic fever. There are pink rings on the trunk which come and go.

## Specific diseases with skin manifestations
### Ulcerative colitis

There may be pyoderma gangrenosum, i.e., ulcers on the back, thigh, and buttocks with a bluish edge.

### Crohn's disease

This is associated with pyoderma gangrenosum and erythema nodosum. There may be perianal and perivulval ulcers.

### Diabetes mellitus

Skin manifestations include recurrent infections, ulcers, necrobiosis lipoidica diabeticorum (shiny area on the shins with a yellowish color and telangiecstasia), granuloma annulare (purplish patches with the skin surface remaining intact), and fat necrosis at the site of injections.

### Celiac disease

Celiac disease is associated with dermatitis herpetiformis. There are pruritic symmetrical clusters of urticarial lesions, particularly in the gluteal region and extensor aspects of the elbows and knees. They progress to vesicles and bullae. There may be secondary bacterial infection. Treatment is with dapsone.

### Hyperthyroidism

Look for pretibial myxedema or red edematous swellings above the lateral malleoli, which progress to thickened edema of the legs and feet.

## Neoplasia

Features may include the following:

- Acanthosis nigricans (especially with gastric carcinoma): these are areas of pigmented rough thickening of the skin in the axillae or groin with warty lesions.
- Dermatomyositis.
- Secondary skin metastases.
- Acquired ichthyosis: dry, scaly skin (vaguely resembling that of a fish), associated with lymphoma.
- Thrombophlebitis migrans (especially with pancreatic carcinoma): successive crops of tender nodules affecting blood vessels throughout the body.
- Chronic myeloid leukemia: skin infiltration.
- Herpes zoster.

Herpes zoster is often present in any debilitating disease or immunosuppressed patient. The appearance is of groups of vesicles on an inflamed base which are painful. It is due to the virus varicella zoster, which remains latent in dorsal root ganglia after infection with chicken pox. Diminished resistance allows reactivation. The lesions heal, leaving scarring and pigmentation. Postherpetic neuralgia may be severe and difficult to treat.

## Liver disease

Look for palmar erythema, spider nevi, gynecomastia, and decrease in secondary sexual hair. For details of this, see Chapters 10 and 32.

## Sarcoidosis

Lupus pernio may be present, i.e., a diffuse bluish plaque with small papules within the swelling, affecting the nose.

## Neurofibromatosis

This condition is autosomal dominant and may include the following features:

- *Café-au-lait* spots (light brown macules).
- Axillary freckling.
- Violaceous dermal neurofibromata.
- Subcutaneous nodules.

## Porphyria

This condition involves light sensitivity and blistering.

## Lyme disease

Cutaneous signs are erythema chronicum migrans. This starts off as a small red papule which gradually enlarges to form a ring with a raised border. It lasts for 2 days to 3 months. Lyme disease is caused by *Borrelia burgdorferi*, a spirochete spread by ticks from deer and rodents. Other features include:

- Malaise.
- Migratory arthralgia.
- Neck stiffness.
- Lymphadenopathy.
- CNS abnormalities (e.g., meningitis and peripheral neuropathies).
- Cardiac disease with conduction disturbances.
- Myopericarditis.

Treatment is with tetracycline, penicillin, or third-generation cephalosporin (e.g., cefotaxime).

## Xanthomatosis

Tendon xanthomata are associated with familial hypercholesterolemia. Eruptive xanthomata occur with greatly elevated serum lipid concentrations. Xanthelasmata are yellow plaques commonly found on the eyelids. They may indicate hyperlipidemia.

## Behçet's disease

This is a recurrent progressive systemic disease of unknown etiology with painful ulceration of the oral and genital regions. Other features of Behçet's disease may include:

- Iritis.
- Keratitis.
- Hypopyon and retinal vein occlusion.
- Arthritis.
- CNS complications (e.g., meningoencephalitis, parkinsonism, dementia, thrombophlebitis).

Treatment is with steroids for ulcers and systemic features. In resistant cases colchicine or cytotoxic drugs (e.g., azathioprine) may be needed.

## Malignant skin tumors

### Basal cell carcinoma

This is the most common skin tumor and is frequently seen in elderly, fair-skinned people. Lesions mainly occur on the face, especially at the side of the nose or periorbital skin. They may be flesh-colored papules or plaques with superficial dilated blood vessels over the surface. There may be central necrosis with ulceration or crusting and a pearly rolled edge. They may also be pigmented or cystic. They tend to be locally invasive (hence the alternative name rodent ulcer) but metastases are rare.

Treatment is by surgical excision, cryotherapy, or radiotherapy. Mohs surgey is often necessary in areas that are difficult to excise, including around the eyes, ears, or nose.

## Squamous cell carcinoma

This tumor arises from the epidermis or skin appendages and is most commonly seen on damaged or chronically irritated skin. Squamous cell carcinoma in situ or without invasion is often referred to as Bowen's disease. It is invasive and can metastasize. Viral disease (e.g., human papilloma virus) may be a predisposing factor. Tumors are hyperkeratotic, crusted, and indurated, and may ulcerate.

Treatment is by excision or radiotherapy. Treatment of Bowen's disease includes topical 5-FU, cryotherapy, or surgical excision. Invasive disease requires surgical excision that may require plastic surgery techniques or Mohs surgery for danger areas around nose, eyes, and ears. Radiation treatments are sometimes also necessary.

## Malignant melanoma

This tumor is increasing in incidence and occurs particularly in fair-skinned people with exposure to UV light, people with more than 5 atypical moles, people with more than 50 moles, people with inability to tan, patients with severe sunburn (typically before age 14 years), and people with a family history of melanoma. Some melanomas arise in pre-existing moles. Malignancy should be expected if a pigmented lesion shows the following:
- Rapid enlargement.
- Bleeding.

- Increasing variegated pigmentation, particularly blue-black or gray.
- Ulceration.
- An indistinct border.
- Persistent itching.
- Small "satellite" lesions around the principal lesion.

The prognosis is related to the thickness of the tumor assessed histologically. All suspicious lesions should be treated with excisional biopsy. For large lesions, punch biopsy is appropriate. The 5-year survival rate for patients with a tumor less than 1 mm thick is greater than 90%. If the thickness is greater than 3.5 mm, the 5-year survival rate is less than 35%.

Sites of malignant melanoma with a poor prognosis are **BANS**: **b**ack of the **a**rm, **n**eck, and **s**calp.

Patients with lesions on the limbs have a better prognosis than those with truncal lesions who, in turn, have a better prognosis than those with facial lesions. Interferon may slow progression of metastases. Currently much work is being done looking at the use of tumor vaccines.

### Management

People should avoid exposure to direct sunlight and should use sunscreen lotions. Self-examination should be practised, and people should be aware of the warning signs and symptoms listed above. Treatment is by wide excision with skin grafting if necessary.

# 37. Hematologic Disorders

## Anemia

Anemia is a common clinical problem as it is the end result of many different pathologic processes. The etiology, clinical evaluation, complications, and investigation policy have been considered in Chapter 25. The general approach to management is outlined first, and then specific conditions are discussed in detail.

## General approach to the management of anemia

### Keep in mind the following

Hemoglobin, hematocrit, and RBC count indicate, respectively, concentrations of the oxygen-carrying component of blood, the percent of blood occupied by RBCs, and the number of RBCs in a given volume. Therefore, these values depend on the fluid status of the patient. Acute blood loss does not change these values, and it often takes 36–48 hours for compensation to occur.

### What is the underlying cause of anemia?

Anemia can be caused by decreased production of RBCs, increased destruction of RBCs, or blood loss. Often laboratory results will influence what additional tests need to be ordered and can help diagnose the cause.

Remember that there may be more than one cause of anemia in any one patient, and this can confuse the unwary! For example, folate and iron deficiencies may both be present in celiac disease.

Fig. 37.1 shows possible causes of anemia in rheumatoid arthritis.

### Treat the underlying cause (when possible)

The anemia will recur if the underlying problem persists (e.g., peptic ulceration or colonic neoplasm).

### Correct the anemia

The method of correction will depend on the type of anemia and presence of complications. In general, iron, vitamin $B_{12}$, and folate should be prescribed only when the patient has been appropriately investigated and shown to have a deficiency.

### Iron replacement

Oral iron replacement therapy (e.g., ferrous sulfate, 200mg t.i.d.) should be continued for 3 months after the hemoglobin returns to normal to replace iron stores (although the hemoglobin should rise 2g/dL in 3 weeks if the anemia is due to iron deficiency). Side effects include nausea, change in bowel habit, and abdominal pain. (Note that stool color becomes very dark or black). If side effects occur, reduce dose to once or twice daily. Intramuscular iron can be given but only in cases of poor patient compliance with oral therapy, severe gastrointestinal (GI) disturbance with oral therapy, or malabsorption.

### Vitamin $B_{12}$ replacement

Most causes of vitamin $B_{12}$ deficiency are due to malabsorption and so vitamin $B_{12}$ is given by intramuscular injection. Stores are replaced by giving hydroxocobalamin, 1mg repeated every 2–3 days for a total of 6 doses. Maintenance therapy is 1mg every 3 months, which needs to be lifelong in most patients.

### Folate replacement

Oral folic acid, 1–5mg daily for 4 months, corrects anemia and replaces folate stores (a higher dose may be needed in malabsorption states). Oral folic acid, 400µg daily, should be given as prophylaxis against neural tube defects to women prior to conception and throughout the first 12 weeks of pregnancy.

It should not be given in malignancy unless essential, as some tumors are dependent on folate, and it should not be given alone in megaloblastic anemia unless vitamin $B_{12}$ status has been shown to be normal, as it can precipitate the neurologic complications of vitamin $B_{12}$ deficiency (subacute combined degeneration of the cord).

### Blood transfusion

Whole blood should be administered only when there is hypovolemia in addition to anemia, as occurs in massive acute hemorrhage. In an emergency, when time does not allow cross-matching, O Rhesus-negative blood can be given safely. In chronic symptomatic anemia, which cannot be corrected by folate, vitamin $B_{12}$, or iron therapy, matched packed red blood cells (RBCs) may be given. Fig. 37.2 summarizes the complications of transfusion.

## Splenectomy

Splenectomy is useful in hereditary spherocytosis and autoimmune hemolytic anemia that is refractory to steroids or immunosuppressive therapy. Other

| Causes of anemia in rheumatoid arthritis |
| --- |
| • anemia of chronic disease |
| • hypersplenism due to splenomegaly (Felty's syndrome if also neutropenic) |
| • chronic blood loss from peptic ulceration due to steroid and NSAID administration |
| • bone marrow suppression by disease modifying drugs such as gold and penicillamine |
| • folate deficiency (increased utilization of folate) |

**Fig. 37.1** Causes of anemia in rheumatoid arthritis. (NSAID, nonsteroidal anti-inflammatory drug.)

indications for splenectomy include trauma, refractory idiopathic thrombocytopenic purpura, and symptomatic splenomegaly, as in myelofibrosis, lymphoma, chronic lymphocytic leukemia (CLL), or chronic myeloid leukemia (CML). Complications of splenectomy include thrombocytosis and increased susceptibility to infection with encapsulated bacteria (pneumococci, meningococci, and *Haemophilus influenzae* type B). Patients should be immunized with vaccines against these three organisms and given penicillin for home use in case of fever. Dental treatment should be covered by antibiotic prophylaxis, and any febrile episode should be treated quickly.

# Sideroblastic anemia
## Etiology

Sideroblastic anemia can be congenital or acquired:
• Congenital: X-linked.
• Acquired: primary—refractory anemia with ring sideroblasts (this is a subgroup of myelodysplasia); secondary—drugs (e.g., isoniazid, pyrazinamide), alcohol, lead poisoning, myeloproliferative disease, connective tissue disease.

| Complications of blood transfusion | |
| --- | --- |
| **Complication** | **Cause** |
| hemolytic reaction | ABO incompatibility (severe), extravascular hemolysis (mild/clinically silent) |
| anaphylaxis | hypersensitivity to plasma proteins |
| febrile reaction | antibodies to white cells |
| volume overload | particularly the elderly and in megaloblastic anemia |
| coagulopathies | platelets and clotting factors are reduced by a dilutional effect in massive transfusion |
| infection | virus (HIV, hepatitis B and C, EBV, CMV) Gram-negative bacteria (uncommon) |
| hemosiderosis | with repeated transfusions |
| alloimmunization | antibodies may develop to red cells, leukocytes, platelets and plasma proteins despite receiving compatible blood; this may cause problems the next time the patient receives a transfusion |
| graft versus host disease | uncommon: preventable by using irradiated blood (important in transplant recipients) |
| air embolism | particularly if given via central lines |
| thrombophlebitis | at cannula site |

**Fig. 37.2** Complications of blood transfusion. (CMV, cytomegalovirus; EBV, Epstein-Barr virus; HIV, human immunodeficiency virus.)

## Pathology
- Heme cannot be incorporated into protoporphyrin to form hemoglobin.
- Erythropoiesis becomes disordered.
- Iron accumulates in the marrow.

## Presentation
- Symptoms and signs of anemia.
- No specific clinical features.

## Complications
- Those of anemia (see Chapter 25).
- Primary refractory anemia with ring sideroblasts may progress to acute myeloid leukemia (AML).
- Hemosiderosis if recurrent transfusions are given.

## Investigations
- Dimorphic RBCs on blood film with normochromic and hypochromic cells.
- Mean corpuscular volume: low, normal, or slightly raised.
- Low mean corpuscular hemoglobin concentration (MCHC) and low mean corpuscular hemoglobin (MCH).
- Ferritin is raised.
- Ring sideroblasts in the marrow (these are erythroblasts in which heme has accumulated in the mitochondria, causing granules which stain with Prussian blue and are situated in a perinuclear ring).

## Treatment
- Withdraw any possible etiologic agents, such as drugs, as the anemia may resolve.
- Pyridoxine, 50–200mg daily given orally, in hereditary sideroblastic anemia.
- Folate orally may also help.
- Blood transfusion.

# Lead poisoning
## Etiology
- In adults, usually due to industrial exposure (e.g., lead smelting).
- Exposure in children is mostly from old toys (as toy paints used to contain lead).

## Pathology
- Absorbed from the lungs or GI tract.
- Most profound effects on bone marrow, nervous system, and kidneys.
- Also deposited in bones, teeth, nails, and hair.

## Presentation
- Nausea, vomiting, and colicky abdominal pain.
- Constipation.
- Altered consciousness level, irritability, and seizures if encephalopathic (more common in children).
- Foot drop or wrist drop (usually adults).
- Burton's line (blue line on the gums).

## Complications
- Peripheral motor neuropathy.
- Encephalopathy.
- Sideroblastic anemia.
- Hemolytic anemia.
- Fanconi's syndrome (lead nephropathy).

## Investigations
- Blood lead levels >50mg/dL. Symptoms may start at 30μg/dL.
- Lead lines on x-ray: dense metaphyseal lines in children (wrists and knees) due to lead and calcium deposition.
- Hypochromic anemia with basophilic stippling of RBCs (RNA deposition).
- May be evidence of hemolysis (see Chapter 25).
- Ring sideroblasts may be present in bone marrow.
- Free RBC protoporphyrin is raised.

## Treatment
- Discuss with CDC poison center.
- Treat with sodium calcium edetate (drug of choice), dimercaprol, or penicillamine.

# Anemia of chronic disease
## Etiology and pathology
For the etiology, see Fig. 25.2. The pathology is multifactorial, with inappropriate erythropoeitin production, poor release of iron from macrophages, and reduced RBC survival.

## Presentation and complications
Presentation is with the symptoms and signs of anemia (see p. 139) and of the primary disease. The complications are those of anemia (see p. 141) and the underlying disease.

## Investigations
Characteristic findings are:
- Normochromic normocytic anemia (may be hypochromic, microcytic).
- Serum iron low.

- Serum ferritin high (can be normal).
- Increased storage iron in bone marrow.
- A raised erythrocyte sedimentation rate (ESR), neutrophil leukocytosis, and thrombocytosis, in addition to the anemia, constitute a "reactive" blood picture reflecting the primary pathology.

## Treatment

- Treat the underlying disease. Iron therapy is usually not beneficial and often results in iron overload.
- If mild and asymptomatic, no treatment is necessary.
- If symptomatic, consider transfusion and rarely recombinant erythropoietin therapy.

# Hereditary spherocytosis

Hereditary spherocytosis is an inherited disease (autosomal dominant), with an incidence of 1 in 5000.

## Pathology

- Deficiency or defect of RBC membrane protein (probably spectrin).
- RBCs are normally shaped when released from the bone marrow.
- Circulating cells lose membrane due to instability of the lipid layer and become dehydrated (increased permeability to sodium).
- RBCs become spherical. They are no longer deformable and become trapped in the spleen where they are hemolyzed.
- Severity is variable.

## Presentation

- Jaundice can develop at any age depending on severity.
- Splenomegaly is usually present.
- Signs of complications may also be present.

## Complications

- Gallstones (pigmented) due to increased unconjugated bilirubin in the bile—directly related to age. Gallstones are uncommon before age 10 years but present in 50% of adults.
- Aplastic crises due to parvovirus infection.
- Megaloblastic anemia due to increased folate utilization, particularly during pregnancy (see Fig. 25.4).

## Investigations

- Anemia, which may not be present if bone marrow compensates for hemolysis.
- Spherocytosis and reticulocytosis (polychromasia) on blood film.
- Mean corpuscular hemoglobin concentration (MCHC) often increased.
- Erythroid hyperplasia in bone marrow (to compensate for increased breakdown).
- Increased unconjugated bilirubin.
- Increased lactate dehydrogenase (LDH).
- Reduced haptoglobin.
- Increased urinary urobilinogen.
- Increased osmotic fragility (RBCs will lyse at a lower osmotic level than normal RBCs).

## Treatment

- No treatment if the hemolysis is mild or if the patient is very young.
- Splenectomy in moderate-to-severe disease. (Before splenectomy is done, patients should be vaccinated against encapsulated pathogens.)
- Folate supplementation.
- Transfusion for separate disease.
- Screen family members.

Note that hereditary elliptocytosis is an autosomal dominant condition with a similar but milder presentation than that of hereditary spherocytosis. The RBCs are elliptical on the blood film. Most cases require no treatment, but the severity is variable. Severe forms may also require splenectomy and folate supplementation.

# Glucose-6-phosphate dehydrogenase deficiency

Glucose-6-phosphate dehydrogenase (G6PD) deficiency occurs in 300 million people worldwide. It is an inherited (X-linked recessive) condition.

## Pathology

- G6PD is an important enzyme in the hexose monophosphate shunt pathway.
- Glutathione is kept in a reduced state by this pathway and provides protection against oxidative stress.
- If erythrocytes deficient in G6PD are exposed to oxidative stress (usually older erythrocytes), hemoglobin becomes oxidized and forms precipitates called Heinz bodies, which stick to the RBC membrane. The cells lose

deformability and become trapped and destroyed in the spleen.

## Presentation
- The disease affects males in the Middle East, South-East Asia, West Africa, the Mediterranean, and Southern Europe.
- The severity of disease varies, being most severe in the Mediterranean type.
- Acute episodes of intravascular hemolysis are precipitated by intercurrent illness (particularly infection), drugs (e.g., antimalarials, nitrofurantoin, sulfonamides), and the ingestion of fava beans (favism).
- The patient is usually completely well between episodes.
- In severe deficiency, chronic hemolysis with splenomegaly may occur.
- Icterus neonatorum may occur and lead to kernicterus.
- Female heterozygotes have improved resistance to *Falciparum* malaria.

## Complications
These include anemia, kernicterus (icterus neonatorum), and shock, which can be fatal (particularly in favism).

## Investigations
- Between episodes: G6PD assays (concentration or activity) show deficiency; other tests are normal.
- During acute episode: the blood film shows "bite" cells, "blister" cells, Heinz bodies, and reticulocytosis. Features of hemolysis will be present: increased unconjugated bilirubin, reduced haptoglobin, and increased urinary urobilinogen.

## Treatment
- Avoiding or stopping precipitating drugs.
- Treating any underlying infection.
- Transfusion for severe, symptomatic anemia.
- Considering exchange transfusion and phototherapy in icterus neonatorum.

## Pyruvate kinase deficiency
This is an inherited condition (autosomal recessive).

## Pathology
- Pyruvate kinase is an important enzyme in the glycolytic (Embden-Meyerhof) pathway.

- In deficiency, ATP production is reduced.
- Abnormal erythrocytes are removed by the spleen.
- 2,3-DPG increases, shifting the oxygen dissociation curve to the right, resulting in better toleration of anemia.

## Presentation
This condition presents with symptoms of anemia, jaundice, and gallstones; splenomegaly is common. Severity is variable.

## Complications
Complications include anemia and gallstones.

## Investigations
- Blood film: poikilocytosis (with "prickle" cells) and reticulocytosis.
- Elevated indirect bilirubin and LDH, decreased haptoglobin.
- Autohemolysis: abnormal.
- Pyruvate kinase: assay demonstrates deficiency.

## Treatment
Treatment is by blood transfusion for severe anemia; consider splenectomy if multiple transfusions are required. During pregnancy intrauterine transfusions may be necessary for severe disease.

## Sickle cell anemia
Sickle cell anemia occurs in 4% of African Americans. It is an inherited (autosomal recessive) condition which most commonly affects blacks but is also found in the Middle East and Mediterranean. Heterozygotes are less susceptible to infection with *Falciparum* malaria.

## Pathology
- A single base mutation in the DNA on chromosome 11 causes substitution of glutamic acid for valine at position 6 in the $\beta$-hemoglobin chain (HbS).
- When HbS becomes deoxygenated, it aggregates in an organized fashion, forming polymers within the RBCs, which are less soluble and less deformable.
- As a result, the erythrocyte shape becomes distorted and changes from a biconcave disc to a sickle shape.
- The sickle cells cannot readily pass through the microcirculation and become trapped in small

vessels (causing infarction) and in the spleen (where they are destroyed—hemolyzed).

## Presentation

In the homozygote, severity is variable, and the disease may present from the third month onward (as hemoglobin F levels fall). There is chronic hemolysis with intermittent crises and complications.

### Types of sickle cell anemia crisis

There are four types of sickle cell anemia crisis:

- Aplastic: due to parvovirus infection of RBC precursors. Profound anemia and reticulocytopenia. Self-limiting, but transfusion may be required.
- Sequestration: sequestration may occur in the spleen, liver, and lungs and can result in hypovolemic shock (mortality rate: 10–15%). The hemoglobin drops rapidly with a compensatory increase in reticulocytes. Splenic sequestration is seen only in children as the spleen is usually infarcted by 6 years old. Exchange transfusion may be required.
- Hemolytic: may be precipitated by infection. Seen particularly in cases with coexistent G6PD deficiency. The hemoglobin drops rapidly with a compensatory increase in reticulocytes.
- Painful: due to vascular occlusion. Can be precipitated by dehydration, hypoxia, infections, and cold exposure. Almost any organ can be affected. Small bones of the hands and feet are most often affected in childhood ("hand-foot syndrome"). In older patients, the lungs, hips, shoulders, and spine are more commonly involved.

## Complications

- Anemia.
- Infection: pneumonia (*Streptococcus pneumoniae*, *H. influenzae*), ostomyelitis (*Salmonella*).
- Vessel occlusion: retinopathy (proliferative with vitreous hemorrhage and retinal detachment), splenic infarction (resulting in predisposition to infection), renal papillary necrosis, priapism, aseptic necrosis of the femoral head, transient ischemic attacks, strokes, placental infarction, and spontaneous abortion.
- Gallstones.
- Leg ulceration.

## Investigations

- Normochromic normocytic anemia.
- Reticulocytosis, sickle cells, and target cells on film (features of hyposplenism may also be present following splenic infarction; Fig. 25.7).
- Elevated unconjugated bilirubin and LDH, decreased haptoglobin).
- Hemoglobin electrophoresis demonstrates HbS.
- Leukocyte and platelet counts may also be raised.
- Prenatal diagnosis can be made using PCR (polymerase chain reaction) techniques on chorionic villous samples.

## Treatment

- Prophylactic folate (increased folate utilization because of hemolysis).
- Immunization against pneumococci, meningococci, and *H. influenzae* (increased risk of these because of hyposplenism secondary to splenic infarction).
- Prophylactic penicillin in children.
- Supportive care during crises.
- Prophylactic exchange transfusions in patients with recurrent crises or significant organ damage.

## Prognosis

There is a 5% mortality rate in the first 10 years of life. Cerebrovascular events are common in sickle cell patients, as is retinopathy. The risk of infection is also increased.

Note that in the sickle cell trait (a heterozygous carrier state) the disease is much milder with no anemia and a normal blood film. Crises may be caused in extreme conditions. The most common complication is renal disease.

## Thalassemia

Normal hemoglobin synthesis is summarized in Fig. 37.3.

### Prevalence and etiology

The prevalence of thalassemia is 2.5–15% in the "thalassemia belt" (see below). It is an inherited condition.

### Pathology

- Reduced production of one or more of the hemoglobin chains (most importantly α or β), which results in a relative excess and accumulation of the other chain (called "imbalanced globin chain synthesis").

---

### Normal hemoglobin synthesis

- normal hemoglobin is composed of four polypeptide chains (tetramer)
- at various stages of development, different polypeptide chains are produced ($\zeta$, $\epsilon$, $\alpha$, $\gamma$, $\delta$ and $\beta$)
- in the embryo (first 8 weeks' gestation), three different hemoglobins are produced by the yolk sac, Hb Gower-1 ($\zeta_2$, $\epsilon_2$), Hb Gower-2 ($\alpha_2$, $\epsilon_2$) and Hb Portland ($\zeta_2$, $\gamma_2$)
- fetal hemoglobin (HbF) is composed of two $\alpha$ chains and two $\gamma$ chains ($\alpha_2$, $\gamma_2$) and is the major hemoglobin of intrauterine life. It declines rapidly around birth and constitutes less than 1% hemoglobin by 6 months of age. HbF is produced predominantly made by the liver until 30 weeks, after which the bone marrow takes over. It has an avid affinity for oxygen
- production of $\beta$ chains increases rapidly at 36 weeks' gestation; 96% adult hemoglobin is HbA ($\alpha_2$, $\beta_2$), 3.5% is HbA$_2$ ($\alpha_2$, $\delta_2$) with the remainder being HbF
- the genes for the globin chains $\alpha$ and $\zeta$ are found clustered on chromosome 16. The genes for the remaining chains are located in a cluster on chromosome 11
- each person has four $\alpha$ genes (two on each chromosome 16) and two $\beta$ genes (one on each chromosome 11)

**Fig. 37.3** Normal hemoglobin synthesis.

---

### Characteristic features of the $\alpha$-thalassemias

| Subtype | Silent carrier | $\alpha$-Thalassemia trait | HbH disease | Hydrops fetalis |
|---|---|---|---|---|
| genetic abnormality | one $\alpha$ gene deleted | two $\alpha$ genes deleted | three $\alpha$ genes deleted | four $\alpha$ genes deleted |
| clinical features | asymptomatic | usually asymptomatic | hemolytic anemia splenomegaly bone changes | hepatosplenomegaly gross edema hypoalbuminemia extramedullary hemopoiesis |
| hematologic findings | no abnormality | hypochromia microcytosis | hypochromia microcytosis reticulocytosis HbH ($\beta_4$) on electrophoresis inclusion bodies with cresyl blue | hypochromia microcytosis reticulocytosis target cells nucleated red cells Hb Bart's ($\gamma_4$) on electrophoresis |
| survival | normal | normal | variable | stillborn or death shortly after birth |

**Fig. 37.4** Characteristic features of the $\alpha$-thalassemias. (HbH, hemoglobin H.)

---

- The unstable hemoglobin precipitates, causing ineffective erythropoiesis and hemolysis.
- There is deficiency of $\alpha$ chains in $\alpha$-thalassemia and of $\beta$ chains in $\beta$-thalassemia.

### Presentation

- $\alpha$-Thalassemia is found in populations in the Mediterranean, Africa, the Middle East and South-East Asia.
- $\beta$-Thalassemia affects those in China, the Mediterranean, the Middle East, and India.
- The clinical presentation is dependent on the underlying defect, as shown in Figs. 37.4 and 37.5.

- Thalassemia provides an advantage in infection with *Falciparum* malaria.

### Treatment

- Transfusion to maintain an adequate hemoglobin (>10g/dL) during childhood to ensure normal growth and development.
- Iron chelation using desferrioxamine to prevent hemosiderosis.
- Oral vitamin C also increases iron excretion.
- Splenectomy can reduce transfusion requirements but should be avoided whenever possible because of the increased susceptibility to infection.

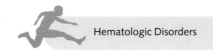
| Characteristic features of the β-thalassemias | | | |
|---|---|---|---|
| Subtype | β-Thalassemia minor | β-Thalassemia intermedia | β-Thalassemia major |
| genetic abnormality | heterozygous abnormality in β globin gene | homozygous or mixed heterozygous abnormality in β globin gene | homozygous abnormality in β globin gene |
| clinical features | usually asymptomatic | variable<br>extramedullary hematopoiesis<br>  hepatosplenomegaly<br>skeletal deformity<br>gallstones<br>leg ulcers | failure to thrive (3–6 months)<br>jaundice<br>extramedullary hematopoiesis<br>  hepatosplenomegaly<br>skeletal deformity<br>hemosiderosis<br>recurrent infections<br>cardiac failure<br>gallstones<br>leg ulcers |
| hemotologic findings | mild anemia<br>microcytosis<br>hypochromia<br>target cells<br>poikilocytosis<br>$HbA_2$ high<br>Hbf may be raised | moderate anemia but not<br>  transfusion dependent<br>microcytosis<br>hypochromia<br>target cells<br>poikilocytosis | transfusion-dependent severe<br>  anemia<br>microcytosis<br>hypochromia<br>target cells<br>anisopoikilocytosis<br>reticulocytosis<br>nucleated RBCs<br>basophilic stippling<br>inclusion bodies on supravital<br>  staining with methyl violet<br>HbA absent or very low<br>HbF high |
| survival | normal | survive to adulthood even<br>  without treatment | death in childhood without<br>  treatment, bone marrow<br>  transplantation may be<br>  curative |

**Fig. 37.5** Characteristic features of the β-thalassemias. (Hb, hemoglobin; RBC, red blood cell.)

- Prophylactic folate supplementation in severe disease (β-thalassemia major).
- Endocrine therapy may be necessary in hemosiderosis.
- Bone marrow transplantation may be curative in some patients with β-thalassemia major.
- Current research emphasis focuses on the prospect of using gene therapy techniques.
- Prenatal diagnosis and genetic counseling should be available.

## Pernicious anemia
### Incidence and etiology
This is an autoimmune condition and has an incidence of 2 per 10,000.

### Pathology
- Immunoglobulin G (IgG) autoantibodies are produced against gastric parietal cells and intrinsic factor.
- This causes gastric mucosal atrophy with loss of parietal cells and achlorhydria.
- Intrinsic factor, necessary for vitamin $B_{12}$ absorption, is not produced.

### Presentation
- The onset is usually insidious and is more common after the age of 50, affecting women more than men.
- Higher prevalence in Scandinavian populations (fair hair and blue eyes).

- Strong association with other autoimmune diseases and blood group A.
- Symptoms include those of anemia and the neurologic complications of vitamin $B_{12}$ deficiency.
- Examination may reveal anemia, glossitis, lemon tint (increased bilirubin due to breakdown of abnormal RBCs), low-grade fever, mild splenomegaly, and neurologic signs.

## Complications
- Complications of anemia (see Chapter 25).
- Neurologic abnormalities from vitamin $B_{12}$ deficiency (dementia, optic atrophy, peripheral neuropathy, subacute combined degeneration of the cord).
- Gastric carcinoma.

## Investigation
- Macrocytic anemia with typical blood film (see Fig. 25.7).
- White cell and platelet counts: may be low.
- Serum vitamin $B_{12}$: low, with abnormal Schilling test.
- Megaloblastic bone marrow.
- Bilirubin: increased.
- LDH: increased (also due to breakdown of abnormal RBCs).
- Parietal cell antibody in 90% (can be seen in normal elderly).
- Intrinsic factor antibody in 50%.
- Thyroid antibodies in 50%.
- Gastroscopy should be performed to exclude gastric carcinoma.

## Treatment
- Lifelong vitamin $B_{12}$ replacement.
- Initial response to treatment can be demonstrated by an increase in reticulocyte count.

# Leukemias

The leukemias are a group of conditions characterized by the malignant proliferation of leukocytes in the bone marrow. The cells spill out into the blood stream and may infiltrate other organs.

In the acute leukemias, there is a proliferation of early lymphoid and myeloid precursors (called blasts) which do not mature. The clinical course is very aggressive and rapidly fatal without treatment.

The chronic leukemias have a more indolent course and are characterized by the proliferation of lymphoid and myeloid cells, which reach maturity (lymphocytes and neutrophils, respectively).

# Acute lymphoblastic leukemia
## Epidemiology and etiology
Acute lymphoblastic leukemia (ALL) is the second most common malignancy in children under 15, accounting for 30% of all childhood cancers. Each year there are between 2500 and 3500 cases of ALL in the U.S. Its etiology is unknown but is probably multifactorial. Known factors include radiation and benzene. In addition, children with Down's syndrome are at increased risk for ALL.

## Pathology
- Lymphoblasts accumulate in the bone marrow and can cause bone marrow failure.
- Lymphoblasts circulate in the blood stream and can infiltrate the lymph nodes, liver, spleen, kidneys, testicles, and central nervous system (CNS).
- Classified according to the French-American-British (FAB) system (Fig. 37.6).

## Presentation
- Peak incidences at age 4 and over 65 years.
- The history is usually short as the disease is so aggressive (days to a few weeks).
- Symptoms are due to rapidly expanding tumor cells in the bone marrow, causing bone pain or bone marrow failure (Fig. 37.7).
- Symptoms on examination include fever, pallor, headache, thrombocytopenia (with increased risk of bleeding and ecchymosis), lymphadenopathy, and hepatosplenomegaly.

| FAB classification of ALL |
| --- |
| • L1: small cells, homogenous, small or absent nucleoli, scanty cytoplasm |
| • L2: large cells, heterogenous, occasional large nucleoli, more cytoplasm |
| • L3: large cells, homogenous, prominent nucleoli, abundant cytoplasm |

**Fig. 37.6** The French-American-British (FAB) classification of acute lymphoblastic leukemia (ALL). Note that ALL may also be classified according to phenotype (B cell, T cell, common, null). (ALL, acute lymphoblastic leukemia.)

| Features of bone marrow failure | | |
|---|---|---|
| **Cells affected** | **Result** | **Manifestation** |
| red cell precursors | anemia | lethargy, dyspnea, pallor |
| white cell precursors | neutropenia | recurrent infections, fever |
| platelet precursors | thrombocytopenia | bleeding, bruising, purpura |

**Fig. 37.7** Features of bone marrow failure.

- Main sites of relapse are bone marrow, CNS, and testes.

## Investigations
- Normochromic normocytic anemia with low reticulocyte count.
- High white cell count due to lymphoblasts; neutropenia may be present.
- Thrombocytopenia: 25% of patients have severe thrombocytopenia (<20,000µL) at diagnosis.
- Bone marrow is hypercellular and dominated by lymphoblasts (usually >50%).
- Cytogenetic abnormalities may be present (e.g. hyperdiploidy or the Philadelphia chromosome [Ph]).
- Urate high.
- LDH high.
- Calcium, potassium, and phosphate may also be raised.
- Mediastinal mass on chest x-ray in T cell-ALL.
- Cerebrospinal fluid examination may show lymphoblasts, increased pressure, and increased protein.

## Treatment
Care should be managed in a specialized unit and includes:
- Supportive care with antibiotics, blood products, and colony-stimulating factors (e.g., G-CSF for neutropenia).
- Allopurinol to prevent tumor lysis syndrome (uric acid nephropathy).
- Cytotoxic chemotherapy (induction, consolidation, maintenance. ALL treatment consists of three areas: induction of remission, consolidation, and maintenance.
  1. Induction of remission is achieved by using the triad of vincristine, prednisone, and anthracycline (not, however, that many different regimens are in use). Exact combinations depend on factors such as age.
  2. Consolidation therapy is done to eradicate any subclinical residual disease during hematologic remission. Without consolidation chemotherapy, patients with ALL usually relapse. This stage of treatment lasts 2–3 years. The numerous consolidation regimens vary in exact duration of therapy and combination of medications used. One regimen includes methotrexate biweekly and 6-mercaptopurine daily.
  3. Maintenance therapy is the standard of care for ALL patients of all ages despite the fact that benefit from such treatment has not been demonstrated in adults. The standard maintenance therapy includes 6-mercaptropurine and methotrexate with vincristine and prednisone, given monthly for 12–36 months.
- CNS prophylaxis (secondary to the propensity for relapse due to CNS sources): cranial irradiation, intrathecal methotrexate.
- Testes: no prophylaxis but often a site of relapse.
- Treat with radiotherapy if relapse occurs.
- Bone marrow transplantation (allogeneic or autonomous) can be curative; it is used in poor risk patients. Transplantation is done during the consolidation phase of therapy with the hope that the pretransplant myeloablative chemotherapy used, with or without whole body irradiation, will eradicate any remaining tumor cells. Currently bone marrow transplantation is recommended during the second remission after a first relapse.

## Prognosis
- Children: 60% 5-year survival rate.
- Adults: 30% 5-year survival rate.
- Poor prognostic indicators include increasing age, increasing white cell count, null-cell or T-cell phenotype, male sex, and abnormal karyotype.

## Acute myeloid leukemia and acute nonlymphocytic leukemia
### Epidemiology
Acute myeloid leukemia (AML) and acute nonlymphocytic leukemia (ANLL) account for 20% of all leukemias and 85% of adult leukemias.

### Etiology
- Genetic predisposition: concordance in twins, Down's syndrome, Bloom's syndrome, Fanconi's anemia, and ataxia telangiectasia.
- Ionizing radiation: survivors of Hiroshima and military personnel involved in nuclear test explosions.
- Chemical exposure: leather and rubber workers (benzene) or cigarette smokers.
- Previous chemotherapy: alkylating agents.
- Other drugs: chloroquine, LSD.
- Predisposing diseases: myeloproliferative diseases, multiple myeloma, aplastic anemia, myelodysplasia.

### Pathology
- Accumulation of immature hemopoietic cells in the bone marrow, which can cause bone marrow failure.
- Blasts can infiltrate the gums, liver, spleen, skin, and, less commonly, the CNS.
- Classified as shown in Fig. 37.8.

### Presentation
- More frequent with increasing age (median age at presentation is 50).

- Symptoms are due to marrow failure (Fig. 37.7, particularly skin infections), infiltration by leukemic cells, or bleeding (epistaxis, ecchymoses gingival bleeding).
- Bone pain, joint pain, and malaise may be prominent symptoms.
- Hepatomegaly and moderate splenomegaly are common.
- Lymphadenopathy is rare except in subtype M5.
- Gingival hypertrophy and skin lesions are features of subtypes M4 and M5.
- When the circulating white cell count is very high, leukostasis may occur, resulting in a cerebrovascular event or acute pulmonary deterioration.

### Investigations
- Normochromic normocytic anemia with low reticulocyte count.
- High white cell count due to circulating blasts; neutropenia may be present.
- Blasts may contain Auer rods.
- Thrombocytopenia.
- Bone marrow is hypercellular and normal marrow is replaced by blast cells.
- Cytogenetic abnormalities may be present in around 50% of patients.
- Urate high.
- LDH high.
- Hypokalemia may occur.
- Calcium and phosphate may also be raised.
- Lumbar puncture for patients with CNS symptoms.

| French–American–British (FAB) classification of AML | | |
|---|---|---|
| **FAB subtype** | **Name (predominant cell type)** | **Specific clinical features** |
| M1 | undifferentiated myeloblastic | — |
| M2 | myeloblastic | most common |
| M3 | promyelocytic | DIC may cause fatal bleeding |
| M4 | myelomonocytic | gingival, skin and meningeal infiltration |
| M5 | monocytic | gingival, skin and meningeal infiltration lymphadenopathy and DIC may occur |
| M6 | erythroleukemia | particularly older patients |
| M7 | megakaryocytic | — |

**Fig. 37.8** The French-American-British (FAB) classification of AML. (AML, acute myeloid leukemia; DIC, disseminated intravascular coagulation.)

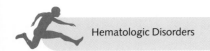

## Treatment
Treatment should be managed in a specialized unit and includes:
- Supportive care with antibiotics and blood products.
- Allopurinol to prevent tumor lysis syndrome and gout.
- Intensive cytotoxic chemotherapy: induction, remission, and consolidation. Induction is most often a combination of cytarabine for 7 days and daunorubicin for 3 days. Consolidation therapy normally uses the same medications as induction therapy, given as 2 cycles of both duanorubicin (2 days per cycle) and cytarabine (5 days per cycle).
- Bone marrow transplantation in some patients. Bone marrow transplantation is recommended during the first remission for patients with AML. While the cure rate with transplantation is 45–65%, many of these patients would have been cured by chemotherapy alone. However, since the survival rate after bone marrow transplantation during a relapse of AML is 35% or less, it is more advantageous to undergo the procedure during the first remission.

## Prognosis
- 25% long-term survivors (may be improved with transplantation).
- Poor prognostic factors include increasing age, very high white cell count, secondary leukemia (e.g., previous myelodysplasia), cytogenetic abnormalities, and the presence of disseminated intravascular coagulation (DIC).

# Chronic lymphocytic leukemia
## Epidemiology and etiology
Chronic lymphocytic leukemia (CLL) is the most common leukemia in the Western Hemisphere (30% of all leukemias). Its etiology is unknown.

## Pathology
- Proliferation of small lymphocytes in bone marrow, blood, and lymphoid tissues.
- These are morphologically mature but functionally abnormal.
- 95–98% of CLL patients have B-cell phenotype (remainder are T cells).

## Incidence and presentation
- The most common type of leukemia in the Western World.
- Uncommon in the Far East.
- Increasing incidence with age (90% cases >50 years).
- More common in males.
- Some patients are asymptomatic; others may describe malaise, weight loss, night sweats, recurrent infections, bleeding, or symptoms of anemia.
- Lymphadenopathy is usually found (60%).
- Hepatosplenomegaly may also be present.

## Investigations
- Monoclonal lymphocytosis with "smear" or "smudge" cells seen on film.
- Anemia may be due to marrow infiltration or autoimmune hemolysis (Coombs positive).
- Thrombocytopenia may be due to marrow infiltration or autoimmune destruction.
- Bone marrow shows accumulation of mature lymphocytes.
- Hypogammaglobulinemia (monoclonal gammopathy may occur).
- Lymph node biopsy: will show mature-looking lymphocytic infiltrate.

## Treatment
- Observe only if asymptomatic mild disease. Currently no data suggest that early treatment increases long-term survival. Current indications to treat include anemia, thrombocytopenia, night sweats, weight loss, painful lymphadenopathy, fever, autoimmune hemolytic anemia, increasing lymphocytosis, and enlarged liver or spleen.
- If there is symptomatic and progressive disease, use oral alkylating agents (e.g., chlorambucil or cyclophosphamide).
- Intravenous fludarabine (antimetabolite) can be used in disease resistant to alkylating agents.
- Autoimmune phenomena are responsive to oral prednisolone.
- Radiotherapy may be beneficial in symptomatic, localized disease.
- Splenectomy is sometimes used in refractory hypersplenism.
- Anti-CD20+ monoclonal antibody (rituximab) can also be used for both untreated and resistant disease.
- Anti-CD52 monoclonal antibody (alemtuzumab) can be used for post-remission therapy or resistant disease.

## Prognosis
- Dependent on extent of disease (survival ranges from 1.5 years to over 12 years).
- In around 10% of CLL, Richter transformation to high-grade lymphoma occurs as a terminal event.

# Chronic myeloid leukemia
## Incidence and etiology
The incidence of CML is 1–2 per 100,000 (20% of all leukemias). It can be due to ionizing radiation in some patients, but often the cause is unknown.

## Pathology
Malignant proliferation of myeloid cells.

## Presentation
- Presents in middle age, most commonly between 40 and 60 years, with a male preponderance. Up to 50% of patients are asymptomatic at presentation.
- Symptoms include lethargy, weight loss, sweats, and left hypochondrial discomfort (enlarging spleen).
- Symptoms of anemia or thrombocytopenia may be present.
- On examination there is splenomegaly, which may be massive.
- Hepatomegaly is present in 50% of cases, but lymphadenopathy is uncommon.
- The natural history is characterized by a chronic phase lasting several years, followed by an acute, aggressive phase (the blast phase, which occurs within 3–5 years of diagnosis).
- Leukostasis may occur in the acute phase.

## Investigations
- High white cell count with full range of immature and mature myeloid cells.
- Anemia may be due to marrow infiltration or hypersplenism.
- Thrombocytosis is common.
- Bone marrow demonstrates accumulation of myeloid cells.
- 95% of patients have a chromosomal translocation called the Philadelphia chromosome (Ph), which is a reciprocal translocation between chromosomes 9 and 22, producing the chimeric bcr/abl gene. Ph can be detected by FISH.
- Neutrophil alkaline phosphatase is low.
- Urate is high.
- LDH is high.
- Serum vitamin $B_{12}$ is high.

## Treatment
- Allopurinol orally.
- Cytotoxic chemotherapy with hydroxyurea (drug of choice) or busulphan.
- α-Interferon achieves good hematologic control and reduction in the presence of Ph.
- Allogeneic bone marrow transplantation may be curative and should be considered in young patients with an HLA-matched sibling.
- Leukopharesis will reduce the white count quickly in leukostasis.
- A new approach to treating CML has come from the understanding of the function of the Philadelphia chromosome. Given that this mutation causes the production of a novel protein via tyrosine kinase, a product was developed that can inhibit this function. ST1–571 (Gleevec) is a tyrosine kinase inhibitor that blocks the function of the bcr/abl gene fusion. Gleevec has been approved for use in CML patients with myeloid blast crisis, those who are in an accelerated phase, those who are in a chronic phase after failure of treatment, and those who have yet to receive any treatment for CML. Gleevec has been shown to be better than interferon therapy plus cytarabine for all endpoints at 18 months and should be considered the first-line therapy. Side effects include nausea, diarrhea, muscle cramp, and skin rash.

## Prognosis
- Chronic phase: median time 2–6 years.
- Acute phase: median survival <3 months.
- Transformation is to AML in two-thirds of patients and to ALL in the remainder.

# Multiple myeloma

## Incidence and etiology
The incidence of multiple myeloma is 4 per 100,000 (1% of all malignancies, 10–15% of all hematologic malignancies). Its etiology is unknown, although exposure to ionizing radiation, benzene, and insectides may be important in some patients.

## Pathology

- Neoplastic proliferation of a single clone of plasma cells (a plasma cell is a terminally differentiated B cell).
- The malignant cells secrete a monoclonal immunoglobulin or light chain and normal immunoglobulin production is suppressed.
- Osteoclast activity is increased resulting in bone reabsorption.
- AL (systemic) amyloidosis affects 10% of cases.

## Presentation

- Disease mainly of the elderly with a peak incidence in the 7th decade.
- Bone pain due to osteolytic lesions and pathologic fractures affect two-thirds of patients. Pain typically involves the back or chest.
- Recurrent infections result from impaired antibody response and hypogammaglobulinemia.
- Symptoms of anemia may be present.
- Examination usually reveals pallor alone.
- Hepatosplenomegaly is occasionally present.
- Peripheral neuropathy occurs with amyloidosis.
- Spinal cord compression and radiculopathy can result from compression by tumor or vertebral collapse.
- Patients occasionally present in acute renal failure.
- Polymerization of the monoclonal antibody occasionally results in hyperviscosity.
- Abnormal bleeding is caused by platelet dysfunction.

## Investigations

- Normochromic normocytic anemia.
- Rouleaux (RBCs sticking together) and background immunoglobulin staining may be seen on the blood film.
- ESR: usually high.
- Serum protein electrophoresis (SPEP) demonstrates a monoclonal pattern.
- Bence Jones protein may be found in the urine.
- Skeletal survey reveals generalized osteopenia, "punched-out" lytic lesions, and pathologic fractures.
- Over 10% of bone marrow cells are plasma cells.
- Calcium is high (increased osteoclastic activity), alkaline phosphatase is normal.
- Urate is high.
- Renal failure may result from a number of factors (Fig. 37.9).

| Causes of renal failure in multiple myeloma |
| --- |
| - hypercalcemia <br> - hyperuricemia <br> - precipitated light chains <br> - amyloidosis <br> - NSAIDs prescribed for bone pain |

Fig. 37.9 Causes of renal failure in multiple myeloma. (NSAID, nonsteroidal anti-inflammatory drug.)

## Treatment

- Observation only in asymptomatic, uncomplicated "smoldering" disease.
- Supportive treatment with antibiotics, blood products, analgesics, and correction of hypercalcemia when necessary.
- Melphalan and prednisolone usually control symptoms and reduce tumor burden.
- Combination cytotoxic chemotherapy can be used in refractory disease.
- High-dose chemotherapy with autologous stem cell rescue can lead to durable remission.
- Radiotherapy may be useful in localized disease causing bony pain.
- The role of α-interferon is not yet defined.

## Prognosis

- Median survival is 3 years.
- Poor prognostic factors include high $\beta_2$-microglobulin levels (most accurate), high urea, low hemoglobin, increasing age, and low albumin.

*Note:* A monoclonal gammopathy may be present in the absence of myeloma in monoclonal gammopathy of uncertain significance (MGUS). These patients should be observed over the long term.

The three principal features of multiple myeloma are:
- Skeletal abnormalities.
- Production of a monoclonal protein.
- Accumulation of plasma cells in the bone marrow.

# Malignant lymphomas

Malignant lymphomas are neoplastic proliferations of lymphocytes which form solid tumors within lymphoid tissue. They are split into two broad categories on the basis of histologic findings: Hodgkin's disease (Reed–Sternberg [RS] cells present) and non-Hodgkin's lymphoma (all others).

## Hodgkin's disease
### Incidence and etiology
The incidence of Hodgkin's disease (HD) is 6 per 100,000 (one of the most common malignancies in young adults). There is a bimodal distribution with peaks in the 20s and 50s. The etiology is unknown, but there is a definite link with Epstein–Barr virus (EBV).

### Pathology
- Characteristic RS cells in a background of inflammatory infiltrate.
- RS cells are large bi- or multinucleated cells with prominent "owl-eyed" nucleoli.
- HD is divided using the Rye classification into four histologic subgroups (Fig. 37.10).

### Presentation
- Bimodal age at presentation with peaks at 20–29 and above 50 years with a male preponderance in children.
- Principally affects white populations and is more common in higher socioeconomic groups.
- Symptoms are due to painless lymph node enlargement (particularly cervical, axillary, and mediastinal) and/or "B symptoms" (Fig. 37.11).
- Lymphadenopathy is supradiaphragmatic in 90% of patients, and mediastinal disease may cause dry cough and exertional dyspnea.
- Some patients describe pruritus and alcohol-induced lymph node pain.
- Affected lymph nodes feel rubbery.
- Pallor and hepatosplenomegaly may also be found on examination.

### Investigations
- The diagnosis is usually made on lymph node biopsy (reviewed by hematopathologist); staging of disease is then performed to determine the extent of disease and is central to planning appropriate treatment (Fig. 37.12).
- Normochromic normocytic anemia, neutrophilia, eosinophilia, and thrombocytosis.
- Alkaline phosphatase raised (serum $Ca^{2+}$ may be high).
- LDH raised in bulky disease (prognostic indicator).
- Urate high.
- ESR may be raised.
- Chest x-ray: mediastinal lymphadenopathy.
- Computed tomography (CT) scan of the thorax, abdomen and pelvis to stage the extent of the disease.
- Bipedal lymphogram may demonstrate pelvic lymphadenopathy not detectable on CT scan (rarely performed).
- Bone marrow examination in some patients usually shows reactive marrow only.
- Staging laparotomy with splenectomy, which used to be performed for early stage disease, is now almost never necessary.

### Treatment
- Localized disease (stage IA–IIA): radiotherapy (usually mantle), either alone or with ABVD (doxorubicin [Adriamycin], bleomycin, vinblastine, and dacarbazine) for 4–6 cycles.
- Stage IIB–IIIA: treatment is controversial (? combined radiotherapy and chemotherapy).

| The Rye classification of Hodgkin's disease | | |
| --- | --- | --- |
| Subtype | Percentage | Prognosis |
| lymphocyte predominant | 10 | excellent |
| mixed cellularity | 30 | intermediate |
| lymphocyte depleted | <5 | poor |
| nodular sclerosis | 60 | variable |

Fig. 37.10 The Rye classification of Hodgkin's disease.

| B symptoms |
| --- |
| <ul><li>weight loss >10% of initial weight over previous 6 months</li><li>drenching night sweats</li><li>fever >38?C</li></ul> |

Fig. 37.11 B symptoms.

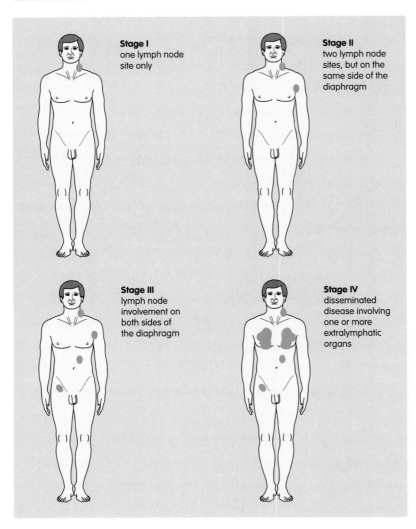

**Fig. 37.12** Ann Arbor staging of malignant lymphomas. Diagram shows stages I to IV. When you stage a patient you give a number (I–IV) and a letter (A or B). The letter A denotes the absence of B symptoms and B denotes the presence of B symptoms. Patients at stage IIA, for example, have stage II lymphoma without B symptoms.

Within figure:

**Stage I**
one lymph node site only

**Stage II**
two lymph node sites, but on the same side of the diaphragm

**Stage III**
lymph node involvement on both sides of the diaphragm

**Stage IV**
disseminated disease involving one or more extralymphatic organs

- Extensive disease (stage IIIB–IVB): chemotherapy (MOPP—mustine, oncovin, procarbazine, and prednisone, which is the gold standard, although other regimens are available).
- Relapse after radiotherapy: chemotherapy as above.
- Relapse after chemotherapy: alternative chemotherapy regimen, high-dose chemotherapy with autologous bone marrow or stem-cell transplant in selected patients.

## Prognosis
- Overall 5-year survival rate is 75%, but this is greatly affected by histologic type and stage of disease at presentation.

- Poor prognostic indicators include B symptoms, high stage, lymphocyte-depleted histology, increasing age, high ESR, and high LDH.
- A series of seven prognostic factors (albumin, hemoglobin, WBC count, male gender, age >45 years, stage IV disease, and lymphocyte count <600/$\mu$L) can predict survival at 5 years. The more factors that are positive, the shorter the survival time).

## Non-Hodgkin's lymphomas
### Incidence and etiology
Non-Hodgkin's lymphomas (NHL) account for 4% of all cancers, and the incidence is increasing for reasons which are unclear. Incidence increases with

age (uncommon before 40; median age is 50), and the condition is more common in males. The etiology is probably multifactorial, including the following:

- Genetic predisposition.
- Immunosuppression (e.g., HIV infection, transplant recipients).
- Viruses (e.g., EBV; particularly Burkitt's lymphoma).
- Ionizing radiation (e.g., survivors of the atomic bomb).

## Pathology

- Neoplastic proliferation of B (usually) or T lymphocytes within the lymphoid system forming solid tumors, which do not have RS cells.
- Heterogenous group of conditions with many different subtypes.
- A number of different classification schemes have been developed in an attempt to identify groups of patients with similar clinical, histological, and genetic features. The most recent scheme is called the REAL (Revised European American Lymphoma) classification.
- In practical terms, NHL can be broadly divided into two groups: low-grade NHL and high-grade NHL.
- Certain diseases are a risk factor for NHL (e.g., celiac disease, *H. pylori* gastritis, Crohn's disease).

## Presentation

- Most common hematologic malignancy.
- Usually presents with painless lymphadenopathy or "B" symptoms (fever, weight loss, night sweats).
- May also involve extranodal sites, including skin, lung, bowel, CNS, and bone.
- Low-grade NHL has an indolent course but is not curable; high-grade NHL presents aggressively but may be cured in up to 40% of patients.
- Lymphadenopathy, hepatosplenomegaly, pallor, and involvement of Waldeyer's ring or extranodal sites should be looked for on examination.

## Investigations

- The diagnosis is usually made on lymph node biopsy (and should be reviewed by a hematopathologist as diagnosis can be difficult); staging investigations should then be performed to

determine the extent of disease using the Ann Arbor system (see Fig. 37.12).

- Normochromic normocytic anemia is often present.
- Circulating lymphoma cells are sometimes seen on the peripheral film.
- Bone marrow is not uncommonly infiltrated by lymphoma cells and may cause bone marrow failure.
- LDH is high in bulk disease.
- Urate is high.
- Chromosomal translocations are characteristic of certain subtypes.
- CT scan of the thorax, abdomen and pelvis: determine the stage of the disease.

## Treatment
### Low-grade NHL

- Asymptomatic: observation only or radiotherapy.
- Localized disease: radiotherapy.
- Symptomatic or progressive disease: oral chemotherapy (chlorambucil or cyclophosphamide).
- Combination chemotherapy can be given in refractory disease.

### High-grade NHL

- Localized lesion: radiotherapy.
- Most patients require cytotoxic chemotherapy. CHOP (cyclophosphamide, hydroxyurea, vincristine [Oncovin], and prednisone) is the gold standard).
- The role of high-dose chemotherapy with autologous bone marrow or stem-cell transplantation is currently under evaluation.

## Prognosis

- Low-grade NHL: median survival is around 8–10 years.
- High-grade NHL: 40% 5-year survival rate.
- Poor prognostic factors include increasing age, high LDH, extensive disease, T-cell phenotype, certain extranodal sites, poor performance status, and low-grade NHL that has transformed into high-grade NHL.

## Bleeding disorders

An increased tendency to bleeding can result from abnormalities of platelets, the coagulation pathway, or blood vessels. The differential diagnosis, clinical findings, and investigation of these disorders are discussed in detail in Chapter 23. Specific conditions and their management are considered here.

# Hemophilia A
## Incidence and etiology
Hemophilia A affects 1 in 5000 males. It is an inherited condition (X-linked recessive).

## Pathology
Decreased plasma factor VIII activity.

## Presentation
- Severity of bleeding correlates with level of factor VIII activity (lower levels correspond to more severe symptoms).
- Bleeding may be spontaneous or secondary to trauma.
- Recurrent hemarthroses and intramuscular hematomas cause long-term disability due to arthopathy and contractures.
- Hematuria and intracranial bleeding may also occur.
- Bleeding from small cuts is usually minor (due to normal platelet function), but easy bruising occurs and bleeding following surgery may be fatal.
- After trauma, bleeding may be delayed as initial hemostasis is maintained by platelets.
- GI bleeding is uncommon.

## Investigations
- aPTT: prolonged.
- PT: normal.
- TT: normal.
- Bleeding time: normal.
- Factor VIII assay: low.

## Treatment
- Usually managed in specialized hemophilia centers.
- When there is bleeding or the patient requires surgery, factor VIII levels can be increased in two ways—mild hemophilia with desmopressin (DDAVP); moderate or severe hemophilia with factor VIII concentrates.
- Other aspects of management include analgesia (avoiding aspirin), joint replacement, synovectomy for arthropathy, regular dental care, and psychosocial support.

## Prognosis
Life expectancy should be normal with current therapies.

## Complications
Complications of receiving factor VIII concentrates include exposure to HIV, hepatitis B and C, and the development of inhibitors to infused factor VIII.

# Hemophilia B (Christmas disease)
## Incidence and etiology
Incidence is 1 per 25,000. It is an inherited condition (X-linked recessive and therefore affects males).

## Pathology
Decreased plasma factor IX activity.

## Presentation
Identical to hemophilia A.

## Investigations
- aPTT: prolonged.
- PT: normal.
- TT: normal.
- Bleeding time: normal.
- Factor IX assay: low.

## Treatment
Treatment is with factor IX concentrates (DDAVP has no effect on factor IX levels). Otherwise treatment is the same as for hemophilia A.

## Prognosis
With current therapies life expectancy should be normal.

# Von Willebrand's disease
## Incidence and etiology
Von Willebrand's disease (VWD) occurs in 1% of the general population. It is an inherited (autosomal dominant) condition, although type III disease is a recessive form. VWD can also be acquired due to antibody formation in lymphoproliferative and autoimmune disorders.

## Pathology
- Deficiency of von Willebrand's factor (VWF).
- VWF is a plasma protein that acts as a cofactor in platelet adherence to the subendothelium and platelet aggregation; it is also a carrier protein for factor VIII.

## Presentation

- Some patients go undiagnosed due to the mild nature of their disease. Severity of disease is variable.
- Both sexes are equally affected.
- Most patients present with mucosal bleeding (epistaxis, bleeding gums, GI bleeding).
- Menorrhagia and bleeding following surgery, dental extractions, trauma, and delivery are common.
- Hemarthroses and intramuscular hematomas are rare.

## Investigations

- aPTT: prolonged (may be normal).
- PT: normal.
- TT: normal.
- Bleeding time: prolonged.
- VWF assays: low.
- Ristocetin platelet aggregation: abnormal.

## Treatment

Treatment is with desmopressin (DDAVP) or concentrates (usually cryoprecipitate) in hemorrhage or perioperatively.

## Prognosis

Usually normal life expectancy.

# Disseminated intravascular coagulation

## Etiology

DIC may be caused by:

- Malignancy: mucus-secreting adenocarcinomas, prostate, pancreatic carcinoma, acute promyelocytic leukemia.
- Infection: gram-negative septicemia, meningococcal septicemia, *Clostridia*, toxic shock syndrome.
- Obstetric: amniotic fluid embolism, placental abruption, eclampsia, septic abortion.
- Tissue damage: rhabdomyolysis, fat embolism, severe trauma, burns.
- Immunologic: incompatible blood transfusion, drug reaction, anaphylaxis.
- Liver disease: acute fatty liver of pregnancy, fulminant liver failure.
- Others: snake bites, acute pancreatitis, aortic aneurysm.

## Pathology

- Intravascular coagulation is precipitated by release of tissue factor or procoagulant substances into the circulation from injured cells, malignant cells, or damaged endothelium.
- Microthrombi form throughout the microcirculation, causing ischemia and infarction.
- Platelets, fibrin, and clotting factors are consumed by the thrombotic process, and the fibrinolytic system becomes activated. These two processes result in a tendency to bleed, and hemorrhage may be significant.

## Presentation

- DIC may be mild and chronic (e.g., adenocarcinoma) or severe and life-threatening.
- Thrombosis can cause ischemia or infarction in the lungs, kidneys, liver, heart, brain, or skin.
- Bleeding is often into the skin or recent venipuncture sites.
- GI and pulmonary hemorrhage may also occur.

## Investigations

- Platelet count: low.
- PT: prolonged.
- aPTT: prolonged.
- TT: prolonged.
- Fibrinogen: low (may be normal as acute-phase reactant).
- D-dimers (fibrin degradation products): high.
- Blood smear: fragmented RBCs due to microangiopathic hemolysis.

## Treatment

- Treatment of the underlying disease usually resolves the DIC.
- Supportive care (e.g., fluids, antibiotics, debridement of gangrene).
- Replacement of platelets and clotting factors (using fresh frozen plasma or cryoprecipitate) may be used if there is hemorrhage or risk of hemorrhage (e.g., in surgery).
- Pharmacologic inhibitors of coagulation or fibrinolysis (e.g., heparin or tranexamic acid) may be beneficial in certain circumstances, but their use is controversial.

## Prognosis

Mortality rate is 80% in severe DIC and is usually due to the underlying disease.

## Thrombotic disorders

### Etiology
Risk factors for venous thrombosis are outlined in Fig. 37.13.

### Pathology
- Venous thrombosis can be caused by abnormal vein walls, venous stasis, or hypercoagulable blood.
- Thrombosis may be precipitated by a specific provoking event, such as surgery, or a physiologic state, such as pregnancy.
- The lower limbs are the most common site of thrombosis.
- Small clots may break off and cause pulmonary embolus or, very rarely, cerebral infarction by paradoxical embolus in patients with a patent foramen ovale.

### Presentation
- Deep vein thrombosis (DVT) causes local pain and swelling.
- The diagnosis can be difficult to make on clinical grounds.
- Pulmonary embolus (PE) causes sudden onset of pleuritic chest pain, dyspnea, and hemoptysis.

- Inherited hypercoagulable states present with recurrent venous thromboses (often at an early age), spontaneous abortions, and warfarin-induced skin necrosis.
- Antiphospholipid syndrome and hyperhomocysteinemia may cause arterial as well as venous thromboses.

### Investigations
- Every effort should be made to confirm the diagnosis of suspected venous thrombosis by radiologic tests as it has important implications for long-term management. These tests include venous Doppler, venogram, ventilation/perfusion scan, and pulmonary angiogram.
- Careful clinical examination should be performed, looking for an underlying cause such as malignancy, and investigated as appropriate.
- If the patient is young, ask if there have been recurrent episodes, recurrent spontaneous abortions, or a family history of thromboembolism, and consider hereditary thrombophilia. Assays are available to detect these abnormalities.
- A baseline platelet count and clotting screen should always be done.

| Risk factors for venous thrombosis | | |
|---|---|---|
| Etiology | Risk factor | Example |
| inherited | antithrombin deficiency<br>protein C deficiency<br>protein S deficiency<br>activated protein C resistance<br>homocysteinuria<br>dysfibrinogenemia | |
| acquired | physiologic | pregnancy and childbirth<br>obesity<br>elderly |
| | provoking events | surgery<br>trauma |
| | pathologic | immobility<br>malignancy<br>venous trauma/obstruction<br>estrogen therapy<br>nephrotic syndrome<br>antiphospholipid syndrome<br>hyperviscosity syndromes |

**Fig. 37.13** Risk factors for venous thrombosis.

## Treatment if thrombosis is proven

- Full anticoagulation with heparin for 5 days (low-molecular-weight heparin can be used for lower limb DVT, unfractionated heparin for PE and other thromboses).
- Oral warfarin should be given simultaneously and monitored using the INR (International Normalized Ratio) which should be maintained between 2 and 3.
- Heparin should be continued until the INR is therapeutic.

## Treatment period

The length of time a patient should be anticoagulated is controversial and currently under review, but as a general rule:

- Lower limb DVT: warfarin for 3 months.
- PE: warfarin for 6 months.
- Two or more unprovoked and documented thromboses: lifelong warfarin.

Infections affecting specific systems have been discussed in the appropriate chapters. This chapter considers in detail two important multisystem infections, human immunodeficiency virus (HIV) and malaria.

## HIV and AIDS

### Epidemiology

In the U.S. 1.1 million cases have been diagnosed; 71% of new cases are in men. New cases reported for HIV infection are affecting African-American and Hispanic populations at a disproportionate rate (54% and 19%, respectively), with Caucasians accounting for 26% of new cases. Given that African-Americans make up only 13% of the population, this statistic is alarming. In fact, among the African-American population AIDS is the leading cause of death in men and the third leading cause of death in women. So far 450,000 people have died from AIDS. In addition, with the rise of antiretroviral therapy, more people are living with AIDS. Through the year 2000, 322,000 people were living with the disease.

Approximately 56 million cases have been reported worldwide, but the true prevalence is likely to be much higher. Eighty per cent of cases are found in the developing countries, particularly Africa.

### Etiology

HIV-1 (i.e., the first type discovered, also once called HTLV-III, for human T-cell lymphotropic virus III, and LAV, for lymphadenopathy-associated virus) is found throughout the world.

HIV-2 (similar to the monkey virus, simian immunodeficiency virus; hence SIV) is uncommon except in West Africa.

The original source of the virus is unknown, but it may have been Central Africa. HIV can be transmitted by sexual, parenteral, or vertical routes (Fig. 38.1).

### Pathology

HIV is a lentivirus, which is a subgroup of the human retroviruses. Its genetic information is stored in a single strand of ribonucleic acid (RNA). Three specific genes produce proteins essential for HIV survival (Fig. 38.2). The virus can infect any cells expressing CD4$^+$, notably T helper cells, lymphocytes central to the immune response. Macrophages and monocytes also express CD4$^+$ and can serve as a reservoir for HIV. CD4$^+$ acts as a receptor for glycoprotein on the virus envelope, allowing the virus to enter the cell.

The enzyme reverse transcriptase makes DNA copies of the virus RNA, which become integrated into the host cell's genome, resulting in constant production of more viruses. The normal function of the infected cells is disrupted, and the host cells are eventually destroyed.

Because the principal cells affected are those of the immune system, HIV infection is characterized by diseases resulting from immunodeficiency (e.g., infections and malignancies).

### Presentation

There are four recognized phases of HIV infection (Fig. 38.3).

#### Seroconversion

Seroconversion usually occurs after 6–8 weeks of incubation, and severity varies significantly. Symptoms include mild "mononucleosis-type" illness, arthralgia, fever, headaches, rash, nausea, diarrhea, generalized lymphadenopathy, and neurologic abnormalities (e.g., headache, meningitis). The illness is self-limiting and usually resolves within 8 weeks.

#### Asymptomatic phase—clinical latent phase

The patient may remain well and asymptomatic for up to 15 years.

| Routes of HIV transmission | |
| --- | --- |
| **Route** | **Examples** |
| sexual | vaginal intercourse, anal intercourse |
| parenteral | intravenous drug abuse, blood transfusion, needlestick injury |
| vertical (i.e. from mother to fetus) | during gestation or delivery, via breast milk |

**Fig. 38.1** Routes of HIV transmission.

| HIV genes and the proteins they encode | |
| --- | --- |
| **Gene** | **Protein** |
| *pol* | reverse transcriptase (makes DNA copies of the viral RNA) |
| *gag* | core protein p24 |
| *env* | external (envelope) glycoprotein (for attachment of HIV to target cells) |

**Fig. 38.2** HIV genes and the proteins they encode.

| Phases of HIV infection | |
| --- | --- |
| **Phase** | **Features** |
| I | seroconversion |
| II | asymptomatic phase |
| III | persistent generalized lymphadenopathy |
| IV | symptomatic infection including AIDS |

**Fig. 38.3** Phases of HIV infection.

### Generalized lymphadenopathy

Rubbery, mobile lymphadenopathy develops in multiple sites for at least 3 months prior to the onset of symptomatic disease. Biopsy shows nonspecific reactive histiocytosis. The CDC cites this as "B symptoms."

### Symptomatic infection

This stage is characterized by constitutional symptoms (weight loss, diarrhea, and fever), recurrent infections, malignancies, and neurologic abnormalities (Fig. 38.4). Specific criteria for the diagnosis of AIDS are based on the development of certain indicator diseases with or without laboratory confirmation of HIV infection. Malignancies seen with increased frequency in HIV infection are often associated with specific viral infections (Fig. 38.5).

## Investigations

All investigations for HIV infection should be performed under the strictest confidentiality. The diagnosis has immense social, financial, health, and psychological implications; counseling prior to testing is very important.

The activity of HIV infection can be assessed by the measurement of viral antigens (p24), the immune response to the infection (anti-HIV antibodies), or the effects of the infection (CD4+ counts). Fig. 38.6 summarizes the findings at the different stages.

In practice, the diagnosis is usually made using HIV antibody tests. Several different methods of detection are now commercially available. In the U.S. the first step in diagnosis is an ELISA. Positive tests are run on a Western block protein electrophoresis. If that is also positive, a further serum sample should be taken and the tests repeated before the diagnosis is confirmed. In this way, false-positive results are reduced to a minimum.

Note that HIV antibodies may be undetectable for up to 3 months after infection and that this is a window for false-negative results.

Once the diagnosis is made, progress can be assessed by monitoring CD4+ counts. Fig. 38.7 lists other illnesses that may reduce the CD4+ count, and it is important to look at the general trend rather than individual counts.

Other tests for detection of HIV include viral culture and polymerase chain reaction detection.

| Features of symptomatic HIV infection | | |
|---|---|---|
| **Organ/ body system** | **Feature** | **Examples** |
| mouth | infection | *Candida*, abscesses, gingivitis, periodontitis |
| | premalignant | hairy leukoplakia |
| | malignancy | **Kaposi's sarcoma** of hard palate |
| | others | aphthous ulceration |
| lungs | infection | *Pneumocystis carinii* pneumonia, pneumococcal pneumonia, *Haemophilus influenzae*, *Staphylococcus aureus*, *Pseudomonas aeruginosa*, *Mycobacterium tuberculosis*, *Mycobacterium avium-intracellulare* complex, fungal pneumonia (*Aspergillus*) |
| | malignancy | **Kaposi's sarcoma**, lymphoma |
| neurologic | infection | **toxoplasmosis** (intracranial abscess, encephalitis), **cryptococcal meningitis**, **cytomegalovirus** (encephalitis, ascending polyradiculopathy, transverse myelitis), herpes simplex (encephalitis), herpes zoster (transverse myelitis), bacterial abscesses, tuberculomas |
| | malignancy | **cerebral lymphoma** |
| | HIV-related | **encephalopathy**, meningitis, myelopathy, peripheral neuropathy (sensory), proximal myopathy, inflammatory demyelinating polyneuropathy (e.g. Guillain-Barré syndrome) |
| gastrointestinal | infection | esophagitis (*Candida*, **herpes simplex, cytomegalovirus**), liver disease (mycobacteria, hepatitis B cytomegalovirus, microsporidia), biliary disease (cytomegalovirus, *Cryptosporidium*, microsporidia), enterocolitis (*Campylobacter, Salmonella, Shigella, Cryptosporidium, Giardia*, **cytomegalovirus**, microsporidia) |
| | malignancy | **Kaposi's sarcoma**, lymphoma |
| | HIV-related | enteropathy, gastropathy, malabsorption |
| skin | infection | viral (**herpes simplex**, herpes zoster, molluscum contagiosum), bacteria (*Staphylococcus*), fungi (*Candida*, tinea cruris, and tinea pedis) |
| | malignancy | **Kaposi's sarcoma**, basal cell carcinoma, squamous carcinoma |
| | others | seborrheic dermatitis, psoriasis |
| eyes | infection | retinitis (**cytomegalovirus**, herpes virus, toxoplasmosis) |
| joints | mono/polyarthropathy | cause unclear |

**Fig. 38.4** Features of symptomatic HIV infection. Conditions seen in AIDS (indicator diseases) are in **bold**.

These may have specific clinical indications, such as in children and after occupational exposure, but are not routinely performed.

Anemia, leukopenia, and thrombocytopenia may be found; $\beta_2$-microglobulin levels may also be raised.

## Treatment

Treatment falls into three broad categories: treatment of opportunistic infections, treatment of malignancies, and treatment of the HIV infection itself. There are many clinical trials currently in progress looking at these different aspects. It is likely that, as the results of these studies become available and with the emergence of drug-resistant organisms, the management of HIV patients will change. Management should be by an infectious disease doctor or a physician with experience treating HIV-positive patients.

## Treatment of opportunistic infections

Treatment of opportunistic infections is summarized in Fig. 38.8.

## Treatment of malignancies

- Kaposi's sarcoma: caused by human herpes virus 8 (HHV-8). The incidence of KS has decreased since the advent of HAART. KS affects the oral mucosa, lungs, and digestive tract, mostly of men. No known cure for KS exists, but local treatment includes camouflage to hide the lesions, vinblastine, or interferon injections into the tumor, and radiotherapy. For widespread disease α-interferon or vincristine plus bleomycin may be given.
- Cerebral lymphoma: associated with EBV infection and usually a B-cell lymphoma. From 2% to 4% of patients with AIDS will develop this type of non-Hodgkin's lymphoma. Whole brain irradiation and corticosteroids achieve a response in 20–50% of patients. With the addition of HAART, patients usually remain symptom-free for 12–18 months. Prognosis is poor.
- Cervical carcinoma: incidence of both invasive and noninvasive disease is higher in HIV-infected women. Cervical carcinoma is caused by HPV. The risk of carcinoma is highest in women with CD4+ counts less than 200. Screening for this population is especially important. CIN is treated with ablation/excision. Invasive carcinoma requires surgery and radiation.
- Non-Hodgkin's lymphoma: unlike KS, HAART has not decreased the incidence of NHL. The risk of NHL increases with the degree of immunosuppression. Local radiotherapy or iCHOP chemotherapy is used for widespread disease. (CHOP = cyclophosphamide, doxorubicin, vincristine [Oncovin], and prednisone.) Like CNS lymphoma, the prognosis is poor.

## Treatment directed at the HIV virus itself: HAART

Treatment for HIV infection should be started when the CD4+ count is below 200/μL or 300/μL, depending on the guideline. Little benefit is seen from starting therapy above 350/μL. Assessment of the viral load and the CD4+ count should be started before initiating highly active anti-retroviral therapy (HAART). Effective treatment is usually with two protease inhibitors and two nucleosides (reverse

| Malignancies seen with increased frequency and associated viruses | |
|---|---|
| **Tumour** | **Associated virus** |
| Kaposi's sarcoma | human herpesvirus 8 |
| cerebral lymphoma | Epstein–Barr virus |
| non-Hodgkin's lymphoma | Epstein–Barr virus |
| Hodgkin's disease | not determined |
| cervical carcinoma | human papillomavirus |
| anal carcinoma | human papillomavirus |

**Fig. 38.5** Malignancies seen with increased frequency and associated viruses.

| Investigation at different stages of HIV infection | | | | |
|---|---|---|---|---|
| **Phase** | **Viral replication** | **p24** | **HIV antibodies** | **CD4+ count** |
| seroconversion | high | detectable until HIV antibodies appear | detectable 3 weeks to 3 months after exposure | transient fall due to high viral load, but returns to normal when HIV antibodies appear |
| asymptomatic phase | low | undetectable as antibody in excess to antigen | detectable | normal |
| symptomatic phase | high | detectable | detectable | falls; when <200 × 10⁶/L risk of infection is very high |

**Fig. 38.6** Investigation at different stages of HIV infection.

transcriptase inhibitors) or two nucleoside analogs. The difficulty with this treatment is the high morbidity associated with it. Patients are often not able to take the overwhelming amount of medications; in addition, they may not be able to adhere to the regimen because of its complexity or the severe GI side effects. Patients who fail to comply with their regimen promote the appearance of drug-resistant strains. Therapy should be adjusted based on CD4+ counts, viral loads, and viral resistance.

The two different classes of drugs currently available are summarized in Fig. 38.9. Combination treatment has been shown to be more effective than monotherapy. Currently the two most commonly used regimens are the following:

- Lopinavir plus lamivudine (3TC) plus either dideoxyinosine (DDI) or stavudine (D4T).
- Efavirenz (EFV) plus 3TC and one of the following three drugs: tenofovir, azidothymidine (AZT), or D4T.

These multidrug therapies consist of two protease inhibitors (lopinavir, tenofovir, lamivudine, efavirenz) and two reverse transcriptase inhibitors (AZT, D4T, DDI).

The role of other drugs is the focus of ongoing clinical trials.

---

| Differential diagnosis of a low CD$^{4+}$ count |
|---|
| • HIV infection |
| • acute viral infections |
| • TB |
| • SLE |
| • sarcoidosis |
| • steroids |

**Fig. 38.7** Differential diagnosis of a low CD4+ count (HIV, human immunodeficiency virus; SLE, systematic lupus erythematosis; TB, tuberculosis.)

---

| Treatment and prophylaxis of opportunistic infections | | | | |
|---|---|---|---|---|
| **Infection** | **Treatment** | **Treatment alternatives** | **Indication for prophylaxis** | **Prophylactic drug regimes** |
| *Pneumocystis carinii* | high-dose intravenous cotrimoxazole, steroids may be beneficial | intravenous pentamidine, or clindamycin + primaquine, or dapsone + trimethoprim | secondary prevention or CD4+ <200 × 10$^6$/L | oral cotrimoxazole, or nebulized pentamidine, or dapsone + pyrimethamine |
| toxoplasmosis | sulphadiazine + pyrimethamine + folate | clindamycin replacing sulphadiazine | secondary prevention or CD4+ <200 × 10$^6$/L positive serology | pyrimethamine + sulphadiazine, or clindamycin, or cotrimoxazole, or dapsone |
| cytomegalovirus | ganciclovir or foscarnet | — | secondary prevention | ganciclovir or foscarnet |
| herpes simplex | aciclovir | valaciclovir or foscarnet | secondary prevention | aciclovir |
| herpes zoster | aciclovir | valaciclovir or foscarnet or famciclovir | — | — |
| cryptococcal meningitis | fluconazole or amphotericin B and/or flucytosine | — | secondary prevention | fluconazole |
| *Mycobacterium avium-intracellulare* | rifampicin + ethambutol + clarithromycin | rifabutin replacing rifampicin | secondary prevention | rifabutin |
| *Candida* | fluconazole | ketoconazole or itraconazole | secondary prevention | fluconazole |

**Fig. 38.8** Treatment and prophylaxis of opportunistic infections.

**Fig. 38.9** Anti-HIV drugs.

| Anti-HIV drugs | | |
|---|---|---|
| **Class** | **Actions** | **Examples** |
| reverse transcriptase inhibitors | DNA copy of viral genome not made and therefore not integrated into the host cell genome | azidothymidine (AZT) dideoxyinosine (DDI) zalcitabine (DDC) stavudine (D4T) |
| protease inhibitors | prevent cleavage of a structural protein, producing defective viruses | efavirenz lopinavir tenofovir lamivudine saquinavir ritonavir indinavir |

## Prevention

As there is no "cure" for HIV infection, preventative measures must remain a high priority. Such measures include education, the provision of clean needles for intravenous drug abusers, the use of condoms, the screening of blood products and organs donated for transplantation, and avoidance of breastfeeding in HIV-positive mothers. In addition, HIV-positive mothers can be treated with antiretrovirals to reduce the transmission of HIV to their newborns.

## Prognosis

HAART regimens have enabled HIV-positive patients to survive with viral loads at undetectable levels. While patients able to receive the proper medication and medical care are doing well, the lack of access to these new medications has resulted in high mortality rates among the untreated. In addition to HAART, prophylaxis against *Pneumocystis carinii* pneumonia and *Mycobacterium avium* infection has also decreased mortality. Prognosis depends on the patient's ability to comply with the HAART regimen, increasing HIV resistance, and the appearance of HIV-associated malignancies.

## Malaria

## Epidemiology

Worldwide, malaria affects over 100 million people each year. It causes around 1 million deaths each year (particularly of children) and is endemic in the tropics and subtropics. It is seen in temperate zones when imported by people who have visited or come from endemic areas. The resurgence of malaria is the result of insecticide resistance of the *Anopheles* mosquito and development of resistance to chloroquine by *Plasmodium falciparum*

## Etiology

The disease is caused by protozoal infection with one of the species of the genus *Plasmodium* (*P. vivax*, *P. ovale*, *P. malariae*, or *P. falciparum*).

## Pathology

Malaria is spread from an infected person to a noninfected person by the female *Anopheles* mosquito. At schizogony the red blood cell bursts, releasing malaria parasites, malaria antigen, malaria pigment, hemoglobin, and other constituents of the red blood cells into the blood stream, causing the typical clinical picture.

This occurs every 72 hours in *P. malariae* (quartan malaria), every 48–72 hours in *P. vivax* and *P. ovale* (tertian malaria), and every 48 hours in *P. falciparum* (subtertian malaria). *P. vivax*, *P. ovale*, and *P. malariae* invade up to 2% of the circulating red blood cells. *P. falciparum* may affect over 10% of cells, producing a more severe clinical picture.

Fig. 38.10 demonstrates the life cycle of malaria.

## Presentation

Malaria is characterized by periodic fevers, sweating, and rigors, which coincide with schizogony. Nausea, vomiting, abdominal pain, headache, cough, and arthralgia may also be present. Splenomegaly is

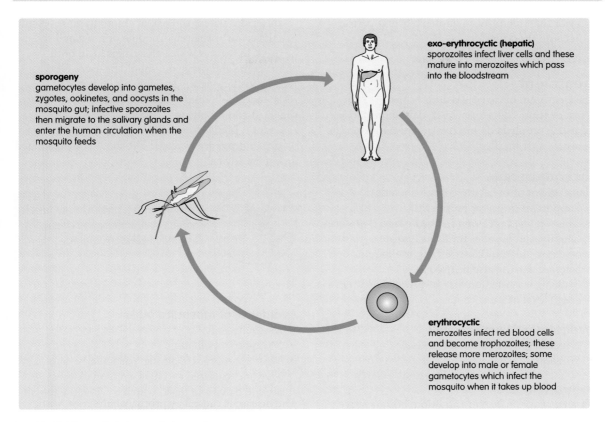

**sporogeny**
gametocytes develop into gametes, zygotes, ookinetes, and oocysts in the mosquito gut; infective sporozoites then migrate to the salivary glands and enter the human circulation when the mosquito feeds

**exo-erythrocyctic (hepatic)**
sporozoites infect liver cells and these mature into merozoites which pass into the bloodstream

**erythrocyctic**
merozoites infect red blood cells and become trophozoites; these release more merozoites; some develop into male or female gametocytes which infect the mosquito when it takes up blood

**Fig. 38.10** The malaria transmission cycle.

commonly found but mild icterus and hepatomegaly may also be present.

P. falciparum can produce severe illness ("malignant" malaria), characterized by a high level of parasitemia, which causes the occlusion of small blood vessels by adherence to their endothelium. The most feared manifestation of the disease is cerebral malaria, which can lead to coma. This is thought to result from the occlusion of small vessels, cytokine release and/or hypoglycemia associated with the infection. Reversible acute renal failure and pulmonary edema can also be associated with infection.

Fig. 38.11 summarizes the complications of P. falciparum malaria.

## Investigations
- Thin and thick blood films stained with Giemsa: thick films allow parasites to be identified, thin films are useful in species identification.

---

**Complications of infection with *Plasmodium falciparum***

- cerebral malaria (hyperpyrexia, coma, death)
- hypoglycemia
- noncardiogenic pulmonary edema
- seizures
- severe intravascular hemolysis with hemoglobinuria "blackwater fever"
- acute tubular necrosis
- hepatic necrosis
- jaundice

**Fig. 38.11** Complications of infection with *Plasmodium falciparum*.

- Anemia, leukocytosis, and thrombocytopenia may occur.
- Coagulopathy: may be a feature of *P. falciparum* infection.

- Liver function tests, including bilirubin, often become abnormal.
- Hyponatremia: *P. falciparum*.

## Treatment

The treatment of malaria is under constant review as resistant strains develop. Up-to-date information regarding prophylaxis and treatment of malaria can be obtained from the CDC.

### The acute episode

Management of the acute episode includes:

- Supportive care as appropriate.
- Chloroquine for *P. vivax*, *P. ovale*, and *P. malaria*.
- Quinine and fansidar for *P. falciparum* as most cases are chloroquine-resistant; mefloquine or halofantrine can also be used.
- Exchange transfusion may be useful when there is a high level of parasitemia.

### Eradication of liver parasites

- Necessary in *P. ovale* and *P. vivax*.
- Primaquine is used.

## Prevention

With the emergence of resistant organisms, the avoidance of mosquito bites and mosquito control take on greater importance.

### Chemoprophylaxis

For chemoprophylaxis, refer to up-to-date information from the CDC. It should be started 1 week prior to travel and continued for at least 4 weeks.

In regions where the risk of chloroquine-resistant malaria is low, either chloroquine or proguanil should be used. In regions where this risk is high, both chloroquine and proguanil should be used. CDC recommendations are available for endemic resistance; mefloquine (Lariam) and doxycycline are the most commonly used drugs in areas with resistant *P. falciparum*.

Other drugs are available but should be prescribed on expert advice.

Even though a patient may take malaria prophylaxis, he or she may still develop malaria.

### Avoidance of mosquito bites

- Mosquito nets.
- Mosquito repellents.
- Wear appropriate clothing, particularly long-sleeved/trousered and light-colored clothes around dawn and dusk, which is when the female *Anopheles* mosquito is most active.
- Spray bedroom with insecticide last thing in the evening.

### Prognosis

Prognosis is excellent with *P. vivax*, *P. ovale*, and *P. malariae* infection, but *P. falciparum* is still a life-threatening condition, especially with high parasite counts.

# 39. Drug Overdose

## Epidemiology

It is estimated that there are between 2 and 5 million poisonings and drug overdoses in the U.S. per year. However, the number may be much higher because the true incidence is unknown.

## Etiology

Overdose may be due to the following:
- Accidental: particularly in children, IV drug abusers.
- Deliberate: self-administration in suicide or near suicide, homicide, or child abuse (e.g., Munchausen's by proxy).
- Iatrogenic: uncommon (e.g., interacting drugs).

## Presentation

### History
Drug overdose in many patients may result in a mild illness requiring little intervention. However, some patients take many tablets or cocktails of drugs, causing a life-threatening state that requires intensive care and may be fatal. Around 80% of patients are conscious and able to provide a history. In all patients, particularly the unconscious, make every effort to talk to family, friends, and the ambulance staff. Always consider overdose in any unconscious patient. Where possible, try to establish the following facts.

### What drugs were taken and when?
It is very common for more than one drug to be taken, and alcohol is often also used. The most common drugs taken for suicide are analgesics, antipsychotics, and sedatives. Remember to ask specifically about illicit drug use. Cocaine, sedatives, marijuana, and opiates are the most common illicit drugs found in psychiatric ED settings. Try to establish which tablets were taken, how many and how long ago in order to establish the likely ongoing risk. However, it is good policy to treat the patient and not the history, which may be unreliable.

### Try to assess the suicidal risk
Has the patient taken an overdose before? What events led to the overdose? Did the patient intend suicide at the time, or was it a reaction to acute stress such as an argument? Was the act premeditated? For example, were tablets collected over a period of time, was a suicide note left, were the tablets taken when the patient expected to be alone for a while? What did the patient do after taking the tablets—did the patient call for a family member or ambulance immediately? Does the patient feel suicidal now? Would the patient do it again?

Often patients present while intoxicated or attempt suicide while intoxicated and no longer have suicidal ideation upon regaining sobriety.

Fig. 39.1 summarizes features indicating a high suicidal risk.

## Examination
The examination should be in three stages: assess how ill the patient is, look for evidence to suggest the likely drug(s) involved, and look for complications of overdose.

### How ill is the patient?
The first priority is ABC—ensure the patient has an adequate airway, breathing (respiration), and circulation. Assessment of coma scale, pulse, blood pressure, temperature, and capillary blood glucose (glucose estimation) should then be assessed.

### Is there any evidence to suggest underlying cause?
Relatives or ambulance staff may have brought bottles from the scene. Look for evidence on the patient such as diabetic cards or medical alert

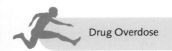

## Features indicating a high suicide risk

- elderly
- male
- previous suicide attempts
- unemployed
- socially isolated (single, living alone)
- chronic debilitating illness (psychiatric or physical)
- drug or alcohol abuse

**Fig. 39.1** Features indicating a high suicide risk.

## Complications of drug overdose

- coma
- respiratory depression
- hypotension or hypertension
- arrhythmias
- seizures
- head injury
- hypothermia or hyperthermia
- aspiration pneumonia
- rhabdomyolysis
- gastric stress ulceration

**Fig. 39.2** Complications of drug overdose.

bracelets (e.g., it may be an insulin overdose). Also look for:

- Pinpoint pupils: opiates, organophosphates, sedatives/benzodiazepines.
- Dilated pupils: tricyclic antidepressants, amphetamines, cocaine.
- Nystagmus: phenytoin, alcohol, PCP.
- Papilledema: carbon monoxide, cocaine-induced hypertension or encephalopathy.
- Burns around the mouth: corrosives, crack pipe use.
- Hyperventilation: aspirin.
- Hypothermia: chlorpromazine.
- Odors: fruity (alcohol, antifreeze), almond (cyanide), garlic (organophosphates, arsenic).
- Needle "track" marks: opiates, benzodiazepines, stimulants.

### Have any complications occurred?

Fig. 39.2 summarizes complications of drug overdose.

## Investigations

- Acetaminophen and salicylate levels should be measured in all patients.
- Metabolic panel, blood glucose, serum osmolarity.
- Baseline clotting and liver function tests in acetaminophen overdose.
- Drug levels can be measured in the blood, gastric contents, and urine, but this is not necessary in the majority of patients.
- Electrocardiogram: if clinically indicated (e.g., arrhythmia). QT prolongation suggests tricyclics, antipsychotics, antihistamines. Ventricular tachycardias suggest cocaine, amphetamines, tricyclics, potassium. Bradycardia suggests sedatives, beta blockers, digoxin, lithium, calcium channel blockers.
- Chest x-ray: if evidence of aspiration.
- Arterial blood gases: in patients with neurologic impairment or lack of respiratory drive.

## Management

The management of drug overdose can be divided into three parts: general measures for all patients, specific measures according to the drug taken, and psychiatric assessment and social input when the patient recovers physically.

### General approach
#### Supportive care

- If the patient is unconscious, clear the airway and give oxygen via a face-mask.
- If the patient has no gag reflex, call an anesthesiologist because the patient may need endotracheal intubation.
- Some patients may require assisted ventilation.
- Gain intravenous access, keep patient with head downward, and give intravenous fluids for hypotension unless there is cardiogenic shock (central venous pressure monitoring may be necessary).
- Nurse the patient in a semiprone position and measure observations regularly—some patients who walk into the ED may deteriorate rapidly.
- Attach cardiac monitor if arrhythmia is suspected or the patient is known to have taken tricyclic antidepressants.

| | Specific measures in the management of drug overdose | |
|---|---|---|
| **Drug** | **Toxic side effects** | **Specific management** |
| opiates | respiratory depression, drowsiness or coma, pinpoint pupils, hypotension, bradycardia, hypothermia, pulmonary edema | naloxone 0.4–2 mg intravenously every 2–3 minutes to a maximum of 10 mg due to its short half-life; can be administered by continuous intravenous infusion |
| benzodiazepines | drowsiness, dysarthria, nystagmus, ataxia, coma, respiratory depression; fairly safe if taken alone but potentiate the effects of other sedative drugs which are often taken at the same time | flumazenil 0.2 mg over 15 seconds, then 100 μg every 60 seconds until response (maximum dose 1 mg); should be used cautiously |
| acetaminophen | nausea and vomiting in the first 24 hours; acute hepatocellular necrosis may develop after 3 days with as few as 20 tablets causing jaundice, encephalopathy, hypoglycemia and abdominal pain; renal tubular necrosis may also occur | monitor prothrombin time, glucose, metabolic panel; check acetaminophen levels from 4 hours onwards (treatment may begin before result is available if significant overdose suspected); use nomogram to determine whether antidote should be given if less than 24 hours since tablets were taken; give acetylcysteine (Parvolex) by intravenous infusion |
| aspirin | nausea, vomiting, tinnitus, deafness, sweating, hyperventilation, tachycardia, delirium, seizures, coma, impaired clotting, hypokalemia, hypoglycemia, metabolic acidosis (respiratory alkalosis initially) | correct dehydration, hypokalemia and hypoglycemia; if plasma salicylate levels >500 mg/L (3.6 mmol/L), the patient should have forced alkaline diuresis under close supervision; in severe poisoning (>700 mg/L or 5.1 mmol/L), hemodialysis may be life-saving |
| iron | usually accidental affecting children causes hemorrhagic enteritis (corrosion) with nausea, vomiting, abdominal pain, hematemesis, bloody diarrhea, acute hepatocellular necrosis, metabolic acidosis, peritonitis, hypotension, coma | desferrioxame by intravenous or intramuscular injection |
| digoxin | nausea, vomiting, diarrhea, hyperkalemia, bradyarrhythmias, tachyarrhythmias, altered color vision, delirium | correct electrolyte disturbance; temporary ventricular pacing in atrioventricular block digoxin-specific antibody fragments (Digibind) in severe overdose |
| β-blockers | bradycardia, hypotension, cardiac failure, convulsions, coma, asystole | atropine intravenously for bradycardia; glucagon intravenously in severe overdose |
| heparin | hemorrhage | intravenous protamine sulfate |
| warfarin | hemorrhage | intravenous vitamin K, intravenous infusion of concentrates of factors II, VII, IX, and X, or fresh frozen plasma |

**Fig. 39.3** Specific measures in the management of drug overdose with certain of the more common drugs.

- In arrhythmia, correct hypoxia, acidosis, or electrolyte balance; antiarrhythmic agents should be used with caution because they can exacerbate the arrhythmia.
- Convulsions should be treated with intravenous benzodiazepines.

## Prevent gastrointestinal absorption

Gastrointestinal absorption may be prevented by either emptying the stomach or preventing bowel adsorption.

### Emptying stomach

- Indications: consider gastric emptying within 4 hours for most drugs; within 6 hours after opiates and anticholinergics; within 12 hours after tricyclic antidepressants, salicylates, and aminophylline.
- Contraindications: ingestion of caustic, corrosive, or petroleum derivatives.
- There are two methods of gastric emptying: induced emesis (vomiting) or gastric lavage:
  1. Induced emesis—syrup of ipecac was used more frequently in the past but has not been proven to be more effective than gastric lavage preventing absorption of substance. It should not be given if the patient is drowsy or likely to become drowsy because of the risks of aspiration. Ipecac may also prevent use of charcoal due to continuous vomiting.
  2. Gastric lavage—used where induced emesis is refused, contraindicated, or unsuccessful (usually in the unconscious patient whose airway is protected by a cuffed endotracheal tube). No longer recommended unless a nasogatric tube can be placed within the first hour.

### Preventing absorption in the bowel

- Activated charcoal binds poisons in the stomach, preventing absorption.
- More effective the sooner it is given.
- Doses may be given every 4 hours to increase the elimination of certain drugs (aspirin, carbamazepine, phenobarbitone, quinine).
- Contraindicated in drowsy patients (risk of aspiration) and patients with bowel perforation/obstruction.

- Ineffective for iron, lithium, potassium, alcohol, and cyanide.

## Increase elimination of drug

Elimination of drugs can be increased using forced alkaline diuresis or dialysis.

### Forced alkaline diuresis

- Done by infusing 0.45 NS to which 50–150mEq of sodium bicarbonate has been added.
- Increases renal drug excretion.
- Used in severe salicylate, phenobarbitone, and amphetamine overdose.
- Can cause fatal fluid overload, electrolyte disturbance, or acid–base disturbance and should be monitored very carefully.

### Dialysis

Dialysis should be used in severe overdose when other methods are contraindicated or unsuccessful. The techniques include peritoneal or hemodialysis and hemoperfusion.

## Specific antidotes

Advice for overdose of any drug or ingestion of any poisons can be obtained 24 hours/day from a number of poisons information centers. Each ED and hospital switchboard will have a list of national numbers.

Fig. 39.3 summarizes the specific management of overdose of some of the more common drugs.

## Psychiatric and social assessment

Once the acute event and medical management is completed, an assessment of the patient's psychiatric state (ongoing suicidal risk) and social circumstances should be made, however trivial the overdose may have appeared. It is important to remember that a patient with psychiatric disturbances may still be intoxicated or in fact going through withdrawal. Where appropriate, psychiatrists and social care workers should be involved.

All suicide threats should be taken seriously.

# Index